HANDBOOK OF
SIGNS & SYMPTOMS

P9-DFT-897

Springhouse Corporation
Springhouse, Pennsylvania

STAFF

Senior Publisher
Matthew Cahill

Editorial Director
Donna O. Carpenter

Clinical Director
Judith Schilling McCann, RN, MSN

Art Director
John Hubbard

Managing Editor
H. Nancy Holmes

Clinical Editors
Carla Roy, RN, BSN, CCRN; Beverly
Ann Tscheschlog, RN

Editorial Project Manager
Doris Weinstock

Copy Editors
Cynthia C. Breuninger (manager),
Karen C. Comerford, Stacey A. Follin,
Brenna H. Mayer, Pamela Wingrod

Designers
Arlene Putterman (associate art direc-
tor), Donald Knauss (project manager),
Jeffrey Sklarow

Manufacturing
Deborah Meiris (director), Patricia K.
Dorshaw (manager), Otto Mezei

Production Coordinator
Stephen Hungerford, Jr.

Editorial Assistant
Beverly Lane

Indexer
Barbara Hodgson

616.047
HAN

Ⓡ A member of the Reed Elsevier plc group

**Library of Congress Cataloging-in-Publica-
tion Data**

Handbook of signs & symptoms.
    p. cm.
    Includes index.
    1. Symptomatology—Handbooks, manuals,
etc.   I. Springhouse Corporation
    [DNLM: 1. Diagnosis handbooks. 2. Thera-
peutics handbooks. WB39 H23663 1998]
RC69.H246 1998
616'.047—dc21
DNLM/DLC   97-51521
ISBN 0-87434-893-5 (alk. paper)   CIP

CONTENTS

CONTRIBUTORS

Sherry L. Altschuler, PhD
Private practice
Audiology–Speech Pathology
Associate, Department of Head and
Neck Surgery
University of Pennsylvania Medical
School
Philadelphia

**Charold L. Baer, RN, PhD, FCCM,
CCRN**
Professor
Oregon Health Sciences University
Portland

Laura P. Barnes, RN, MSN, CNAA
Nursing Director of Critical Care
Services
East Tennessee Children's Hospital
Knoxville

**Roxanne Aubol Batterden, RN, MS,
CCRN**
Nurse Educator, Care Coordinator
Johns Hopkins Medical Center
Baltimore

Jack M. Becker, MD
Chief, Allergy Services
St. Christopher's Hospital for Children
Assistant Professor of Pediatrics
Allegheny University of the Health
Sciences
Philadelphia

John M. Bertoni, MD, PhD
Chairman and Professor
Department of Neurology
Creighton University
Omaha

Heather Boyd-Monk, RN, SRN, BSN
Assistant Director of Nursing for
Education Programs
Wills Eye Hospital
Philadelphia

**Barbara Gross Braverman, RN, MSN,
CS**
Geropsychiatric Clinical Nurse Specialist
Abington (Pa.) Memorial Hospital

Sally A. Brozenec, RN, MS, PhD
Assistant Professor
Rush University College of Nursing
Chicago

**Laura J. Burke, RN, MSN, PhD,
CNAA**
Director of Nursing Research
St. Luke's Medical Center
Milwaukee

**Dorothea Caldwell-Brown, RN, NP,
BSN, MPH, JD**
Law Clerk, U.S. District Court
Southern District of New York

**Paul L. Carmichael, MD, MSc(Med),
FAAO, FACS, FICS**
Retired from private practice
Ophthalmology
Lansdale, Pa.

Robert B. Cooper, MD
Clinical Assistant Professor of Medicine
Assistant Attending Physician
New York Hospital–Cornell University
Medical College

Jerome M. Cotler, MD, FAAOS, FACS
Everett J. and Marian Gordon Professor
of Orthopedic Surgery
Jefferson Medical College of Thomas
Jefferson University
Philadelphia

Mary Helen Davis, MD
Associate Professor
Department of Psychiatry
University of Louisville School of
Medicine

Nancy Davis, RN, MSN, CRNP
Surgical First Assistant
Cardiovascular and Chest Surgical
Associates
Boise, Idaho

Gloria Donnelly, RN, PhD, FAAN
Dean and Professor
Allegheny University of the Health
Sciences
Philadelphia

Brian B. Doyle, MD
Co-Director
Psychopharmacology Research Division
Clinical Professor of Psychiatry
Department of Psychiatry
Georgetown University School of
Medicine
Washington, D.C.

Stephen C. Duck, MD
Associate Professor of Pediatrics
Northwestern University Medical
School
Evanston (Ill.) Hospital

Kenneth H. Einhorn, MD
Private practice
Otolaryngology
Abington, Pa.

**Mary Jo Sagaties Farmer, RN,C, MS,
PhD**
Medical student
Tufts University School of Medicine
Boston

Susan Gauthier, RN, MSN, PhD
Associate Professor
Department of Nursing
College of Allied Health Professions
Temple University
Philadelphia

Jalal K. Ghali, MD
Associate Professor of Medicine
Louisiana State University School
of Medicine
Shreveport

**Roslyn M. Gleeson, RN,C, MSN, APN,
CS, CRNP**
Clinical Nurse Specialist
Pediatric–Spinal Dysfunction Program
Alfred I. Du Pont Institute
Wilmington, Del.

Kelly J. Henrickson, MD
Associate Professor of Pediatrics
Medical College of Wisconsin
Milwaukee

**Barbara S. Henzel, RN, BSN, CCRC,
CGRN**
Clinical Research Coordinator
Division of Gastroenterology
University of Pennsylvania
Philadelphia

Denise A. Hess, RN
Boynton Beach, Fla.

Marcia J. Hill, RN, MSN
Director of Nursing
Polly Ryon Memorial Hospital
Richmond, Tex.

Esther Holzbauer, RN,C, BS, MSN
Assistant Professor of Nursing
Mount Marty College
Yankton, S. Dak.

Sheila Scannell Jenkins, RN, MSN
Instructor
Bridgeport (Conn.) Hospital School of
Nursing

Lee Ann Kelly, RN, MS, PNP
Head Nurse
Antepartum-Postpartum
Hermann Hospital
Houston

Robert L. Klaus, MD, FACS
Urologist
Milford (Del.) Memorial Hospital

**Karen A. Landis, RN, MSN, CCRN,
CRNP**
Family Nurse Practitioner
McGarry and Neumann Family Practice
Allentown, Pa.

Gizell Rosetti Larson, MD
Chairman, Neuroscience Division
LaSalle Clinic
Menasha, Wis.

Herbert A. Luscombe, MD
Professor Emeritus of Dermatology
Jefferson Medical College of Thomas
Jefferson University
Philadelphia

Neil MacIntyre, MD
Professor of Medicine
Duke University Medical Center
Durham, N.C.

Steven Margulis, MD, FACP
Assistant Clinical Professor of Medicine
New York Hospital–Cornell University
Medical College

Margaret E. Miller, RN, MSN
Oncology Head and Neck, Lung
Clinical Specialist
Northwestern Medical Faculty
Foundation
Chicago

Chris Platt Moldovanyi, RN, MSN
Nurse Consultant
Phillips and Mille Co. LPA
Middleburg Heights, Ohio

Mary Lou Moore, RN,C, PhD, FAAN, FACCE
Research Assistant Professor
Department of Obstetrics and
Gynecology
Wake Forest University School of
Medicine
Winston-Salem, N.C.

Roger M. Morrell, MD, PhD, FACP
Private practice
Neurology
Lathrup Village, Mich.

Frances W. Quinless, RN, PhD
Dean, School of Nursing
University of Medicine and Dentistry of
New Jersey
Newark

Patricia L. Radzewicz, RN, BSN
Associate Claim Manager
University of Illinois Office of
University Counsel
Chicago

Amy Perrin Ross, RN, MSN, CNRN
Neuroscience Program Coordinator
Loyola University Medical Center
Maywood, Ill.

Grannum R. Sant, MD
Chairman, Department of Urology
Tufts University School of Medicine
Boston

Kristine A. Scordo, RN, PhD
Assistant Professor
Wright State University
Dayton, Ohio
Clinical Nurse Specialist
The Cardiology Center of Cincinnati

Ellen Shapiro, MD
Professor of Urology
New York University School of
Medicine

Harrison J. Shull, Jr., MD
Gastroenterologist
Vanderbilt University Medical Center
Nashville, Tenn.

Eric Silfen, MD, MSHA
Physician Liaison, Quality and Planning
Reston (Va.) Hospital Center

Carol E. Smith, RN, PhD
Professor
School of Nursing
Kansas University Medical Center
Kansas City

June Stark, RN, BSN, MEd
Critical Care Nurse Educator
St. Elizabeth Medical Center
Boston

Frances J. Storlie, RN, PhD, CANP
Director, Personal Health Services
Southwest Washington Health District
Vancouver

Richard W. Tureck, MD
Professor of Obstetrics and Gynecology
Hospital of the University of
Pennsylvania
Philadelphia

**Dharmapuri Vidyasagar, MD, MSc,
FCCM**
Professor of Pediatrics
Director of Neonatology
University of Illinois Hospital–Michael
Reese Hospital
Chicago

Naomi Walpert, RN, MS, CDE
Endocrine Clinical Nurse Specialist
Sinai Hospital
Baltimore

Maryann Banko Wee, RN, BSN
Risk Management Consultant
Virginia Professional Underwriters, Inc.
Jackson, Miss.

John K. Wiley, MD, FACES
Neurosurgeon
Chief of Staff
Miami Valley Hospital
Dayton, Ohio

Sandi Wind, RN, CETN
Enterostomal Nurse
Allegheny University of the Health
Sciences
Philadelphia

Janette R. Yanko, RN, MN, CNRN
Neuroscience Advanced Practice Nurse
Allegheny General Hospital
Pittsburgh

Joseph A. Zeccardi, MD, FACEP
Director, Division of Emergency
Medicine
Thomas Jefferson University Hospital
Philadelphia

FOREWORD

Diagnosing and managing medical problems begins with an assessment of the patient's physical signs and presenting symptoms. Indeed, it is this assessment that sets into motion the specific tests, procedures, and therapeutic plans for the patient. Moreover, changes in signs and symptoms are often used to monitor the effects of therapy and can serve as important outcome measurements of the therapy's success. Because of this pivotal role of signs and symptoms assessment in the management of patients, all health care workers need to be skilled at eliciting a good history, clarifying that history, and then detecting the important clinical signs. Imprecise assessment of signs and symptoms can lead not only to inappropriate diagnostic plans but also to inappropriate therapies and an inability to monitor the course of treatment.

Handbook of Signs & Symptoms discusses in-depth more than 250 important signs and symptoms in a concise handbook format that can be carried with the clinician to the patient's bedside. This up-to-date and easy-to-use reference is arranged in alphabetical order, making it exceptionally convenient for the busy clinician. Each entry contains sections on history and physical examination, common and other medical causes, special considerations and, where appropriate, pediatric pointers. Numerous illus-trations enhance the text by showing how to recognize or elicit certain signs.

In addition, numerous symbols throughout the book highlight especially useful information. For example, "Emergency interventions" provides instructions for taking immediate action in response to a life-threatening finding. "Elder tip" calls your attention to the implications of certain signs and symptoms in the older patient, including the effects of different medications on this population. "Alternative therapy" discusses nontraditional approaches to management, such as biofeedback, yoga, and herbal remedies. Finally, a comprehensive appendix briefly describes another 250 less common signs and symptoms.

Handbook of Signs & Symptoms combines the authoritative information of a comprehensive signs and symptoms review with the convenience of a handbook that can be carried into the clinical arena. I believe it will become a valuable companion for any health care professional involved in patient assessment.

Neil R. MacIntyre, MD
Professor of Medicine
Duke University
Durham, N.C.

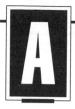

ABDOMINAL DISTENTION

Abdominal distention refers to increased abdominal girth—the result of increased intra-abdominal pressure forcing the abdominal wall outward. Distention may be mild or severe, depending on the amount of pressure. It may be localized or diffuse and may occur gradually or suddenly. Acute abdominal distention may signal life-threatening peritonitis or acute bowel obstruction.

Abdominal distention results from accumulation of fluid or gas (or both) within the lumen of the GI tract or peritoneal cavity. Both fluid and gas are normally present in the GI tract, but not in the peritoneal cavity. However, if fluid and gas are unable to pass freely through the GI tract, abdominal distention occurs. In the peritoneal cavity, distention may reflect acute bleeding, accumulation of ascitic fluid, or air from perforation of an abdominal organ.

Abdominal distention doesn't always signal pathology. For example, in anxious patients or those with digestive distress, localized distention in the left upper quadrant can result from aerophagia—the unconscious swallowing of air. Generalized distention can result from ingestion of fruits or vegetables with large amounts of unabsorbable carbohydrates (such as legumes) or from abnormal food fermentation by microbes.

Emergency interventions

 If the patient displays abdominal distention, quickly check for signs of hypovolemia, such as pallor, diaphoresis, hypotension, and a rapid, thready pulse. Ask the patient if he's experiencing severe abdominal pain or difficulty breathing. Find out about any recent accidents and observe the patient for signs of trauma and of peritoneal bleeding such as a bluish tinge around the umbilicus (Cullen's sign). Then auscultate all abdominal quadrants, noting rapid and high-pitched, diminished, or absent bowel sounds. (If you don't hear bowel sounds immediately, listen for at least 5 minutes.) *Gently* palpate the abdomen for rigidity. Remember that deep or extensive palpation may increase pain.

If you detect abdominal distention, pain, and rigidity along with abnormal bowel sounds, begin emergency interventions. Place the patient in a supine position, administer oxygen, and insert an I.V. line for fluid replacement. Prepare to insert a nasogastric tube to relieve acute intraluminal distention. Reassure the patient and prepare him for surgery.

History and physical examination

If the patient's abdominal distention is not acute, ask about the onset and duration of distention and its associated signs. The patient with localized distention may report a sensation of pressure, fullness, or tenderness in the affected area. The patient with generalized distention may report a bloated feeling, a pounding heart, and difficulty breathing deeply or when lying flat.

1

ABDOMINAL DISTENTION: COMMON CAUSES AND ASSOCIATED FINDINGS

CAUSES	MAJOR ASSOCIATED SIGNS AND SYMPTOMS							
	Abdominal mass	Abdominal pain	Abdominal rigidity	Anorexia	Bowel sounds, absent	Bowel sounds, hyperactive	Bowel sounds, hypoactive	Constipation
Abdominal trauma		●	●		●		●	
Cirrhosis		●		●				●
Heart failure		●						
Irritable bowel syndrome		●						●
Large-bowel obstruction		●				●		●
Nephrotic syndrome				●				
Ovarian cysts	●	●						
Paralytic ileus		●			●		●	●
Peritonitis		●	●		●		●	
Small-bowel obstruction		●			●			●

The patient may also feel unable to bend at his waist. Be sure to ask about abdominal pain, fever, nausea, vomiting, anorexia, altered bowel habits, and weight gain or loss.

Obtain a medical history, noting GI or biliary disorders that may cause peritonitis or ascites, such as cirrhosis, hepatitis, or inflammatory bowel disease. Also note chronic constipation. Has the patient recently had abdominal surgery, which might lead to abdominal distention? Also ask about recent accidents, even minor ones, like falling off a stepladder.

Next, perform a physical examination. Stand at the foot of the bed and observe the recumbent patient for abdominal asymmetry to determine if distention is localized or generalized. Then assess abdominal contour by stooping at his side. Inspect for tense, glistening skin and bulging flanks, which may indicate ascites. Note the umbilicus. An everted umbilicus may indicate ascites or umbilical hernia. An inverted umbilicus may indicate gas distention; it's also common in obesity. Inspect the abdomen for signs of inguinal or femoral hernia and for incisions that may point to adhesions. Both may lead to intestinal obstruction. Then

	Diarrhea	Edema	Fever	Hepatomegaly	Hypotension	Jaundice	Jugular vein distention	Nausea	Oliguria	Rebound tenderness	Succussion splash	Tachycardia	Tachypnea	Urinary frequency	Vomiting	Weight change
					•										•	
	•	•	•	•		•		•							•	•
			•		•			•	•			•			•	
	•							•								
															•	
			•						•							
															•	
				•		•		•		•		•			•	
								•		•					•	

auscultate for bowel sounds, abdominal friction rubs (indicating peritoneal inflammation), and bruits (indicating an aneurysm). Listen for succession splash—a splashing sound normally heard in the stomach when the patient moves or when palpation disturbs the viscera. However, an abnormally loud splash indicates fluid accumulation, suggesting gastric dilation or obstruction.

Next, percuss and palpate the abdomen to determine if distention results from air, fluid, or both. A tympanic note in the left lower quadrant suggests an air-filled descending or sigmoid colon. A tympanic note throughout a generally distended abdomen suggests an air-filled peritoneal cavity. A dull percussion note throughout a generally distended abdomen suggests a fluid-filled peritoneal cavity. Remember that obesity also causes a dull note throughout the abdomen.

Palpate the abdomen for tenderness, noting if it's localized or generalized. Finally, measure abdominal girth for a baseline. Mark the flanks with a felt-tip pen as a reference for subsequent measurements.

Common medical causes
• *Abdominal trauma.* When brisk internal bleeding accompanies trauma, ab-

dominal distention may be acute and dramatic. Associated signs of this life-threatening disorder include abdominal rigidity with guarding, decreased or absent bowel sounds, vomiting, tenderness, and abdominal bruising. Pain may occur over the trauma site, or over the scapula if abdominal bleeding irritates the phrenic nerve. Signs of hypovolemic shock, such as hypotension and rapid, thready pulse, will appear with significant blood loss.

● *Cirrhosis.* In this disorder, ascites causes generalized distention and is confirmed by a fluid wave, shifting dullness, and a puddle sign. (See *Detecting ascites.*) Umbilical eversion and caput medusae (dilated veins around the umbilicus) are common. The patient may report a feeling of fullness or weight gain. Associated findings include vague abdominal pain, fever, anorexia, nausea, vomiting, constipation or diarrhea, bleeding tendencies, severe pruritus, palmar erythema, spider angiomas, leg edema, and possibly splenomegaly. Jaundice is usually a late sign. Hepatomegaly occurs initially, but the liver may not be palpable in advanced disease.

● *Heart failure.* Generalized abdominal distention caused by ascites is confirmed by shifting dullness and a fluid wave. Accompanying the distention are the hallmarks of heart failure: peripheral edema, jugular vein distention, dyspnea, and tachycardia. Common associated signs include nausea, vomiting, productive cough, crackles, cool extremities, cyanotic nail beds, and hepatomegaly, which may cause right upper quadrant pain.

● *Irritable bowel syndrome.* This disorder may produce intermittent, localized distention—the result of periodic intestinal spasms. Lower abdominal pain or cramping typically accompanies these spasms. The pain is usually relieved by defecation or by passage of intestinal gas and is aggravated by stress. Other possible signs and symptoms include diarrhea that may alternate with constipation or

normal bowel function, nausea, dyspepsia, and small, mucus-streaked stools.

● *Large-bowel obstruction.* Dramatic abdominal distention is characteristic in this life-threatening disorder; loops of the large bowel may even become visible on the abdomen. Constipation precedes the distention and may be the only symptom for days. Associated findings may include tympany, high-pitched bowel sounds, and sudden onset of colicky lower abdominal pain that becomes persistent. Fecal vomiting is a late sign.

● *Ovarian cysts.* Typically, large ovarian cysts produce lower abdominal distention accompanied by umbilical eversion. Because they're thin-walled and fluid-filled, these cysts produce a fluid wave and shifting dullness—signs that mimic ascites. Lower abdominal pain and a palpable mass may be present.

● *Paralytic ileus.* This disorder produces generalized distention with a tympanic percussion note. It's accompanied by absent or hypoactive bowel sounds and, occasionally, mild abdominal pain and vomiting. The patient may be severely constipated or may pass flatus and small, liquid stools.

● *Peritonitis.* In this life-threatening disorder, abdominal distention may be localized or generalized, depending on the extent of peritonitis. Fluid accumulates first within the peritoneal cavity and then within the bowel lumen, causing a fluid wave and shifting dullness. Typically, distention is accompanied by sudden and severe abdominal pain that worsens with movement, rebound tenderness, and abdominal rigidity.

The skin over the patient's abdomen may appear taut. Associated signs and symptoms usually include hypoactive or absent bowel sounds, fever, chills, hyperalgesia, nausea, and vomiting. Signs of shock, such as tachycardia and hypotension, will appear with significant fluid loss into the abdomen.

● *Small-bowel obstruction.* Abdominal distention is characteristic in this life-

DETECTING ASCITES

To differentiate ascites from other causes of distention, check for shifting dull-ness, fluid wave, or puddle sign, as described below.

Shifting dullness

With the patient supine, percuss from the umbilicus outward to the flank. Draw a line on the patient's skin to mark the change from tympany to dullness.

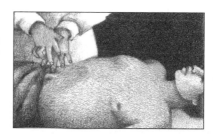

Turn the patient onto his side, which causes ascitic fluid to shift. Percuss again and mark the change from tympany to dull-ness. Any difference between these lines can indicate ascites.

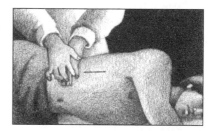

Fluid wave

Have another person press deeply into the patient's midline to prevent vibration from traveling along the abdominal wall. Place one of your palms on one of the patient's flanks. Strike the oppo-site flank with your other hand. If you feel the blow in the opposite palm, ascitic fluid is present.

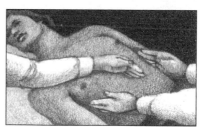

Puddle sign

Position the patient on his elbows and knees, which causes ascitic fluid to pool in the most depen-dent part of the abdomen. Per-cuss the abdomen from the flank to the midline. The percussion note becomes louder at the edge of the puddle, or ascitic pool.

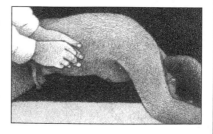

threatening disorder. It's most pronounced in late obstruction, especially in the distal small bowel. Auscultation reveals hypoactive or hyperactive bowel sounds, whereas percussion produces a tympanic note. Accompanying distention are colicky periumbilical pain, constipation, nausea, and vomiting; the higher the obstruction, the earlier and more severe the vomiting. Rebound tenderness reflects intestinal strangulation with ischemia. Associated signs and symptoms may include drowsiness, malaise, and signs of dehydration. Signs of hypovolemic shock will appear with progressive dehydration and plasma loss.

Special considerations

Position the patient comfortably, using pillows for support. Place him on his left side to help flatus escape. Or, if he has ascites, elevate the head of the bed to ease his breathing. If the patient's anxiety triggers air swallowing or deep breathing that causes discomfort, advise him to take slow breaths. Administer drugs to relieve pain, and offer emotional support. If the patient has an obstruction or ascites, explain food and fluid restrictions. Stress good oral hygiene to prevent dry mouth.

Prepare the patient for diagnostic tests, such as abdominal X-rays, endoscopy, laparoscopy, ultrasonography, computed tomography, or possibly paracentesis.

Pediatric pointers

Because the young child's abdomen is normally rounded, distention may be difficult to observe. Fortunately, though, the abdominal wall is less developed than an adult's, making palpation easier. When percussing the abdomen, remember that children normally swallow air when eating and crying, resulting in louder than normal tympany. Minimal tympany with abdominal distention may result from fluid accumulation or solid masses. To check for abdominal fluid, test for shifting dullness instead of for a fluid wave. (In a child, air swallowing and incomplete abdominal muscle development make the fluid wave hard to interpret.)

In the neonate, ascites usually results from GI or urinary perforation; in an older child, it may result from heart failure, cirrhosis, or nephrosis. Besides ascites, congenital malformations of the GI tract (such as intussusception and volvulus) may cause abdominal distention. A hernia may cause distention if it produces an intestinal obstruction. In addition, overeating and constipation can also cause distention.

ABDOMINAL MASS

Commonly detected on routine physical examination, an abdominal mass is a localized swelling in one of the abdominal quadrants. Typically, this sign develops insidiously and may represent an enlarged organ, a neoplasm, an abscess, a vascular defect, or a fecal mass. (See *Abdominal mass: Locations and common causes.*)

Distinguishing an abdominal mass from normal structures requires skillful palpation. At times, palpation must be repeated with the patient in a different position or performed by a second examiner to verify initial findings. A palpable abdominal mass is an important clinical sign and usually represents a serious—and perhaps life-threatening—disorder.

Emergency interventions

 If the patient has a pulsating midabdominal mass and severe abdominal pain, suspect an aortic aneurysm. Quickly take his vital signs. Because the patient may require emergency surgery, withhold food or fluids until the patient is examined. Prepare to administer oxygen and to start an I.V. infusion for fluid and blood replacement. Obtain routine preoperative tests, and

ABDOMINAL MASS: LOCATIONS AND COMMON CAUSES

The location of an abdominal mass provides an important clue to the causative disorder. Here are the disorders responsible for abdominal masses and the quadrants where the masses occur.

Right upper quadrant
- Aortic aneurysm (epigastric area)
- Cholecystitis or cholelithiasis
- Gallbladder, gastric, hepatic carcinoma
- Hepatomegaly
- Hydronephrosis
- Pancreatic abscess or pseudocysts
- Renal cell carcinoma

Left upper quadrant
- Aortic aneurysm (epigastric area)
- Gastric carcinoma (epigastric area)
- Hydronephrosis
- Pancreatic abscess (epigastric area)
- Pancreatic pseudocysts (epigastric area)
- Renal cell carcinoma
- Splenomegaly

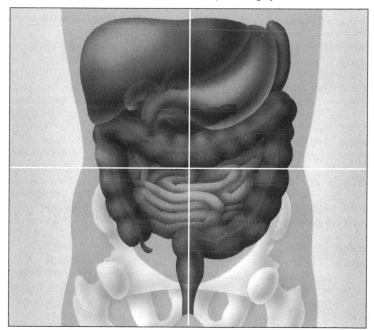

Right lower quadrant
- Bladder distention (suprapubic area)
- Colon cancer
- Crohn's disease
- Ovarian cyst (suprapubic area)
- Uterine leiomyomas (suprapubic area)

Left lower quadrant
- Bladder distention (suprapubic area)
- Colon cancer
- Diverticulitis
- Ovarian cyst (suprapubic area)
- Uterine leiomyomas (suprapubic area)
- Volvulus

prepare the patient for angiography. Frequently monitor blood pressure, pulse, respirations, and urine output.

Be alert for signs of shock, such as tachycardia, hypotension, and cool, clammy skin, which may indicate significant blood loss.

History and physical examination

If the patient's abdominal mass doesn't suggest an aortic aneurysm, continue with a detailed history. Ask the patient if the mass is painful. If so, ask if the pain is constant or if it occurs only on palpation. Is it localized or generalized? Determine if the patient was already aware of the mass. If he was, find out if the patient noticed any change in the mass's size or location.

Next, review the patient's medical history, paying special attention to GI disorders. Ask the patient about GI signs and symptoms, such as constipation, diarrhea, rectal bleeding, abnormally colored stools, vomiting, and a change in appetite. If the patient is female, ask about the regularity of her menstrual cycles.

Begin the physical examination by auscultating for bowel sounds in each quadrant. Listen for bruits or friction rubs, and check for enlarged veins. Palpate the abdomen, first lightly then deeply, assessing any painful or suspicious areas last. Be sure to note the patient's position when you locate the mass. Some masses can only be detected with the patient supine; others require a side-lying position.

Estimate the size of the mass in centimeters. Determine its shape. Is it round or sausage-shaped? Describe its contour as smooth, rough, sharply defined, nodular, or irregular.

Further, determine the consistency of the mass. Is it doughy, soft, solid, or hard? Also, percuss the mass: A dull sound indicates a fluid-filled mass; a tympanic sound indicates an air-filled mass.

Next, determine if the mass moves with your hand or in response to respiration. Is the mass free-floating or attached to intra-abdominal structures? To determine whether the mass is located in the abdominal wall or the abdominal cavity, ask the patient to lift his head and shoulders off the examination table, thereby contracting his abdominal muscles. While these muscles are contracted, try to palpate the mass. If you can, the mass is in the abdominal wall; if you can't, the mass is within the abdominal cavity.

Common medical causes

• *Abdominal aortic aneurysm.* This disorder may persist for years, producing only a pulsating periumbilical mass with a systolic bruit over the aorta. However, it may become life-threatening if the aneurysm expands and its walls weaken. In such cases, the patient initially reports constant upper abdominal pain or, less commonly, low back or dull abdominal pain. If the aneurysm ruptures, he'll report severe abdominal and back pain. And after rupture, the aneurysm no longer pulsates.

Associated signs and symptoms may include mottled skin below the waist, absent femoral and pedal pulses, lower blood pressure in the legs than in the arms, mild to moderate tenderness with guarding, and abdominal rigidity. Signs of shock—such as tachycardia and cool, clammy skin—will appear with significant blood loss.

• *Cholecystitis.* Deep palpation below the liver border may detect a smooth, firm, sausage-shaped mass. However, in acute inflammation, the gallbladder is usually too tender to palpate. Cholecystitis can cause severe right upper quadrant pain that may radiate to the right shoulder, chest, or back; abdominal rigidity and tenderness; fever; pallor; diaphoresis; anorexia; and nausea and vomiting.

• *Colon cancer.* A right lower quadrant mass may occur in cancer of the right colon, which may also cause occult bleeding and abdominal aching, pressure, or dull cramps. Associated findings include weakness, fatigue, exertional dyspnea, vertigo, and signs of intestinal obstruction, such as obstipation and vomiting.

Occasionally, cancer of the left colon also causes a palpable mass. Usually, though, it produces rectal bleeding, intermittent abdominal fullness or cramping, and rectal pressure. Later, the patient develops obstipation, diarrhea, or pencil-shaped, grossly bloody, or mucus-streaked stools. Typically, defecation relieves pain.

● *Crohn's disease.* In this disorder, tender, sausage-shaped masses are usually palpable in the right lower quadrant and, at times, in the left lower quadrant. Attacks of colicky right lower quadrant pain and diarrhea are common. Associated signs and symptoms include fever, anorexia, weight loss, hyperactive bowel sounds, nausea, and abdominal tenderness with guarding.

● *Diverticulitis.* Most common in the sigmoid colon, this disorder may produce a left lower quadrant mass. It also produces intermittent abdominal pain that's relieved by defecation or passage of flatus. Other findings may include alternating constipation and diarrhea, nausea, and a low-grade fever.

● *Hepatomegaly.* This produces a firm, blunt, irregular mass in the epigastric region or below the right costal margin. Associated signs and symptoms depend on the causative disorder but commonly include ascites, right upper quadrant pain and tenderness, anorexia, nausea, vomiting, leg edema, jaundice and, possibly, splenomegaly.

● *Hydronephrosis.* Enlarging one or both kidneys, this disorder produces a smooth, boggy mass in one or both flanks. Other findings vary with the degree of hydronephrosis. There may be severe colicky renal pain or dull flank pain that radiates to the groin. There may also be hematuria, pyuria, dysuria, alternating oliguria and polyuria, nausea, and vomiting.

● *Ovarian cyst.* A large ovarian cyst may produce a smooth, rounded, fluctuant mass resembling a distended bladder, in the suprapubic region. Large or multiple cysts may also cause mild pelvic discomfort, low back pain, and menstrual irregularities. A twisted or ruptured cyst may cause abdominal tenderness, distention, and rigidity.

● *Splenomegaly.* Lymphomas, leukemias, hemolytic anemias, and inflammatory diseases are among the many disorders that may cause splenomegaly. Typically, the smooth edge of the enlarged spleen is palpable in the left upper quadrant. Associated signs and symptoms vary with the causative disorder but commonly include a feeling of abdominal fullness, left upper quadrant pain and tenderness, splenic friction rub, splenic bruits, and low-grade fever.

● *Uterine leiomyomas (fibroids).* If large enough, these common, benign uterine tumors produce a round, multinodular mass in the suprapubic region. The patient's chief complaint is usually menorrhagia, but she also may experience a feeling of heaviness in the abdomen. Pressure on surrounding organs may cause back pain, constipation, and urinary frequency or urgency.

Special considerations

Discovery of an abdominal mass typically causes anxiety. Offer emotional support to the patient and his family as they await the diagnosis. Position the patient comfortably, and administer drugs for pain or anxiety, as needed.

Carefully explain diagnostic tests, which may include blood and urine studies, abdominal X-rays, barium enema, computed tomography, ultrasonography, radioisotope scans, and gastroscopy or sigmoidoscopy. A pelvic or rectal examination may be indicated.

If an abdominal mass causes bowel obstruction, watch for symptoms of peritonitis—abdominal pain and rebound tenderness—and for signs of shock, such as tachycardia and hypotension.

Pediatric pointers

Detecting an abdominal mass in an infant can be quite a challenge. However, these tips will make palpation easier for you: Allow an infant to suck on his bottle or pacifier to prevent crying, which causes abdominal rigidity and interferes with palpation. Avoid tickling him because laughter also causes abdominal rigidity. Also reduce his apprehension by distracting him with cheerful conversation. Rest your hand on his abdomen for a few moments before palpation. If he remains sensitive, place his hand under yours as you palpate.

In newborns, most abdominal masses result from renal disorders, such as polycystic kidney disease or congenital hydronephrosis. In older infants and children, abdominal masses usually result from enlarged organs, such as the liver and spleen.

Other common causes include Wilms' tumor, neuroblastoma, intussusception, volvulus, Hirschsprung's disease, pyloric stenosis, and abdominal abscess.

ABDOMINAL PAIN

Usually, abdominal pain results from GI disorders, but it can also result from reproductive, genitourinary (GU), musculoskeletal, and vascular disorders; drug use; and the effects of toxins. At times, abdominal pain signals life-threatening complications.

Abdominal pain arises from the abdominopelvic viscera, the parietal peritoneum, or the capsules of the liver, kidney, or spleen. It may be acute or chronic, diffuse or localized. Visceral pain develops slowly into a dull, aching pain that's poorly localized in the epigastric, periumbilical, or lower midabdominal region.

In contrast, somatic pain produces a bright, sharp, more intense, and well-localized discomfort that rapidly follows the insult. Movement or coughing aggravates this pain.

Pain may also be referred to the abdomen from another site with the same or similar nerve supply. This sharp, well-localized, referred pain is felt in skin or deeper tissues and may coexist with skin hyperesthesia and muscle hyperalgesia.

Mechanisms that produce abdominal pain include stretching or tension of the gut wall, traction on the peritoneum or mesentery, vigorous intestinal contraction, inflammation, ischemia, or sensory nerve irritation. (See *Abdominal pain: Types and location.*)

Emergency interventions

 If the patient is experiencing sudden and severe abdominal pain, quickly take his vital signs and palpate pulses below the waist. Be alert for signs of hypovolemic shock, such as tachycardia and hypotension.

Emergency surgery may be required if the patient also exhibits mottled skin below the waist and a pulsating epigastric mass, or rebound tenderness and rigidity.

History and physical examination

If the patient has no life-threatening signs or symptoms, take his history. Ask the patient if the pain is constant or intermittent and when the pain began. Constant, steady abdominal pain suggests organ perforation, ischemia, or inflammation or blood in the peritoneal cavity. Intermittent, cramping abdominal pain suggests the patient may have obstruction of a hollow organ.

If pain is intermittent, find out the duration of a typical episode. In addition, ask the patient where the pain is located and if it radiates to other areas.

ABDOMINAL PAIN: TYPES AND LOCATION

AFFECTED ORGAN	VISCERAL PAIN	PARIETAL PAIN	REFERRED PAIN
Appendix	Periumbilical area	Right lower quadrant	Right lower quadrant
Distal colon	Hypogastrium and left flank for descending colon	Over affected site	Left lower quadrant and back (rare)
Gallbladder	Middle epigastrium	Right upper quadrant	Right subscapular area
Ovaries, fallopian tubes, and uterus	Hypogastrium and groin	Over affected site	Inner thighs
Pancreas	Middle epigastrium and left upper quadrant	Middle epigastrium and left upper quadrant	Back and left shoulder
Proximal colon	Periumbilical area and right flank for ascending colon	Over affected site	Right lower quadrant and back (rare)
Small intestine	Periumbilical area	Over affected site	Midback (rare)
Stomach	Middle epigastrium	Middle epigastrium and left upper quadrant	Shoulders
Ureters	Costovertebral angle	Over affected site	Groin, scrotum in men, labia in women (rare)

Find out if movement, coughing, exertion, vomiting, eating, elimination, or walking worsens or relieves the pain. The patient may report abdominal pain as indigestion or gas pain, so have him describe it in detail.

Ask the patient about drug and alcohol use and any history of vascular, GI, GU, or reproductive disorders. As appropriate, ask the female patient about the date of her last menses, changes in her menstrual pattern, or dyspareunia.

Ask the patient about appetite changes. In addition, ask him about the onset and frequency of nausea or vomiting. Find out about any changes in bowel habits, such as constipation, diarrhea, and changes in stool consistency. When was the last bowel movement? Ask about urinary frequency, urgency, or pain. Is the urine cloudy or pink?

Perform a physical examination. You should take the patient's vital signs and assess skin turgor and mucous membranes. Inspect his abdomen for distention or visible peristaltic waves and, if indicated, measure his abdominal girth.

Auscultate for bowel sounds and characterize their motility. Percuss all quadrants, carefully noting the percussion sounds. Palpate the entire abdomen for masses, rigidity, and tenderness. Check specifically for costovertebral angle (CVA) tenderness, abdominal tenderness with guarding, and rebound tenderness.

Common medical causes

● *Abdominal aortic aneurysm (dissecting).* Initially, this life-threatening disorder may produce dull abdominal, low back, or severe chest pain. More commonly, it produces constant upper abdominal pain, which may worsen when the patient lies down and abate when he leans forward or sits up. Palpation may reveal an epigastric mass that pulsates before rupture but not after it. Other findings may include mottled skin below the waist, absent femoral and pedal pulses, lower blood pressure in the legs than in the arms, mild to moderate abdominal tenderness with guarding, and abdominal rigidity. Signs of shock appear, such as tachycardia and tachypnea.

● *Abdominal trauma.* Generalized or localized abdominal pain occurs with possible ecchymoses on the abdomen, abdominal tenderness, vomiting and, with hemorrhage into the peritoneal cavity, abdominal rigidity.

● *Adrenal crisis.* Severe abdominal pain appears early, along with nausea, vomiting, weakness, anorexia, and fever. Later signs are progressive loss of consciousness, hypotension, tachycardia, oliguria, and cool, clammy skin.

● *Appendicitis.* In this life-threatening disorder, dull discomfort in the epigastric or umbilical region typically precedes anorexia, nausea, and vomiting. Pain localizes at McBurney's point in the right lower quadrant, accompanied by abdominal rigidity, increasing tenderness (especially over McBurney's point), rebound tenderness, and retractive respirations. Later signs and symptoms include constipation (or diarrhea), slight fever, and tachycardia.

● *Cholelithiasis.* Patients may suffer sudden, severe, and paroxysmal pain in the right upper quadrant lasting several minutes to several hours. The pain may radiate to the epigastrium, back, or shoulder blades. The pain is accompanied by anorexia, nausea, vomiting (sometimes bilious), diaphoresis, restlessness, and abdominal tenderness with guarding over the gallbladder or biliary duct.

● *Cirrhosis.* Dull abdominal aching occurs early, and this is usually accompanied by anorexia, indigestion, nausea, vomiting, constipation, or diarrhea. Subsequent right upper quadrant pain worsens when the patient sits up or leans forward. Associated signs include fever, ascites, leg edema, weight gain, hepatomegaly, jaundice, severe pruritus, bleeding tendencies, palmar erythema, and spider angiomas.

● *Crohn's disease.* An *acute* attack causes severe, cramping pain in the lower abdomen, typically preceded by weeks or months of milder, cramping pain. It may also cause diarrhea or constipation, bloody stools, hyperactive bowel sounds, high fever, abdominal tenderness with guarding, and possibly a palpable mass in a lower quadrant.

Milder *chronic* symptoms include right lower quadrant pain with diarrhea, steatorrhea, and weight loss.

● *Duodenal ulcer.* Localized abdominal pain—described as steady, gnawing, burning, aching, or hungerlike—may occur high in the midepigastrium or slightly off center, usually on the right. It usually does not radiate unless pancreatic penetration occurs. Commonly, pain begins 2 to 4 hours after meals and may cause nocturnal awakening. Ingestion of food or antacids brings relief until the cycle starts again but also may produce weight gain. Other symptoms include changes in bowel habits, and heartburn or retrosternal burning.

• *Ectopic pregnancy.* Lower abdominal pain may be sharp, dull, or cramping, and constant or intermittent in this potentially life-threatening disorder. Vaginal bleeding, nausea, and vomiting may occur, along with urinary frequency, a tender adnexal mass, and a 1- to 2-month history of amenorrhea. Rupture of the fallopian tube produces sharp lower abdominal pain, which may radiate to the shoulders and neck and become extreme with cervical or adnexal palpation. Signs of shock, such as pallor, tachycardia, and hypotension, may also appear.

• *Endometriosis.* Constant, severe pain in the lower abdomen usually begins 5 to 7 days before menstruation begins and may be aggravated by defecation. Depending on the location of the ectopic tissue, the pain may be accompanied by constipation, abdominal tenderness, dysmenorrhea, dyspareunia, and deep sacral pain.

• *Gastric ulcer.* Diffuse, gnawing, burning pain in the left upper quadrant or epigastric area commonly occurs 1 to 2 hours after meals and may be relieved by food or antacids. Vague bloating and nausea after eating are common. Indigestion, weight change, anorexia, and episodes of GI bleeding also occur.

• *Heart failure.* Right upper quadrant pain commonly accompanies this disorder's hallmarks: neck vein distention, dyspnea, tachycardia, and peripheral edema. Other findings may include nausea, vomiting, ascites, productive cough, crackles, cool extremities, and cyanotic nail beds.

• *Hepatitis.* Liver enlargement from any type of hepatitis will cause discomfort or dull pain and tenderness in the right upper quadrant. Associated findings may include dark urine, clay-colored stools, nausea, vomiting, anorexia, jaundice, and pruritus.

• *Intestinal obstruction.* Short episodes of intense, colicky, cramping pain alternate with pain-free intervals in this life-threatening disorder. Accompanying signs and symptoms may include abdominal distention, tenderness, and guarding; visible peristaltic waves; high-pitched, tinkling, or hyperactive sounds proximal to obstruction and hypoactive or absent sounds distally; obstipation; and pain-induced agitation. In jejunal and duodenal obstruction, nausea and bilious vomiting occur early. In distal small-bowel or large-bowel obstruction, nausea and vomiting are often feculent. Complete obstruction produces absent bowel sounds. Late-stage obstruction produces signs of hypovolemic shock, such as hypotension and tachycardia.

• *Ovarian cyst.* Torsion or hemorrhage causes pain and tenderness in the right or left lower abdominal quadrant. Sharp and severe if the patient suddenly stands or stoops, the pain becomes brief and intermittent if the torsion self-corrects, or dull and diffuse after several hours if it doesn't. Pain is accompanied by slight fever, mild nausea and vomiting, abdominal tenderness and a palpable mass, and possibly amenorrhea. Abdominal distention may occur with large cysts. Peritoneal irritation, or rupture and peritonitis, causes high fever and severe nausea and vomiting.

• *Pancreatitis.* Life-threatening *acute pancreatitis* produces fulminating, continuous upper abdominal pain that may radiate to both flanks and to the back. To relieve this pain, the patient may bend forward, draw his knees to his chest, or move restlessly about. Early findings include abdominal tenderness, nausea, vomiting, fever, pallor, tachycardia and, in some patients, abdominal rigidity, rebound tenderness, and hypoactive bowel sounds. Grey Turner's or Cullen's sign signals hemorrhagic pancreatitis. As inflammation subsides, jaundice may occur.

Chronic pancreatitis produces severe left upper quadrant or epigastric pain that radiates to the back. Abdominal tender-

ABDOMINAL PAIN: COMMON CAUSES AND ASSOCIATED FINDINGS

CAUSES	Abdominal distention	Abdominal mass	Abdominal rigidity	Abdominal tenderness	Amenorrhea	Anorexia	Bowel sounds, absent	Bowel sounds, hyperactive	Bowel sounds, hypoactive	Breath odor, fruity	
Abdominal aortic aneurysm		●	●	●							
Abdominal cancer	●	●				●					
Adrenal crisis						●					
Appendicitis			●	●		●					
Cholelithiasis		●		●							
Cirrhosis	●					●					
Crohn's disease		●		●				●			
Diabetic ketoacidosis										●	
Diverticulitis		●	●								
Duodenal ulcer											
Ectopic pregnancy		●			●						
Endometriosis				●							
Gastric ulcer						●					
Gastroenteritis								●			
Heart failure	●										
Hepatic abscess				●		●					
Hepatitis				●		●					
Herpes zoster				●							
Intestinal obstruction	●			●			●	●	●		
Ovarian cyst	●	●		●	●						
Pancreatitis			●	●					●		
Pelvic inflammatory disease		●		●							

MAJOR ASSOCIATED SIGNS AND SYMPTOMS

Chest pain	Constipation	Costovertebral angle tenderness	Cough	Diarrhea	Dyspnea	Fever	Kussmaul's respirations	Nausea	Oliguria or anuria	Skin lesions	Skin mottling	Tachycardia	Tachypnea	Urinary frequency	Vomiting	Weakness	Weight change
•											•	•	•				
																•	•
						•		•	•			•			•	•	
	•			•		•		•				•			•		
						•		•							•		
	•			•		•		•							•		•
	•			•		•											•
							•					•					
	•							•									
•	•			•													•
								•						•	•		
	•																
								•									
				•				•							•		
•			•		•			•				•			•		
				•		•		•							•		
								•							•		
						•				•							
•	•							•				•	•		•		
				•				•							•		
				•				•				•			•		
				•				•							•		

(continued)

ABDOMINAL PAIN: COMMON CAUSES AND ASSOCIATED FINDINGS *(continued)*

	MAJOR ASSOCIATED SIGNS AND SYMPTOMS									
CAUSES	Abdominal distention	Abdominal mass	Abdominal rigidity	Abdominal tenderness	Amenorrhea	Anorexia	Bowel sounds, absent	Bowel sounds, hyperactive	Bowel sounds, hypoactive	Breath odor, fruity
Perforated ulcer			●	●			●			
Peritonitis	●		●	●			●		●	
Pneumothorax										
Prostatitis										
Pyelonephritis				●						
Renal calculi										
Sickle cell crisis										
Ulcerative colitis				●		●		●		

ness, a midepigastric mass, jaundice, fever, and splenomegaly may occur. Steatorrhea and weight loss are common.

● *Pelvic inflammatory disease.* Pain in the right or left lower quadrant ranges from vague discomfort worsened by movement to deep, severe, and progressive pain. Sometimes, metrorrhagia precedes or accompanies the onset of pain. Extreme pain accompanies cervical or adnexal palpation. Associated findings may include abdominal tenderness, a palpable abdominal or pelvic mass, fever, occasional chills, nausea, vomiting, and abnormal vaginal bleeding.

● *Perforated ulcer.* In this life-threatening disorder, sudden, severe, and prostrating epigastric pain may radiate through the abdomen to the back. Other signs and symptoms include boardlike abdominal rigidity, tenderness with guarding, generalized rebound tenderness, absent bowel sounds, grunting and shallow respirations and, in many cases, fever, tachycardia, and hypotension.

● *Peritonitis.* In this life-threatening disorder, sudden and severe pain can be diffuse or localized in the area of the underlying disorder; movement worsens the pain. The degree of abdominal tenderness usually depends on the disease's extent. Typical findings include fever, chills, nausea, vomiting, hypoactive or absent bowel sounds, rebound tenderness and guarding, hyperalgesia, tachycardia, hypotension, tachypnea, and abdominal tenderness, distention, and rigidity.

● *Prostatitis.* Vague abdominal pain or discomfort in the lower abdomen, groin, perineum, or rectum may develop. Other findings may include dysuria, urinary frequency and urgency, fever, chills, lower back pain, myalgia, and arthralgia.

● *Pyelonephritis (acute).* Progressive lower quadrant pain in one or both sides, flank pain, and CVA tenderness charac-

Chest pain	Constipation	Costovertebral angle tenderness	Cough	Diarrhea	Dyspnea	Fever	Kussmaul's respirations	Nausea	Oliguria or anuria	Skin lesions	Skin mottling	Tachycardia	Tachypnea	Urinary frequency	Vomiting	Weakness	Weight change
						•						•					
						•		•				•	•		•		
•						•						•	•	•			
						•											
		•				•		•						•	•		
		•				•		•							•		
•						•										•	
				•		•		•							•		•

terize this disorder. Pain may radiate to the lower midabdomen or to the groin. Additional signs and symptoms may include abdominal and back tenderness, high fever, shaking chills, nausea, vomiting, and urinary frequency and urgency.

• *Renal calculi.* Depending on the location of calculi, severe abdominal or back pain may occur. However, the classic symptom is severe, colicky pain that travels from the CVA to the flank, the suprapubic region, and the external genitalia. The pain may be excruciating or dull and constant. Pain-induced agitation, nausea, vomiting, abdominal distention, fever, chills, and urinary urgency may occur.

• *Splenic infarction.* Fulminating pain in the left upper quadrant occurs along with chest pain that may worsen on inspiration. Pain commonly radiates to the left shoulder with splinting of the left diaphragm, abdominal guarding, and occasionally a splenic friction rub.

• *Ulcerative colitis.* This disorder may begin with vague abdominal discomfort that leads to cramping lower abdominal pain. As the disorder progresses, pain can become steady and diffuse, increasing with movement and coughing. The most common symptom—recurrent and possibly severe diarrhea with blood, pus, and mucus—may relieve the pain. The abdomen may feel soft, squashy, and extremely tender. High-pitched, infrequent bowel sounds may accompany nausea, vomiting, anorexia, weight loss, and mild, intermittent fever.

Other causes

• *Drugs.* Salicylates and nonsteroidal anti-inflammatory drugs commonly cause burning, gnawing pain in the left upper quadrant or epigastric area, along with nausea and vomiting.

Special considerations

Help the patient find a comfortable position, if possible, to ease his distress, and monitor him closely, because abdominal pain can signal a life-threatening disorder. Especially important indications include tachycardia, hypotension, clammy skin, abdominal rigidity, rebound tenderness, a change in the pain's location or intensity, or a sudden relief from pain.

Withhold analgesics from the patient because they may mask symptoms. Also withhold food and fluids because surgery may be needed. Prepare for I.V. infusion and insertion of a nasogastric or other intestinal tube. Peritoneal lavage or abdominal paracentesis may be required.

You may have to prepare patients for diagnostic procedures. These may include pelvic or rectal examination, X-rays, barium studies, ultrasonography, endoscopy, biopsy, or blood, urine, and stool tests.

Pediatric pointers

Because a child commonly has difficulty describing abdominal pain, pay close attention to nonverbal cues—wincing, lethargy, or unusual positioning (such as a side-lying position with knees flexed to the abdomen).

In children, abdominal pain can signal a disorder with greater severity or different associated signs than in adults. Appendicitis, for example, has a higher rupture rate and mortality in children, and vomiting may be the only other sign. Acute pyelonephritis may cause abdominal pain, vomiting, and diarrhea, but not the classic urologic signs found in adults. Peptic ulcer, which is becoming increasingly common in teenagers, causes nocturnal pain and colic that, unlike peptic ulcer in adults, may not be relieved by food.

Abdominal pain in children can also result from lactose intolerance, volvulus, Meckel's diverticulum, intussusception, mesenteric adenitis, diabetes mellitus, juvenile rheumatoid arthritis, and many uncommon disorders such as heavy metal poisoning. Remember, too, that a child's complaint of abdominal pain may reflect an emotional need, such as a wish to avoid school or to gain adult attention.

ABDOMINAL RIGIDITY
[Abdominal muscle spasm, involuntary guarding]

Detected by palpation, abdominal rigidity refers to abnormal muscle tension or inflexibility of the abdomen. Rigidity may be voluntary or involuntary. Voluntary rigidity reflects the patient's fear or nervousness upon palpation, while involuntary rigidity reflects potentially life-threatening peritoneal irritation or inflammation. (See *Recognizing voluntary rigidity*.)

Involuntary rigidity usually results from GI disorders but may also result from pulmonary and vascular disorders and from the effects of insect toxins. It typically occurs with nausea, vomiting, fever, and abdominal tenderness, distention, and pain.

Emergency interventions

 After palpating abdominal rigidity, quickly take the patient's vital signs. Even though the patient may not appear gravely ill or have markedly abnormal vital signs, his abdominal rigidity calls for emergency interventions.

Prepare to administer oxygen and to insert an I.V. line for fluid and blood replacement. The patient may require drugs to support blood pressure. Also prepare the patient for catheterization, and monitor intake and output.

An intestinal tube may have to be inserted to relieve abdominal distention. Because emergency surgery may be necessary, the patient should be prepared for laboratory tests and X-rays.

History and physical examination

If the patient's condition allows further assessment, take a brief history. Find out when the abdominal rigidity began. Is it associated with abdominal pain? If so, did the pain begin at the same time? Determine whether abdominal rigidity is localized or generalized. Is it always present? Has its site changed or remained constant? Next ask about aggravating or alleviating factors, such as position changes, coughing, vomiting, elimination, and walking.

Then explore other signs and symptoms. Inspect the abdomen for peristaltic waves, which may be visible in thin patients. Also check for a visible distended bowel loop. Next, auscultate bowel sounds. Perform light palpation to locate the rigidity and determine its severity. Avoid deep palpation, which may exacerbate abdominal pain. Finally, check for poor skin turgor and dry mucous membranes, indicating dehydration.

Common medical causes

● *Abdominal aortic aneurysm (dissecting).* Mild to moderate abdominal rigidity occurs in this life-threatening disorder. Typically, it's accompanied by constant upper abdominal pain that may radiate to the lower back. The pain may worsen when the patient lies down and may be relieved when he leans forward or sits up. Before rupture, the aneurysm may produce a pulsating mass in the epigastrium, accompanied by a systolic bruit over the aorta. However, the mass stops pulsating after rupture. Associated signs and symptoms may include mottled skin below the waist, absent femoral and pedal pulses, lower blood pressure in the legs than in the arms, and mild to moderate tenderness with guarding. Significant blood loss causes signs of shock, such as tachycardia, tachypnea, and cool, clammy skin.

● *Insect toxins.* Insect stings and bites, especially black widow spider bites, release toxins that can produce general-

EXAMINATION TIP

RECOGNIZING VOLUNTARY RIGIDITY

Distinguishing voluntary and involuntary abdominal rigidity is a must for accurate assessment. Review this comparison so that you can quickly tell the two apart.

Voluntary rigidity is:
● usually symmetrical
● more rigid on inspiration (expiration causes muscle relaxation)
● eased by relaxation techniques, such as positioning the patient comfortably and talking to him in a calm, soothing manner
● painless when the patient sits up using his abdominal muscles alone.

Involuntary rigidity is:
● usually asymmetrical
● equally rigid on inspiration and expiration
● unaffected by relaxation techniques
● painful when the patient sits up using his abdominal muscles alone.

ized, cramping abdominal pain usually accompanied by rigidity. These toxins may also cause low-grade fever, nausea, vomiting, tremors, and burning sensations in the hands and feet.

● *Mesenteric artery ischemia.* In this life-threatening disorder, 2 to 3 days of persistent, low-grade abdominal pain and diarrhea precede abdominal rigidity. Rigidity occurs in the central or periumbilical region and is accompanied by severe abdominal tenderness, fever, and signs of shock, such as tachycardia and hypotension. Other findings may include vomiting, anorexia, diarrhea, and constipation.

● *Peritonitis.* Depending on the cause of peritonitis, abdominal rigidity may be localized or generalized. For example, if an inflamed appendix causes local peritonitis, rigidity may be localized in the right lower quadrant. If a perforated ulcer causes widespread peritonitis, rigidity may be generalized and, in severe cases, boardlike.

Peritonitis also causes sudden and severe abdominal pain that can be localized or generalized. It can also produce abdominal tenderness and distention, rebound tenderness, guarding, hyperalgesia, hypoactive or absent bowel sounds, nausea, and vomiting. Usually, the patient also displays fever, chills, tachycardia, tachypnea, and hypotension.

● *Pneumonia.* In lower lobe pneumonia, severe upper abdominal pain and tenderness accompany rigidity that diminishes with inspiration. Associated signs and symptoms include a dry, hacking cough, blood-tinged or rusty sputum, dyspnea, achiness, headache, fever, and sudden onset of chills.

Special considerations
Continue to monitor the patient closely for signs of shock. Position him as comfortably as possible. Because analgesics may mask symptoms, withhold them until a tentative diagnosis has been made. Because emergency surgery may be required, withhold food and fluids and administer I.V. antibiotics. Prepare the patient for diagnostic tests, which may include chest and abdominal X-rays, peritoneal lavage, gastroscopy or colonoscopy, and blood, urine, and stool studies. A pelvic or rectal examination may also be done.

Pediatric pointers
Voluntary rigidity may be difficult to distinguish from involuntary rigidity if associated pain makes the child restless, tense, or apprehensive. However, in any child with suspected involuntary rigidity, your priority is early detection of dehydration and shock, which can rapidly become life-threatening.

Abdominal rigidity in the child can stem from gastric perforation, hypertrophic pyloric stenosis, duodenal obstruction, meconium ileus, intussusception, cystic fibrosis, celiac disease, and appendicitis.

ACCESSORY MUSCLE USE

When breathing requires extra effort, the accessory muscles—the sternocleidomastoid, scalene, pectoralis major, trapezius, internal intercostals, and abdominal muscles—stabilize the thorax during respiration. (See *Reviewing accessory muscle location and function.*) Some accessory muscle use normally takes place during such activities as singing, talking, coughing, defecating, and exercising. However, more pronounced use of these muscles may signal acute respiratory distress, diaphragmatic weakness, or fatigue. It may also result from chronic respiratory disease. Typically, the extent of accessory muscle use reflects the severity of the underlying cause.

Emergency interventions

 If the patient displays increased accessory muscle use, immediately look for signs of acute respiratory distress. These include decreased level of consciousness, shortness of breath when speaking, tachypnea, intercostal and sternal retractions, cyanosis, external breath sounds like wheezing or stridor, diaphoresis, nasal flaring, and extreme apprehension or agitation. Quickly auscultate for abnormal, diminished, or absent breath sounds. Check for airway obstruction and, if detected, attempt to restore airway patency. Insert an airway or intubate the patient. Then begin suctioning and manual or mechanical ventilation. Administer oxygen; if the patient has chronic obstructive pulmonary

REVIEWING ACCESSORY MUSCLE LOCATION AND FUNCTION

Physical exertion and pulmonary disease commonly increase the work of breathing, taxing the diaphragm and external intercostal muscles. When this happens, accessory muscles provide the extra effort needed to maintain respirations. The upper accessory muscles assist with inspiration, while the upper chest, the sternum, the internal intercostal muscles, and the abdominal muscles assist with expiration.

In inspiration, the scalene muscles elevate, fix, and expand the upper chest. The sternocleidomastoid muscles raise the sternum, expanding the chest's anteroposterior and longitudinal dimensions. The pectoralis majors elevate the chest, increasing its anteroposterior size, and the trapezius muscles raise the thoracic cage.

In expiration, the internal intercostals depress the ribs, decreasing the chest size. The abdominal muscles pull the lower chest down, depress the lower ribs, and compress the abdominal contents, which exerts pressure on the chest.

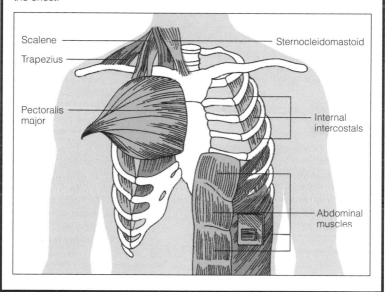

disease (COPD), use a low flow rate. An I.V. line may be required.

History and physical examination

If the patient's condition allows, examine him more closely. Ask him about the onset, duration, and severity of associated symptoms, such as dyspnea, chest pain, cough, or fever.

Explore his medical history, focusing on respiratory disorders, such as infection or COPD. Ask about cardiac disorders such as heart failure, which may lead to pulmonary edema, and about neuromuscular disorders such as amyotrophic lateral sclerosis, which may affect respiratory muscle function. Note a history of allergies or asthma. Because collagen

ACCESSORY MUSCLE USE: COMMON CAUSES AND ASSOCIATED FINDINGS

CAUSES	Barrel chest	Chest pain	Cough	Crackles	Cyanosis	Diaphoresis	Dyspnea	Fever	Muscle weakness	Paralysis	Stridor	Tachycardia	Tachypnea	Wheezing
Adult respiratory distress syndrome			•	•		•	•					•	•	
Airway obstruction			•		•		•				•	•	•	•
Asthma	•		•	•	•	•	•					•	•	•
Emphysema	•		•		•		•					•		
Pneumonia		•	•	•	•	•	•	•				•	•	
Pulmonary edema			•	•	•		•					•	•	•
Pulmonary embolism		•	•	•	•		•	•				•	•	•
Spinal cord injury									•	•				

vascular diseases can cause diffuse infiltrative lung disease, ask about such conditions as rheumatoid arthritis and lupus erythematosus.

Ask about recent trauma, especially to the spine or chest. Determine if the patient has recently undergone pulmonary function tests or received respiratory therapy. Ask about smoking, which can aggravate respiratory disorders, and about occupational exposure to chemical fumes or mineral dusts such as asbestos, which can cause diffuse infiltrative lung disease. Explore the family history for such disorders as cystic fibrosis and neurofibromatosis, which can cause diffuse infiltrative lung disease.

Perform a detailed chest examination, noting abnormal respiratory rate, rhythm, or depth. Assess the color, temperature, and turgor of the patient's skin, and check for clubbing.

Common medical causes
● *Adult respiratory distress syndrome.* In this life-threatening disorder, accessory muscle use increases in response to hypoxia. It's accompanied by intercostal, supracostal, and sternal retractions on inspiration and by grunting on expiration. Other characteristics include tachypnea, dyspnea, diaphoresis, diffuse crackles, and a cough with pink, frothy sputum. Worsening hypoxia produces anxiety, tachycardia, and mental sluggishness.
● *Airway obstruction.* Acute upper airway obstruction can be life-threatening—fortunately, most obstructions are subacute or chronic. Typically, this disorder increases accessory muscle use. Its most

telling sign, however, is inspiratory stridor. Associated signs and symptoms commonly include dyspnea, tachypnea, gasping, wheezing, coughing, intercostal retractions, cyanosis, and tachycardia.

● *Asthma.* During acute asthmatic attacks, the patient usually displays increased accessory muscle use. Accompanying it are severe dyspnea, tachypnea, wheezing, productive cough, nasal flaring, and cyanosis. Auscultation reveals faint or possibly absent breath sounds, musical crackles, and rhonchi. Other signs and symptoms include tachycardia, diaphoresis, and apprehension caused by air hunger. Chronic asthma may also cause barrel chest.

● *Emphysema.* Increased accessory muscle use occurs with progressive dyspnea on exertion and minimally productive cough in this form of COPD. The patient will display pursed-lip breathing and tachypnea. Associated signs and symptoms include peripheral cyanosis, anorexia, weight loss, malaise, barrel chest, and clubbing. Auscultation reveals distant heart sounds, percussion detects hyperresonance.

● *Pneumonia.* Bacterial pneumonia most commonly produces increased accessory muscle use. Initially, this infection produces sudden high fever with chills. Its associated signs and symptoms include chest pain, productive cough, dyspnea, tachypnea, tachycardia, expiratory grunting, cyanosis, diaphoresis, and fine crackles.

● *Pulmonary edema.* In acute pulmonary edema, increased accessory muscle use is accompanied by dyspnea, tachypnea, orthopnea, crepitant crackles, wheezing, and a cough with pink, frothy sputum. Other findings include restlessness, tachycardia, ventricular gallop, and cool, clammy, cyanotic skin.

● *Pulmonary embolism.* Although signs and symptoms vary with the size, number, and location of the emboli, this life-threatening disorder may cause increased accessory muscle use. Commonly, it produces dyspnea and tachypnea that may be accompanied by pleuritic or substernal chest pain. Other signs include restlessness, tachycardia, productive cough, low-grade fever and, with a large embolus, hemoptysis, cyanosis, syncope, neck vein distention, scattered crackles, or focal wheezing.

● *Spinal cord injury.* Increased accessory muscle use may occur, depending on the location and severity of injury. Injury below L1 typically doesn't affect the diaphragm or accessory muscles, whereas injury between C3 and C5 affects only the upper respiratory muscles and diaphragm, causing increased accessory muscle use.

Associated signs and symptoms of spinal cord injury may include unilateral or bilateral Babinski's reflex; hyperactive deep tendon reflexes; spasticity; and variable or total loss of pain and temperature sensation, proprioception, and motor function. Horner's syndrome (unilateral ptosis, pupillary constriction, facial anhidrosis) may occur with lower cervical cord injury

Other causes

● *Diagnostic tests and treatments.* Pulmonary function tests, incentive spirometry, and widely used intermittent positive-pressure breathing can increase accessory muscle use.

Special considerations

Because labored breathing can make the patient apprehensive, provide emotional support. If the patient is alert, elevate the head of the bed to make his breathing as easy as possible. Allow him to get plenty of rest, and encourage fluid intake to liquefy secretions. Administer oxygen. Prepare him for such tests as pulmonary function studies, chest X-rays, lung scans, arterial blood gas analysis, complete blood count, and sputum culture.

If appropriate, stress how smoking endangers the patient's health, and refer him to an organized program to stop smoking. Also teach him how to prevent infection. Explain the purpose of prescribed drugs, such as bronchodilators and mucolytics, and make sure he knows their dosage and schedule.

Pediatric pointers
Because an infant or child tires sooner than an adult, respiratory distress can more rapidly precipitate respiratory failure. Upper airway obstruction—caused by edema, bronchospasm, or a foreign object—most commonly produces respiratory distress and increased accessory muscle use. Disorders associated with airway obstruction include acute epiglottitis, croup, pertussis, cystic fibrosis, and asthma.

AGITATION

Agitation refers to a state of hyperarousal, increased tension, and irritability that can lead to confusion, hyperactivity, and overt hostility. This common sign can result from various disorders, pain, fever, anxiety, drug use and withdrawal, and hypersensitivity reactions. It can arise gradually or suddenly and last for minutes or months. Whether it's mild or severe, agitation worsens with increased fever, pain, stress, or external stimuli.

Agitation alone merely signals a change in the patient's condition. But it's a useful indicator of a developing disorder when considered with his history, current status, and other findings.

History and physical examination
Determine the severity of the patient's agitation by examining the number and quality of agitation-induced behaviors, such as emotional lability, confusion, memory loss, hyperactivity, and hostility. Obtain a history from the patient or a family member, including diet and known allergies.

Ask if the patient is being treated for any illnesses. Has the patient had any recent infections, trauma, stress, or changes in sleep patterns? You should ask the patient about prescribed or over-the-counter drug use. Check for signs of drug abuse, such as needle tracks or dilated pupils. Ask about alcohol intake. You will need to obtain baseline data for future comparison and check and record the patient's vital signs and neurologic status.

Common medical causes
● *Affective disturbance.* Agitation may occur in both depressed and manic phases of this disorder. In its depressive form, chronic anxiety occurs with varying severity. The hallmark is depression upon awakening, which eases during the day. Psychomotor agitation may be characterized by an inability to sit still, handwringing, pacing, and irritability. Other findings in manic states may include decreased sleep, pressured speech, and grandiosity.

● *Alcohol withdrawal syndrome.* Mild to severe agitation occurs with hyperactivity, tremors, and anxiety. In *delirium tremens*, the potentially life-threatening stage of alcohol withdrawal, severe agitation accompanies visual hallucinations, insomnia, diaphoresis, and depression. Pulse rate and temperature rise as withdrawal progresses; status epilepticus, cardiac exhaustion, and shock can occur.

● *Chronic renal failure.* Moderate to severe agitation occurs here, marked especially by confusion and memory loss. The agitation is accompanied by diverse signs and symptoms, such as nausea, vomiting, anorexia, mouth ulcers, ammonia breath odor, GI bleeding, pallor, edema, dry skin, and uremic frost.

● *Dementia.* Mild to severe agitation can result from many common syndromes, such as Alzheimer's disease and Huntington's chorea. The patient may display a decrease in memory, attention span, problem-solving ability, and alertness. Hypoactivity, wandering behavior, hallucinations, aphasia, and insomnia may also occur.

● *Drug withdrawal syndrome.* Mild to severe agitation occurs. Related findings vary with the drug but may include anxiety, abdominal cramps, diaphoresis, and anorexia. In narcotic or barbiturate withdrawal, a decreased level of consciousness (LOC) can occur as well as seizures and elevated blood pressure, heart, and respiratory rates.

● *Hypersensitivity reaction.* Moderate to severe agitation appears, possibly as the first sign of a reaction. Depending on the reaction's severity, agitation may be accompanied by urticaria, pruritus, and facial and dependent edema.

In *anaphylactic shock,* a potentially life-threatening reaction, agitation occurs rapidly along with apprehension, urticaria or diffuse erythema, paresthesia, pruritus, edema, dyspnea, wheezing, stridor, hypotension, tachycardia, and warm, moist skin. Abdominal cramps, vomiting, and diarrhea can also occur.

● *Hypoxemia.* Beginning as restlessness, agitation rapidly worsens. The patient may be confused and have impaired judgment and motor coordination. He may also have tachycardia, tachypnea, dyspnea, and cyanosis.

● *Increased intracranial pressure (ICP).* Agitation usually precedes other symptoms. Other early indicators may include headache, nausea, and vomiting. Increased ICP produces respiratory changes, such as Cheyne-Stokes, cluster, ataxic, or apneustic breathing; sluggish, nonreactive, or unequal pupils; widening pulse pressure; tachycardia; decreased LOC; seizures; and motor changes, such as decerebrate or decorticate posture.

● *Post-head-trauma syndrome.* Shortly after or even years after injury, mild to severe agitation develops, characterized by disorientation, loss of concentration, angry outbursts, and emotional lability. Other findings include fatigue, wandering behavior, and poor judgment.

● *Vitamin B$_6$* deficiency. Agitation can range from mild to severe. Other effects include seizures, peripheral paresthesia, and dermatitis. Oculogyric crisis may also occur.

Other causes

● *Drugs.* Mild to moderate agitation, commonly dose-related, develops as an adverse effect of central nervous system stimulants—especially sympathomimetic drugs such as ephedrine; caffeine; theophylline; and appetite suppressants, such as amphetamines and amphetamine-like drugs.

● *Radiographic contrast media.* Reaction to the contrast medium injected during various diagnostic tests produces moderate to severe agitation along with other signs of hypersensitivity.

Special considerations

Because agitation can be an early sign of diverse disorders, you will need to continue to monitor the patient's vital signs and neurologic status while the cause is being determined. Eliminate stressors, which can increase agitation. Provide adequate lighting, maintain a calm environment, and allow the patient ample time to sleep. Ensure a balanced diet, and provide vitamin supplements.

Remain calm, nonjudgmental, and nonargumentative. Use restraints sparingly because they tend to increase agitation.

If appropriate, prepare the patient for diagnostic tests, such as computed tomography scanning, skull X-rays, magnetic resonance imaging, and blood studies.

Elder tip

 If your elderly patient is agitated, consider which medications he may be taking. Certain classes of drugs may have adverse effects that are the opposite of those intended; for example, antihistamines, benzodiazepines, and sleeping pills can all cause agitation in elderly patients.

Pediatric pointers
A common sign in children, agitation accompanies the expected childhood diseases as well as more severe disorders that can lead to brain damage: hyperbilirubinemia, phenylketonuria, vitamin A deficiency, hepatitis, frontal lobe syndrome, increased ICP, and lead poisoning. In neonates, agitation can stem from alcohol or drug withdrawal if the mother abused these substances.

When evaluating the agitated child, remember to use words that he can understand and to look for nonverbal cues. For instance, if you suspect that pain is causing agitation, ask him to tell you where it hurts, but be sure to watch for other indicators, such as wincing, crying, or moving away.

AMENORRHEA

The absence of menstrual flow, amenorrhea can be classified as primary or secondary. In *primary amenorrhea,* menstruation fails to begin before the age of 16. In *secondary amenorrhea,* it begins at an appropriate age but later ceases for 3 or more months in the absence of normal physiologic causes, such as pregnancy, lactation, and menopause.

Pathologic amenorrhea results from anovulation or physical obstruction to menstrual outflow, such as from an imperforate hymen, cervical stenosis, or intrauterine adhesions. Anovulation itself may result from hormonal imbalance, debilitating disease, stress or emotional disturbances, strenuous exercise, malnutrition, obesity, and anatomic abnormalities, such as congenital absence of the ovaries or uterus. Amenorrhea may also result from drug or hormonal treatments. (See *How amenorrhea develops,* pages 28 and 29.)

History and physical examination
Begin by determining whether the amenorrhea is primary or secondary. If it's primary, ask the patient at what age her mother first menstruated, because age of menarche is fairly consistent in families. Form an overall impression of the patient's physical, mental, and emotional development because these factors as well as heredity and climate may delay menarche until after the age of 16.

If menstruation began at an appropriate age but has since ceased, determine the frequency and duration of the patient's previous menstrual cycles. Ask her about the onset and nature of any changes in her normal menstrual pattern, and determine the date of her last menstruation. Find out if she has noticed any related signs, such as breast swelling or weight changes.

Determine when the patient last had a physical examination. Review her health history, noting especially any long-term illnesses, such as anemia, or use of oral contraceptives. Ask about exercise habits, especially running, and stress on the job or at home. Probe the patient's eating habits, including number and size of daily meals and snacks, and recent weight gain.

Observe the patient's appearance for secondary sex characteristics or signs of virilization.

If you're responsible for performing a pelvic examination, check for anatomic aberrations of the outflow tract, such as cervical adhesions, fibroids, or an imperforate hymen.

Common medical causes
● *Adrenal tumor.* Amenorrhea may be accompanied by acne, thinning scalp hair, hirsutism, increased blood pressure, truncal obesity, and psychotic changes.
● *Adrenocortical hyperplasia.* Amenorrhea precedes characteristic cushingoid

signs, such as truncal obesity, moon face, buffalo hump, bruises, purple striae, and widened pulse pressure. Acne, thinning scalp hair, and hirsutism typically appear.

• *Adrenocortical hypofunction.* Besides amenorrhea, this disorder may cause fatigue, irritability, weight loss, skin color changes, nausea, vomiting, and orthostatic hypotension.

• *Amenorrhea-lactation disorders.* These disorders, such as Forbes-Albright and Chiari-Frommel syndromes, produce secondary amenorrhea accompanied by lactation in the absence of breast-feeding. Associated features may include large, engorged breasts and vaginal atrophy.

• *Anorexia nervosa.* This psychological disorder can cause either primary or secondary amenorrhea. Related findings commonly include significant weight loss, a thin or emaciated appearance, compulsive behavior patterns, blotchy or sallow complexion, constipation, reduced libido, decreased pleasure in once-enjoyable activities, dry skin, loss of scalp hair, skeletal muscle atrophy, and sleep disturbances.

• *Congenital absence of the ovaries.* This anomaly results in primary amenorrhea and absence of secondary sex characteristics.

• *Congenital absence of the uterus.* Primary amenorrhea occurs with this disorder.

• *Corpus luteum cysts.* Commonly causing sudden amenorrhea, these cysts may also produce acute abdominal pain and breast swelling. An examination may reveal a tender adnexal mass as well as vaginal and cervical hyperemia.

• *Hypothalamic tumor.* In addition to amenorrhea, a hypothalamic tumor can cause endocrine and visual field defects, gonadal underdevelopment or dysfunction, and short stature.

• *Hypothyroidism.* Deficient thyroid hormone levels can cause primary or secondary amenorrhea. Typically vague early findings include fatigue, forgetfulness, cold intolerance, unexplained weight gain, and constipation. Subsequent signs include bradycardia; decreased mental acuity; dry, flaky, inelastic skin; puffy face, hands, and feet; hoarseness; periorbital edema; ptosis; dry, sparse hair; and thick, brittle nails. Other common findings include anorexia, abdominal distention, decreased libido, ataxia, intention tremor, nystagmus, and delayed reflex relaxation time, especially in the Achilles tendon.

• *Ovarian insensitivity to gonadotropins.* This hormonal disturbance leads to amenorrhea and an absence of secondary sex characteristics.

• *Pituitary tumor.* Amenorrhea may be the first sign of a pituitary tumor. Associated findings may include headache, acromegaly, and visual disturbances such as bitemporal hemianopia. Cushingoid signs include moon face, buffalo hump, hirsutism, hypertension, truncal obesity, bruises, purple striae, and widened pulse pressure.

• *Polycystic ovary syndrome.* Typically, menarche occurs at a normal age, followed by irregular menstrual cycles, oligomenorrhea, and secondary amenorrhea. Or periods of profuse bleeding may alternate with periods of amenorrhea. Obesity, hirsutism, slight deepening of the voice, and enlarged, "oyster-like" ovaries may also accompany this disorder.

• *Pseudoamenorrhea.* An anatomic anomaly such as imperforate hymen obstructs menstrual flow, causing primary amenorrhea and possibly abdominal cramps. Examination may reveal a pink or blue bulging hymen.

• *Pseudocyesis.* Amenorrhea may be accompanied by lordosis, abdominal distention, nausea, and breast enlargement in this disorder.

• *Testicular feminization.* Primary amenorrhea may signal this form of male pseudohermaphroditism. The patient, outwardly female but genetically male, shows breast and external genital development, but scant or absent pubic hair.

HOW AMENORRHEA DEVELOPS

A disruption at any point in the menstrual cycle can produce amenorrhea, as illustrated in the flowchart below.

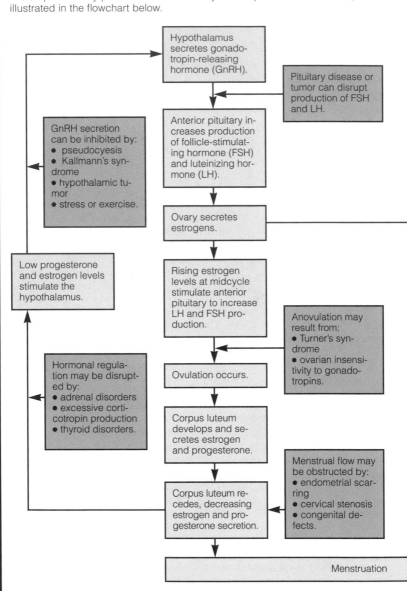

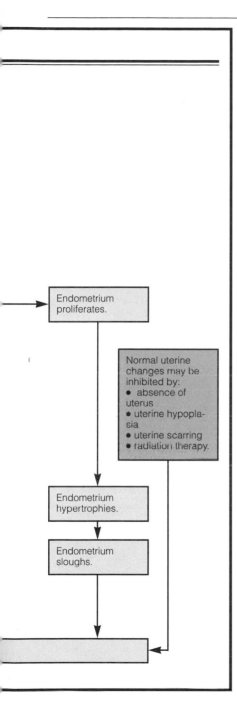

Endometrium proliferates.

Normal uterine changes may be inhibited by:
● absence of uterus
● uterine hypoplasia
● uterine scarring
● radiation therapy.

Endometrium hypertrophies.

Endometrium sloughs.

● **Turner's syndrome.** Primary amenorrhea and failure to develop secondary sex characteristics may signal this syndrome of genetic ovarian dysgenesis. Typical features include short stature, webbing of the neck, low nuchal hairline, a broad chest with widely spaced nipples and poor breast development, underdeveloped genitalia, and edema of the legs and feet.

● **Uterine hypoplasia.** Primary amenorrhea results from underdevelopment of the uterus, which is detectable on physical examination.

Other causes

● **Drugs.** Busulfan, chlorambucil, cyclophosphamide, and phenothiazines may cause amenorrhea. Oral contraceptives may cause anovulation and amenorrhea after discontinuation.

Special considerations

In patients with secondary amenorrhea, physical and pelvic examinations must rule out pregnancy before diagnostic testing begins. Typical tests include progestin withdrawal, serum hormone and thyroid function studies, and endometrial biopsy.

After diagnosis, answer the patient's questions about the type of treatment that will be provided and its expected outcome. Because amenorrhea can cause severe emotional distress, provide emotional support. Be sure to encourage the patient to discuss her fears; if necessary, refer her for psychological counseling.

Pediatric pointers

Adolescent girls are especially prone to amenorrhea caused by emotional upsets, typically stemming from school, social, or family problems.

AMNESIA

Amnesia—a disturbance in or loss of memory—may be partial or complete, and anterograde or retrograde. Anterograde amnesia denotes memory loss for events that occurred *after* onset of the causative trauma or disease; retrograde amnesia denotes memory loss for events that occurred *before* onset. Depending on the cause, amnesia may arise suddenly or slowly and may be temporary or permanent.

Organic, or *true, amnesia* results from temporal lobe dysfunction and characteristically spares patches of memory. A common symptom in patients with seizures and head trauma, organic amnesia can also be an early indicator of Alzheimer's disease. *Hysterical amnesia* has a psychogenic origin and characteristically causes complete memory loss. *Treatment-induced amnesia* is usually transient.

History and physical examination

Because many patients aren't aware that they have amnesia, you'll usually need help gathering information from family members or friends. Throughout your assessment, notice the patient's general appearance, behavior, mood, and train of thought. Ask when the amnesia first appeared and what types of things the patient can't remember. Can he learn new information? How long does he remember it? Does the amnesia encompass a recent or a remote time period?

Test the patient's recent memory by asking him to identify and repeat three items. Retest him after 3 minutes. Test his intermediate memory by asking, "Who was the president before this one?" and "What was the last type of car you bought?" Test remote memory with such questions as "How old are you?" and "Where were you born?"

Take the patient's vital signs and assess his level of consciousness (LOC). Check his pupils: They should be equal in size and should constrict quickly when exposed to direct light. Also assess his extraocular movements. Test motor function by having the patient move his arms and legs through their range of motion. Evaluate sensory function with pinpricks on the patient's skin.

Common medical causes

• *Alzheimer's disease.* This disease usually begins with retrograde amnesia, which progresses slowly over many months or years to include anterograde amnesia, producing severe and permanent memory loss. Associated findings include agitation, inability to concentrate, disregard for personal hygiene, confusion, irritability, and emotional lability. Later signs and symptoms include aphasia, dementia, incontinence, and muscle rigidity.

• *Head trauma.* Depending on the trauma's severity, amnesia may last for minutes, hours, or longer. Amnesia for the event usually persists and may be accompanied by brief retrograde and longer anterograde amnesia. Severe head trauma can cause permanent amnesia or difficulty in retaining recent memories. Related findings may include altered respirations and LOC, headache, dizziness, confusion, visual disturbances, and motor and sensory disturbances, such as hemiparesis and paresthesia, on the side of the body opposite the injury.

• *Hysteria.* Hysterical amnesia, a complete and long-lasting memory loss, begins and ends abruptly. It's commonly accompanied by apparent confusion.

• *Seizure.* In temporal lobe seizures, amnesia occurs suddenly and lasts for several seconds to minutes. The patient may recall an aura or nothing at all.

An irritable focus on the left side of the brain primarily causes amnesia for verbal memories, whereas an irritable focus on the right side of the brain causes

AMNESIA: COMMON CAUSES AND ASSOCIATED FINDINGS

CAUSES	MAJOR ASSOCIATED SIGNS AND SYMPTOMS												
	Agitation	Ataxia	Confusion	Decreased level of consciousness	Diplopia	Dizziness	Emotional lability	Headache	Nausea	Paresthesia	Vertigo	Visual blurring	Vomiting
Alzheimer's disease	●		●				●						
Cerebral hypoxia	●		●	●			●	●		●			
Head trauma	●	●	●	●	●	●	●	●	●	●	●	●	●
Hysteria			●				●						
Vertebrobasilar circulatory disorders		●	●		●	●		●	●	●	●		●
Wernicke-Korsakoff syndrome		●	●	●	●			●		●			

graphic *and* nonverbal amnesia. Associated signs may include decreased LOC during the seizure, confusion, abnormal mouth movements, and visual, olfactory, and auditory hallucinations.

● *Wernicke-Korsakoff syndrome.* Retrograde and anterograde amnesia can become permanent if this syndrome is not treated. Accompanying clinical findings include apathy, an inability to concentrate or to put events into sequence, and confabulation to fill memory gaps. The syndrome may also cause diplopia, decreased LOC, headache, ataxia, and symptoms of peripheral neuropathy, such as numbness and tingling.

Other causes

● *Drugs.* Anterograde amnesia can be precipitated by general anesthetics, especially fentanyl, halothane, and isoflurane; barbiturates, most commonly thiopental and pentobarbital; and certain benzodiazepines, especially triazolam.

● *Electroconvulsive therapy.* Sudden onset of retrograde or anterograde amnesia occurs with electroconvulsive therapy. Typically, the amnesia lasts for several minutes to several hours, but severe, prolonged amnesia occurs when treatments are given frequently over a prolonged period.

● *Temporal lobe surgery.* Usually performed on only one lobe, this surgery causes brief, slight amnesia. However, removal of both lobes leaves permanent amnesia.

Special considerations

Prepare the patient for diagnostic tests, such as computed tomography scan, EEG, and cerebral angiography.

Provide reality orientation for the patient with retrograde amnesia, and encourage his family members to help by supplying familiar photos, objects, or music.

Adjust your patient-teaching techniques for the patient with anterograde amnesia because he can't acquire new information. Include his family in teaching sessions. In addition, write down all instructions—particularly medication dosages and schedules—so the patient won't have to rely on his memory.

Consider basic needs, such as safety, elimination, and nutrition, for the patient with severe amnesia. If necessary, arrange for placement in an extended-care facility.

Pediatric pointers
A child who suffers amnesia during seizures may be mistakenly labeled as "learning disabled." To prevent this mislabeling, stress the importance of adhering to the prescribed medication schedule, and discuss ways that the child, his parents, and his teachers can cope with amnesia.

ANALGESIA

The absence of sensitivity to pain, analgesia is an important symptom of central nervous system disease, commonly indicating a specific type and location of spinal cord lesion. It always occurs with loss of temperature sensation (thermanesthesia) because these sensory nerve impulses travel together in the spinal cord. It can also occur with other sensory deficits, such as paresthesia, loss of proprioception and vibratory sense, and tactile anesthesia in various disorders involving the peripheral nerves, spinal cord, and brain. However, when accompanied only by thermanesthesia, analgesia points to an incomplete lesion of the spinal cord.

Analgesia can be partial or total below the level of the lesion, and unilateral or bilateral, depending on the cause and level of the lesion. Its onset may be slow and progressive with a tumor or abrupt with trauma. In many cases, analgesia is transient and resolves spontaneously.

Emergency interventions
 If the patient complains of unilateral or bilateral analgesia over a large body area, accompanied by paralysis, suspect spinal cord injury. Immobilize his spine in proper alignment, using a cervical collar and a long backboard if possible. If a collar or backboard isn't available, position the patient supine on a flat surface, and place sandbags around his head, neck, and torso. Use correct technique and extreme caution when moving him, to prevent exacerbating spinal injury. Continuously monitor respiratory rate and rhythm, and observe for accessory muscle use because a complete lesion above the T6 level may cause diaphragmatic and intercostal muscle paralysis. Have an artificial airway and a handheld resuscitation bag on hand, and be prepared to initiate emergency resuscitation measures in case of respiratory failure.

History and physical examination
Once you're satisfied that the patient's spine and respiratory status are stabilized—or if the analgesia is less severe and isn't accompanied by signs of spinal cord injury—perform a physical examination and baseline neurologic evaluation. First, take the patient's vital signs and assess his level of consciousness. Then test pupillary, corneal, cough, and gag reflexes to rule out brain stem and cranial nerve involvement. If the patient is conscious, evaluate his speech and ability to swallow.

If possible, observe the patient's gait and posture, and assess his balance and coordination. Evaluate muscle tone and strength in all extremities. Test for other sensory deficits over all dermatomes (individual skin segments innervated by a specific spinal nerve) by applying light tactile stimulation with a tongue depressor or cotton swab. Repeat a more thorough check of pain sensitivity, if necessary, using a pin. Also test temperature sensation over all dermatomes, using two test tubes—one filled with hot water, the other with cold water. In each arm and leg, test vibration sense (using a tuning fork), proprioception, and both superficial and deep tendon reflexes. Check for increased muscle tone by extending and flexing the patient's elbows and knees as he tries to relax.

Focus your history taking on the onset of analgesia—sudden or gradual—and on any recent trauma, such as a fall, a sports injury, or automobile accident. Obtain a complete medical history, noting especially any incidence of cancer in the patient or his family.

Common medical causes

• *Anterior cord syndrome.* In this syndrome, analgesia and thermanesthesia occur bilaterally below the level of the lesion, along with flaccid paralysis and hypoactive deep tendon reflexes (DTRs).

• *Central cord syndrome.* Typically, analgesia and thermanesthesia occur bilaterally in several dermatomes, commonly extending in a capelike fashion over the arms, back, and shoulders. Early weakness in the hands progresses to weakness and muscle spasms in the arms and shoulder girdle. Hyperactive DTRs and spastic weakness of the legs may develop. However, if the lesion affects the lumbar spine, hypoactive DTRs and flaccid weakness may persist in the legs.

With brain stem involvement, additional findings may include facial analgesia and thermanesthesia, vertigo, nystagmus, atrophy of the tongue, and dysarthria. The patient may also have dysphagia, urine retention, anhidrosis, decreased intestinal motility, and hyperkeratosis.

• *Spinal cord hemisection.* Contralateral analgesia and thermanesthesia occur below the level of the lesion. In addition, loss of proprioception, spastic paralysis, and hyperactive DTRs develop ipsilaterally. The patient may experience urine retention with overflow incontinence.

Other causes

• *Drugs.* Analgesia may occur with use of topical and local anesthetics, although numbness and tingling are more common.

Special considerations

Prepare the patient for spinal X-rays, and maintain spinal alignment and stability during transport to the laboratory.

Focus your care on preventing further injury to the patient because analgesia can mask injury or developing complications. Prevent formation of decubitus ulcers through meticulous skin care, massage, use of lamb's wool pads, and frequent repositioning, especially when significant motor deficits hamper the patient's movement. Guard against scalding by testing the patient's bathwater temperature before he bathes; advise him to test it at home using a thermometer or a body part with intact sensation.

Elder tip

Because an older person may be unable to sense heat as well or as quickly as a younger person, he is more prone to burns or scalding. Instruct such a patient to follow directions on heating pads and warming blankets to avoid burns and not to use a heating pad or hot water bottle while he's sleeping. To prevent accidents in the home, tell him to set household hot water temperatures at 115° F (46° C) or less. Conversely, when using ice therapy to reduce pain or swelling, an elderly patient is more susceptible to hypothermic skin damage. Instruct him to apply cold packs intermittently for short periods of time and to inspect the area between applications.

Pediatric pointers
Because a child may have difficulty describing analgesia, observe him carefully during the assessment for nonverbal clues to pain—facial expressions, crying, retraction from stimulus. Remember that pain thresholds are high in infants, so your assessment findings may not be reliable. Also remember to test bathwater carefully for a child who's too young to test it himself.

ANOREXIA

Anorexia, a lack of appetite in the presence of a physiologic need for food, is a common symptom of GI and endocrine disorders. It's also characteristic of certain severe psychological disturbances. Anorexia can result from such factors as anxiety, chronic pain, poor oral hygiene, increased blood temperature due to hot weather or fever, and changes in taste or smell that normally accompany aging. It also can result from drug therapy or abuse. Short-term anorexia rarely jeopardizes health, but chronic anorexia can lead to life-threatening malnutrition.

History and physical examination
Take the patient's vital signs and weigh him. Find out his previous minimum and maximum weights. Explore dietary habits, such as when and what he eats. Ask what foods he likes and dislikes, and why. The patient may identify tastes and smells that nauseate him and cause loss of appetite. Ask about dental problems that interfere with chewing, such as poor-fitting dentures. Ask if he has difficulty or pain when swallowing or if he vomits or has diarrhea after meals. Also ask how frequently and intensely he exercises.

Check for a history of stomach or bowel disorders, which can interfere with the ability to digest, absorb, or metabolize nutrients. Find out about changes in bowel habits. Ask about alcohol use and drug use and dosage.

If the medical history doesn't reveal an organic basis for anorexia, consider psychological factors. Ask the patient if he knows what's causing his decreased appetite. Situational factors, such as a death in the family or problems at school or on the job, can lead to depression and subsequent loss of appetite. Be alert for signs of malnutrition, consistent refusal of food, and a 7% to 10% loss of body weight in the last month. (See *Is your patient malnourished?*)

Common medical causes
• *Acquired immunodeficiency syndrome.* An infection or Kaposi's sarcoma affecting the GI or respiratory tract may lead to anorexia. Other findings may include fatigue, afternoon fevers, night sweats, diarrhea, cough, bleeding, lymphadenopathy, and skin disorders.
• *Adrenocortical hypofunction.* In this disorder, anorexia may begin slowly and subtly, causing gradual weight loss. Other common signs and symptoms include nausea and vomiting, abdominal pain, diarrhea, weakness, fatigue, malaise, vitiligo, bronze-colored skin, and purple striae on the breasts, abdomen, shoulders, and hips.
• *Alcoholism.* Chronic anorexia commonly accompanies alcoholism, leading to malnutrition. Other findings include signs of liver damage (jaundice, spider angiomas, ascites, edema), paresthesias, tremors, increased blood pressure, bruising, GI bleeding, and abdominal pain.
• *Anorexia nervosa.* Chronic anorexia begins insidiously and leads to life-threatening malnutrition, as evidenced by skeletal muscle atrophy, loss of fatty tissue, constipation, amenorrhea, dry and blotchy or sallow skin, alopecia, sleep disturbances, distorted self-image, an-

IS YOUR PATIENT MALNOURISHED?

When assessing a patient with anorexia, be sure to check for these common signs of malnutrition.

Hair. Dull, dry, thin, fine, straight, and easily plucked; areas of lighter or darker spots and hair loss

Face. Generalized swelling; dark areas on cheeks and under eyes; lumpy or flaky skin around the nose and mouth; enlarged parotid glands

Eyes. Dull appearance; dry and either pale or red membranes; triangular, shiny gray spots on conjunctivae; red and fissured eyelid corners; bloodshot ring around cornea

Lips. Red and swollen, especially at corners

Tongue. Swollen, purple, and raw-looking, with sores or abnormal papillae

Teeth. Missing, or emerging abnormally; visible cavities or dark spots; spongy, bleeding gums

Neck. Swollen thyroid gland

Skin. Dry, flaky, swollen, and dark, with lighter or darker spots, some resembling bruises; tight and drawn, with poor skin turgor

Nails. Spoon-shaped, brittle, and ridged

Musculoskeletal system. Muscle wasting, knock-knee or bowlegs, bumps on ribs, swollen joints, musculoskeletal hemorrhages

Cardiovascular system. Heart rate above 100 beats/minute; arrhythmias; elevated blood pressure

Abdomen. Enlarged liver and spleen

Reproductive system. Decreased libido; amenorrhea

Nervous system. Irritability; confusion; paresthesia in hands and feet; loss of proprioception; decreased ankle and knee reflexes

---

hedonia, and decreased libido. Paradoxically, many patients exhibit extreme restlessness and vigor and exercise avidly.

• *Appendicitis.* Anorexia closely follows the abrupt onset of generalized or localized epigastric pain, nausea, and vomiting. It can continue as pain localizes in the right lower quadrant (McBurney's point) and other signs appear: abdominal rigidity, rebound tenderness, constipation (or diarrhea), slight fever, and tachycardia.

• *Cancer.* Chronic anorexia occurs, with possible weight loss, weakness, apathy, and cachexia.

• *Chronic renal failure.* Chronic anorexia is common and insidious in this disorder. It's accompanied by changes in all body systems, such as nausea, vomiting, mouth ulcers, ammonia breath odor, GI bleeding, constipation or diarrhea, drowsiness, confusion, tremors, pallor, dry and scaly skin, pruritus, alopecia, purpuric lesions, and edema.

• *Cirrhosis.* Anorexia occurs early and may be accompanied by weakness, nausea, vomiting, constipation or diarrhea, and dull abdominal pain. It continues after these early signs subside and is accompanied by lethargy, slurred speech, bleeding tendencies, ascites, severe pruritus, dry skin, poor skin turgor, hepatomegaly, fetor hepaticus, jaundice, edema of the legs, and right upper quadrant pain.

• *Crohn's disease.* Chronic anorexia causes marked weight loss. Associated signs vary according to the site and extent of the lesion and may include diarrhea, abdominal pain, fever, abdominal mass, weakness and, rarely, clubbing of the fingers. Acute inflammatory symptoms—right lower quadrant pain, cramping, tenderness, flatulence, fever, nausea, diarrhea, and bloody stools—mimic appendicitis.

● *Gastritis.* In *acute gastritis,* the onset of anorexia may be sudden. The patient may experience postprandial epigastric distress after a meal, accompanied by nausea, vomiting (commonly with hematemesis), fever, belching, and malaise.

● *Hepatitis.* In *viral hepatitis (hepatitis A, B, C, or D),* anorexia begins in the preicteric phase, accompanied by fatigue, malaise, headache, arthralgia, myalgia, photophobia, nausea and vomiting, mild fever, hepatomegaly, and lymphadenopathy. It may continue throughout the icteric phase, along with mild weight loss, dark urine, clay-colored stools, jaundice, right upper quadrant pain and, possibly, irritability and severe pruritus.

In *nonviral hepatitis,* anorexia and its accompanying signs usually resemble those of viral hepatitis but may vary depending on the causative agent and the extent of liver damage.

● *Hypothyroidism.* Anorexia is common and usually insidious. Early findings include fatigue, forgetfulness, cold intolerance, unexplained weight gain, and constipation. Subsequent findings include decreased mental stability; dry, flaky, and inelastic skin; edema of the face, hands, and feet; ptosis; hoarseness; thick, brittle nails; coarse, broken hair; and signs of decreased cardiac output such as bradycardia. Other common findings include abdominal distention, menstrual irregularities, decreased libido, ataxia, intention tremor, nystagmus, and slow reflex relaxation time.

● *Ketoacidosis.* Anorexia usually arises gradually and is accompanied by dry, flushed skin; fruity breath odor; polydipsia; hypotension; weak, rapid pulse; dry mouth; abdominal pain; and vomiting.

Other causes

● *Drugs.* Anorexia results from the use of chemotherapeutic agents, amphetamines, sympathomimetics such as ephedrine, and some antibiotics. It also signals digitalis toxicity.

● *Radiation therapy.* Radiation treatments can cause anorexia, possibly due to metabolic disturbances.

● *Total parenteral nutrition (TPN).* Maintenance of blood glucose levels by I.V. therapy may cause anorexia.

Special considerations

Because the causes of anorexia are diverse, diagnostic procedures may include thyroid function studies, endoscopy, upper GI series, gallbladder series, barium enema, liver and kidney function tests, hormone assays, computed tomography scans, ultrasonography, and blood studies to assess nutritional status.

Promote protein and caloric intake by providing high-calorie snacks or frequent, small meals. Encourage the patient's family to supply his favorite foods to help stimulate his appetite. Take a 24-hour diet history daily. Because the patient may consistently exaggerate his food intake (a common occurrence in anorexia nervosa), you'll need to maintain strict calorie and nutrient counts for his meals. In severe malnutrition, provide supplemental nutritional support, such as TPN or oral nutritional supplements.

Because anorexia and poor nutrition increase susceptibility to infection, monitor the patient's vital signs and white blood cell count and closely observe any wounds.

Pediatric pointers

In children, anorexia accompanies many illnesses but usually resolves promptly. However, in preadolescent and adolescent girls, be alert for the often subtle signs of anorexia nervosa.

ANURIA

Clinically defined as urine output of less than 75 ml daily, anuria indicates either urinary tract obstruction or acute renal failure due to various mechanisms. Fortunately, anuria is rare; even in renal failure, the kidneys usually produce at least 75 ml of urine daily.

Because urine output is easily measured, anuria rarely goes undetected. However, without immediate treatment, anuria can rapidly cause uremia and other complications of urine retention.

Emergency interventions

 After detecting anuria, your priorities are to determine if urine formation is occurring and to intervene appropriately. Prepare to catheterize the patient to relieve any lower urinary tract obstruction and to check for residual urine. You may find that an obstruction hinders catheter insertion and that urine return is cloudy and foul-smelling. If you collect more than 75 ml of urine, suspect lower urinary tract obstruction; less than 75 ml, renal dysfunction or obstruction higher in the urinary tract.

History and physical examination

Take the patient's vital signs and obtain a complete history. First ask about any changes in voiding pattern. Determine the amount of fluid normally ingested each day, the amount of fluid ingested in the last 24 to 48 hours, and the time and amount of his last urination. Review his medical history, noting especially previous kidney disease, urinary tract obstruction or infection, prostate enlargement, renal calculi, neurogenic bladder, or congenital abnormalities. Ask about drug use and about any abdominal, renal, or urinary tract surgery.

Inspect and palpate the abdomen for asymmetry, distention, or bulging. Inspect the flank area for edema or erythema, and percuss and palpate the bladder. Palpate the kidneys both anteriorly and posteriorly, and percuss them at the costovertebral angle. Auscultate over the renal arteries, listening for bruits.

Common medical causes

- *Acute tubular necrosis.* Prolonged (up to 2 weeks) anuria or, more commonly, oliguria is a typical finding in this disorder. It precedes the onset of diuresis, which is heralded by polyuria. Associated findings reflect the underlying cause and may include signs and symptoms of hyperkalemia (muscle weakness and cardiac arrhythmias), uremia (anorexia, nausea, vomiting, confusion, lethargy, twitching, seizures, pruritus, uremic frost, and Kussmaul's respirations), and heart failure (edema, jugular vein distention, crackles, and dyspnea).
- *Cortical necrosis (bilateral).* This disorder is characterized by a sudden change from oliguria to anuria, along with gross hematuria, flank pain, and fever.
- *Glomerulonephritis (acute).* This disorder produces anuria or oliguria. Related effects include mild fever, malaise, flank pain, hematuria, facial and generalized edema, elevated blood pressure, headache, nausea, vomiting, abdominal pain, and signs of pulmonary congestion (crackles and dyspnea).
- *Hemolytic-uremic syndrome.* Anuria commonly occurs in the initial stages of this disorder and may last from 1 to 10 days. The patient may have vomiting, diarrhea, abdominal pain, hematemesis, melena, purpura, fever, elevated blood pressure, hepatomegaly, ecchymoses, edema, hematuria, and pallor. He may also show signs of upper respiratory tract infection.
- *Renal artery occlusion (bilateral).* This disorder produces anuria or severe oliguria, commonly accompanied by nausea and vomiting, decreased bowel

sounds, fever up to 102° F (39° C), and severe, continuous upper abdominal and flank pain.

• *Urinary tract obstruction.* Severe obstruction can produce acute and sometimes total anuria, alternating with or preceded by burning and pain on urination, overflow incontinence or dribbling, increased urinary frequency and nocturia, voiding of small amounts, or altered urinary stream. Associated findings may include bladder distention, pain and a sensation of fullness in the lower abdomen and groin, upper abdominal and flank pain, nausea and vomiting, and signs and symptoms of secondary infection, such as fever, chills, malaise, and cloudy, foulsmelling urine.

Other causes

• *Diagnostic tests.* Contrast media used in radiographic studies can cause nephrotoxicity, producing oliguria and, rarely, anuria.

• *Drugs.* Many classes of drugs can cause anuria or, more commonly, oliguria through their nephrotoxic effects. Antibiotics, especially the aminoglycosides, are the most commonly seen nephrotoxins. Anesthetic agents, heavy metals, and organic solvents can also be nephrotoxic. Adrenergic and anticholinergic drugs can cause anuria by affecting the nerves and muscles of micturition to produce urine retention.

Special considerations

If catheterization fails to initiate urine flow, prepare the patient for diagnostic studies, such as ultrasonography, cystoscopy, retrograde pyelography, and renal scan, to detect possible obstruction higher in the urinary tract. If these tests reveal an obstruction, prepare him for immediate surgery to remove the obstruction, and insert a nephrostomy or ureterostomy tube to drain the urine. If these tests fail to reveal an obstruction, prepare the patient for further kidney function studies.

Carefully monitor the patient's vital signs and intake and output, initially saving any urine for inspection. Restrict daily fluid allowance to 600 ml more than the previous day's total urine output. Restrict foods and juices high in potassium and sodium, and make sure the patient maintains a balanced diet with controlled protein levels. Provide low-sodium hard candy to help decrease thirst. Record fluid intake and output, and weigh the patient daily.

Pediatric pointers

Anuria in neonates is clinically defined as the absence of urine output for 24 hours. It can be classified as primary or secondary. Primary anuria results from bilateral renal agenesis, aplasia, or multicystic dysplasia. Secondary anuria, associated with edema or dehydration, results from renal ischemia, renal vein thrombosis, or congenital anomalies of the genitourinary tract.

ANXIETY

A subjective reaction to a real or imagined threat, anxiety is a nonspecific feeling of uneasiness or dread. It may be mild, moderate, or severe. Mild anxiety may cause slight physical or psychological discomfort. Severe anxiety may be incapacitating or even life-threatening.

Everyone experiences anxiety from time to time—it's a normal response to actual danger, prompting the body (through stimulation of the sympathetic and parasympathetic nervous systems) to purposeful action. It's also a normal response to physical and emotional stress, which can be produced by virtually any illness. In addition, anxiety can be precipitated or exacerbated by many nonpathologic factors, including lack of sleep, poor diet, and excessive intake of caffeine or other stimulants. However, excessive, unwarranted anxiety may indicate an underlying psychological problem.

History and physical examination

If the patient displays acute, severe anxiety, quickly take his vital signs and determine his chief complaint. This will determine how you proceed. For example, if the patient's anxiety is accompanied by chest pain and shortness of breath, you may suspect myocardial infarction and act accordingly. While examining the patient, try to keep him as calm as possible. Suggest relaxation techniques, and talk to him in a reassuring, soothing voice. Uncontrolled anxiety can alter vital signs and exacerbate the causative disorder.

If the patient displays mild or moderate anxiety, ask about its duration. Is the anxiety constant or sporadic? Did he notice any precipitating factors? Find out if the anxiety is exacerbated by stress, lack of sleep, or excessive caffeine intake and alleviated by rest, tranquilizers, or exercise.

Obtain a complete medical history, especially noting drug use. Then perform a physical examination, focusing on any complaints that may trigger or be aggravated by anxiety.

If the patient's anxiety isn't accompanied by significant physical signs, suspect a psychological basis. Determine the patient's level of consciousness (LOC) and observe his behavior. If appropriate, refer him for psychiatric evaluation.

Common medical causes

● *Anaphylactic shock.* Acute anxiety usually signals the onset of this shock state. It's accompanied by urticaria, angioedema, pruritus, and shortness of breath. Soon, other signs and symptoms develop: light-headedness, hypotension, tachycardia, nasal congestion, sneezing, wheezing, dyspnea, barking cough, abdominal cramps, vomiting, diarrhea, and urinary urgency and incontinence.

● *Angina pectoris.* Acute anxiety may either precede or follow an attack of angina pectoris. An attack produces sharp and crushing substernal or anterior chest pain that may radiate to the back, neck, arms, or jaw. The pain is commonly relieved by nitroglycerin or rest, which eases anxiety.

● *Asthma.* In allergic asthma attacks, acute anxiety occurs with dyspnea, wheezing, productive cough, accessory muscle use, hyperresonant lung fields, diminished breath sounds, coarse crackles, cyanosis, tachycardia, and diaphoresis.

● *Cardiogenic shock.* In this disorder, acute anxiety is accompanied by tachycardia, weak and thready pulse, tachypnea, ventricular gallop, crackles, neck vein distention, decreased urine output, hypotension, narrowing pulse pressure, peripheral edema, and cool, pale, clammy skin.

● *Chronic obstructive pulmonary disease.* Acute anxiety, dyspnea on exertion, cough, wheezing, crackles, hyperresonant lung fields, tachypnea, and accessory muscle use characterize this disorder.

● *Heart failure.* In this disorder, acute anxiety is commonly the first symptom of inadequate oxygenation. Associated findings include restlessness, shortness of breath, tachypnea, decreased LOC, edema, crackles, ventricular gallop, hypotension, diaphoresis, and cyanosis.

● *Hyperthyroidism.* Acute anxiety may be an early symptom of this disorder. Classic signs include heat intolerance, weight loss despite increased appetite, nervousness, tremor, palpitations, sweating, an enlarged thyroid, and diarrhea. Exophthalmos also may occur.

● *Mitral valve prolapse.* Panic may occur in patients with this valvular disorder, also referred to as the click-murmur syndrome. The disorder also may cause paroxysmal palpitations accompanied by sharp, stabbing, or aching precordial pain.

ALTERNATIVE THERAPY

RELIEVING ANXIETY WITH YOGA

Yoga is a form of mind-body exercise that uses certain postures, coordinated breathing techniques, and meditation to achieve physical and mental self-discipline. The postures help the person develop strength and flexibility by using all the muscles in the body, increasing circulation, and stretching and aligning the spinal column. Breathing exercises and meditation help reduce stress and anxiety.

Its hallmark is a midsystolic click, followed by an apical systolic murmur.

● *Mood disorder.* In the depressive phase of a mood disorder, chronic anxiety occurs with varying severity. The hallmark is depression upon awakening, which abates during the day. Associated findings may include dysphoria, anger, insomnia or hypersomnia, appetite disturbance, multiple somatic complaints, suicidal thoughts, and decreased libido, interest, energy, and concentration.

● *Myocardial infarction.* In this life-threatening disorder, acute anxiety commonly occurs with persistent, crushing substernal pain that may radiate to the left arm, jaw, neck, or shoulder blades. It can be accompanied by shortness of breath, nausea, vomiting, diaphoresis, and cool, pale skin.

● *Obsessive-compulsive disorders.* Chronic anxiety occurs in this disorder along with recurrent, unshakable thoughts or impulses to perform ritualistic acts. The patient recognizes these acts as irrational but can't control them. Anxiety builds if he can't perform these acts and diminishes after he does.

● *Pheochromocytoma.* Acute, severe anxiety accompanies this disorder's cardinal sign—persistent or paroxysmal hypertension. Common associated signs and symptoms include tachycardia, diaphoresis, postural hypotension, tachypnea, flushing, severe headache, palpitations, nausea, vomiting, epigastric pain, and paresthesia.

● *Phobic disorder.* In this disorder, chronic anxiety occurs with persistent fear of an object, activity, or situation that results in a compelling desire to avoid it. The patient recognizes the fear as irrational but can't suppress it.

● *Pneumothorax.* Acute anxiety occurs in moderate to severe pneumothorax associated with profound respiratory distress. It's accompanied by sharp pleuritic pain, coughing, shortness of breath, cyanosis, asymmetrical chest expansion, weak and rapid pulse, pallor, and neck vein distention.

● *Posttraumatic stress disorder.* This disorder produces chronic anxiety of varying severity. It's accompanied by intrusive, vivid memories and thoughts of the traumatic event. The patient also relives the event in dreams and nightmares. Insomnia, depression, and feelings of numbness and detachment are common.

● *Pulmonary edema.* In this disorder, acute anxiety occurs with dyspnea, orthopnea, cough with frothy sputum, tachycardia, tachypnea, crackles, ventricular gallop, hypotension, and thready pulse. The patient's skin may be cool, clammy, and cyanotic.

● *Pulmonary embolism.* Acute anxiety is usually accompanied by dyspnea, tachypnea, chest pain, tachycardia, blood-tinged sputum, and low-grade fever.

● *Rabies.* Anxiety signals the beginning of the acute phase of this rare disorder. It's commonly accompanied by painful laryngeal spasms associated with difficulty swallowing and, as a result, hydrophobia.

● *Somatoform disorder.* Most common in adolescents and young adults, this disorder is characterized by chronic anxiety and various somatic complaints that have no physiologic basis. Anxiety and depression may be prominent or hidden by dramatic, flamboyant, or seductive behavior.

Other causes
• *Drugs.* Many drugs cause anxiety, especially sympathomimetics and central nervous system stimulants. In addition, many antidepressants may cause paradoxical anxiety.

Special considerations
In many cases, supportive care can help relieve anxiety. Provide a calm, quiet atmosphere. Make the patient comfortable. Encourage him to express his feelings and concerns freely. If it helps, take a short walk with him while you're talking. Or try anxiety-reducing measures, such as distraction, relaxation techniques, yoga, or biofeedback. (See *Relieving anxiety with yoga.*)

Pediatric pointers
Anxiety in children usually results from painful physical illness or inadequate oxygenation. Its autonomic signs tend to be more common and dramatic than in adults.

APHASIA
[Dysphasia]

Aphasia, impaired expression or comprehension of written or spoken language, reflects disease or injury of the brain's language centers. (See *Where language originates,* page 42.) Depending on its severity, aphasia may slightly impede communication or make it impossible. It can be classified as Broca's, Wernicke's, anomic, or global aphasia. (See *Identifying types of aphasia,* page 43.) Anomic aphasia eventually resolves in more

than 50% of patients, but global aphasia is commonly irreversible.

Emergency interventions
 Quickly look for signs of increased intracranial pressure (ICP), such as pupillary changes, decreased level of consciousness (LOC), vomiting, seizures, bradycardia, widening pulse pressure, and irregular respirations. If you detect signs of increased ICP, you will need to administer mannitol I.V. to decrease cerebral edema. In addition, you should make sure that emergency resuscitation equipment is readily available to support respiratory and cardiac function, if necessary. You may have to prepare the patient for emergency surgery.

History and physical examination
If the patient doesn't display signs of increased ICP, or if his aphasia has developed gradually, perform a thorough neurologic examination, starting with the patient history. You'll probably need to obtain this history from the patient's family or companion because of the patient's impairment. Ask about a history of headaches, hypertension, or seizure disorders and about drug use. Also ask about the patient's ability to communicate and to perform routine activities before aphasia began.

Check for obvious signs of neurologic deficit, such as ptosis or fluid leakage from the nose and ears. Take the patient's vital signs and assess his LOC. Recognize, though, that assessing LOC can be difficult because the patient's verbal responses may be unreliable. Also recognize that dysarthria (impaired articulation due to weakness or paralysis of the muscles necessary for speech) may accompany aphasia; so speak slowly and distinctly, and allow the patient ample time to respond. Assess the patient's pupillary response, eye movements, and motor function, especially his mouth and tongue movement, swallowing ability, and spontaneous movements and ges-

WHERE LANGUAGE ORIGINATES

Aphasia reflects damage to one or more of the brain's primary language centers, which, in most persons, are located in the left hemisphere. *Broca's area* lies next to the region of the motor cortex that controls the muscles necessary for speech. *Wernicke's area* is the center of auditory, visual, and language comprehension. It lies between *Heschl's gyrus,* which is the primary receiver of auditory stimuli, and the *angular gyrus,* a "way station" between the brain's auditory and visual regions. Connecting Wernicke's and Broca's areas is a large nerve bundle, the *arcuate fasciculus,* which enables repetition of speech.

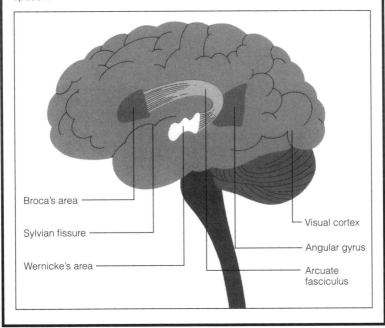

Broca's area

Sylvian fissure

Wernicke's area

Visual cortex

Angular gyrus

Arcuate fasciculus

---

tures. To best assess motor function, first demonstrate the motions and then have the patient imitate them.

Common medical causes

● *Alzheimer's disease.* In this degenerative disease, anomic aphasia may begin insidiously and then progress to severe global aphasia. Associated signs and symptoms typically include behavioral changes, loss of memory, poor judgment, restlessness, myoclonus, and muscle rigidity. Incontinence is usually a late sign.

● *Brain abscess.* Any type of aphasia may occur in brain abscess. Usually, aphasia develops insidiously and may be accompanied by hemiparesis, ataxia, facial weakness, and signs of increased ICP.

● *Brain tumor.* This may cause any type of aphasia. As the tumor enlarges, other aphasias may occur along with behavioral changes, memory loss, motor weakness, seizures, auditory hallucinations, visual field deficits, and increased ICP.

IDENTIFYING TYPES OF APHASIA

TYPE	LOCATION OF LESION	CLINICAL FINDINGS
Broca's (expressive) aphasia	Broca's area; usually in third frontal convolution of the left hemisphere	Patient's understanding of written and spoken language is relatively spared, but speech is nonfluent, evidencing word-finding difficulty, jargon, paraphasias, limited vocabulary, and simple sentence construction. He can't repeat words and phrases. If Wernicke's area is intact, the patient recognizes speech errors and shows frustration. He is commonly hemiparetic.
Wernicke's (receptive) aphasia	Wernicke's area; usually in posterior or superior temporal lobe	Patient has difficulty understanding written and spoken language. He can't repeat words or phrases or follow directions. His speech is fluent but may be rapid and rambling, with paraphasias. He has difficulty naming objects (anomia) and is unaware of speech errors.
Anomic aphasia	Temporoparietal area; may extend to angular gyrus, but sometimes poorly localized	Patient's understanding of written and spoken language is relatively unimpaired. His speech, though fluent, lacks meaningful content. Word-finding difficulty and circumlocution are characteristic. Rarely, the patient also displays paraphasias.
Global aphasia	Broca's and Wernicke's areas	Patient has profoundly impaired receptive and expressive ability. He can't repeat words or phrases and can't follow directions. His occasional speech is marked by paraphasias or jargon.

• **Cerebrovascular accident.** The most common cause of aphasia, this disorder may produce Wernicke's, Broca's, or global aphasia. Associated findings usually include decreased LOC, right-sided hemiparesis, homonymous hemianopia, paresthesia, and loss of sensation. (These symptoms may appear on the left side if the right hemisphere contains the language centers.)

• **Head trauma.** Any type of aphasia may accompany severe head trauma; typically, it occurs suddenly and may be transient or permanent, depending on the extent of brain damage. Associated signs and symptoms may include blurred or double vision, headache, pallor, diaphoresis, numbness and paresis, cerebrospinal otorrhea or rhinorrhea, altered respirations, tachycardia, disorientation, behavioral changes, and signs of increased ICP.

• **Transient ischemic attack (TIA).** This disorder can produce any type of aphasia. Usually, aphasia occurs suddenly and resolves within 24 hours of the TIA. Associated symptoms include transient hemiparesis, hemianopia, and paresthesia (all usually right-sided), dizziness, and confusion.

• **Seizures.** Seizures and the postictal state may cause a transient aphasia if the seizures involve the language centers.

Special considerations
Immediately after aphasia develops, the patient may become confused or disoriented. Help to restore a sense of reality by frequently telling him what has happened, where he is and why, and the date. Carefully explain diagnostic tests, such as skull X-rays, computed tomography scan, angiography, and EEG. Later, expect periods of depression as the patient recognizes his disability. Help him to communicate by providing a relaxed, accepting environment with a minimum of distracting stimuli.

Be alert for sudden outbursts of profanity by the patient. This common behavior usually reflects intense frustration with his impairment. Deal with such outbursts as gently as possible to ease embarrassment.

When you speak to the patient, don't assume that he understands you. He may simply be interpreting subtle clues to meaning, such as social context, facial expressions, and gestures. To help avoid misunderstanding, use nonverbal techniques, speak to him in simple phrases, and use demonstration to clarify your verbal directions.

Remember that aphasia is a *language* disorder, not an emotional or auditory one, so speak to the patient in a normal tone of voice. Make sure he has necessary aids, such as eyeglasses or dentures, to facilitate communication.

Refer the patient to a speech pathologist early to help him cope with his aphasia.

Pediatric pointers
Recognize that the term *childhood aphasia* is sometimes mistakenly applied to children who fail to develop normal language skills but who aren't considered mentally disabled or developmentally delayed. Aphasia refers solely to loss of previously developed communication skills.

Brain damage associated with aphasia in children most commonly follows anoxia—the result of near-drowning or airway obstruction.

APNEA

Apnea is the cessation of spontaneous respiration. Occasionally, it's temporary and self-limiting, as occurs during Cheyne-Stokes and Biot's respirations. In most cases, though, it's a life-threatening emergency that requires immediate intervention to prevent death.

Apnea usually results from one or more of six pathophysiologic mechanisms, each of which has numerous causes. Its most common causes include trauma, cardiac arrest, neurologic disease, aspiration of foreign objects, bronchospasm, and drug overdose. (See *Common causes of apnea.*)

Emergency interventions
 If you detect apnea, first establish and maintain a patent airway. Position the patient supine and open his airway using the head-tilt, chin-lift technique. (*Caution:* Use the jaw-thrust technique on a patient with an obvious or suspected head or neck injury to prevent hyperextending the neck.) Next, quickly look, listen, and feel for spontaneous respiration; if it's absent, begin artificial ventilation until it occurs or until mechanical ventilation can be initiated.

Because apnea may result from cardiac arrest (or may cause it), be sure to assess the patient's carotid pulse imme-

COMMON CAUSES OF APNEA

Airway obstruction
- Asthma
- Bronchospasm
- Chronic bronchitis
- Foreign body aspiration
- Hemothorax or pneumothorax
- Mucus plug
- Obstruction by tongue or tumor
- Obstructive sleep apnea
- Secretion retention
- Tracheal/bronchial rupture

Brain stem dysfunction
- Brain abscess
- Brain stem injury
- Brain tumor
- Central nervous system depressants
- Central sleep apnea
- Cerebral hemorrhage
- Cerebral infarction
- Encephalitis
- Head trauma
- Increased intracranial pressure
- Meningitis
- Pontine or medullary hemorrhage or infarction
- Transtentorial herniation

Neuromuscular failure
- Amyotrophic lateral sclerosis
- Botulism
- Diphtheria
- Guillain-Barré syndrome
- Myasthenia gravis
- Phrenic nerve paralysis
- Rupture of the diaphragm
- Spinal cord injury

Parenchymal disease
- Adult respiratory distress syndrome
- Diffuse pneumonia
- Emphysema
- Near drowning
- Pulmonary edema
- Pulmonary fibrosis
- Secretion retention

Pleural pressure gradient disruption
- Flail chest
- Open chest wounds

Pulmonary capillary perfusion decrease
- Arrhythmias
- Cardiac arrest
- Myocardial infarction
- Pulmonary embolism
- Pulmonary hypertension
- Shock

diately after you've established a patent airway. Or, if the patient is an infant or small child, assess the brachial pulse instead. If you can't palpate a pulse, begin cardiac compression.

History and physical examination
When the patient's respiratory and cardiac status is stable, investigate the underlying cause of apnea. Ask him (or, if he's unable to answer, anyone who witnessed the episode) about the onset of apnea and events immediately preceding it. The cause may become readily apparent, as in trauma.

Take a patient history, noting especially any reports of headache, chest pain, muscle weakness, sore throat, or dyspnea. Ask about any history of respiratory, cardiac, or neurologic disease and about allergies and drug use.

Inspect the head, face, neck, and trunk for soft-tissue injury, hemorrhage, or skeletal deformity. Don't overlook obvious clues, such as oral and nasal secretions reflecting fluid-filled airways and alveoli or facial soot and singed nasal hair suggesting thermal injury to the tracheobronchial tree.

Auscultate over all lung lobes for adventitious breath sounds, particularly crackles and rhonchi, and percuss the lung fields for increased dullness or hyperresonance. Move on to the heart, auscultating for murmurs, pericardial friction rub, and arrhythmias. Check for cyanosis, pallor, jugular vein distention, and edema. If appropriate, perform a neurologic assessment. Evaluate level of consciousness (LOC), orientation, and mental status; test cranial nerve function and motor function, sensation, and reflexes in all extremities.

Common medical causes

• *Airway obstruction.* Occlusion or compression of the trachea, central airways, or smaller airways can cause sudden apnea by blocking the patient's airflow and producing acute respiratory failure.

• *Brain stem dysfunction.* Primary or secondary brain stem dysfunction can cause apnea by destroying the brain stem's ability to initiate respirations. Apnea may arise suddenly (as in trauma, hemorrhage, or infarction) or gradually (as in degenerative disease or tumor). Apnea may be preceded by a decreased LOC and by various motor and sensory deficits.

• *Neuromuscular failure.* Trauma or disease can disrupt the mechanics of respiration, causing sudden or gradual apnea. Associated findings may include diaphragmatic or intercostal muscle paralysis from injury, or respiratory weakness or paralysis from acute or degenerative disease.

• *Parenchymal lung disease.* An accumulation of fluid within the alveoli produces apnea by interfering with pulmonary gas exchange and producing acute respiratory failure. Apnea may arise suddenly, as in near drowning and acute pulmonary edema, or gradually, as in emphysema. Apnea also may be preceded by crackles and labored respirations with accessory muscle use.

• *Pleural pressure gradient disruption.* Conversion of normal negative pleural air pressure to positive pressure by chest wall injuries (such as flail chest) causes lung collapse, producing respiratory distress and, if untreated, apnea. Associated signs include an asymmetrical chest wall and asymmetrical or paradoxical respirations.

• *Pulmonary capillary perfusion decrease.* Apnea can stem from obstructed pulmonary circulation, most commonly due to heart failure or lack of circulatory patency. It occurs suddenly in cardiac arrest, massive pulmonary embolism, and most cases of severe shock. In contrast, it occurs progressively in septic shock and pulmonary hypertension. Related findings include hypotension, tachycardia, and edema.

Other causes

• *Drugs.* Hypoventilation and apnea may be caused by central nervous system (CNS) depressants. Benzodiazepines may cause respiratory depression and apnea when given I.V. along with other CNS depressants to elderly or acutely ill patients.

Neuromuscular blocking agents— such as curariform drugs and anticholinesterase inhibitors—may produce sudden apnea because of respiratory muscle paralysis.

• *Sleep-related apneas.* These repetitive apneas occur during sleep due to airflow obstruction or brain stem dysfunction.

Special considerations

Closely monitor the apneic patient's cardiac and respiratory status to prevent further apneic episodes.

Pediatric pointers

Premature infants are especially susceptible to periodic apneic episodes due to CNS immaturity. Other common causes of apnea in infants include sepsis, intraventricular and subarachnoid hemorrhage, seizures, bronchiolitis, and sudden infant death syndrome.

In toddlers and older children, the primary cause of apnea is acute airway obstruction from aspiration of foreign objects. Other causes include acute epiglottitis, croup, asthma, and systemic disorders, such as muscular dystrophy and cystic fibrosis.

APNEUSTIC RESPIRATIONS

This irregular breathing pattern is characterized by prolonged, gasping inspiration, with a pause at full inspiration. It's an important localizing sign of severe brain stem damage.

Involuntary breathing is primarily regulated by groups of neurons located in respiratory centers in the medulla oblongata and the pons. In the medulla, neurons react to impulses from the pons and other areas to regulate respiratory rate and depth. In the pons, two respiratory centers regulate respiratory rhythm by interacting with the medullary respiratory center to smooth the transition from inspiration to expiration and back. The apneustic center in the pons stimulates inspiratory neurons in the medulla to precipitate inspiration. These inspiratory neurons, in turn, stimulate the pneumotaxic center in the pons to precipitate expiration. Destruction of neural pathways by pontine lesions disrupts normal regulation of respiratory rhythm, causing apneustic respirations.

Apneustic respirations must be differentiated from bradypnea and hyperpnea (disturbances in rate and depth, but not in rhythm), Cheyne-Stokes respirations (rhythmic alterations in rate and depth, followed by periods of apnea), and Biot's respirations (irregularly alternating periods of hyperpnea and apnea).

Emergency interventions

 Your first priority for the patient with apneustic respirations is to ensure adequate ventilation.

You'll need to insert an artificial airway and administer oxygen until mechanical ventilation can begin. Next, thoroughly evaluate the patient's neurologic status, using a standardized tool such as the Glasgow Coma Scale. In addition, obtain a brief patient history from a family member or companion, if possible.

Common medical causes
• *Pontine lesions.* Apneustic respirations usually result from extensive damage to the upper or lower pons, whether due to infarction, hemorrhage, herniation, severe infection, tumor, or trauma. Typically, these respirations are accompanied by profound stupor or coma; pinpoint midline pupils; ocular bobbing (a spontaneous downward jerk, followed by a slow drift up to midline); quadriplegia or, less commonly, hemiplegia with the eyes pointing toward the weak side; a positive Babinski's reflex; negative oculocephalic and oculovestibular reflexes; and possibly decorticate posture.

Special considerations
Constantly monitor the patient's neurologic and respiratory status. Watch for prolonged apneic periods or signs of neurologic deterioration. Monitor the patient's arterial blood gas levels. If appropriate, prepare him for neurologic tests, such as electroencephalography and computed tomography.

Pediatric pointers
In young children, avoid using the Glasgow Coma Scale because it requires verbal responses and assumes a certain level of language development.

ARM PAIN

Usually, arm pain results from musculoskeletal disorders, but it can also result from neurovascular or cardiovascular dis-

COMMON CAUSES OF LOCAL PAIN

Various disorders cause hand, wrist, elbow, or shoulder pain. In some disorders, pain may radiate from the injury site to other areas.

Hand pain
Arthritis
Buerger's disease
Carpal tunnel syndrome
Dupuytren's contracture
Elbow tunnel syndrome
Fracture
Ganglion
Infection
Occlusive vascular disease
Radiculopathy
Raynaud's disease
Shoulder-hand syndrome
Sprain or strain
Thoracic outlet syndromes
Trigger finger

Wrist pain
Arthritis
Carpal tunnel syndrome
Fracture
Ganglion
Sprain or strain
Tenosynovitis (de Quervain's disease)

Elbow pain
Arthritis
Bursitis

Dislocation
Fracture
Lateral epicondylitis (tennis elbow)
Tendinitis

Shoulder pain
Acromioclavicular separation
Acute pancreatitis
Adhesive capsulitis
Angina pectoris
Arthritis
Bursitis
Cholecystitis or cholelithiasis
Clavicle fracture
Diaphragmatic pleurisy
Dislocation
Dissecting aortic aneurysm
Gastritis
Humeral neck fracture
Infection
Pancoast's syndrome
Perforated ulcer
Pneumothorax
Ruptured spleen (left shoulder)
Shoulder-hand syndrome
Subphrenic abscess
Tendinitis

orders. (See *Common causes of local pain*.) Its location, onset, and character provide clues to its cause. The pain may affect the entire arm or only the upper arm or forearm. It may arise suddenly or gradually and be constant or intermittent. Arm pain can be described as sharp or dull, burning or numbing, shooting or penetrating. Diffuse arm pain, though, may be difficult to describe, especially if it isn't associated with injury.

History and physical examination
If the patient reports arm pain after an injury, take a brief history of the injury from the patient or his companion. Then quickly assess for severe injuries requiring immediate treatment. If you've ruled out severe injuries, check pulses, capillary refill time, sensation, and movement distal to the affected area because circulatory impairment or nerve injury may require immediate surgery. Inspect the arm for deformity, assess the level of pain, and immobilize the arm to prevent further injury.

If the patient reports generalized or intermittent arm pain, ask him to describe the pain and relate when it began. Is pain associated with repetitive or specific movements or positions? Ask him to point out other painful areas because arm pain may be referred. For example, arm pain may accompany the characteristic chest pain of myocardial infarction. Ask him if the pain worsens in the morning or in the evening, if it prevents him from performing his job, or if it restricts any movements. Also ask if heat, rest, or drugs relieve it. Finally, ask about any preexisting illnesses, a family history of gout or arthritis, and current drug therapy.

Next, perform a focused examination. Observe the way the patient walks, sits, and holds his arm. Inspect the entire arm, comparing it to the opposite arm for symmetry, movement, and muscle atrophy. Palpate the entire arm for swelling, nodules, and tender areas. In both arms, compare active range of motion, muscle strength, and reflexes.

If the patient reports numbness or tingling, check his sensation to vibration and pinprick. Compare bilateral hand grasps and shoulder strength to detect weakness.

If a patient has a cast, splint, or restrictive dressing, check for circulation, sensation, and mobility distal to the dressing. Ask the patient about edema and if the pain has worsened within the last 24 hours. Also ask what activities he has been performing.

Common medical causes

• **Angina.** This disorder may cause inner arm pain as well as chest and jaw pain. Typically, the pain follows exertion and persists for a few minutes. Accompanied by dyspnea, diaphoresis, and apprehension, the pain is relieved by rest or vasodilators such as nitroglycerin.

• **Biceps rupture.** Rupture of the biceps after excessive weight lifting or osteoarthritic degeneration of bicipital tendon insertion at the shoulder can cause pain in the upper arm. Forearm flexion and supination aggravate the pain. Other signs and symptoms include muscle weakness, deformity, and edema.

• **Cellulitis.** Typically, this disorder affects the legs, but it can also affect the arms. It produces pain as well as redness, tenderness, edema and, at times, fever, chills, tachycardia, headache, and hypotension.

• **Cervical nerve root compression.** Compression of the cervical nerves supplying the upper arm produces chronic arm and neck pain, which may worsen with movement or prolonged sitting. The patient may also experience muscle weakness, paresthesia, and decreased reflex response may also occur.

• **Compartment syndrome.** Severe pain with passive muscle stretching is the cardinal symptom of this syndrome. It may also impair distal circulation and cause muscle weakness, decreased reflex response, paresthesia, and edema. Ominous signs include paralysis and absent pulse.

• **Fractures.** In fractures of the cervical vertebrae, humerus, scapula, clavicle, radius, or ulna, pain can occur at the injury site and radiate throughout the entire arm. Pain at a fresh fracture site is intense and worsens with movement. Associated signs and symptoms include crepitus, felt and heard from bone ends rubbing together (do not attempt to elicit this sign); deformity, if bones are unaligned; local ecchymosis and edema; impaired distal circulation; paresthesia; and decreased sensation distal to the injury site.

• **Muscle contusion.** This disorder may cause generalized pain in the area of injury. It may also cause local swelling and ecchymosis.

• **Muscle strain.** Acute or chronic muscle strain causes mild to severe pain with movement. The resultant reduction in arm movement may cause muscle weakness and atrophy.

• **Myocardial infarction.** In this life-threatening disorder, the patient may complain of left arm pain as well as the characteristic deep and crushing chest pain. He may display weakness, pallor, nausea, vomiting, diaphoresis, altered blood pressure, tachycardia, dyspnea, and feelings of apprehension or impending doom.

ARM PAIN: COMMON CAUSES AND ASSOCIATED FINDINGS

CAUSES	MAJOR ASSOCIATED SIGNS AND SYMPTOMS											
	Chest pain	Crepitus	Decreased motion	Decreased reflex response	Deformity	Ecchymosis	Edema	Impaired circulation	Muscle weakness	Nausea	Paresthesia	Vomiting
Angina	●											
Biceps rupture					●		●		●			
Cellulitis							●					
Cervical nerve root compression				●					●		●	
Compartment syndrome				●			●	●	●		●	
Fractures		●	●		●	●	●	●			●	
Muscle contusion						●	●					
Muscle strain			●						●			
Myocardial infarction	●									●		●
Neoplasms of the arm							●	●			●	
Osteomyelitis			●				●					

● **Neoplasms of the arm.** This disorder produces continuous, deep, and penetrating arm pain that worsens at night. Occasionally, redness and swelling accompany arm pain; later, skin breakdown, impaired circulation, and paresthesia may occur.

● **Osteomyelitis.** This disorder typically begins with the sudden onset of localized arm pain and fever. It's accompanied by local tenderness, painful and restricted movement and, later, swelling. Associated findings include malaise and tachycardia.

Special considerations
If you suspect a fracture, apply a sling or a splint to immobilize the arm, and monitor for worsening pain, numbness, or decreased circulation distal to the injury site. Also monitor vital signs, and be alert for tachycardia, hypotension, and diaphoresis. Withhold food, fluids, and analgesics until potential fractures are evaluated. Promote the patient's comfort by elevating his arm and applying ice. Clean abrasions and lacerations and apply dry, sterile dressings, if necessary.

Also prepare the patient for X-rays or other diagnostic tests.

Pediatric pointers

In children, arm pain commonly results from fractures, muscle sprain, muscular dystrophy, or rheumatoid arthritis. In young children especially, the exact location of the pain may be difficult to establish. Watch for nonverbal clues, such as wincing or guarding.

If the child has a fracture or sprain, obtain a complete account of the injury. Closely observe interactions between the child and his family, and don't rule out the possibility of child abuse.

ASTERIXIS
[Liver flap, flapping tremor]

A bilateral, coarse movement, asterixis is characterized by sudden relaxation of muscle groups holding a sustained posture. This elicited sign is most commonly observed in the wrists and fingers but also may appear during any sustained voluntary action. Typically, it signals hepatic, renal, and pulmonary disease.

To elicit asterixis, have the patient extend his arms, dorsiflex his wrists, and spread his fingers (or do this for him, if necessary). Briefly observe for asterixis. Alternately, if the patient has a decreased level of consciousness (LOC) but can follow verbal commands, ask him to squeeze two of your fingers. Consider rapid clutching and unclutching positive for asterixis. Or elevate the patient's leg off the bed and dorsiflex the foot. Briefly observe for asterixis in the ankle. If the patient can tightly close his eyes and mouth, observe for irregular tremulous movements of the eyelids and corners of the mouth. If he can stick out his tongue, watch for continuous quivering.

Emergency interventions

 Because asterixis may signal serious metabolic deterioration, quickly evaluate the patient's neurologic status and vital signs. Compare these data to the patient's baseline. Watch carefully for acute changes. Continue to monitor neurologic status, vital signs, and urine output closely.

Watch for signs of respiratory insufficiency, and be prepared to provide endotracheal intubation and ventilatory support. Also be alert for complications of end-stage hepatic, renal, or pulmonary disease.

If the patient has hepatic disease, assess for early signs of hemorrhage, including restlessness, tachypnea, and cool, moist, pale skin. (If the patient is jaundiced, check for pallor in the conjunctiva and mucous membranes of the mouth.)

It is important to recognize that hypotension, oliguria, hematemesis, and melena are late signs of hemorrhage. Prepare to insert a large-bore I.V. catheter for fluid and blood replacement. Position the patient flat in bed with his legs elevated 20 degrees. Begin or continue to administer oxygen.

If the patient has renal disease, ask what type of therapy he has received. If he's on dialysis, ask about the frequency of treatments to help gauge the severity of disease. Ask a relative if the patient's LOC is significantly decreased.

Then assess for hyperkalemia and metabolic acidosis. Look for tachycardia, nausea, diarrhea, abdominal cramps, muscle weakness, hyperreflexia, and Kussmaul's respirations (deep, gasping breaths). Prepare to administer sodium bicarbonate, calcium gluconate, dextrose, insulin, or Kayexalate.

If the patient has pulmonary disease, assess for labored respirations, tachypnea, accessory muscle use, and cyanosis, which are critical signs. Prepare to provide ventilatory support via nasal cannula, mask, or intubation and mechanical ventilation.

Common medical causes
● *Hepatic encephalopathy.* A life-threatening disorder, hepatic encepha-

lopathy initially causes slight personality changes and a slight tremor. This tremor progresses into asterixis—a hallmark of hepatic encephalopathy—and is accompanied by lethargy, aberrant behavior, and apraxia. Eventually, the patient becomes stuporous and displays hyperventilation. When he slips into coma, hyperactive reflexes, a positive Babinski's reflex, and fetor hepaticus are characteristic signs. The patient also may experience bradycardia, decreased respirations, and seizures.

• *Uremic syndrome.* This life-threatening disorder initially causes lethargy, somnolence, confusion, disorientation, behavior changes, and irritability. Eventually, though, signs and symptoms appear in diverse body systems. Asterixis is accompanied by stupor, paresthesias, muscle twitching, fasciculations, and footdrop. Other signs and symptoms include polyuria and nocturia followed by oliguria and, then, anuria; elevated blood pressure; signs of heart failure and pericarditis; Kussmaul's respirations; anorexia; nausea; vomiting; diarrhea; GI bleeding; weight loss; ammonia breath odor; and metallic taste.

Other causes
• *Drugs.* Certain drugs, such as phenytoin, may cause asterixis.

Special considerations
Provide simple patient comfort measures such as frequent rest periods to minimize fatigue. Elevate the head of the bed to relieve dyspnea and orthopnea. Administer oil baths and avoid soap to relieve itching caused by jaundice and uremia. Provide emotional support to the patient and his family.

Provide enteral or parenteral nutrition if the patient is intubated or has a decreased LOC. Closely monitor serum and urine glucose levels to evaluate hyperalimentation. Because the patient will probably be on bed rest, reposition him at least once every 2 hours to prevent skin breakdown. Also, recognize that his debilitated state makes him prone to infection.

Observe strict hand washing and aseptic technique when changing dressings and caring for invasive lines.

Pediatric pointers
End-stage hepatic, renal, and pulmonary disease may cause asterixis in children.

ATAXIA

Classified as cerebellar or sensory, ataxia refers to incoordination and irregularity of voluntary, purposeful movements. *Cerebellar ataxia* results from disease of the cerebellum and its pathways to and from the cerebral cortex, brain stem, and spinal cord. It causes gait, trunk, limb, and possibly speech disorders. *Sensory ataxia* results from impaired position sense (proprioception) caused by interruption of afferent nerve fibers in the peripheral nerves, posterior roots, posterior columns of the spinal cord, or medial lemnisci, or occasionally by a lesion in both parietal lobes. It causes gait disorders. (See *Identifying ataxia.*)

Ataxia occurs in acute and chronic forms. *Acute ataxia* may result from hemorrhage or a large tumor in the posterior fossa. In this life-threatening condition, the cerebellum may herniate downward through the foramen magnum behind the cervical spinal cord or upward through the tentorium upon the cerebral hemispheres. Herniation may also compress the brain stem. Acute ataxia may also result from drug toxicity or poisoning. *Chronic ataxia* can be progressive and, at times, can result from acute disease. It can also occur in metabolic and chronic degenerative neurologic disease.

Emergency interventions
 If ataxic movements suddenly develop, examine the patient for signs of increased intracranial pressure and impending herniation. De-

IDENTIFYING ATAXIA

Ataxia may be observed in the patient's speech, in the movements of his trunk and limbs, or in his gait.

In **speech ataxia,** a form of dysarthria, the patient typically speaks slowly and stresses usually unstressed words and syllables. Speech content is not affected.

In **truncal ataxia,** a disturbance in equilibrium, the patient cannot sit or stand without falling. Also, his head and trunk may bob and sway (titubation). If he's able to walk, his gait is reeling.

In **limb ataxia,** the patient loses the ability to gauge distance, speed, and power of movement, resulting in poorly controlled, variable, and inaccurate voluntary movements. He may move too quickly or too slowly, or his movements may break down into component parts, giving him the appearance of a puppet or a robot. Other effects include a coarse, irregular tremor in purposeful movement (but not at rest) and reduced muscle tone.

In **gait ataxia,** the patient's gait is wide-based, unsteady, and irregular. In cerebellar ataxia, the patient may stagger or lurch in zigzag fashion, turn with extreme difficulty, and lose his balance when his feet are together. In sensory ataxia, the patient moves abruptly and stomps or taps his feet. This occurs because he throws his feet forward and outward, then brings them down first on the heels, then on the toes. The patient also fixes his eyes on the ground, watching his steps. However, if he's unable to watch them, staggering worsens. When he stands with his feet together, he sways or loses balance.

---

termine his level of consciousness (LOC) and be alert for pupillary changes, motor weakness or paralysis, neck stiffness or pain, and vomiting. Check vital signs, especially respirations; abnormal respiratory patterns may quickly lead to respiratory arrest. Elevate the head of the bed. Have emergency resuscitation equipment readily available. Prepare the patient for computed tomography scanning or surgery.

History and physical examination

If the patient isn't in distress, review his history. Ask about previous cerebrovascular accident, multiple sclerosis, diabetes, central nervous system infection, neoplastic disease, and family history of ataxia. Also ask about chronic alcohol abuse or prolonged exposure to industrial toxins such as mercury. Ask if the ataxia arose suddenly or gradually.

If necessary, perform Romberg's test to help distinguish cerebellar from sensory ataxia. Instruct the patient to stand with his feet together and his arms at his side. Note his posture and balance, first with his eyes open, then closed. Test results may indicate normal posture and balance (minimal swaying), cerebellar ataxia (swaying and inability to maintain balance with eyes open or closed), or sensory ataxia (increased swaying and inability to maintain balance with eyes closed). Stand near the patient during this test to prevent his falling.

If you test for gait and limb ataxia, be aware that motor weakness may mimic ataxic movements, so check motor strength, too. Gait ataxia may be severe, even when there is minimal limb ataxia. In gait ataxia, ask the patient if he tends to fall to one side or if falling usually occurs at night. In truncal ataxia, remember that the patient's inability to walk or stand, combined with the absence of other signs while he's lying down, may give the impression of hysteria or drug or alcohol intoxication.

Common medical causes

● *Cerebellar abscess.* This disorder commonly causes limb ataxia on the same side of the lesion, as well as gait and truncal ataxia. Typically, the initial symptom is headache localized behind the ear or in the occipital region, followed by ocular motor palsy, fever, vomiting, altered LOC, and coma.

● *Cerebrovascular accident (CVA).* In CVA, occlusions in the vertebrobasilar arteries halt blood flow to cause infarction in the medulla, pons, or cerebellum that may lead to ataxia. Ataxia may occur at the onset of CVA and remain as a residual deficit. Worsening ataxia during the acute phase may indicate extension of the CVA or severe swelling. Ataxia may be accompanied by unilateral or bilateral motor weakness, possible altered LOC, sensory loss, vertigo, nausea, vomiting, ocular motor palsy, and dysphagia.

● *Diabetic neuropathy.* Peripheral nerve damage caused by diabetes mellitus may cause sensory ataxia as well as extremity pain, slight leg weakness, skin changes, and bowel and bladder dysfunction.

● *Diphtheria.* Within 4 to 8 weeks of the onset of symptoms, a life-threatening neuropathy can produce sensory ataxia. Diphtheria can be accompanied by fever, paresthesia, and paralysis of the limbs and, sometimes, the respiratory muscles.

● *Friedreich's ataxia.* This progressive familial disorder affects the spinal cord and cerebellum. It causes gait ataxia, followed by truncal, limb, and speech ataxia. Other features include pes cavus, kyphoscoliosis, cranial nerve palsy, and motor and sensory deficits. A positive Babinski's reflex may appear.

● *Hepatocerebral degeneration.* Some patients who survive hepatic coma are left with residual neurologic defects, including mild cerebellar ataxia with a wide-based, unsteady gait. Ataxia may be accompanied by altered LOC, dysarthria, rhythmic arm tremors, and choreoathetosis of the face, neck, and shoulders.

● *Multiple sclerosis (MS).* Nystagmus and cerebellar ataxia commonly occur in this disorder, but they aren't always accompanied by limb weakness and spasticity. Speech ataxia (especially scanning) may occur as well as sensory ataxia from spinal cord involvement. During remissions, ataxia may subside or even disappear. During exacerbations, it may reappear, worsen, or even become permanent.

MS also causes optic neuritis, optic atrophy, numbness and weakness, diplopia, dizziness, and bladder dysfunction.

● *Olivopontocerebellar atrophy.* This disease produces gait ataxia and, later, limb and speech ataxia. Rarely, it produces intention tremor. It's accompanied by choreiform movements, dysphagia, and loss of sphincter tone.

● *Poisoning.* Chronic *arsenic* poisoning may cause sensory ataxia, along with headache, seizures, altered LOC, motor deficits, and muscle aching. Chronic *mercury* poisoning causes gait ataxia and limb ataxia, principally of the arms. It also causes tremors of the extremities, tongue, and lips; mental confusion; mood changes; and dysarthria.

● *Polyneuropathy.* Carcinomatous and myelomatous polyneuropathy may occur before detection of the primary tumor in cancer, multiple myeloma, or Hodgkin's disease. Signs and symptoms include ataxia, severe motor weakness, muscle atrophy, and sensory loss in the limbs. Pain and skin changes may also occur.

● *Posterior fossa tumor.* Gait, truncal, or limb ataxia is an early sign and may worsen as the tumor enlarges. It's accompanied by vomiting, headache, papilledema, vertigo, ocular motor palsy, decreased LOC, and motor and sensory impairment on the side of the lesion.

● *Spinocerebellar ataxia.* In this disorder, the patient may initially experience fatigue, followed by stiff-legged gait ataxia. Eventually, limb ataxia, dysarthria, static tremor, nystagmus, cramps, paresthesias, and sensory deficits occur.

- **Wernicke's disease.** The result of thiamine deficiency, this disease produces gait ataxia and, rarely, intention tremor or speech ataxia. In severe ataxia, the patient may be unable to stand or walk. Ataxia decreases with thiamine therapy. Associated signs and symptoms include nystagmus, diplopia, ocular palsies, confusion, tachycardia, exertional dyspnea, and postural hypotension.

Other causes
- **Drugs.** Toxic levels of anticonvulsants, especially phenytoin, may result in gait ataxia. Toxic levels of anticholinergics and tricyclic antidepressants may also result in ataxia. Aminoglutethimide causes ataxia in about 10% of patients; however, this effect usually disappears 4 to 6 weeks after cessation of drug therapy.

Special considerations
Prepare the patient for laboratory studies, such as blood tests for toxic drug levels and radiologic tests. Then focus on helping the patient adapt to his condition. Promote goals of rehabilitation and help ensure the patient's safety. For example, instruct the patient with sensory ataxia to move slowly, especially when turning or getting up from a chair. Provide a cane or walker for extra support. Ask the patient's family to check his home for hazards, such as uneven surfaces or the absence of hand rails on stairs. If appropriate, refer the patient with progressive disease for counseling.

Pediatric pointers
In children, ataxia occurs in acute and chronic forms, resulting from congenital or acquired disease. Acute ataxia may stem from febrile infection, brain tumors, mumps, and other disorders. Chronic ataxia may stem from Gaucher's disease, Refsum's disease, and other inborn errors of metabolism.

When assessing a child for ataxia, consider his level of motor skills and emotional state. Your examination may be limited to observing the child in spontaneous activity and carefully questioning his parents about changes in his motor activity, such as increased unsteadiness or falling. If you suspect ataxia, refer the child for neurologic evaluation to rule out brain tumor.

AURA

An aura is a sensory or motor phenomenon, idea, or emotion that marks the initial stage of a seizure or the approach of a classic migraine headache. It may be classified as cognitive, affective, psychosensory, or psychomotor.

When associated with a seizure, an aura stems from an irritable focus in the brain that spreads throughout the cortex. Although an aura was once considered a sign of impending seizure, it's now considered the first stage of a seizure. Typically, it occurs seconds to minutes before the ictal phase. Its intensity, duration, and type depend on the origin of the irritable focus. For example, an aura of bitter taste often accompanies a frontal lobe lesion. Unfortunately, an aura is difficult to describe because the postictal phase of a seizure temporarily alters the patient's level of consciousness, impairing his memory of the event.

The aura associated with classic migraine headache results from cranial vasoconstriction. Diagnostically important, it helps distinguish classic migraine from other types of headache. Typically, the aura lasts from 10 to 30 minutes and varies in intensity and duration. If the patient recognizes the aura as a warning sign, he may be able to prevent the headache by taking appropriate drugs.

Emergency interventions
 When an aura rapidly progresses to the ictal phase of a seizure, quickly evaluate the seizure and

TYPES OF AURAS

Determining whether an aura marks the patient's thought processes, emotions, or sensory or motor function often requires keen observation. Auras are typically difficult to describe and only dimly remembered when associated with seizures. The types of auras and their manifestations are listed below.

Cognitive auras
- Déjà vu (familiarity with unfamiliar events or environments)
- Jamais vu (unfamiliarity with a known event)
- Time standing still
- Flashback of past events

Affective auras
- Fear
- Paranoia
- Other emotions

Psychosensory auras
- Visual: flashes of light or scintillations
- Olfactory: foul odors
- Gustatory: acidic, metallic, or bitter tastes
- Auditory: buzzing or ringing in the ears
- Tactile: numbness or tingling
- Vertigo

Psychomotor auras
- Automatisms (inappropriate, repetitive movements): lip smacking, chewing, swallowing, grimacing, picking at clothes, climbing stairs

History and physical examination
Later, obtain a thorough history of the patient's headaches, asking him to describe any sensory or motor phenomena that precede each headache. (See *Types of auras.*) Find out how long each headache typically lasts. Does anything make it worse, such as bright lights, noise, or caffeine? Does anything make it better? Ask the patient about drugs for pain relief.

Common medical causes
• *Classic migraine headache.* This is preceded by a vague premonition and then, usually, a visual aura involving flashes of light. The aura lasts 10 to 30 minutes and may intensify until it completely obscures the patient's vision. A classic migraine may cause numbness or tingling of lips, face, or hands; slight confusion; and dizziness before the characteristic unilateral, throbbing headache appears. It slowly intensifies; when it peaks, it may cause photophobia, nausea, and vomiting.

Special considerations
Advise the patient to keep a diary of factors that precipitate each headache as well as associated symptoms to evaluate the effectiveness of drug therapy and recommended lifestyle changes.

Pediatric pointers
In children, auras usually herald seizure activity, not a classic migraine headache. Watch for nonverbal clues that may be associated with an aura, such as rubbing the eyes, coughing, and spitting.

When taking the seizure history, recognize that children—like adults—tend to forget the aura. Ask simple, direct questions, such as: "Do you see anything funny before the seizure?" and "Do you get a bad taste in your mouth?" Give the child ample time to respond because he may have difficulty describing the aura.

be alert for life-threatening complications such as apnea. When an aura heralds a classic migraine, make the patient as comfortable as possible. Place him in a dark, quiet room and administer drugs to prevent headache.

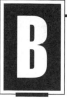

BABINSKI'S REFLEX
[Extensor plantar reflex]

Babinski's reflex—dorsiflexion of the great toe with extension and fanning of the other toes—is an abnormal reflex elicited by firmly stroking the lateral aspect of the sole of the foot with a blunt object. (See *How to elicit Babinski's reflex,* page 58.) In some patients, this reflex can be triggered by noxious stimuli, such as pain, noise, or even bumping of the bed. An indicator of corticospinal damage, Babinski's reflex may occur unilaterally or bilaterally. It may also be temporary or permanent. A temporary Babinski's reflex commonly occurs during the postictal phase of a seizure, whereas a permanent Babinski's reflex occurs with corticospinal damage. A positive Babinski's reflex is normal in neonates and in infants less than 12 months old.

History and physical examination
After eliciting a positive Babinski's reflex, evaluate the patient for other neurologic signs. Evaluate muscle strength in each extremity by having the patient push or pull against your resistance. Passively flex and extend the extremity to assess muscle tone.

Intermittent resistance to flexion and extension indicates spasticity, and a lack of resistance indicates flaccidity. Next, check for evidence of incoordination by asking the patient to perform a repetitive activity.

Test deep tendon reflexes in the patient's elbow, antecubital area, wrist, knee, and ankle by striking the tendon with a reflex hammer. An exaggerated muscle response indicates hyperactive deep tendon reflexes; little or no muscle response indicates hypoactivity. Then evaluate pain sensation and proprioception in the feet. As you move the patient's toes up and down, ask the patient to identify the direction in which the toes have been moved without looking at his feet.

Common medical causes
● *Amyotrophic lateral sclerosis (ALS).* In this progressive motor neuron disorder, bilateral Babinski's reflex may occur with hyperactive deep tendon reflexes and spasticity. Typically, ALS produces fasciculations accompanied by muscle atrophy and weakness. Incoordination makes carrying out activities of daily living difficult for the patient. Associated signs and symptoms include impaired speech; difficulty chewing, swallowing, and breathing; urinary frequency and urgency; and, occasionally, choking and excessive drooling. Although his mental status remains intact, the patient's poor prognosis may cause periodic depression. Progressive bulbar palsy involves the brain stem and may cause episodes of crying or inappropriate laughter.
● *Brain tumor.* When it involves the corticospinal tract, a brain tumor may produce Babinski's reflex. The reflex may be accompanied by hyperactive deep tendon reflexes (unilateral or bilateral), spasticity, seizures, cranial nerve dysfunction, hemiparesis or hemiplegia, de-

HOW TO ELICIT BABINSKI'S REFLEX

To elicit Babinski's reflex, stroke the lateral aspect of the sole of the patient's foot with your thumbnail or another moderately sharp object. Normally, this elicits flexion of all toes (a negative Babinski's reflex), as shown at left. In a positive Babinski's reflex, the great toe dorsiflexes and the other toes fan out, as shown at right.

NEGATIVE BABINSKI'S REFLEX

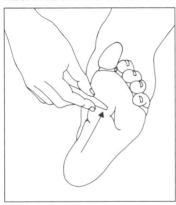

POSITIVE BABINSKI'S REFLEX

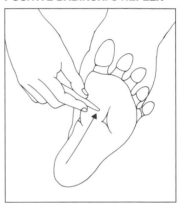

creased pain sensation, unsteady gait, incoordination, headache, emotional lability, and decreased level of consciousness (LOC).

● *Cerebrovascular accident (CVA).* Babinski's reflex varies with the site of the CVA. If the CVA involves the cerebrum, it produces unilateral Babinski's reflex, commonly accompanied by hemiplegia or hemiparesis, unilateral hyperactive deep tendon reflexes, hemianopia, and aphasia. If it involves the brain stem, it produces bilateral Babinski's reflex accompanied by bilateral weakness or paralysis, bilateral hyperactive deep tendon reflexes, cranial nerve dysfunction, incoordination, and unsteady gait. Generalized signs and symptoms of CVA may include headache, vomiting, fever,

disorientation, nuchal rigidity, seizures, and coma.

● *Head trauma.* Unilateral or bilateral Babinski's reflex may occur as the result of primary corticospinal damage or secondary injury associated with increased intracranial pressure. Hyperactive deep tendon reflexes and spasticity commonly occur with Babinski's reflex. The patient may also have weakness and incoordination. Other signs and symptoms vary with the type of head trauma and may include headache, vomiting, behavior changes, altered vital signs, and decreased LOC with abnormal pupillary size and response to light.

● *Hepatic encephalopathy.* Babinski's reflex occurs late in this disorder when the patient slips into a coma. It's accompanied by hyperactive reflexes and fetor hepaticus.

• *Rabies.* Bilateral Babinski's reflex— possibly elicited by nonspecific noxious stimuli alone—appears in the excitation phase of rabies. This phase occurs 2 to 10 days after the onset of prodromal symptoms, such as fever, malaise, and irritability. (These symptoms occur 30 to 40 days after an animal bite.) It's characterized by marked restlessness and extremely painful pharyngeal muscle spasms. Difficulty swallowing causes excessive drooling and hydrophobia in about 50% of affected patients. Seizures and hyperactive deep tendon reflexes may also occur.

• *Spinal cord injury.* In acute injury, spinal shock temporarily erases all reflexes. As shock resolves, Babinski's reflex occurs—unilaterally when injury affects only one side of the spinal cord (Brown-Séquard's syndrome), bilaterally when injury affects both sides. Rather than signaling the return of neurologic function, this reflex confirms corticospinal damage. It's accompanied by hyperactive deep tendon reflexes, spasticity, and variable or total loss of pain and temperature sensation, proprioception, and motor function. Horner's syndrome, marked by unilateral ptosis, pupillary constriction, and facial anhidrosis, may occur with lower cervical cord injury.

• *Spinal cord tumor.* Unilateral or bilateral Babinski's reflex occurs with variable loss of pain and temperature sensation, proprioception, and motor function. Spasticity, hyperactive deep tendon reflexes, absent abdominal reflexes, and incontinence are also characteristic. Diffuse pain may occur at the level of the tumor.

• *Spinal paralytic poliomyelitis.* Unilateral or bilateral Babinski's reflex occurs 5 to 7 days after the onset of fever in this disorder. It's accompanied by progressive weakness, paresthesia, muscle tenderness, spasticity, irritability and, later,

atrophy. Resistance to neck flexion is characteristic, as are Hoyne's, Kernig's, and Brudzinski's signs.

• *Syringomyelia.* In this disorder, bilateral Babinski's reflex occurs with muscle atrophy and weakness that may progress to paralysis. It's accompanied by spasticity, ataxia and, occasionally, deep pain. Deep tendon reflexes may be hypoactive or hyperactive. Cranial nerve dysfunction, such as dysphagia and dysarthria, commonly appears late in the disorder.

Special considerations

Babinski's reflex usually occurs with incoordination, weakness, and spasticity, all of which increase the patient's risk of injury. To prevent injury, assist the patient with activity and keep his environment free from obstructions.

Procedures that may be required include a computed tomography scan of the brain or spine, an angiogram or myelogram, or possibly a lumbar puncture to clarify or confirm the cause of Babinski's reflex. Prepare the patient, as necessary.

Pediatric pointers

Babinski's reflex occurs normally in children under age 2 and reflects immaturity of the corticospinal tract. After age 2, Babinski's reflex is pathologic and may result from hydrocephalus or any of the causes more commonly seen in adults.

BACK PAIN

Back pain affects an estimated 80% of the population; in fact, it's second only to the common cold for lost time from work. Although this symptom may herald a spondylogenic disorder, it may also result from genitourinary, GI, cardiovascular, or neoplastic disorders. Postural imbalance associated with pregnancy may also cause back pain.

The onset, location, and distribution of pain and its response to activity and rest provide important clues about the causative disorder. Pain may be acute or chronic, constant or intermittent. It may remain localized in the back or radiate along the spine or down one or both legs. Pain may be exacerbated by activity— most commonly, bending, stooping, or lifting—and alleviated by rest, or it may be unaffected by both.

Intrinsic back pain results from muscle spasm, nerve root irritation, fracture, or a combination of these mechanisms. It most commonly occurs in the lower back, or lumbosacral area. Back pain may also be referred from the abdomen or flank, possibly signaling life-threatening perforated ulcer, acute pancreatitis, or dissecting abdominal aortic aneurysm.

Emergency interventions

 If the patient reports *acute, severe back pain,* quickly take his vital signs; then perform a rapid evaluation to rule out life-threatening causes. Ask him when the pain began. Can he relate it to any causes? For example, did the pain occur after eating? After falling on the ice? Have the patient describe the pain. Is it burning, stabbing, throbbing, or aching? Is it constant or intermittent? Does it radiate to the buttocks or legs? Is there any leg weakness? Or does the pain seem to originate in the abdomen and radiate to the back? What makes it better or worse? Is it affected by activity or rest? Is it worse in the morning or evening? Typically, visceral-referred back pain is unaffected by activity and rest. In contrast, pain of spondylogenic origin worsens with activity and improves with rest. Pain of neoplastic origin is commonly relieved by walking and worsens at night.

If the patient describes *deep lumbar pain unaffected by activity,* palpate for a pulsating epigastric mass. If this sign is present, suspect dissecting abdominal aortic aneurysm. Withhold food and fluid in anticipation of emergency surgery. Prepare for I.V. fluid replacement and oxygen administration.

If the patient describes *severe epigastric pain that radiates through the abdomen to the back,* assess for absent bowel sounds and for abdominal rigidity and tenderness. If these occur, suspect perforated ulcer or acute pancreatitis. Start an I.V. line for fluids and drugs, administer oxygen, and insert a nasogastric tube.

History and physical examination

If life-threatening causes of back pain are ruled out, continue with a more complete history and physical examination. Be aware of the patient's expressions of pain as you do so. Obtain a medical history, including past injuries and illnesses, and a family history. Ask about diet and alcohol intake. Also take a drug history, including past and present prescriptions and over-the-counter drugs.

Next, perform a thorough physical examination. Observe skin color, especially in the patient's legs, and palpate skin temperature. Palpate femoral, popliteal, posterior tibial, and pedal pulses. Ask about unusual sensations in the legs, such as numbness and tingling. Observe the patient's posture if pain doesn't prohibit standing. Does he stand erect or tend to lean toward one side? Observe the level of the shoulders and pelvis and the curvature of the back. Ask the patient to bend forward, backward, and from side to side while you palpate for paravertebral spasms. Note rotation of the spine on the trunk. Palpate the back for tenderness. Then ask the patient to walk first on his heels, then on his toes. Protect him from falling as he does so. Weakness may reflect a muscular disorder or spinal nerve root irritation. Place the patient in a sitting position to evaluate and compare patellar tendon (knee), Achilles tendon, and Babinski's reflex. Evaluate the strength of the extensor hallucis longus by asking the patient to hold up his big toe against resistance. Measure leg length and hamstring and quadriceps muscles bilaterally. Note a difference of more than ³/₈″ (1 cm) in muscle size, especially in the calf.

To reproduce leg and back pain, position the patient supine on the examining table. Grasp his heel and slowly lift his leg. If he feels pain, note its exact location and the angle between the table and his leg when it occurs. Repeat this maneuver with the opposite leg. Pain along the sciatic nerve may indicate disk herniation or sciatica. Also note range of motion of the hip and knee.

Common medical causes

• *Abdominal aortic aneurysm (dissecting).* Life-threatening dissection of this aneurysm may initially cause low back pain or dull abdominal pain. Usually, it produces constant upper abdominal pain. A pulsating abdominal mass may be palpated in the epigastrium; after rupture, though, it no longer pulses. Aneurysmal dissection can also cause mottled skin below the waist, absent femoral and pedal pulses, lower blood pressure in the legs than in the arms, mild to moderate tenderness with guarding, and abdominal rigidity. Signs of shock, such as cool, clammy skin, will appear if blood loss is significant.

• *Ankylosing spondylitis.* This chronic, progressive disorder causes sacroiliac pain, which radiates up the spine and is aggravated by lateral pressure on the pelvis. The pain is usually most severe in the morning or after a period of inactivity and isn't relieved by rest. Abnormal rigidity of the lumbar spine with forward flexion is also characteristic. This disorder can also cause local tenderness, fatigue, fever, anorexia, weight loss, and occasional iritis.

• *Appendicitis.* In this life-threatening disorder, a vague and dull discomfort in the epigastric or umbilical region migrates to McBurney's point in the right lower quadrant. In retrocecal appendicitis, pain may also radiate to the back. The shift in pain is preceded by anorexia and nausea. It's accompanied by fever, occasional vomiting, abdominal tenderness (especially over McBurney's point), and rebound tenderness. Some patients also have painful, urgent urination.

• *Cholecystitis.* This disorder produces severe pain in the right upper quadrant that may radiate to the right shoulder, chest, or back. The pain may arise suddenly or may increase gradually over several hours. Accompanying signs and symptoms include anorexia, fever, nausea, vomiting, right upper quadrant tenderness, abdominal rigidity, pallor, and diaphoresis.

• *Chordoma.* A slow-developing malignant tumor, chordoma causes persistent pain in the lower back, sacrum, and coccyx. As the tumor expands, pain may be accompanied by constipation and bowel and bladder incontinence.

• *Endometriosis.* This disorder causes deep sacral pain and severe, cramping pain in the lower abdomen. The pain worsens just before or during menstruation and may be aggravated by defecation. It's accompanied by constipation, abdominal tenderness, dysmenorrhea, and dyspareunia.

• *Intervertebral disk rupture.* This disorder produces gradual or sudden low back pain with or without leg pain (sciatica). In rare cases, it produces leg pain alone. Usually, pain begins in the back and radiates to the buttocks and leg. The pain is exacerbated by activity, coughing, and sneezing and is eased by rest. It's accompanied by paresthesia (usually numbness or tingling in the lower leg and foot), paravertebral muscle spasm, and decreased reflexes on the affected side. This disorder also affects posture and gait. The patient's spine is slightly flexed and he leans toward the painful side. He walks slowly and rises from a sitting to standing position with extreme difficulty.

• *Lumbosacral sprain.* This disorder causes aching, localized pain and tenderness associated with muscle spasm on lateral motion. The recumbent patient will typically flex his knees and hips to help ease pain. Flexion of the spine intensifies pain, whereas rest helps relieve it.

• *Metastatic tumors.* These tumors commonly spread to the spine, causing low back pain in at least 25% of patients. Typically, the pain begins abruptly, is accompanied by cramping muscular pain, and isn't relieved by rest.

• *Myeloma.* Back pain caused by this primary malignant tumor commonly begins abruptly and worsens with exercise. It may be accompanied by arthritic symptoms, such as achy joints, joint swelling, and tenderness. Other clinical effects include fever, malaise, peripheral paresthesia, and weight loss.

• *Pancreatitis (acute).* This life-threatening disorder usually produces fulminating, continuous upper abdominal pain that may radiate to both flanks and to the back. To relieve this pain, the patient may bend forward, draw his knees to his chest, or move restlessly about.

Early associated signs and symptoms include abdominal tenderness, nausea, vomiting, fever, pallor, tachycardia and, in some patients, abdominal guarding, rigidity, rebound tenderness, and hypoactive bowel sounds. A late sign may be jaundice. Occurring as inflammation subsides, Grey Turner's sign or Cullen's sign signals hemorrhagic pancreatitis.

• *Perforated ulcer.* In some patients, perforation of a duodenal or gastric ulcer causes sudden, prostrating epigastric pain that may radiate throughout the abdomen and to the back. This life-threatening disorder also causes boardlike abdominal rigidity, tenderness with guarding, generalized rebound tenderness, the absence of bowel sounds, and grunting, shallow respiration. Associated signs commonly include fever, tachycardia, and hypotension.

• *Prostatic carcinoma.* Chronic, aching back pain may be the only symptom of prostatic carcinoma. This disorder may also produce hematuria.

• *Pyelonephritis (acute).* This disorder produces progressive flank and lower abdominal pain accompanied by back pain or tenderness (especially over the costovertebral angle). Pyelonephritis may also produce high fever and chills, nausea and vomiting, flank and abdominal tenderness, and urinary frequency and urgency.

• *Renal calculi.* The colicky pain of this disorder usually results from irritation of the ureteral lining, and increases the frequency and force of peristaltic contractions. The pain travels from the costovertebral angle to the flank, suprapubic region, and external genitalia. Its intensity varies but may become excruciating if calculi travel down a ureter. If calculi are in the renal pelvis and calyces, dull and constant flank pain may occur. Renal calculi also cause nausea, vomiting, urinary urgency (if a calculus lodges near the bladder), hematuria, and agitation due to pain.

• *Spinal neoplasm (benign).* Typically, this disorder causes severe, localized back pain and scoliosis.

• *Spinal stenosis.* Resembling a ruptured intervertebral disk, this disorder produces back pain with or without sciatica. Sciatica commonly affects both legs and is accompanied by claudication. The pain may progress to numbness or weakness unless the patient rests for relief.

• *Spondylolisthesis.* A major structural disorder characterized by forward slippage of one vertebra onto another, spondylolisthesis may be asymptomatic or cause low back pain with or without nerve root involvement. Associated symptoms of nerve root involvement include paresthesias, buttock pain, and pain radiating down the leg. Palpation of the lumbar spine may reveal a "step-off" of the spinous process. Flexion of the spine may be limited.

- **Transverse process fracture.** This fracture causes severe localized back pain with muscle spasm and hematoma.
- **Vertebral compression fracture.** Initially, this fracture may be painless. Several weeks later, it causes back pain aggravated by weight bearing and local tenderness. Fracture of a thoracic vertebra may cause referred pain in the lumbar area.
- **Vertebral osteomyelitis.** Initially, this disorder causes insidious back pain. As it progresses, the pain may become constant, more pronounced at night, and aggravated by spinal movement. Accompanying symptoms include vertebral and hamstring spasms, tenderness of the spinous processes, fever, and malaise.
- **Vertebral osteoporosis.** This disorder causes chronic, aching back pain that is aggravated by activity and somewhat relieved by rest. Tenderness may also occur.

Other causes

- **Neurologic tests.** Lumbar puncture and myelography can produce transient back pain.

Special considerations

If back pain suggests a life-threatening cause, monitor the patient closely. Be alert for increasing pain, altered neurovascular status in the legs, loss of bowel or bladder control, altered vital signs, diaphoresis, and cyanosis.

Until a tentative diagnosis is made, withhold analgesics, which may mask symptoms. In addition, withhold food and fluids in case surgery is necessary. Make the patient as comfortable as possible by elevating the head of the bed and placing a pillow under the patient's knees. Encourage relaxation techniques such as deep breathing. Prepare the patient for a rectal or pelvic examination. The patient also may require routine blood tests; urinalysis; X-rays of the chest, abdomen, and spine; computed tomography scan; and appropriate biopsies.

If the patient has chronic back pain, reinforce instructions regarding bed rest, analgesics, anti-inflammatory drugs, and exercise. Also suggest that the patient take daily warm baths to help relieve pain. Help the patient to recognize and make necessary lifestyle changes; for example, advise him to lose weight or correct poor posture.

Fit the patient for a corset or lumbosacral support. Instruct the patient not to wear this in bed. The patient may require heat or cold therapy, a backboard, a convoluted foam mattress, or pelvic traction. Explain these pain-relief measures to the patient. Teach the patient about alternatives to analgesic drugs, such as biofeedback and transcutaneous electrical nerve stimulation.

Be aware that back pain is notoriously associated with malingering. Refer the patient to other professionals, such as a physical therapist, occupational therapist, or psychologist, when indicated.

Pediatric pointers

Because a child may have difficulty describing back pain, be alert for nonverbal clues, such as wincing or refusal to walk. Closely observe family dynamics during history taking for clues suggesting child abuse.

Back pain in the child may stem from intervertebral disk inflammation (diskitis), neoplasms, idiopathic juvenile osteoporosis, and spondylolisthesis. Disk herniation typically doesn't cause back pain. Scoliosis, a common disorder in adolescents, also rarely causes back pain.

BATTLE'S SIGN

Battle's sign—ecchymosis over the mastoid process of the temporal bone—is commonly the only outward sign of basilar skull fracture. In fact, this type of fracture may go undetected by skull X-rays. If left untreated, it can be fatal because of associated injury to the nearby cranial nerves and brain stem as well as to blood vessels and the meninges.

Appearing behind one or both ears, Battle's sign is easily overlooked or even hidden by the patient's hair. Also, during emergency care of the trauma victim, it may be overshadowed by imminently life-threatening or more apparent injuries.

Force exerted on the head great enough to fracture the base of the skull causes Battle's sign by damaging supporting tissues of the mastoid area. Or the sign may result from seepage of blood from the fracture site to the mastoid. Battle's sign usually develops 24 to 36 hours after the fracture and may persist for several days to weeks.

History and physical examination

Perform a complete neurologic examination. Begin with the history. Ask the patient about recent trauma to the head. Did the patient sustain a severe blow to the head? Was he involved in a motor vehicle accident? Note level of consciousness as the patient responds. Does the patient respond quickly or slowly? Are his answers appropriate or does he appear confused?

Check the patient's vital signs; be alert for widening pulse pressure and bradycardia, signs of increased intracranial pressure. Assess cranial nerve function in nerves II, III, IV, VI, VII, and VIII. Evaluate pupillary size and response to light as well as motor and verbal responses. Relate this data to the Glasgow Coma Scale. Also note cerebrospinal fluid (CSF) leakage from the nose or ears. Ask about postnasal drip, which may reflect CSF drainage down the throat. Also look for the halo sign—a bloodstain encircled by a yellowish ring—on bed linens or dressings. To confirm that drainage is CSF, test it with glucose reagent strips; CSF is positive for glucose, whereas mucus is not. Follow up the neurologic examination with a complete physical examination to detect other injuries associated with basilar skull fracture.

Common medical causes

• **Basilar skull fracture.** Battle's sign may be the only outward sign of this fracture. Or it may be accompanied by periorbital ecchymosis (raccoon eyes), conjunctival hemorrhage, nystagmus, ocular deviation, epistaxis, anosmia, a bulging tympanic membrane (from CSF or blood accumulation), visible fracture lines on the external auditory canal, tinnitus, hearing difficulty, facial paralysis, and vertigo.

Special considerations

Expect the patient with basilar skull fracture to be on bed rest for several days to weeks. Keep him flat to decrease pressure on dural tears and minimize CSF leakage. Monitor neurologic status closely. Avoid nasogastric intubation and nasopharyngeal suction, which may cause cerebral infection. Also caution the patient against blowing his nose, which may worsen a dural tear.

The patient may need skull X-rays and a computed tomography scan to help confirm basilar skull fracture and to evaluate the severity of head injury. Typically, basilar skull fracture and any associated dural tears heal spontaneously within several days to weeks. However, if the patient has a large dural tear, a craniotomy may be necessary to repair the tear with a graft patch.

Pediatric pointers

Many children who are victims of abuse sustain basilar skull fractures from severe blows to the head. As in adults, Battle's sign may be the only outward sign of fracture and, perhaps, the only clue to child abuse. If you suspect child abuse, follow hospital protocol for reporting the incident.

BIOT'S RESPIRATIONS
[Ataxic respirations]

A late and ominous sign of neurologic deterioration, Biot's respirations are characterized by irregular and unpredictable periods of apnea alternating with periods in which four or five breaths of identical depth are taken. (See *Identifying Biot's respirations*.) This rare breathing pattern may appear abruptly and reflect increased pressure on the medulla coinciding with brain stem compression.

Emergency interventions

 Observe the patient's breathing pattern for several minutes to avoid confusing Biot's respirations with other respiratory patterns. Prepare to intubate the patient and provide mechanical ventilation. Next, take vital signs, noting especially increased systolic pressure.

Common medical causes

● ***Brain stem compression.*** Biot's respirations are characteristic in this neurologic emergency. Rapidly enlarging lesions may cause ataxic respirations but commonly lead to complete respiratory arrest.

Special considerations

Monitor vital signs frequently. Elevate the head of the patient's bed 30 degrees to help reduce intracranial pressure.

Prepare the patient for emergency surgery to relieve pressure on the brain stem. Computed tomography scans or magnetic resonance imaging may confirm the cause of brain stem compression.

Because Biot's respirations typically reflect a grave prognosis for the patient, give the patient's family information and emotional support.

Pediatric pointers

Biot's respirations are rarely seen in children.

IDENTIFYING BIOT'S RESPIRATIONS

Biot's respirations, also known as ataxic respirations, have an irregular pattern. Deep breaths alternate with abrupt periods of apnea. Both shallow and deep breaths occur randomly. There are haphazard, irregular pauses. The respiratory rate tends to be slow and may progressively decelerate to apnea.

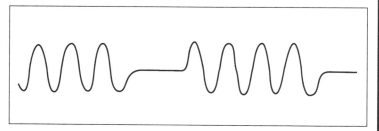

BLADDER DISTENTION: COMMON CAUSES AND ASSOCIATED FINDINGS

CAUSES	**MAJOR ASSOCIATED SIGNS AND SYMPTOMS**											
	Ataxia	Constipation	Dysuria	Fatigue	Fever	Hematuria	Muscle weakness	Myalgia	Nausea	Nocturia	Pain, buttock and sacral	Pain, flank
Benign prostatic hyperplasia		•				•				•		
Bladder calculi			•			•						
Bladder neoplasms			•			•	•			•	•	•
Multiple sclerosis	•						•					
Prostatic neoplasms		•	•	•						•		
Prostatitis (acute)			•	•	•	•		•	•			
Prostatitis (chronic)			•			•						
Urethral calculi											•	
Urethral strictures			•									

BLADDER DISTENTION

Bladder distention—the abnormal enlargement of the bladder—results from an inability to excrete urine, causing its accumulation. Distention can result from mechanical and anatomic obstructions, neuromuscular disorders, and drugs. Relatively common in all ages and both sexes, it usually occurs in older men with prostate disorders, leading to urine retention.

Distention usually develops gradually but occasionally appears suddenly. Gradual distention usually remains asymptomatic until stretching of the bladder produces discomfort. Acute distention produces suprapubic fullness, pressure, and pain. If severe distention isn't corrected promptly by catheterization or massage, the bladder rises within the abdomen, its walls become thin, and renal function can be impaired.

Bladder distention is aggravated by intake of caffeine, alcohol, large quantities of fluid, and diuretics.

Emergency interventions

 If the patient has *severe distention,* insert an indwelling urinary catheter to help relieve discomfort and prevent bladder rupture.

Pain, lower back	Pain, pelvic	Pain, penile	Pain, perineal	Pain, vulvar	Prostatic enlargement	Prostatic rigidity	Pyuria	Suprapubic fullness	Urethral discharge	Urinary frequency	Urinary stream changes	Urinary urgency	Vomiting
			●		●			●		●	●		
		●	●							●		●	
●								●		●		●	●
			●			●				●			
			●		●			●		●	●	●	●
	●	●	●		●		●	●	●	●	●		
		●	●	●				●					
							●		●	●	●	●	

History and physical examination

If distention isn't severe, begin by reviewing the patient's voiding patterns. Find out the time and amount of his last voiding and the amount of fluid consumed since then. Ask if he has difficulty urinating. Does he use Valsalva's or Credé's maneuver to initiate it? Also ask if urination occurs with urgency or without warning and if it's painful or irritating. Ask about force and continuity of the urine stream and if he feels that his bladder is empty after voiding.

Explore the patient's history for urinary tract obstruction or infections; venereal disease; neurologic, intestinal, or pelvic surgery; lower abdominal or urinary tract trauma; and systemic or neurologic disorders. Note drug history, including use of over-the-counter preparations.

Take the patient's vital signs, and percuss and palpate the bladder. (Remember that if the bladder is empty, it can't be palpated through the abdominal wall.) Inspect the urethral meatus and measure its diameter, and describe the appearance and amount of any discharge. Finally, test for perineal sensation and anal sphincter tone, and in the male patient examine the prostate gland.

Common medical causes

● *Benign prostatic hyperplasia.* In this disorder, bladder distention gradually develops as the prostate enlarges. Occasionally, its onset is acute. Initially, the patient experiences urinary hesitancy, straining, frequency, reduced force of his urinary stream, nocturia, and postvoiding dribbling. As the disorder progresses, it produces prostatic enlargement, sensations of suprapubic fullness and incomplete bladder emptying, perineal pain, constipation, and hematuria.

• *Bladder calculi.* This disorder may produce bladder distention but more commonly produces pain as its only symptom. The pain is usually referred to the tip of the penis or the vulvar area. It worsens during walking or exercise and abates when the patient lies down. It can be accompanied by urinary frequency and urgency, hematuria, and dysuria.

• *Bladder neoplasms.* By blocking the urethral orifice, neoplasms can cause bladder distention. Associated signs and symptoms include hematuria (most common), urinary frequency and urgency, nocturia, dysuria, pyuria, vomiting, diarrhea, sleeplessness, and pain in the bladder, rectum, pelvis, flank, back, or legs.

• *Multiple sclerosis.* In this neuromuscular disorder, urine retention and bladder distention result from interruption of upper motor neuron control of the bladder. Associated signs and symptoms include optic neuritis, paresthesias, impaired position and vibratory senses, diplopia, nystagmus, dizziness, abnormal reflexes, dysarthria, muscle weakness, emotional lability, Lhermitte's sign (transient, electric-like shocks that spread down the body when the head is flexed), and ataxia.

• *Prostatic neoplasms.* This disorder eventually causes bladder distention in approximately 25% of patients. The usual clinical features include dysuria, urinary frequency and urgency, nocturia, weight loss, fatigue, perineal pain, constipation, and a rigid, irregular prostate. Some patients exhibit urine retention and bladder distention as their only signs.

• *Prostatitis.* In *acute prostatitis,* bladder distention occurs rapidly along with perineal discomfort and suprapubic fullness. Other signs and symptoms include perineal pain, enlarged prostate, decreased libido, impotence, decreased force of the urine stream, dysuria, hematuria, and urinary frequency and urgency. Other findings include fatigue, malaise, myalgia, fever, chills, nausea, and vomiting.

In *chronic prostatitis,* bladder distention is rare. However, it may be accompanied by sensations of perineal discomfort and suprapubic fullness, prostatic tenderness, decreased libido, urinary frequency and urgency, dysuria, pyuria, hematuria, persistent urethral discharge, and dull pain radiating to the lower back, buttocks, penis, or perineum.

• *Urethral calculi.* In this disorder, urethral obstruction leads to bladder distention. This obstruction causes pain radiating to the penis or vulva and referred to the perineum or rectum. It may also produce a palpable stone and urethral discharge.

• *Urethral stricture.* This disorder results in urine retention and bladder distention with chronic urethral discharge (most common symptom), urinary frequency (also common), dysuria, urgency, decreased force and diameter of the urine stream, and pyuria.

Other causes

• *Drugs.* Parasympatholytics and anticholinergics, ganglionic blockers, sedatives, anesthetics, and opiates can produce urine retention and bladder distention.

• *Catheterization.* Using an indwelling urinary catheter can result in urine retention and bladder distention. While the catheter is in place, inadequate drainage due to kinked tubing or an occluded lumen may lead to urine retention.

In addition, a misplaced urinary catheter or irritation from catheter removal may cause edema, thereby blocking urine outflow.

Special considerations

Monitor the patient's vital signs and the extent of bladder distention. Encourage the patient to change positions to alleviate discomfort. He may require analgesics.

If he doesn't require immediate urinary catheterization, provide privacy and suggest that he assume the normal voiding position. Teach him to perform Valsalva's maneuver, or gently perform Credé's maneuver. You can also stroke or intermittently apply ice to the inner thigh or help him relax in a warm tub or sitz bath. Use the power of suggestion to stimulate voiding. For example, run water in the sink, pour warm water over his perineum, place his hands in warm water, or play tapes of aquatic sounds.

Prepare the patient for diagnostic tests (such as endoscopy and radiologic studies) to determine the cause of bladder distention. Or prepare him for surgery if interventions fail to relieve bladder distention and obstruction prevents catheterization.

Pediatric pointers

Look for urine retention and bladder distention in any infant who fails to void normal amounts. (In the first 48 hours of life, an infant excretes about 60 ml of urine; during the next week, he excretes about 300 ml of urine daily.) In males, posterior urethral valves, meatal stenosis, phimosis, spinal cord anomalies, bladder diverticuli, and other congenital defects may cause a urinary tract obstruction and resultant bladder distention.

BLOOD PRESSURE DECREASE

[Hypotension]

Low blood pressure refers to inadequate blood pressure to perfuse or oxygenate the body's tissues. Although commonly linked to shock, this sign may also result from cardiovascular, respiratory, neurologic, and metabolic disorders. Low blood pressure may be drug-induced or may accompany diagnostic tests—usually, those using contrast media. It may stem from stress or change of position—specifically, rising abruptly from a supine or sitting position to a standing position (postural hypotension).

Normal blood pressure varies considerably; what may qualify as low blood pressure for one person may be perfectly normal for another. Consequently, every blood pressure reading must be compared against the patient's baseline. Typically, a reading below 90/60 mm Hg or a drop of 30 mm Hg from the baseline is considered low blood pressure. (See *Ensuring accurate blood pressure measurement,* page 70.)

Low blood pressure can reflect an expanded intravascular space (as in vasodilatation), reduced intravascular volume (as in dehydration and hemorrhage), or decreased cardiac output (as in impaired cardiac muscle contractility). However, because the body's pressure-regulating mechanisms are complex and interrelated, a combination of these factors usually contributes to low blood pressure.

Emergency interventions

 If the patient's systolic pressure is less than 80 mm Hg, or 30 mm Hg below his baseline, suspect shock immediately. To confirm shock, quickly evaluate for decreased level of consciousness. Check apical pulse for tachycardia and respirations for tachypnea. Also inspect for cool, clammy skin. Elevate the patient's legs above the level of his heart. Then start an I.V. line to replace fluids and blood or to administer drugs. Prepare to administer oxygen with mechanical ventilation, if necessary.

EXAMINATION TIP

 # ENSURING ACCURATE BLOOD PRESSURE MEASUREMENT

When taking your patient's blood pressure, begin by applying the cuff properly, as shown here.

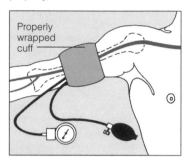

Properly wrapped cuff

Then, be alert for these common pitfalls to avoid recording an inaccurate blood pressure measurement.

• *Wrong-sized cuff.* Confirm that the cuff size is appropriate for the patient. This ensures that adequate pressure is applied to compress the brachial artery during cuff inflation. If the cuff bladder is too narrow, the reading will be falsely high. If it's too wide, the reading will be falsely low. The cuff bladder width should be about 40% of the circumference of the midpoint of the limb; bladder length should be twice the width. If the arm circumference is less than 33 cm, select a regular-sized cuff; if it's between 33 and 41 cm, a large-sized cuff; if it's more than 41 cm, a thigh cuff. Pediatric cuffs are also available.

• *Slow cuff deflation, causing venous congestion in the extremity.* Don't deflate the cuff slower than 2 mm Hg/heartbeat or you'll get a spuriously high reading.

• *Cuff wrapped too loosely, reducing its effective width.* Tighten the cuff to avoid a falsely elevated reading.

• *Mercury column not read at eye level.* Read the mercury column at eye level. If the column is below eye level, you may record a falsely low reading; if it's above eye level, a falsely high reading.

• *Tilted mercury column.* Keep the mercury column vertical to avoid a falsely high reading.

• *Poorly timed measurement.* Don't measure blood pressure if the patient appears anxious or has just eaten or ambulated; you'll get a falsely high reading.

• *Incorrect position of the arm.* Keep the patient's arm level with his heart to avoid a falsely low reading.

• *Cuff overinflation, causing venospasm or pain.* Don't overinflate the cuff or you'll get a falsely high reading.

• *Failure to notice an auscultatory gap.* Sound fades out for 10 to 15 mm Hg, then returns). To avoid missing the top Korotkoff sound, estimate systolic pressure by palpation first. Then inflate the cuff rapidly—at a rate of 2 to 3 mm Hg/second—to about 30 mm Hg above the palpable systolic pressure.

• *Inaudibility of feeble sounds.* Before reinflating the cuff, have the patient raise his arm to reduce venous pressure and amplify low-volume sounds. After inflating the cuff, lower the patient's arm. Then deflate the cuff and listen. Or, with the patient's arm positioned at heart level, inflate the cuff and have the patient make a fist. Have him rapidly open and close his hand 10 times before you begin to deflate the cuff. Then listen. Be sure to document that the blood pressure reading was augmented.

Monitor the patient's intake and output; insert an indwelling urinary catheter for accurate measurement of urine output. Also insert a central venous line or a pulmonary artery catheter to evaluate fluid status. Prepare for cardiac monitoring to evaluate cardiac rhythm. Be ready to insert a nasogastric tube to prevent aspiration in the comatose patient. Throughout emergency interventions, keep the patient's spinal column immobile until spinal cord trauma is ruled out.

History and physical examination

If the patient is conscious, ask him about associated symptoms. For example, does he feel unusually weak or fatigued? Is his vision blurred? Is his gait unsteady? Does he have chest or abdominal pain or difficulty breathing? Has he had episodes of dizziness or fainting? Do these episodes occur when he stands up suddenly? If so, take blood pressure with the patient lying down, sitting, and then standing; compare readings. A drop in systolic or diastolic pressure of 10 to 20 mm Hg or more between position changes suggests postural hypotension.

Next, continue with a physical examination. Inspect the skin for pallor, diaphoresis, and clamminess. Palpate peripheral pulses. Note paradoxical pulse—an accentuated fall in systolic pressure during inspiration—which suggests pericardial tamponade. Then auscultate for abnormal heart sounds (gallops, murmurs), rates (bradycardia, tachycardia), or rhythms. Auscultate the lungs for abnormal breath sounds (diminished sounds, crackles, wheezing), rates (bradypnea, tachypnea), or rhythms (agonal respirations, Cheyne-Stokes respirations). Look for signs and symptoms of hemorrhage, including visible bleeding and palpable masses, bruising, and tenderness. Assess for abdominal rigidity and rebound tenderness; auscultate for abnormal bowel sounds.

Common medical causes

• *Acute adrenal insufficiency.* Postural hypotension is characteristic in this disorder. Accompanying it are fatigue, weakness, nausea, vomiting, abdominal discomfort, weight loss, fever, and tachycardia. Hyperpigmentation of fingers, nails, nipples, scars, and body folds; pale, cool, clammy skin; restlessness; decreased urine output; tachypnea; and coma may also occur.

• *Anaphylactic shock.* Following exposure to an allergen, such as penicillin or insect venom, a dramatic fall in blood pressure and narrowed pulse pressure signal this severe allergic reaction. Initially, anaphylactic shock causes anxiety, restlessness, a feeling of doom, intense itching (especially of the hands and feet), and a pounding headache. Later, it may also produce coughing, difficulty breathing, nausea, abdominal cramps, involuntary defecation, seizures, flushing, change or loss of voice due to laryngeal edema, urinary incontinence, and tachycardia.

• *Cardiac arrhythmias.* In arrhythmias, blood pressure may fluctuate between normal and low readings. Dizziness, light-headedness, weakness, fatigue, and palpitations may also occur. Auscultation typically reveals a pulse rate greater than 100 beats/minute or less than 60 beats/minute, or an irregular rhythm.

• *Cardiac tamponade.* An accentuated fall in systolic pressure (greater than 10 mm Hg) during inspiration, known as pulsus paradoxus, is characteristic in cardiac tamponade. This disorder also causes cyanosis, tachycardia, neck vein distention, muffled heart sounds, dyspnea, and Kussmaul's respirations.

• *Cardiogenic shock.* In this disorder, systolic pressure falls to less than 80 mm Hg, or 30 mm Hg less than the patient's baseline. Accompanying low blood pressure are narrowed pulse pressure, diminished Korotkoff sounds, peripheral cyanosis, and pale, cool, clammy skin. Cardiogenic shock also causes restlessness and anxiety, which may progress to disorientation and confusion. Associated signs and symptoms include anginal pain, dyspnea, neck vein distention, oliguria, ventricular gallop, tachypnea, and weak, rapid pulse.

• *Diabetic ketoacidosis.* Hypovolemia triggered by osmotic diuresis in hyperglycemia is responsible for low blood pressure in this disorder. It also commonly produces polydipsia, polyuria, polyphagia, dehydration, weight loss, abdominal pain, nausea, vomiting, Kussmaul's respirations, tachycardia, seizures, and stupor that may progress to coma.

• *Hyperosmolar hyperglycemic nonketotic coma.* This disorder decreases blood pressure—at times dramatically, if the patient loses significant fluid from diuresis. It also produces dry mouth, poor skin turgor, tachycardia, confusion progressing to coma and, occasionally, focal grand mal seizures.

• *Hypovolemic shock.* In this disorder, systolic pressure falls to less than 80 mm Hg, or 30 mm Hg less than the patient's baseline. Accompanying it are diminished Korotkoff sounds, narrowed pulse pressure, and rapid, weak, and occasionally irregular pulse. Peripheral vasoconstriction causes cyanosis of the extremities and pale, cool, clammy skin. Other signs and symptoms include oliguria, confusion, disorientation, restlessness, and anxiety.

• *Myocardial infarction (MI).* In this life-threatening disorder, blood pressure may be low or high. However, a precipitous drop in blood pressure may signal cardiogenic shock. Associated signs and symptoms of MI include chest pain that may radiate to the jaw, shoulder, arm, or epigastrium; dyspnea; anxiety; nausea or vomiting; diaphoresis; and cool, pale, or cyanotic skin. Auscultation reveals an atrial gallop, murmur and, occasionally, irregular pulse.

• *Neurogenic shock.* The result of sympathetic denervation due to cervical injury or anesthesia, neurogenic shock produces low blood pressure and bradycardia. However, the patient's skin remains warm and dry because of cutaneous vasodilation and sweat gland denervation. Depending on the cause of shock, there may also be motor weakness of the limbs and diaphragm.

• *Pulmonary embolism.* This disorder causes sudden chest pain and dyspnea accompanied by cyanosis and, occasionally, fever. Low blood pressure occurs with narrowed pulse pressure and diminished Korotkoff sounds. Associated signs include tachycardia, tachypnea, neck vein distention, and hemoptysis.

• *Vasovagal syncope.* This transient attack is characterized by low blood pressure, pallor, cold sweats, nausea, slowed heart rate, and weakness.

Other causes

• *Diagnostic tests.* These include the gastric acid stimulation test using histamine and X-ray studies using contrast media. The latter may trigger an allergic reaction, which causes low blood pressure.

• *Drugs.* Calcium channel blockers, diuretics, vasodilators, antihypertensives, general anesthetics, narcotic analgesics, monoamine oxidase inhibitors, antianxiety agents (such as benzodiazepines), tranquilizers, and most I.V. antiarrhythmics (especially bretylium tosylate) can cause low blood pressure.

Special considerations

Check the patient's vital signs frequently to determine if low blood pressure is constant or intermittent. If blood pressure is extremely low, an arterial catheter may be inserted to allow close monitoring of pressures. Or use a Doppler flowmeter.

Place the patient on bed rest. Keep the side rails of the bed up. If the patient is ambulatory, assist him, as necessary. To avoid falls, don't leave a dizzy patient

GUIDE TO PEDIATRIC BLOOD PRESSURE

AGE	NORMAL SYSTOLIC PRESSURE	NORMAL DIASTOLIC PRESSURE
Birth to 3 months	40 to 80 mm Hg	Not detectable
3 months to 1 year	80 to 100 mm Hg	Not detectable
1 to 4 years	100 to 108 mm Hg	60 mm Hg
4 to 12 years	Add 2 mm Hg for every year to 100 mm Hg	60 to 70 mm Hg

unattended when he's sitting or walking. If the patient has postural hypotension, instruct him to stand up slowly. Evaluate his need for a cane or walker.

Prepare the patient for laboratory tests, which may include urinalysis, routine blood studies, electrocardiogram, and chest, cervical, and abdominal X-rays.

Pediatric pointers

Normal blood pressure in children is lower than in adults. (See *Guide to pediatric blood pressure*.)

Because accidents commonly occur in children, suspect trauma or shock first as a possible cause of low blood pressure. Remember that low blood pressure typically doesn't accompany head injury in adults because intracranial hemorrhage is insufficient to cause hypovolemia. However, it does accompany head injury in infants and young children; their expandable cranial vaults allow significant blood loss into the cranial space, resulting in hypovolemia.

Another common cause of low blood pressure in children is dehydration—the result of failure to thrive or of persistent diarrhea and vomiting for as little as 24 hours.

BLOOD PRESSURE INCREASE
[Hypertension]

Elevated blood pressure—an intermittent or sustained increase in blood pressure exceeding 140/90 mm Hg—strikes more men than women and twice as many blacks as whites. By itself, this common sign is easily ignored by the patient; after all, he can't see or feel it. However, its causes can be life-threatening.

Elevated blood pressure may develop suddenly or gradually. A sudden, severe rise in blood pressure (exceeding 200/120 mm Hg) indicates life-threatening hypertensive crisis. However, even a less dramatic rise may be equally significant if it heralds dissecting aortic aneurysm, increased intracranial pressure, eclampsia, or thyrotoxicosis.

Most commonly associated with essential hypertension, elevated blood pressure may also result from renal and endocrine disorders, treatments that affect fluid status (such as dialysis), and the adverse effects of certain drugs. Ingestion of large amounts of certain foods, such as black licorice and cheddar cheese, may temporarily elevate blood pressure.

PATHOPHYSIOLOGY OF ELEVATED BLOOD PRESSURE

Blood pressure—the force blood exerts on vessels as it flows through them—depends on cardiac output, peripheral resistance, and blood volume. A brief review of its regulating mechanisms—nervous system control, capillary fluid shifts, kidney excretion, and hormonal changes—will help you understand how elevated blood pressure develops.

• *Nervous system control* involves the sympathetic division, chiefly baroreceptors and chemoreceptors, which promotes moderate vasoconstriction to maintain normal blood pressure. When this system responds inappropriately, increased vasoconstriction enhances peripheral resistance, resulting in elevated blood pressure.

• *Capillary fluid shifts* regulate blood volume by responding to arterial pressure. Increased pressure forces fluid into the interstitial space; decreased pressure allows it to be drawn back into the arteries by osmosis. However, this fluid shift may take several hours to adjust blood pressure.

• *Kidney excretion* also helps regulate blood volume by increasing or decreasing urine formation. Normally, an arterial pressure of about 60 mm Hg maintains urine output. When pressure drops below this

reading, urine formation ceases, thereby increasing blood volume. Conversely, when arterial pressure exceeds this reading, urine formation increases, thereby reducing blood volume. Like capillary fluid shifts, this mechanism may take several hours to adjust blood pressure.

• *Hormonal changes* reflect stimulation of the kidney's renin-angiotensin system in response to low arterial pressure. This system causes vasoconstriction, which increases arterial pressure, and stimulates aldosterone release, which regulates sodium retention—a key determinant of blood volume.

Elevated blood pressure signals the breakdown or inappropriate response of these pressure-regulating mechanisms. Its associated signs and symptoms concentrate in the target organs and tissues illustrated above.

(See *Pathophysiology of elevated blood pressure.*)

Unfortunately, elevated blood pressure may simply reflect inaccurate blood pressure measurement. However, careful measurement alone doesn't ensure a clinically useful reading. To be useful, each blood pressure reading must be compared to the patient's baseline. Also, serial readings may be necessary to establish elevated blood pressure.

History and physical examination

If you detect sharply elevated blood pressure, you'll need to quickly rule out pos-

sible life-threatening causes. (See *Managing elevated blood pressure,* page 76.)

After ruling out life-threatening causes of elevated blood pressure, complete a history and physical examination. Ask about a family history of high blood pressure (a likely finding in essential hypertension), pheochromocytoma, and polycystic kidney disease. Then ask about its onset. Did high blood pressure appear abruptly? Also find out the patient's age. Sudden onset in middle-aged or elderly patients suggests renovascular stenosis.

Although essential hypertension may begin in childhood, it typically isn't diagnosed until near age 35. Pheochromocytoma and primary aldosteronism usually occur between ages 40 and 60. If you suspect either, check for postural hypotension. Take blood pressures with the patient in a supine position, then sitting and standing. Normally, systolic pressure falls and diastolic pressure rises on standing. In postural hypotension, both pressures fall.

Note headaches, palpitations, blurred vision, and sweating. Ask about urinary burning or frequency, which suggests pyelonephritis, and about wine-colored urine and decreased urine output, which suggest glomerulonephritis.

Obtain a drug history, including past and present prescription and over-the-counter drugs. If the patient is already taking antihypertensive drugs, determine how well he complies with the regimen. Determine his perception of elevated blood pressure. How serious does he believe it is? Does he expect drug therapy to help?

Follow the history with the physical examination. Using a funduscope, check for intraocular hemorrhage, exudate, and papilledema, which characterize severe hypertension. Perform a thorough cardiovascular assessment. Check for carotid bruits and neck vein distention. Assess skin color, temperature, and turgor. Palpate peripheral pulses. Auscultate for abnormal heart sounds (gallops, murmurs), rate (bradycardia, tachycardia), or rhythm. Then auscultate for abnormal breath sounds (crackles, wheezing), rate (bradypnea, tachypnea), or rhythm.

Palpate the abdomen for tenderness, masses, or liver enlargement. Auscultate for abdominal bruits. Renal artery stenosis produces bruits over the upper abdomen or in the costovertebral angles. Easily palpable, enlarged kidneys and a large, tender liver suggest polycystic kidney disease. Obtain a urine sample to check for microscopic hematuria.

Common medical causes

● *Aortic aneurysm (dissecting).* Initially, this life-threatening disorder causes a sudden rise in systolic pressure, but no change in diastolic pressure. But this increase is brief. The body's ability to compensate fails, resulting in hypotension. Other signs vary, depending on whether the aneurysm is abdominal or thoracic aortic aneurysms. An *abdominal aneurysm* may cause persistent abdominal and back pain, weakness, sweating, tachycardia, dyspnea, a pulsating abdominal mass, restlessness, confusion, and cool, clammy skin. A *thoracic aneurysm* may cause a ripping or tearing sensation in the chest, which may radiate to the neck, shoulders, lower back, or abdomen; pallor; syncope; blindness; loss of consciousness; sweating; dyspnea; tachycardia; cyanosis; leg weakness; murmur; and absent radial and femoral pulses.

● *Atherosclerosis.* In this disorder, systolic pressure rises while diastolic pressure remains normal. The patient may show no other signs or he may have weak pulse, flushed skin, tachycardia, anginal pain, and claudication.

● *Cushing's syndrome.* Twice as common in females as in males, this disorder causes elevated blood pressure and widened pulse pressure. It may also produce truncal obesity, moon face, and other cushingoid signs.

● *Hypertension. Essential hypertension* develops insidiously and is characterized by a gradual increase in blood pressure from decade to decade. Except for this rise in blood pressure, the patient may be asymptomatic or may complain of suboccipital headache, light-headedness, tinnitus, and fatigue.

In *malignant hypertension,* diastolic pressure suddenly increases above 120 mm Hg, and systolic pressure may exceed 200 mm Hg. Typical findings include pulmonary edema marked by neck vein distention, dyspnea, tachypnea, tachycardia, and coughing of pink, frothy

MANAGING ELEVATED BLOOD PRESSURE

Elevated blood pressure can signal various life-threatening disorders. However, if blood pressure exceeds 200/120 mm Hg, the patient is experiencing hypertensive crisis and requires prompt treatment. Maintain a patent airway in case the patient vomits, and institute seizure precautions. Prepare to administer I.V. antihypertensive drugs and diuretics. You'll need to insert an indwelling urinary catheter to accurately monitor urine output.

If blood pressure is less severely elevated, continue to rule out other life-threatening causes. If the patient is pregnant, suspect preeclampsia or eclampsia. Place her on bed rest and insert an I.V. line. Administer magnesium sulfate (to decrease neuromuscular irritability) and antihypertensive drugs. Monitor vital signs closely for the next 24 hours. If diastolic blood pressure continues to exceed 100 mm Hg despite drug therapy, prepare the patient for induced labor and delivery or for cesarean section. Offer emotional support if the patient must face delivery of a premature infant.

If the patient isn't pregnant, quickly observe for equally obvious clues. Assess for exophthalmos and an enlarged thyroid gland. If these signs are present, ask about a history of hyperthyroidism. Then look for other associated signs, including tachycardia, widened pulse pressure, palpitations, severe weakness, diarrhea, fever exceeding 100° F (37.8° C), and nervousness.

Prepare to administer antithyroid drugs orally or by nasogastric tube, if necessary. Also evaluate fluid status; look for signs of dehydration such as poor skin turgor. Prepare for I.V. fluid replacement and temperature control by hypothermia blanket, if necessary.

If the patient shows signs of increased intracranial pressure (such as decreased level of consciousness and fixed or dilated pupils), ask him or his companion about recent head trauma. Then check for increased respiratory rate and bradycardia. You'll need to maintain a patent airway in case the patient vomits, and institute seizure precautions. Prepare to give I.V. diuretics. Insert an indwelling urinary catheter, and monitor intake and output. Check vital signs every 15 minutes until they're stable.

If the patient has absent or weak peripheral pulses, ask about chest pressure or pain, which suggests dissecting aortic aneurysm. Enforce bed rest until a diagnosis has been established. As appropriate, administer I.V. antihypertensive drugs or prepare the patient for surgery.

---

sputum. Other characteristic signs and symptoms include severe headache, confusion, tinnitus, epistaxis, muscle twitching, nausea, and vomiting.

• *Increased intracranial pressure (ICP).* Initially, this condition causes an increased respiratory rate. Then, systolic pressure rises and pulse pressure widens. Increased ICP affects heart rate last, causing bradycardia. Associated signs and symptoms include headache, projectile vomiting, decreased level of consciousness, and fixed or dilated pupils.

• *Myocardial infarction.* This life-threatening disorder may cause high or low blood pressure. Common findings include crushing chest pain that may radiate to the jaw, shoulder, arm, or epigastrium. Other findings include dyspnea, anxiety, nausea, vomiting, weakness, diaphoresis, atrial gallop, and murmurs.

● *Pheochromocytoma.* Paroxysmal or sustained elevated blood pressure characterizes pheochromocytoma and may be accompanied by postural hypotension. Associated signs and symptoms include anxiety, diaphoresis, palpitations, tremors, pallor, nausea, weight loss, and headache.

● *Polycystic kidney disease.* Elevated blood pressure is typically preceded by flank pain. Other signs include enlarged kidneys; enlarged, tender liver; and intermittent gross hematuria.

● *Preeclampsia or eclampsia.* Potentially life-threatening to both mother and fetus, this disorder characteristically increases blood pressure. It's defined as a reading of 140/90 mm Hg or more in the first trimester, a reading of 130/80 mm Hg or more in the second or third trimester, an increase of 30 mm Hg above the patient's baseline systolic pressure, or an increase of 15 mm Hg above the patient's baseline diastolic pressure. Accompanying elevated blood pressure are generalized edema, sudden weight gain of 3 lb (1.5 kg) or more per week during the second or third trimester, severe frontal headache, blurred or double vision, decreased urine output or oliguria, midabdominal pain, neuromuscular irritability, nausea, and possibly seizures (eclampsia).

● *Pyelonephritis (chronic).* In some patients, this disorder produces no overt signs until severely elevated systolic and diastolic pressures develop. In others, it may produce recurrent, abrupt episodes of malaise, backache, chills, fever, and pain in one or both loins. Within 24 hours of such episodes, the patient experiences urinary frequency, burning and, occasionally, hematuria.

● *Renovascular stenosis.* This disorder produces abruptly elevated systolic and diastolic pressure. Other characteristic signs and symptoms include bruits over the upper abdomen or in the costovertebral angles, hematuria, and acute flank pain.

● *Thyrotoxicosis.* Accompanying elevated systolic pressure in this potentially life-threatening disorder are widened pulse pressure, tachycardia, bounding pulse, pulsations in the capillary nail beds, palpitations, weight loss, exophthalmos, an enlarged thyroid gland, weakness, diarrhea, fever (over 100° F [37.8° C]), and warm, moist skin. The patient may appear nervous and emotionally unstable, displaying occasional outbursts or even psychotic behavior. Heat intolerance, exertional dyspnea and, in females, decreased or absent menses may also occur.

Other causes

● *Drugs.* Central nervous system stimulants (such as amphetamines), sympathomimetics, corticosteroids, oral contraceptives, monoamine oxidase inhibitors, and cocaine abuse can increase blood pressure.

● *Treatments.* Kidney dialysis and transplantation cause transient elevation of blood pressure.

Special considerations

If routine screening detects elevated blood pressure, stress to the patient the need for follow-up diagnostic tests. Then prepare him for routine blood tests and urinalysis. Depending on the suspected cause of the increased blood pressure, radiographic studies, especially of the kidneys, may be necessary.

If the patient has essential hypertension, explain the importance of long-term control of elevated blood pressure and the purpose, dosage, schedule, route, and adverse effects of prescribed antihypertensive drugs. Reassure him that there are other drugs he can take if the one he's taking isn't effective or causes intolerable adverse effects. Encourage him to report adverse reactions; the drug dosage or schedule may simply need adjustment.

Encourage the patient to lose weight, if necessary, and to restrict dietary sodium. Suggest that he participate in an exercise or stress management program as well. Then teach him how to monitor his blood pressure so that he can evaluate the effectiveness of drug therapy and lifestyle changes. Have him record blood pressure readings and symptoms, and ask him to share this information on his return visits.

Pediatric pointers

Normally, blood pressure in children is lower than in adults, an essential point to recognize when assessing for elevated blood pressure.

Elevated blood pressure in children may result from lead or mercury poisoning, essential hypertension, renovascular stenosis, chronic pyelonephritis, coarctation of the aorta, patent ductus arteriosus, glomerulonephritis, adrenogenital syndrome, and neuroblastoma.

Treatment typically begins with drug therapy. Surgery may then follow in patent ductus arteriosus, coarctation of the aorta, neuroblastoma, and some cases of renovascular stenosis. Diuretics and antibiotics are used to treat glomerulonephritis and chronic pyelonephritis; hormonal therapy, to treat adrenogenital syndrome.

BOWEL SOUNDS, ABSENT

[Silent abdomen]

Absent bowel sounds refers to the inability to hear any bowel sounds through a stethoscope after listening for at least 5 minutes in each abdominal quadrant.

Bowel sounds cease when mechanical or vascular obstruction or neurogenic inhibition halts peristalsis. When peristalsis halts, gas from bowel contents and fluid secreted from the intestinal walls accumulate and distend the lumen, leading to life-threatening complications, such as perforation, peritonitis and sepsis, or hypovolemic shock.

Simple mechanical obstruction, resulting from adhesions, hernia, or tumor, causes loss of fluids and electrolytes and induces dehydration. Vascular obstruction cuts off circulation to the intestinal walls, leading to ischemia, necrosis, and shock. Neurogenic inhibition, affecting innervation of the intestinal wall, may result from infection, bowel distention, or trauma. It may also follow mechanical or vascular obstruction or metabolic derangement such as hypokalemia.

Abrupt cessation of bowel sounds, when accompanied by abdominal pain, rigidity, and distention, signals a life-threatening crisis requiring immediate intervention. Absent bowel sounds following a period of hyperactivity are equally ominous and may indicate strangulation of a mechanically obstructed bowel.

Emergency interventions

 If you fail to detect bowel sounds and the patient reports sudden, severe abdominal pain and cramping or exhibits severe abdominal distention, prepare to insert a nasogastric (NG) or intestinal tube to suction lumen contents and decompress the bowel. Administer I.V. fluids and electrolytes to offset any dehydration and imbalances caused by the dysfunctioning bowel.

Because the patient may require surgery to relieve an obstruction, withhold oral intake. Take the patient's vital signs, and be alert for signs of shock, such as hypotension, tachycardia, and cool, clammy skin. Measure abdominal girth as a baseline for gauging subsequent changes.

History and physical examination

If the patient's condition permits, proceed with a brief history. Start with abdominal pain: When did it begin? Has it become worse? Where does he feel it? Ask about a sensation of bloating and about flatulence. Find out if the patient has had diarrhea or passed pencil-thin stools—possible signs of a developing luminal obstruction. The patient may have had no bowel movements at all—a possible sign of complete obstruction or paralytic ileus.

Ask about conditions that commonly lead to mechanical obstruction, such as abdominal tumors, hernias, and adhesions from past surgery. Determine if the patient was involved in an accident—even a seemingly minor one such as falling off a stepladder—that may have caused vascular clots. Check for a history of acute pancreatitis, diverticulitis, or gynecologic infection, which may have led to intra-abdominal infection and bowel dysfunction. Be sure to ask about previous toxic conditions, such as uremia, and about spinal cord injury, which can lead to paralytic ileus.

If the patient's pain isn't severe or accompanied by other life-threatening signs, obtain a detailed medical and surgical history and then examine the abdomen.

Start by inspecting the patient's abdominal contour. Stoop at the recumbent patient's side and then at the foot of his bed to detect localized or generalized distention. Percuss and palpate the abdomen gently. Listen for dullness over fluid-filled areas and tympany over pockets of gas. Palpate for abdominal rigidity and guarding, suggesting peritoneal irritation that can lead to paralytic ileus. (See *Are bowel sounds really absent?*)

Common medical causes
● **Complete mechanical intestinal obstruction.** Absent bowel sounds follow a period of hyperactive bowel sounds in this potentially life-threatening disorder. This silence accompanies acute, colicky abdominal pain that arises in the quadrant of obstruction and may radiate to the

---

EXAMINATION TIP

 ## ARE BOWEL SOUNDS REALLY ABSENT?

Before concluding that your patient has absent bowel sounds, ask yourself these three questions:
● Did you use the diaphragm of your stethoscope to auscultate for the bowel sounds?
   The diaphragm detects high-frequency sounds, such as bowel sounds, whereas the bell detects low-frequency sounds, such as a vascular bruit or a venous hum.
● Did you listen for bowel sounds in the same spot for at least 5 minutes?
   Normally, bowel sounds occur every 5 to 15 seconds, but the duration of a single sound may be less than 1 second.
● Did you listen for bowel sounds in all quadrants?
   Bowel sounds may be absent in one quadrant, but present in another.

---

flank or lumbar regions. Associated signs and symptoms include abdominal distention and bloating, constipation, and nausea and vomiting (the higher the blockage, the earlier and more severe the vomiting). In late stages, signs of shock may occur with fever, rebound tenderness, and abdominal rigidity.

● **Mesenteric artery occlusion.** In this life-threatening disorder, bowel sounds disappear after a brief period of hyperactive sounds. Sudden, severe mid-epigastric or periumbilical pain occurs next, followed by abdominal distention and possible bruits, vomiting, constipation, and signs of shock. Fever is common. Abdominal rigidity may appear late.

• *Paralytic (adynamic) ileus.* The cardinal sign is absent bowel sounds. In addition to abdominal distention, associated signs and symptoms of paralytic ileus include generalized discomfort and constipation or passage of small, liquid stools. If paralytic ileus follows acute abdominal infection, the patient may also experience fever and abdominal pain.

Other causes

• *Abdominal surgery.* Bowel sounds are normally absent after abdominal surgery—the result of anesthetics and surgical manipulation.

Special considerations

After you've inserted an NG tube or an intestinal tube, elevate the head of the patient's bed at least 30 degrees, and turn the patient to facilitate passage of the tube through the GI tract. Remember not to tape an intestinal tube to the patient's face. Assure tube patency by checking for drainage and for properly functioning suction devices, and irrigate accordingly.

Continue I.V. fluids and electrolytes and make sure that you send a serum specimen to the laboratory for electrolyte analysis at least once a day. You should recognize that the patient may need X-ray studies and further blood work to determine the cause of absent bowel sounds.

After mechanical obstruction and intra-abdominal sepsis have been ruled out as the causes of absent bowel sounds, patients should be given drugs to control pain and stimulate peristalsis.

Pediatric pointers

Absent bowel sounds in children may result from Hirschsprung's disease or intussusception, both of which can lead to life-threatening obstruction.

BOWEL SOUNDS, HYPERACTIVE

Sometimes audible without a stethoscope, hyperactive bowel sounds reflect increased intestinal motility (peristalsis). They're commonly characterized as rapid, rushing, gurgling waves of sounds. They may stem from life-threatening bowel obstruction or GI hemorrhage. However, hyperactive sounds may also stem from GI infection, inflammatory bowel disease (which usually follows a chronic course), food allergies, and stress.

Emergency interventions

 After detecting hyperactive bowel sounds, quickly check vital signs and ask the patient about associated signs and symptoms, such as abdominal pain, vomiting, and diarrhea. If he reports cramping abdominal pain or vomiting, continue to auscultate for bowel sounds. If bowel sounds stop abruptly, suspect complete bowel obstruction and prepare to assist with GI suction and decompression and to give I.V. fluids and electrolytes. Prepare the patient for surgery.

If he has diarrhea, record its frequency, amount, color, and consistency. If you detect excessive watery diarrhea or bleeding, prepare to administer antidiarrheal drugs, I.V. fluids and electrolytes, and possibly blood transfusions.

History and physical examination

If you've ruled out life-threatening conditions, obtain a detailed medical and surgical history. Be sure to ask the patient about hernia and abdominal surgery because they may cause mechanical intestinal obstruction. Does the patient have a history of inflammatory bowel disease? Also ask about recent eruptions

HYPERACTIVE BOWEL SOUNDS: COMMON CAUSES AND ASSOCIATED FINDINGS

CAUSES	Abdominal distention	Abdominal pain	Anorexia	Constipation	Diarrhea	Fever	Nausea	Perianal lesions	Rectal bleeding	Tenesmus	Vomiting	Weight loss
Crohn's disease	●	●	●		●	●		●				●
Food hypersensitivity					●		●				●	
Gastroenteritis		●			●	●	●				●	
GI hemorrhage	●	●			●				●			
Mechanical intestinal obstruction	●	●		●			●				●	
Ulcerative colitis (acute)			●	●	●	●	●		●	●	●	●

Column group header: **MAJOR ASSOCIATED SIGNS AND SYMPTOMS**

of gastroenteritis among family members, friends, or coworkers. If the patient has traveled recently, even within the United States, was he aware of any endemic illnesses?

In addition, you'll need to determine whether stress may have contributed to the patient's problem. Ask about food allergies and recent ingestion of unusual foods or fluids. Check for fever, which suggests infection. Having already auscultated, now gently inspect, percuss, and palpate the abdomen.

Common medical causes

• **Crohn's disease.** Hyperactive bowel sounds usually arise insidiously. Associated signs and symptoms include diarrhea, cramping abdominal pain, anorexia, low-grade fever, abdominal distention and tenderness, and commonly a fixed mass in the right lower quadrant. Peri-anal lesions are common. With progression of the disorder, muscle wasting, weight loss, and signs of dehydration may occur.

• **Food hypersensitivity.** Malabsorption—typically lactose intolerance—may cause hyperactive bowel sounds. Associated findings include diarrhea and, possibly, nausea and vomiting.

• **Gastroenteritis.** Hyperactive bowel sounds follow sudden nausea and vomiting and accompany "explosive" diarrhea. Abdominal cramping or pain is common. Fever may occur, depending on the causative organism.

• **GI hemorrhage.** Hyperactive bowel sounds provide the most immediate indication of persistent upper GI bleeding. Other findings may include abdominal distention, bloody diarrhea, rectal passage of bright red clots and jellylike material or melena, and pain during bleeding. Decreased urine output, tachycardia, and hypotension accompany blood loss.

• *Mechanical intestinal obstruction.* Hyperactive bowel sounds occur simultaneously with cramping abdominal pain every few minutes in this potentially life-threatening disorder; bowel sounds may later become hypoactive and then disappear. In small-bowel obstruction, nausea and vomiting occur earlier and with greater severity than in large-bowel obstruction. In complete bowel obstruction, hyperactive sounds are also accompanied by abdominal distention and constipation, although the bowel distal to the obstruction may continue to empty for up to 3 days.

• *Ulcerative colitis (acute).* Hyperactive bowel sounds arise abruptly in this disorder. They're accompanied by bloody diarrhea, anorexia, abdominal pain, nausea, vomiting, fever, and tenesmus. Weight loss may occur.

Special considerations

Prepare the patient for diagnostic tests. These may include endoscopy to view a suspected lesion, barium X-rays, or stool analysis.

Explain prescribed dietary changes to the patient. These may vary from complete food and fluid restrictions to a liquid or bland diet. Because stress commonly precipitates or aggravates bowel hyperactivity, teach the patient relaxation techniques such as deep breathing. Encourage rest and restrict the patient's physical activity.

Pediatric pointers

Hyperactive bowel sounds in children usually result from gastroenteritis, erratic eating habits, excessive ingestion of certain foods (such as unripened fruit), or food allergy.

BOWEL SOUNDS, HYPOACTIVE

Hypoactive bowel sounds, detected by auscultation, are diminished in regularity, tone, or loudness from normal bowel sounds. In themselves, hypoactive bowel sounds don't herald an emergency; in fact, they're considered normal during sleep. However, they may portend the absence of bowel sounds, which can indicate a life-threatening disorder.

Hypoactive bowel sounds result from decreased peristalsis, which, in turn, can result from a developing bowel obstruction. Such obstruction may be mechanical (as from hernia, tumor, or twisting), vascular (as from an embolism or thrombosis), or neurogenic (as from mechanical, ischemic, or toxic impairment of bowel innervation).

Hypoactive bowel sounds can also result from certain drugs and from abdominal surgery and irradiation.

History and physical examination

After detecting hypoactive bowel sounds, you should look for related symptoms. Ask the patient about the location, onset, duration, frequency, and severity of any pain. Cramping or colicky abdominal pain usually indicates a mechanical bowel obstruction, whereas diffuse abdominal pain usually indicates intestinal distention in paralytic ileus.

Ask the patient about recent vomiting: When did it begin? How often does it occur? Does the vomitus look bloody? Also ask the patient about any changes in bowel habits: Does he have a history of constipation? When was the last time he had a bowel movement or expelled gas?

Obtain a detailed medical and surgical history of any conditions that may cause mechanical bowel obstruction, such as an abdominal tumor or hernia. Does the patient have a history of conditions that can cause paralytic ileus, such as pancreatitis; bowel inflammation or gynecologic infection, which may produce peritonitis; toxic conditions such as uremia; severe pain; or trauma? Has he recently had radiation therapy or abdominal surgery, or ingested drugs such as opiates, which can decrease peristalsis and cause hypoactive bowel sounds?

Once the patient's history is complete, perform a careful physical examination. Inspect the abdomen for distention, noting surgical incisions and obvious masses. Gently percuss and palpate the abdomen for masses, gas, fluid, tenderness, and rigidity. Measure abdominal girth to detect any subsequent increase in distention. Also check for poor skin turgor, hypotension, narrowed pulse pressure, and other signs of dehydration and electrolyte imbalance, which may result from paralytic ileus.

Common medical causes

• *Mechanical intestinal obstruction.* Bowel sounds may become hypoactive after a period of hyperactivity. The patient may also have acute colicky abdominal pain in the quadrant of obstruction, possibly radiating to the flank or lumbar regions; nausea and vomiting (the higher the obstruction, the earlier and more severe the vomiting); constipation; and abdominal distention and bloating. If the obstruction becomes complete, signs of shock may occur.

• *Mesenteric artery occlusion.* After a brief period of hyperactivity, bowel sounds become hypoactive and then quickly disappear, signifying a life-threatening crisis. Associated signs and symptoms include fever, sudden and severe midepigastric or periumbilical pain followed by abdominal distention and possible bruits, vomiting, constipation, and signs of shock. Abdominal rigidity may appear late.

• *Paralytic (adynamic) ileus.* Bowel sounds in this disorder are hypoactive and may become absent. Associated signs and symptoms include abdominal distention, generalized discomfort, and constipation or passage of flatus and small, liquid stools. If the disorder follows acute abdominal infection, fever and abdominal pain may occur.

Other causes

• *Drugs.* Certain classes of drugs reduce intestinal motility and thus produce hypoactive bowel sounds. These include opiates such as codeine, anticholinergics such as propantheline, phenothiazines such as chlorpromazine, and vinca alkaloids such as vincristine. General or spinal anesthetics produce transient hypoactive sounds.

• *Radiation therapy.* Hypoactive bowel sounds and abdominal tenderness may occur following irradiation of the abdomen.

• *Surgery.* Hypoactive bowel sounds may occur after manipulation of the bowel. Motility and bowel sounds in the small intestine usually resume in 24 hours; colonic bowel sounds in 3 to 5 days.

Special considerations

Frequently evaluate the patient with hypoactive bowel sounds for indications of shock (thirst; anxiety; restlessness; cool, clammy skin; tachycardia; weak, thready pulse), which can develop if peristalsis continues to diminish and fluid is lost from the circulation.

Be alert for sudden absence of bowel sounds, especially in postoperative and hypokalemic patients because those patients are at increased risk for paralytic ileus. Monitor the patient's vital signs and auscultate for bowel sounds every 2 to 4 hours.

Severe pain, abdominal rigidity, guarding, and fever, accompanied by hypoactive bowel sounds, may indicate paralytic ileus from peritonitis. Prepare for emergency interventions (see "Bowel sounds, absent").

The patient with hypoactive bowel sounds may require GI suction and decompression, using a nasogastric or intestinal tube. If so, be sure to restrict the patient's oral intake. Then you should elevate the head of the bed at least 30 degrees, and turn the patient to facilitate passage of the tube through the GI tract.

Remember not to tape an intestinal tube to the patient's face. Ensure tube patency by watching for drainage and for properly functioning suction devices. You'll need to irrigate the tube and closely monitor drainage.

Continue I.V. fluids and electrolytes, and send a serum specimen to the laboratory for electrolyte analysis at least once a day. Recognize that the patient may need X-ray studies, endoscopic procedures, and further blood work to determine the cause of hypoactive bowel sounds.

Provide comfort measures as needed. Semi-Fowler's position offers the best relief for the patient with paralytic ileus. Sometimes, walking can reactivate the sluggish bowel. However, if the patient can't tolerate ambulation, range-of-motion exercises or turning from side to side may stimulate peristalsis. Turning from side to side will also help move gas through the intestines.

Pediatric pointers
Hypoactive bowel sounds in a child may simply be due to bowel distention from excessive swallowing of air while the child is eating or crying. However, be sure to observe the child for further signs of illness. As with an adult, sluggish bowel sounds in a child may signal the onset of paralytic ileus or peritonitis.

BRADYCARDIA

Bradycardia, a heart rate of less than 60 beats/minute, occurs normally in young adults, trained athletes, elderly people, and during sleep. It's also a normal response to vagal stimulation caused by coughing, vomiting, or straining during defecation. When bradycardia results from these causes, the heart rate rarely drops below 40 beats/minute. However, when it results from pathologic causes (such as cardiovascular disorders), the heart rate may be slower.

By itself, bradycardia is a nonspecific sign. But in conjunction with such symptoms as chest pain, dizziness, syncope, and shortness of breath, it can signal a life-threatening disorder.

History and physical examination
After detecting bradycardia, check for related signs of life-threatening disorders. (See *Managing severe bradycardia.*) If the patient's bradycardia is *not* accompanied by untoward signs, ask the patient if he or a family member has a history of slow pulse rate because this may be inherited. Find out if the patient has an underlying metabolic disorder such as hypothyroidism, which can precipitate bradycardia. Ask which medications he's taking and if he's complying with the prescribed schedule and dosage.

Common medical causes
• *Cardiac arrhythmia.* Depending on the type of arrhythmia and the patient's tolerance of it, bradycardia may be transient or sustained, benign or life-threatening. Related findings may include hypotension, palpitations, dizziness, weakness, syncope, and fatigue.
• *Cardiomyopathy.* This potentially life-threatening disorder may cause transient or sustained bradycardia and is usually associated with tachycardia. Other findings include dizziness, syncope, edema, fatigue, jugular vein distention, orthopnea, dyspnea, and peripheral cyanosis.
• *Hypothermia.* Bradycardia usually appears when core temperature drops below 89.6° F (32° C). It's accompanied by

EMERGENCY INTERVENTIONS

 ## MANAGING SEVERE BRADYCARDIA

Bradycardia can signal a life-threatening disorder when accompanied by pain, shortness of breath, dizziness, syncope, or other symptoms; prolonged exposure to cold; or head or neck trauma. In such patients, quickly take vital signs. Connect the patient to a cardiac monitor, and insert an I.V. line. Depending on the cause of bradycardia, you'll need to administer fluids, atropine, steroids, or thyroid medication. If indicated, insert an indwelling urinary catheter. Intubation, mechanical ventilation, or placement of a pacemaker may be necessary if the patient's respiratory rate falls.

If appropriate, perform a focused evaluation to help locate the cause of bradycardia. For example, ask about pain. Viselike pressure or crushing or burning chest pain that radiates to the arms, back, or jaw may indicate acute myocardial infarction (MI); a severe headache may signal increased intracranial pressure. Also ask about nausea, vomiting, or shortness of breath—symptoms associated with acute MI and cardiomyopathy. Observe the patient for peripheral cyanosis, edema, or neck vein distention, which may indicate cardiomyopathy. Look for a thyroidectomy scar because severe bradycardia may result from hypothyroidism caused by failure to take thyroid hormone replacements.

If the cause of bradycardia is evident, you'll need to provide supportive care. For example, keep the hypothermic patient warm by applying blankets, and monitor his core temperature until it reaches 99° F (37.2° C). Or stabilize the head and neck of a trauma patient until cervical spinal injury is ruled out.

---

shivering, peripheral cyanosis, confusion leading to stupor, muscle rigidity, and bradypnea.

- *Hypothyroidism.* This disorder causes severe bradycardia along with fatigue, constipation, unexplained weight gain, and sensitivity to cold. Related signs include confusion leading to stupor; cool, dry, thick skin; sparse, dry hair; facial swelling; periorbital edema; and thick, brittle nails.
- *Myocardial infarction (MI).* Sinus bradycardia is the most common arrhythmia found in acute MI. Accompanying signs and symptoms include an aching, burning, or viselike pressure in the chest that may radiate to the jaw, shoulder, arm, back, or epigastric area; nausea and vomiting; cool, clammy, and either pale or cyanotic skin; anxiety; and dyspnea. Blood pressure may be elevated or depressed. Auscultation may reveal abnormal heart sounds.

Other causes
- *Diagnostic tests.* Cardiac catheterization and electrophysiologic studies can induce temporary bradycardia.
- *Drugs.* Beta-adrenergic and some calcium channel blockers, digitalis glycosides, topical miotics (such as pilocarpine), protamine sulfate, quinidine and other antiarrhythmics, and sympatholytics may cause transient bradycardia. Failure to take thyroid replacements may cause bradycardia.
- *Invasive treatments.* Suctioning can induce hypoxia and vagal stimulation, causing bradycardia. Cardiac surgery can cause edema or damage to conduction tissues, causing bradycardia.

Special considerations

Continue to monitor vital signs frequently. Be especially alert for changes in cardiac rhythm, respiratory rate, and level of consciousness.

Prepare the patient for laboratory tests, which can include complete blood count; cardiac enzyme, serum electrolyte, blood glucose, and thyroid function tests; arterial blood gas and blood urea nitrogen levels; and a 12-lead electrocardiogram. If appropriate, prepare the patient for 24-hour Holter monitoring.

Pediatric pointers

Heart rates are normally higher in children than in adults. Fetal bradycardia— a heart rate of fewer than 120 beats/minute—may occur during prolonged labor or complications of delivery, such as compression of the umbilicus, partial abruptio placentae, and placenta previa. Intermittent bradycardia, sometimes accompanied by apnea, commonly occurs in premature infants. Bradycardia rarely occurs in full-term infants or children. However, it can result from congenital heart defects, acute glomerulonephritis, and transient or complete heart block associated with cardiac catheterization or cardiac surgery.

BRADYPNEA

Commonly preceding life-threatening apnea or respiratory arrest, bradypnea is a pattern of regular respirations with a rate of fewer than 12 breaths/minute. This sign results from neurologic and metabolic disorders and drug overdose, which depress the brain's respiratory control centers. (See *Neurologic control of breathing.*)

NEUROLOGIC CONTROL OF BREATHING

The mechanical aspects of breathing are regulated by *respiratory centers,* groups of discrete neurons in the medulla and pons that function as a unit. In the medullary respiratory center, neurons associated with inspiration and neurons associated with expiration interact to control respiratory rate and depth. In the pons, two additional centers interact with the medullary center to regulate rhythm: The *apneustic center* stimulates inspiratory neurons in the medulla to precipitate inspiration; these, in turn, stimulate the *pneumotaxic center* to inhibit inspiration, allowing passive expiration to occur.

Normally, the breathing mechanism is stimulated by increased carbon dioxide levels and decreased oxygen levels in the blood. Chemoreceptors in the medulla and in the carotid and aortic bodies respond to changes in partial pressure of arterial carbon dioxide ($PaCO_2$), partial pressure of arterial oxygen, and pH, signaling respiratory centers to adjust respiratory rate and depth.

Respiratory depression occurs when decreased cerebral perfusion inactivates respiratory center neurons, when changes in $PaCO_2$ and pH affect chemoreceptor responsiveness, or when neuron responsiveness to $PaCO_2$ changes is reduced—for example, because of narcotic overdose.

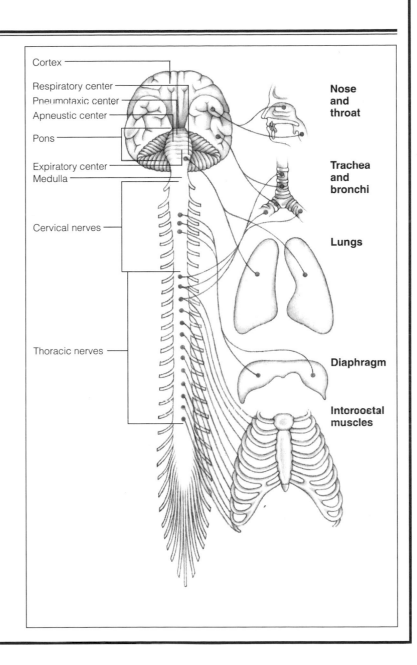

Cortex
Respiratory center
Pneumotaxic center
Apneustic center
Pons
Expiratory center
Medulla
Cervical nerves
Thoracic nerves

Nose and throat

Trachea and bronchi

Lungs

Diaphragm

Intercostal muscles

RESPIRATORY RATES IN CHILDREN

This graph shows normal respiratory rates in children, which are higher than normal rates in adults. Accordingly, bradypnea in children is defined by the age of the child.

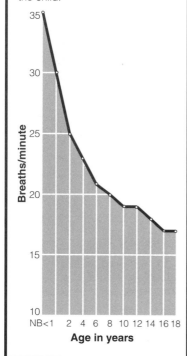

Age in years

Breaths/minute

his ability to move extremities. Place the patient on an apnea monitor, keep emergency airway equipment available, and be prepared to assist with intubation and mechanical ventilation if spontaneous respirations cease. To prevent aspiration, position the patient on his side and clear his airway with suction or finger-sweeps, if necessary.

History and physical examination
Obtain a brief history from the patient, if possible, or whoever accompanied him to the hospital. Ask if the patient may have had a drug overdose; if so, try to determine which drug(s) the patient took, how much, when, and by what route. Check his arms for needle marks, indicating possible drug abuse. You may need to administer I.V. naloxone, a narcotic antagonist.

If you rule out drug overdose, ask about chronic illnesses, such as diabetes and renal failure. Check for medical identification jewelry or an I.D. card that identifies an underlying condition. Also ask whether the patient has a history of head trauma, brain tumor, neurologic infection, or stroke.

Common medical causes
• *Diabetic ketoacidosis.* Bradypnea occurs late in severe, uncontrolled diabetes. Associated signs and symptoms include decreased LOC, fatigue, weakness, fruity breath odor, and oliguria.
• *Hepatic failure.* Occurring in end-stage hepatic failure, bradypnea may be accompanied by coma, hyperactive reflexes, asterixis, a positive Babinski's sign, fetor hepaticus, and other signs.
• *Increased intracranial pressure.* A late sign of this life-threatening condition, bradypnea is preceded by decreased LOC, deteriorated motor function, and fixed, dilated pupils. The triad of bradypnea, bradycardia, and hypertension is a classic sign of late medullary strangulation.

Emergency interventions
 Depending on the degree of central nervous system (CNS) depression, the patient with severe bradypnea may require constant stimulation to breathe. If he seems excessively sleepy, try to arouse him by shaking and instructing him to breathe. Quickly take the patient's vital signs. Assess his neurologic status by checking pupil size and reactions and by evaluating his level of consciousness (LOC) and

• *Respiratory failure.* Bradypnea occurs in end-stage respiratory failure. Its accompanying signs include cyanosis, diminished breath sounds, tachycardia, mildly increased blood pressure, and decreased LOC.

Other causes
• *Drugs.* An overdose of narcotic analgesics and, less commonly, sedatives, barbiturates, phenothiazines, and other CNS depressants can cause bradypnea. Use of any of these drugs with alcohol can also cause bradypnea.

Special considerations
Because the patient with bradypnea may develop apnea, check his respiratory status frequently and be prepared to give ventilatory support if necessary. Don't leave the patient unattended, especially if his LOC is decreased. Keep his bed in the lowest position and raise the side rails. Obtain blood for arterial blood gas analysis, electrolyte studies, and a possible drug screen. Prepare the patient for chest and skull X-rays and, possibly, a computed tomography scan.

Administer drugs and oxygen. Avoid giving CNS depressants to the patient because these drugs exacerbate bradypnea. Similarly, give oxygen judiciously to a patient with chronic carbon dioxide retention, which may occur in chronic obstructive pulmonary disease.

Pediatric pointers
Because respiratory rates are higher in children than in adults, bradypnea in children is defined according to age. (See *Respiratory rates in children.*)

BREAST DIMPLING

Breast dimpling—the puckering or retraction of skin on the breast—results from the abnormal attachment of the skin

---

IDENTIFYING BREAST DIMPLING

Dimpling usually suggests an inflammatory or malignant mass beneath the skin's surface. This illustration shows breast dimpling and nipple retraction caused by a malignant mass above the areola.

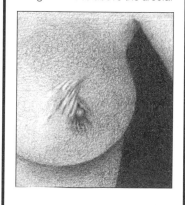

---

to underlying tissue. It suggests an inflammatory or malignant mass beneath the surface of the skin and usually represents a late sign of breast cancer; benign lesions usually don't produce this effect. Dimpling usually affects women over age 40 but also occasionally occurs in males.

Because breast dimpling occurs over a mass or induration, the patient usually discovers other signs before becoming aware of dimpling. However, a thorough breast examination may reveal dimpling and may alert the patient and nurse to a breast problem. (See *Identifying breast dimpling.*)

History and physical examination
Obtain a medical, reproductive, and family history, noting factors that place the patient at a high risk for breast cancer. Ask about her pregnancy history because women who don't experience a full-term

pregnancy until after age 30 are at a higher risk for developing breast cancer. How old was the patient when she began menstruation? How old was she at menopause? More than 30 years of menstrual activity increases the risk of breast cancer.

Has her mother or a sister had breast cancer? Has she herself had cancer before, especially in the other breast? Ask about her dietary habits because a high-fat diet predisposes women to breast cancer.

Ask your patient if she's noticed any changes in the shape of her breast. Is any area painful or tender, and is the pain cyclical? If she's lactating, has she recently experienced high fever, chills, malaise, muscle aches, fatigue, or other flulike symptoms? Can she remember sustaining any traumatic injury to the breast?

Carefully inspect the dimpled area. Is it swollen, red, or warm to the touch? Are bruises or contusions present? Ask the patient to tense her pectoral muscles by pressing her hips with both hands or by raising her hands over her head. Does puckering increase? Gently pull the skin upward toward the clavicle. Is dimpling exaggerated?

Observe the breast for nipple retraction. Do both nipples point in the same direction? Are the nipples flattened or inverted? Does the patient report nipple discharge? If so, ask her to describe the color and character of the discharge. Observe the contour of both breasts. Are they symmetrical?

Examine both breasts with the patient supine, sitting, and leaning forward. Does the skin move freely over both breasts? If you can palpate a lump, describe its size, location, consistency, mobility, and delineation. What relation does the lump have to breast dimpling? Gently mold the breast skin around the lump. Is dimpling exaggerated? Also examine breast and axillary lymph nodes, noting any enlargement.

Common medical causes

● *Breast cancer.* Breast dimpling is an important but somewhat *late* sign of a malignant tumor. A neoplasm that causes dimpling is usually close to the skin and at least $3/8''$ (1 cm) in diameter; it feels irregularly shaped and fixed to underlying tissue. Other signs of breast cancer may include peau d'orange; changes in breast symmetry or size; nipple retraction; and a unilateral, spontaneous, nonmilky nipple discharge that is serous or bloody. (Bloody nipple discharge in the presence of a lump is a classic sign of breast cancer.) Axillary lymph nodes may be enlarged. Pain may be present but isn't a reliable symptom of breast cancer. A breast ulcer may appear as a late sign.

● *Fat necrosis.* Breast dimpling from fat necrosis follows inflammation and trauma to fatty tissue of the breast. Tenderness, erythema, bruising, and contusions may occur, although many patients can't remember an incident of breast injury or trauma. Findings include a hard, indurated, poorly delineated lump, which is fibrotic and fixed to underlying tissue or overlying skin as well as signs of nipple retraction.

● *Mastitis.* Breast dimpling may signal bacterial mastitis, which usually results from duct obstruction and milk stasis during lactation. Heat, erythema, swelling, induration, pain, and tenderness usually accompany mastitis. Dimpling is more likely to occur with diffuse induration than with a single hard mass. The skin on the breast may feel fixed to underlying tissue. Other possible findings include nipple retraction, nipple cracks, a puslike discharge, and enlarged axillary lymph nodes. Flulike signs and symptoms, such as fever, malaise, fatigue, and aching, commonly occur.

Special considerations

Remember that any breast problem can arouse fears of mutilation, loss of sexuality, and death. Allow the patient to express her feelings.

Provide a clear explanation of diagnostic tests that may be ordered, such as mammography, thermography, ultrasound, cytology of nipple discharge, and biopsy.

Discuss breast self-examination, and provide follow-up teaching when the patient expresses a readiness to learn. Advise the lactating mother with mastitis to pump her breasts to prevent further milk stasis, to discard the milk, and to substitute formula until the breast infection responds adequately to antibiotics.

Pediatric pointers

Because breast cancer, the most likely cause of dimpling, is extremely rare in children, consider trauma as a likely cause. As in the adult, breast dimpling may occur in an adolescent as a result of fatty tissue necrosis due to trauma.

BREAST NODULE
[Breast lump]

A commonly reported gynecologic sign, breast nodules have two chief causes: benign breast disease and cancer. Benign breast disease, the leading cause of nodules, can stem from cyst formation in obstructed and dilated lactiferous ducts, hypertrophy or tumor formation in the ductal system, inflammation, or infection.

Although fewer than 20% of breast nodules are malignant, the clinical signs of breast cancer aren't easily distinguished from those of benign breast disease.

Breast cancer is a leading cause of death among women but can occur occasionally in men, with signs and symptoms mimicking those found in women. Thus, breast nodules in both sexes should always be evaluated.

ALTERNATIVE THERAPY

FATTY ACIDS AND CANCER PREVENTION

Omega-3 fatty acids, polyunsaturated fats thought to be essential for cell function, are believed to have some beneficial effects in preventing breast cancer. Soybeans, linseed oil, and cold water fish, such as herring, salmon, and sardines, are rich in omega-3 fatty acids.

Breast cancer prevention is a mainstream focus for researchers today. Research studies have shown that alternative therapy, such as diet modification with specific foods have been linked to cancer prevention. (See *Fatty acids and cancer prevention.*)

Part of breast cancer prevention includes breast self-examination. A woman who's familiar with the feel of her breasts and performs a monthly breast self-examination can detect a nodule 6 mm or less in size, considerably smaller than the 1-cm nodule that's readily detectable by an experienced examiner. However, a woman may not report a nodule because of fear of breast cancer.

History and physical examination

If your patient reports a lump, ask her how and when she discovered it. Does the size and tenderness of the lump vary with her menstrual cycle? Has the lump changed since she first noticed it? Is she aware of any other breast signs, such as discharge or nipple changes?

Find out if the patient has noticed a change in breast shape, size, or contour. Is she lactating? Does she have fever, chills, fatigue, or other flulike signs and symptoms? Ask her to describe any pain or tenderness associated with the lump. Is the pain in one breast only? Has she sustained recent trauma to the breast?

Explore the patient's medical and family history for factors that increase her risk of breast cancer. These include a high-fat diet, having a mother or sister with breast cancer, or having a history of other cancers, especially cancer in the other breast. Other risk factors include nulliparity, a first pregnancy after age 30, and early menarche or late menopause.

Next, perform a thorough breast examination. Pay special attention to the upper outer quadrant of each breast, where half the ductal tissue is located. This is the most common site of malignant breast tumors.

Carefully palpate a suspected breast nodule, noting its location, shape, size, consistency, mobility, and delineation. Does the nodule feel soft, rubbery, and elastic, or hard? Is it mobile, slipping away from your fingers as you palpate it, or firmly fixed to adjacent tissue? Does the nodule seem to limit the mobility of the entire breast? Note the nodule's delineation. Are the borders clearly defined or indefinite? Or does the area feel more like a hardness or diffuse induration than a nodule with definite borders?

Do you feel one nodule or several small ones? Is the shape round, oval, lobular, or irregular? Inspect and palpate the skin over the nodule for warmth, redness, and edema. Palpate the lymph nodes of the breast and axilla for enlargement.

Observe the contour of your patient's breasts, looking for asymmetry and irregularities. Be alert for signs of retraction, such as skin dimpling and nipple deviation, retraction, or flattening. (To exaggerate dimpling, have your patient raise her arms over her head or press her hands against her hips.) Gently pull the breast skin toward the clavicle. Is dimpling evident? Mold the breast skin and again observe for dimpling.

Be alert for nipple discharge that's spontaneous, unilateral, and nonmilky (serous, bloody, or purulent). Be careful not to confuse it with the grayish discharge that can be elicited from the nipples of a woman who has been pregnant.

Common medical causes

● *Adenofibroma.* The extremely mobile or "slippery" feel of this benign neoplasm helps distinguish it from other breast nodules. The nodule usually occurs singly and characteristically feels firm, elastic, and round or lobular, with well-defined margins. It doesn't cause pain or tenderness, can vary from pinhead size to very large, commonly grows rapidly, and usually lies around the nipple or on the lateral side of the upper outer quadrant.

● *Areolar gland abscess.* Tender, palpable abscesses on the periphery of the areola follow inflammation of the sebaceous glands of Montgomery. Fever may also be present.

● *Breast abscess.* A localized, hot, tender, fluctuant mass with erythema and peau d'orange typifies *acute abscess.* Associated signs and symptoms commonly include fever, chills, malaise, and generalized discomfort. In *chronic abscess,* the nodule is nontender, irregular, and firm and may feel like a thick wall of fibrous tissue. It's commonly accompanied by skin dimpling, peau d'orange, and nipple retraction and sometimes by axillary lymphadenopathy.

● *Breast cancer.* A hard, poorly delineated nodule that is fixed to the skin or underlying tissue suggests breast cancer. Malignant nodules commonly cause breast dimpling, nipple deviation or retraction, or flattening of the nipple or breast contour. Of all malignant nodules, 40% to 50% occur in the upper outer quadrant.

Nodules usually occur singly, although satellite nodules may surround the main one. Nipple discharge may be serous or bloody. (Bloody nipple discharge in the presence of a nodule is a classic sign of breast cancer.) Additional findings may

BREAST NODULE: COMMON CAUSES AND ASSOCIATED FINDINGS

KEY CAUSES	MAJOR ASSOCIATED SIGNS AND SYMPTOMS							
	Breast dimpling	Breast pain or tenderness	Erythema	Fever	Lymphadenopathy	Nipple discharge	Nipple retraction signs	Peau d'orange
Areolar gland abscess		•	•					
Breast abscess (acute)		•	•	•				•
Breast abscess (chronic)	•					•	•	•
Breast cancer	•	•	•		•	•	•	•
Mastitis	•	•	•	•			•	•
Proliferative breast disease		•				•		

include edema of the skin overlying the mass, peau d'orange, erythema, tenderness, and axillary lymphadenopathy. A breast ulcer may occur as a late sign. Breast pain, an unreliable symptom, may be present.

• *Mastitis.* In this disorder, breast nodules feel firm and indurated or tender, flocculent, and discrete. Gentle palpation defines the area of maximum purulent accumulation. Skin dimpling and nipple deviation, retraction, or flattening may be present, and the nipple may show a crack or abrasion. Accompanying signs and symptoms include breast warmth, erythema, tenderness, and edema, peau d'orange, plus high fever, chills, malaise, and fatigue.

• *Paget's disease.* This slow-growing intraductal carcinoma begins as a scaling, eczematoid nipple lesion. Later, the nipple becomes reddened and excoriated; complete destruction of the structure may result. The process extends along the skin as well as in the ducts, usually progressing to a deep seated mass.

• *Proliferative breast disease.* The most common cause of breast nodules, this fibrocystic condition produces smooth, round, slightly elastic nodules, which increase in size and tenderness just before menstruation. The nodules may occur in fine, granular clusters in both breasts or as widespread, well-defined lumps of varying sizes. A thickening of adjacent tissue may be palpable.

Cystic nodules are mobile, which helps differentiate them from malignant ones. Because cystic nodules aren't fixed to underlying breast tissue, they don't produce retraction signs, such as nipple deviation or dimpling. A clear, watery (serous), or sticky nipple discharge may appear in one or both breasts. Signs and symptoms of premenstrual syndrome, such as headache, irritability, bloating, nausea, vomiting, and abdominal cramping, may also be present.

Special considerations

Even though many women associate a breast lump with breast cancer, most nodules are benign. As a result, try to avoid alarming your patient further. Provide a simple explanation of your examination, and encourage the patient to express her feelings.

Prepare the patient for diagnostic tests, which may include transillumination, mammography, thermography, needle aspiration or open biopsy of the nodule for tissue examination, and cytologic examination of nipple discharge.

Postpone teaching the patient how to perform breast self-examination until she overcomes her initial anxiety at discovering a nodule. Regular breast self-examination is especially important for women who've had cancer previously, who have a family history of breast cancer, who are nulliparous or had their first child after age 30, and who had an early menarche or late menopause.

Although most nodules occurring during lactation result from mastitis, the possibility of cancer demands careful evaluation. Advise the lactating mother with mastitis to pump her breasts to prevent further milk stasis, to discard the milk, and to substitute formula until the infection responds to antibiotics.

Pediatric pointers

Most nodules in children and adolescents reflect the normal response of breast tissue to hormonal fluctuations. For instance, the breasts of young teenage girls may normally contain cord-like nodules that become tender just before menstruation.

A transient breast nodule in young boys (as well as in women between ages 20 and 30) may result from juvenile mastitis. Signs of inflammation are present in a firm mass beneath the nipple. Usually, one breast is affected.

BREAST PAIN
[Mastalgia]

An unreliable indicator of cancer, this symptom commonly results from benign breast disease. It may occur during rest or movement and may be aggravated by manipulation or palpation. (Breast *tenderness* refers to pain *elicited* by physical contact.)

Breast pain may be unilateral or bilateral; cyclic, intermittent, or constant; and dull or sharp. It may result from surface cuts, furuncles, contusions, and similar lesions (superficial pain); nipple fissures and inflammation in the papillary ducts and areolae (severe, localized pain); stromal distention in the breast parenchyma; a tumor that affects nerve endings (severe, constant pain); or inflammatory lesions that not only distend the stroma but also irritate sensory nerve endings (severe pain). Breast pain may radiate to the back, the arms, and sometimes the neck.

Women may experience breast tenderness before menstruation and during pregnancy. Before menstruation, breast pain or tenderness stems from increased mammary blood flow resulting from hormonal changes. During pregnancy, breast tenderness and throbbing, tingling, or pricking sensations are also influenced by hormonal changes.

In men, breast pain may stem from gynecomastia (especially during puberty and senescence), reproductive tract anomalies, and organic disease of the liver or pituitary, adrenal cortex, and thyroid glands.

History and physical examination

Begin by asking the patient if breast pain is constant or intermittent. For either type, ask about onset and character. If the pain is intermittent, determine the relationship of pain to the phase of the menstrual cycle. Determine if the patient is a nursing mother. If not, ask her if she has any nipple discharge and have her describe it. Is she pregnant? Has she reached menopause? Has she recently experienced any flulike symptoms or sustained any injury to the breast? Has she noticed any change in breast shape or contour?

Ask the patient to describe the pain. She may describe it as sticking, stinging, shooting, stabbing, throbbing, or burning. Determine if the pain affects one breast or both, and ask the patient to point to the painful area.

Instruct the patient to place her arms at her sides, and inspect the breasts. Note their size, symmetry, and contour, and the appearance of the skin. Remember that breast shape and size vary widely and that breasts normally change during the menstrual cycle, pregnancy, and lactation and with aging. Are the breasts red or edematous? Are the veins prominent?

Note the size, shape, and symmetry of the nipples and areolae. Is ecchymosis, rash, ulceration, or discharge present? Do the nipples point in the same direction? Do you see signs of retraction, such as skin dimpling or nipple inversion or flattening?

Repeat your inspection, first with the patient's arms raised above her head and then with her hands pressed against her hips.

Palpate the breasts, first with the patient seated and then with her lying down and a pillow placed under her shoulder on the side being examined. Use the pads of your fingers to compress breast tissue against the chest wall. Proceed systematically from the sternum to the midline and from the axilla to the midline, noting any warmth, tenderness, nodules, masses, or irregularities. Palpate the nipple, noting tenderness and nodules, and check for discharge. Palpate axillary lymph nodes, noting any enlargement.

Common medical causes

• *Areolar gland abscess.* Tender, palpable abscesses on the periphery of the areola follow inflammation of the sebaceous glands of Montgomery. Fever may also occur.

• *Breast abscess (acute).* In the affected breast, local pain, tenderness, erythema, peau d'orange, and warmth are associated with a nodule. Malaise, fever, and chills may also occur.

• *Breast cyst.* A breast cyst that enlarges rapidly may cause acute, localized, and usually unilateral pain. A palpable breast nodule may be present.

• *Mammary duct ectasia.* Burning pain and itching around the areola may occur, although ectasia is commonly asymptomatic at first. The history may include one or more episodes of inflammation with pain, tenderness, erythema, and acute fever, or with pain and tenderness alone, which develop and then subside spontaneously within 7 to 10 days. Other findings may include a rubbery, subareolar breast nodule; swelling and erythema around the nipple; nipple retraction; a bluish green discoloration or edema of the skin overlying the nodule; peau d'orange, a thick, sticky, multicolored nipple discharge; and possible axillary lymphadenopathy. Breast ulcer may occur in late stages.

• *Mastitis.* Unilateral pain may be severe, particularly when the inflammation occurs near the skin surface. Breast skin is commonly red and warm at the inflammation site and may have an orange-peel appearance (peau d'orange). Palpation reveals a firm area of induration. Skin retraction signs, such as breast dimpling and nipple deviation, inversion, or flattening, may be present. Systemic signs and symptoms, such as high fever, chills, malaise, and fatigue, may also be present.

BREAST PAIN: COMMON CAUSES AND ASSOCIATED FINDINGS

CAUSES	MAJOR ASSOCIATED SIGNS AND SYMPTOMS							
	Breast nodule	Erythema	Fever	Lymphadenop- athy	Nipple discharge	Nipple retraction signs	Peau d'orange	Pruritis
Areolar gland abscess	●		●					
Breast abscess (acute)	●	●	●				●	
Mammary duct ectasia	●	●		●	●	●	●	●
Mastitis	●	●	●			●	●	
Proliferative breast disease	●				●			
Sebaceous cyst (infected)	●	●						

● **Proliferative (fibrocystic) breast disease.** In this common cause of breast pain, cysts may cause pain before menstruation and be asymptomatic after it. Later in the disease's course, pain and tenderness may persist throughout the cycle. The cysts feel firm, mobile, and well defined; they're commonly bilateral and found in the upper outer quadrant of the breast but may also be unilateral and generalized. A clear, watery nipple discharge may be present in one or both breasts. Signs and symptoms of premenstrual syndrome (headache, irritability, bloating, nausea, vomiting, and abdominal cramping) may also be present.

● **Sebaceous (infected) cyst.** This cutaneous cyst may produce breast pain;. a small, well-delineated nodule; localized erythema; and induration.

Special considerations
Administer pain medication if needed. Suggest that the patient wear a well-fitting brassiere for support, especially if her breasts are large or pendulous.

Provide emotional support for the patient and, when appropriate, emphasize the importance of monthly breast self-examination. Teach the patient how to perform this examination, and instruct her to call the doctor immediately if she detects any breast changes.

Prepare the patient for diagnostic tests, such as mammography, thermography, cytology of nipple discharge, biopsy, or culture of any aspirate.

Pediatric pointers
Transient gynecomastia can cause breast pain in males during puberty.

BREAST ULCER

Appearing on the nipple, areola, or the breast itself, an ulcer indicates destruction of the skin and subcutaneous tissue. A breast ulcer is usually a late sign of cancer, appearing well after confirming diagnosis. However, it may be the presenting sign of breast cancer in men, who are more apt to dismiss earlier breast changes. Breast ulcer can also result from trauma, infection, or radiation. (See *Identifying a breast ulcer.*)

History and physical examination
Begin the history by asking when the patient first noticed the ulcer and if it was preceded by other breast changes, such as nodules, edema, or nipple discharge, deviation, or retraction. Has she noticed any change in breast shape? Does the ulcer seem to be getting better or worse? Does it cause pain or produce drainage? Has the patient noticed a skin rash? If she has been treating the ulcer at home, find out how.

Review the patient's personal and family history for factors that increase the risk of breast cancer. Ask, for example, about previous cancer, especially of the breast, and mastectomy. Determine if the patient's mother or sister has had breast cancer. Ask the patient's age at menarche and menopause because more than 30 years of menstrual activity increases the risk of breast cancer. Also ask about pregnancy because nulliparity or birth of a first child after age 30 also increases the risk of breast cancer.

If the patient recently gave birth, ask if she breast-feeds her infant or has recently weaned him. Ask if she's currently taking any oral antibiotics and if she's diabetic. All these factors predispose the patient to candidal infections.

Inspect the patient's breasts, noting any asymmetry or flattening. Look for a

IDENTIFYING A BREAST ULCER

Skin irritations and cancer can cause ulcers on the breast, nipple, or areola. The area of tissue destruction can vary in size.

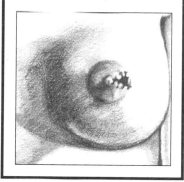

rash, scaling, cracking, or red excoriation on the nipples, areola, and inframammary fold. Check especially for skin changes, such as warmth, erythema, edema, peau d'orange. Palpate the breasts for masses, noting any induration beneath the ulcer. Then carefully palpate for tenderness or nodules around the areola and the axillary lymph nodes.

Common medical causes
● *Breast cancer.* A breast ulcer that does not heal within a month usually indicates cancer. Ulceration along a mastectomy scar may indicate metastatic cancer; a nodule beneath the ulcer may be a late sign of a fulminating tumor.

Other signs include a palpable breast nodule, skin dimpling, nipple retraction, bloody or serous nipple discharge, erythema, peau d'orange, and enlarged axillary lymph nodes.
● *Breast trauma.* Tissue destruction with inadequate healing may produce breast ulcers. Associated signs depend on the type of trauma but may include ecchy-

mosis, lacerations, abrasions, swelling, and hematoma.

● **Candida albicans *infection.*** A severe candidal infection can cause maceration of breast tissue followed by ulceration. Well-defined, red papular patches (often with scaly borders) characterize the infection, which can develop in the breast folds. In breast-feeding women, cracked nipples predispose to infection.

● ***Paget's disease.*** Bright red nipple excoriation can extend to the areola and ulcerate. Serous or bloody nipple discharge and extreme nipple itching may occur.

Other causes

● ***Radiation therapy.*** After treatment, the breasts appear sunburned. Subsequently, the skin ulcerates and the surrounding area becomes red and tender.

Special considerations

Because breast ulcers become infected easily, teach the patient how to apply topical antifungal ointment or cream. Instruct her to keep the ulcer dry to reduce chafing and to wear loose-fitting undergarments.

If breast cancer is suspected, provide emotional support and prepare the patient for diagnostic tests, such as ultrasonography, thermography, mammography, nipple discharge cytology, and breast biopsy. If a candidal infection is suspected, prepare her for skin or blood cultures.

BREATH WITH AMMONIA ODOR
[Uremic fetor]

The odor of ammonia on the breath—described as urinous or "fishy" breath—typically occurs in end-stage chronic renal failure. This sign improves slightly after hemodialysis and persists throughout the disorder's course, but it isn't of great concern.

Ammonia breath odor reflects the long-term metabolic and biochemical abnormalities associated with uremia and end-stage chronic renal failure. This odor is produced by metabolic end products blown off by the lungs and breakdown of urea in the saliva to ammonia. But a specific uremic toxin has not yet been identified. In animals, breath odor analysis has revealed toxic metabolites, such as dimethylamine and trimethylamine, which contribute to the "fishy" odor. The source of these amines may be intestinal bacteria acting on dietary chlorine.

History and physical examination

When you detect ammonia breath odor, the diagnosis of chronic renal failure will probably already be well established. But look for associated GI symptoms so that palliative care and support can be individualized.

Inspect the patient's oral cavity for bleeding, swollen gums or tongue, and for ulceration with drainage. Ask the patient if he has experienced a metallic taste, loss of smell, increased thirst, heartburn, difficulty swallowing, or loss of appetite at the sight of food. Ask about early morning vomiting. Because GI bleeding is common in chronic renal failure, ask about bowel habits, noting especially melenous stools or constipation.

Take the patient's vital signs. Watch for any signs of hypertension (the patient with end-stage chronic renal failure is usually somewhat hypertensive) or hypotension. Be alert for other signs of shock (tachycardia, tachypnea, and cool, clammy skin) and altered mental status. Any significant changes can indicate complications, such as massive GI bleeding or pericarditis with tamponade.

Common medical causes

● ***End-stage chronic renal failure.*** Ammonia breath odor is a late finding. Accompanying signs and symptoms include anuria, skin pigmentation changes and excoriation, brown arcs under the nail margins, tissue wasting, Kussmaul's respirations, neuropathy, lethargy, somnolence, confusion, disorientation, behavior changes with irritability, and mood lability. Later neurologic signs that signal impending uremic coma include muscle twitching and fasciculation, asterixis, paresthesias, and footdrop.

Cardiovascular findings may include hypertension and signs of congestive heart failure and pericarditis. GI findings include anorexia, nausea, heartburn, vomiting, constipation, hiccups, and a metallic taste, with oral manifestations such as stomatitis, gum ulceration and bleeding, and a coated tongue. Weight loss is common. Uremic frost, pruritus, and signs of hormonal changes, such as impotence or amenorrhea, also appear.

Special considerations

Ammonia breath odor is offensive to others, but the patient may become accustomed to it. As a result, remind him to perform frequent mouth care, particularly before meals because reducing foul mouth taste and odor may stimulate his appetite. A half-strength hydrogen peroxide mixture or lemon juice gargle helps neutralize the ammonia; the patient may also want to use commercial lozenges or breath sprays or to suck on hard candy. Advise him to use a soft toothbrush or sponge to prevent trauma. If the patient is unable to perform mouth care, do it for him and teach his family members how to assist him.

Maximize dietary intake by offering the patient frequent small meals of his favorite foods, within dietary limitations. Encourage him to take the ordered antacids.

Pediatric pointers

Ammonia breath odor occurs in the child with end-stage chronic renal failure. Provide hard candies to relieve bad mouth taste and odor. If the child is able to gargle, try mixing hydrogen peroxide with flavored mouthwashes.

BREATH WITH FECAL ODOR

Fecal breath odor may follow an episode of prolonged vomiting associated with long-standing intestinal obstruction or gastrojejunocolic fistula. It is an important late diagnostic clue to a potentially life-threatening GI disorder because complete obstruction of any part of the bowel, if untreated, can cause death within hours from vascular collapse and shock.

When an obstructed or adynamic intestine attempts self-decompression by regurgitating its contents, vigorous peristaltic waves propel bowel contents backward into the stomach. When the stomach fills with intestinal fluid, further reverse peristalsis results in vomiting. The odor of feculent vomitus lingers in the mouth.

In addition, fecal breath odor may occur in the patient with a nasogastric (NG) or intestinal tube. The odor is detected only while the underlying disorder persists and abates soon after its resolution.

Emergency interventions

 Because fecal breath odor signals a potentially life-threatening intestinal obstruction, you'll need to quickly evaluate your patient's condition. Monitor vital signs and be alert for signs of shock, such as hypotension, tachycardia, narrowed pulse pressure, and cool, clammy skin.

Ask the patient if he's experiencing nausea and if he has vomited. Also ask about the frequency of vomiting and have him describe the color, odor, amount, and consistency of the vomitus. Have an emesis basin nearby to collect and accurately measure any vomitus.

Anticipating possible surgery to relieve an obstruction or repair a fistula, withhold all food and fluids. Be prepared to insert an NG or intestinal tube for GI

FECAL BREATH ODOR: COMMON CAUSES AND ASSOCIATED FINDINGS

S&S CAUSES	MAJOR ASSOCIATED SIGNS AND SYMPTOMS									
	Abdominal distention	Abdominal pain	Anorexia	Constipation	Diarrhea	Hyperactive bowel sounds	Hypoactive or absent bowel sounds	Nausea	Vomiting	Weight loss
Distal small-bowel obstruction	●	●		●	●	●		●	●	●
Gastrojejunocolic fistula	●	●	●		●				●	●
Large-bowel obstruction	●	●		●				●	●	

tract decompression. Insert a peripheral I.V. line for vascular access, or assist with central line insertion for large-bore access and central venous pressure monitoring. Obtain a blood sample and send it to the laboratory for complete blood count and electrolyte analysis because large fluid losses and shifts can produce electrolyte imbalances. Maintain adequate hydration and support circulatory status with additional fluids. Give a physiologic solution, such as lactated Ringer's, normal saline, or Plasmanate, to prevent metabolic acidosis from gastric losses and metabolic alkalosis from intestinal fluid losses.

History and physical examination
If the patient's condition permits, ask about previous abdominal surgery because adhesions can cause an obstruction. Also ask about loss of appetite. Determine if the patient is experiencing abdominal pain and have him describe its onset, duration, and location. Ask if the pain is intense, persistent, or spasmodic. Have the patient describe his normal

bowel habits, noting especially constipation, diarrhea, or leakage of stool. Ask when his last bowel movement occurred, and have him describe its color and consistency.

Auscultate for bowel sounds—hyperactive, high-pitched sounds may indicate *impending* bowel obstruction, whereas hypoactive or absent sounds occur *late* in obstruction and paralytic ileus. Inspect the abdomen, noting contour and any surgical scars. Measure abdominal girth to provide baseline data for subsequent assessment of distention. Palpate for tenderness, distention, and rigidity. Percuss for tympany, indicating a gas-filled bowel, and dullness, indicating fluid.

Common medical causes
● *Distal small-bowel obstruction*. In late obstruction, nausea is present although vomiting may be delayed. Initially, vomitus is gastric contents, changing to bilious and then to fecal contents with resultant fecal breath odor. Accompanying symptoms may include achiness, malaise, drowsiness, and polydipsia.

Bowel changes range from diarrhea to constipation and occur with abdominal distention, persistent epigastric or periumbilical colicky pain, and hyperactive bowel sounds and borborygmi, changing to hypoactive or absent sounds in later stages as the obstruction becomes complete. Fever, hypotension, tachycardia, and rebound tenderness may indicate strangulation or perforation.

• *Gastrojejunocolic fistula.* In this disorder, symptoms may be variable and intermittent because of temporary plugging of the fistula. Fecal vomiting with resulting fecal breath odor may occur. Diarrhea is the most common presenting sign, and abdominal pain commonly occurs. Related GI findings include anorexia, weight loss, and abdominal distention.

• *Large-bowel obstruction.* Vomiting is usually absent at first, but fecal vomiting with resultant fecal breath odor occurs as a late sign. Symptoms typically develop more slowly than in small-bowel obstruction. Colicky abdominal pain appears suddenly, followed by continuous hypogastric pain. Marked abdominal distention and tenderness occur, and loops of large bowel may be visible through the abdominal wall. Although constipation develops, defecation may continue for up to 3 days after complete obstruction because of stool remaining in the bowel below the obstruction. Leakage of stool is common with partial obstruction.

Special considerations

After an NG or intestinal tube has been inserted, keep the head of the bed elevated at least 30 degrees and turn the patient to facilitate gravity passage of the intestinal tube through the GI tract. Don't tape the intestinal tube to the patient's face. Ensure tube patency by monitoring drainage and watching that suction devices function properly. Irrigate as required. Monitor GI drainage losses, and send serum specimens to the laboratory for electrolyte analysis at least once a day. Prepare the patient for diagnostic tests, such as abdominal X-rays, barium enema, and proctoscopy.

Encourage the patient to brush his teeth and gargle with a flavored mouthwash or half-strength hydrogen peroxide mixture to minimize offensive breath odor. Assure him that the fecal odor is temporary and will abate after treatment for the underlying cause.

Pediatric pointers

Carefully monitor the child's fluid and electrolyte status. Children can rapidly become dehydrated from persistent vomiting.

BREATH WITH FRUITY ODOR

Fruity breath odor results from respiratory elimination of excess acetone. This sign characteristically occurs in ketoacidosis—a potentially life-threatening condition that requires immediate treatment to prevent severe dehydration, irreversible coma, and death.

Ketoacidosis results from the excessive catabolism of fats for cellular energy in the absence of usable carbohydrates. This occurs when insulin levels are insufficient to transport glucose into the cells, as in diabetes mellitus, or when glucose is unavailable and hepatic glycogen stores are depleted, as in low-carbohydrate diets and malnutrition. Lacking glucose, the cells burn fat faster than enzymes can handle the ketones, the acidic end products. As a result, the ketones (acetone, beta-hydroxybutyric acid, and acetoacetic acid) accumulate in the blood and urine. To compensate for increased acidity, Kussmaul's respirations expel carbon dioxide with enough acetone to flavor the breath. Eventually, this compensatory mechanism fails, producing ketoacidosis.

Emergency interventions

 When you detect fruity breath odor, check for Kussmaul's respirations and examine the patient's level of consciousness. Check vital signs and skin turgor. Be alert for fruity breath odor that accompanies rapid, deep respirations, stupor, and poor skin turgor. Try to obtain a brief history, noting especially diabetes mellitus, nutritional problems such as anorexia nervosa, and fad diets with little or no carbohydrate.

Obtain venous and arterial blood samples for glucose, electrolyte, acetone, complete blood count, and arterial blood gas (ABG) studies. Obtain a urine specimen, and test for glucose and acetone. Give I.V. fluids and electrolytes to maintain hydration and electrolyte balance and, in diabetic ketoacidosis, regular insulin to reduce blood glucose levels.

If the patient is obtunded, you'll need to insert endotracheal and nasogastric (NG) tubes. Suction the tubes as needed. Insert an indwelling urinary catheter and monitor intake and output. Insert central venous pressure and arterial lines to monitor the patient's fluid status and blood pressure. Place the patient on a cardiac monitor, monitor vital signs and neurologic status, and draw blood hourly for glucose, acetone, electrolyte, and ABG studies.

History and physical examination

If the patient isn't in severe distress, obtain a thorough history. Ask about the onset and duration of fruity breath odor. Find out about any changes in breathing pattern. Ask about increased thirst, frequent urination, weight loss, fatigue, and abdominal pain. Ask the female patient if she has had monilial vaginitis or has vaginal secretions with itching. If the patient has a history of diabetes mellitus, ask about stress, infections, and non-compliance with therapy—the most common causes of ketoacidosis in the known diabetic. For the patient with suspected severe weight loss, obtain a dietary and weight history.

Common medical causes

● **Ketoacidosis.** Fruity breath odor accompanies *alcoholic ketoacidosis*, which usually occurs in females with a history of alcohol abuse. It typically follows cessation of drinking after a marked increase in alcohol consumption has caused severe vomiting. Kussmaul's respirations begin abruptly and accompany dehydration, abdominal pain and distention, and absent bowel sounds. In *diabetic ketoacidosis,* fruity breath odor commonly occurs as the ketoacidosis develops over 1 to 2 days. Other findings include polydipsia, polyuria, weak and rapid pulse, hunger, weight loss, weakness, fatigue, nausea, vomiting, and abdominal pain. Eventually, Kussmaul's respirations, orthostatic hypotension, dehydration, tachycardia, confusion, and stupor occur. Symptoms may lead to coma.

Starvation ketoacidosis is a potentially life-threatening disorder that develops gradually. Besides fruity breath odor, typical findings include signs of cachexia and dehydration, decreased level of consciousness, bradycardia, and a history of severely limited food intake.

Other causes

● **Drugs.** Any drug known to cause metabolic acidosis, such as nitroprusside, can result in fruity breath odor.

Special considerations

Provide emotional support for the patient and his family. Explain tests and treatments clearly.

When the patient is more alert and his condition stabilizes, remove any NG tube and start him on an appropriate diet. Switch the diabetic's insulin from I.V. to the subcutaneous route.

Provide appropriate patient teaching and referrals. For example, teach the patient with uncontrolled diabetes mellitus to recognize the signs of hyperglycemia and to wear a medical identification bracelet. Refer the patient with starvation ketoacidosis to a psychologist or a support group, and inform him that he may need long-term follow-up care.

Pediatric pointers
Fruity breath odor in an infant or a child usually stems from uncontrolled diabetes mellitus. Ketoacidosis, however, develops rapidly in this age-group because of low glycogen reserves. As a result, prompt administration of insulin and correction of fluid and electrolyte imbalance is necessary to prevent shock and death.

BRUDZINSKI'S SIGN

A positive Brudzinski's sign (flexion of the hips and knees in response to passive flexion of the neck) signals meningeal irritation. Passive flexion of the neck stretches the nerve roots, causing pain and involuntary flexion of the knees and hips.

Brudzinski's sign is a common and important early indicator of life-threatening meningitis and subarachnoid hemorrhage. It can be elicited in children as well as adults, although more reliable indicators of meningeal irritation exist for infants.

Testing for Brudzinski's sign isn't usually part of a routine examination unless meningeal irritation is suspected. (See *Testing for Brudzinski's sign*, page 104.)

Emergency interventions
 If the patient is alert, ask him about headache, neck pain, nausea, and visual disturbances (blurred or double vision and photophobia)—all symptoms of increased intracranial pressure (ICP). Next, observe for signs and symptoms of increased ICP, such as altered level of consciousness ([LOC] restlessness, irritability, confusion, lethargy, personality changes, and coma), pupillary changes, bradycardia, widened pulse pressure, irregular respiratory patterns (Cheyne-Stokes or Kussmaul's respirations), vomiting, and moderate fever.

Keep artificial airways, intubation equipment, a handheld resuscitation bag, and suction equipment on hand because your patient's condition may deteriorate suddenly. Elevate the head of the bed 30 to 60 degrees to promote venous drainage. Administer an osmotic diuretic such as mannitol to reduce cerebral edema.

Monitor ICP and be alert for ICP that continues to rise. You may have to provide mechanical ventilation and administer barbiturates and additional doses of diuretics. Also, cerebrospinal fluid (CSF) may have to be drained.

History and physical examination
Continue your neurologic examination by evaluating the patient's cranial nerve function and noting any motor or sensory deficits. Also, look for Kernig's sign (resistance to knee extension after flexion of the hip), a further sign of meningeal irritation. In addition, look for signs of central nervous system infection, such as fever and nuchal rigidity.

Ask the patient or his family, if necessary, about a history of hypertension, spinal arthritis, or recent head trauma. Ask about recent dental work and any abscessed teeth (a possible cause of meningitis) and about open head injury, endocarditis, and I.V. drug abuse. Also ask about sudden onset of headaches, which may be associated with subarachnoid hemorrhage.

Common medical causes
• *Arthritis.* In severe spinal arthritis, a positive Brudzinski's sign can occasionally be elicited. The patient may also report back pain (especially after weight bearing) and limited mobility.

TESTING FOR BRUDZINSKI'S SIGN

Here's how to test for Brudzinski's sign when you suspect meningeal irritation:

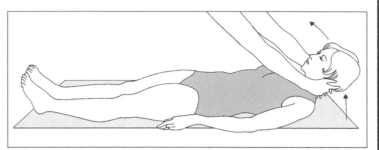

With the patient in a supine position, place your hands behind her neck and lift her head toward her chest.

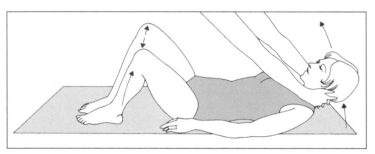

If your patient has meningeal irritation, she'll flex her hips and knees in response to the passive neck flexion.

● **Meningitis.** A positive Brudzinski's sign can usually be elicited 24 hours after the onset of this life-threatening disorder. Accompanying findings may include headache, a positive Kernig's sign, nuchal rigidity, irritability or restlessness, deep stupor or coma, vertigo, fever (which may be high or low, depending on the severity of the infection), chills, malaise, hyperalgesia, muscular hypotonia, opisthotonos, symmetrical deep tendon reflexes, papilledema, photophobia, diplopia, ocular and facial palsies, nausea, vomiting, and unequal, sluggish pupils. As ICP rises, arterial hypertension, bradycardia, widened pulse pressure, Cheyne-Stokes or Kussmaul's respirations, and coma may appear.

● **Subarachnoid hemorrhage.** Brudzinski's sign may be elicited within minutes after initial bleeding in this life-threatening disorder. Other signs and symptoms include sudden onset of severe headache, nuchal rigidity, altered LOC, dizziness, photophobia, cranial nerve palsies (indicated by ptosis, pupil dilation, and limited extraocular muscle movement), nausea and vomiting, fever, and a positive Kernig's sign. Focal signs and symptoms, such as hemiparesis, visual disturbances, and aphasia, may also occur. As ICP rises, arterial hypertension, bradycardia, widened pulse pressure, Cheyne-Stokes or Kussmaul's respirations, and coma may occur.

Special considerations

The patient with a positive Brudzinski's sign is usually critically ill and needs constant ICP monitoring and frequent neurologic checks, along with intensive assessment and monitoring of vital signs, intake and output, and cardiorespiratory status. To promote patient comfort, maintain low lights and minimal noise, and elevate the head of the bed. The patient usually won't receive narcotic analgesics because they may mask signs of increased ICP.

Prepare the patient for diagnostic tests. These may include blood, urine, and sputum cultures to identify bacteria; lumbar puncture to assess CSF and relieve pressure; and computed tomography scan, magnetic resonance imaging, cerebral angiography, and spinal X-rays to locate a hemorrhage.

Pediatric pointers

Brudzinski's sign may not be useful as an indicator of meningeal irritation in infants because more reliable signs (bulging fontanels, weak cry, fretfulness, vomiting, and poor feeding) appear early.

BRUITS

A common indicator of life- or limb-threatening vascular disease, bruits are swishing sounds caused by turbulent blood flow. They're characterized by location, duration, intensity, pitch, and time of onset in the cardiac cycle. Loud bruits produce intense vibration and a palpable thrill. A thrill, however, does not provide any further clue to the causative disorder or to its severity.

Bruits are most significant when heard over the abdominal aorta; the renal, carotid, femoral, popliteal, and subclavian arteries; and the thyroid gland. They're also significant when heard consistently despite changes in patient position and when heard during diastole.

History and physical examination

If you detect bruits over the abdominal aorta, check for a pulsating mass or a bluish discoloration around the umbilicus (Cullen's sign). Either of these signs—or severe, tearing pain in the abdomen, flank, or lower back—may signal life-threatening dissection of an aortic aneurysm. (See *Auscultating bruits,* page 106.)

If you suspect dissection, monitor the patient's vital signs constantly, and withhold food and fluids until a definitive diagnosis is made. Watch for signs and symptoms of hypovolemic shock, such as thirst; hypotension; tachycardia; weak, thready pulse; tachypnea; altered level of consciousness (LOC); mottled knees and elbows; and cool, clammy skin.

If you detect bruits over the thyroid gland, ask the patient if he has a history of hyperthyroidism. Watch for signs and symptoms of life-threatening thyroid storm: tremor, restlessness, diarrhea, abdominal pain, and hepatomegaly.

If you detect carotid artery bruits, be alert for signs and symptoms of a transient ischemic attack (TIA): dizziness, diplopia, slurred speech, and syncope. These findings may indicate an impending cerebrovascular accident (CVA). Evaluate the patient frequently for changes in LOC and muscle function.

If you detect bruits over the femoral, popliteal, or subclavian arteries, watch for signs and symptoms of decreased or absent peripheral circulation—edema, weakness, and paresthesia. Frequently check distal pulses and skin color and temperature. Also watch for pallor, coolness, or sudden absence of pulse, which may indicate a threat to the affected limb.

EXAMINATION TIP

AUSCULTATING BRUITS

To detect a bruit, an abnormal sound caused by turbulent blood flow in the vessels, assess the arteries. Auscultate the carotid, femoral, and popliteal arteries and the abdominal aorta by following these steps.

First, ask the client to hold his breath while you auscultate. Then assess the carotid arteries by auscultating with the bell of the stethoscope on both sides of the trachea, as shown. To evaluate the femoral and popliteal arteries, place the bell of the stethoscope over the pulse sites that were palpated earlier in the assessment. Finally, auscultate the abdominal artery by listening to the epigastric area.

Normally, auscultation should detect no vascular sounds.

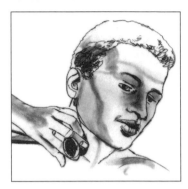

If you detect a bruit, be sure to check for further vascular damage and perform a thorough cardiac assessment.

Common medical causes

● *Abdominal aortic aneurysm.* A pulsating periumbilical mass accompanied by a systolic bruit over the aorta characterizes this disorder. Associated findings may include a rigid, tender abdomen, mottled skin, diminished peripheral pulses, and claudication. Sharp, tearing pain in the abdomen, flank, or lower back signals imminent dissection.

● *Abdominal aortic atherosclerosis.* Loud systolic bruits in the epigastric and midabdominal areas are common. They may be accompanied by leg weakness, numbness, paresthesias, or paralysis; leg pain; and decreased or absent femoral, popliteal, and pedal pulses. Abdominal pain is rarely present.

● *Anemia.* Increased cardiac output causes increased blood flow. In severe anemia, short systolic bruits may be heard over both carotid arteries. They

may be accompanied by headache, fatigue, dizziness, pallor, jaundice, palpitations, mild tachycardia, dyspnea, nausea, anorexia, and glossitis.

● *Carotid artery stenosis.* Systolic bruits can be heard over one or both carotid arteries. Other signs and symptoms may be absent. However, dizziness, vertigo, headache, syncope, aphasia, dysarthria, vision loss, hemiparesis, or hemiparalysis signal TIA and may herald CVA.

● *Carotid cavernous fistula.* Continuous bruits heard over the eyeballs and temples, visual disturbances, and protruding, pulsating eyeballs are typical.

● *Peripheral vascular disease.* This condition characteristically produces bruits over the femoral artery and other arteries in the legs. It can also cause diminished or absent femoral, popliteal, or pedal pulses; intermittent claudication; numbness, weakness, pain, and cramping in the legs, feet, and hips; and cool, shiny skin and hair loss on the affected extremity.

● *Renal artery stenosis.* Systolic bruits commonly are heard over the abdominal midline and flank on the affected side. Hypertension, stenosis, headache, palpitations, tachycardia, anxiety, dizziness, retinopathy, and mental sluggishness may also appear.

• ***Thyrotoxicosis.*** A systolic bruit is commonly heard over the thyroid gland. Other characteristic signs and symptoms include thyroid enlargement, fatigue, nervousness, tachycardia, heat intolerance, sweating, tremor, diarrhea, and weight loss despite increased appetite. Exophthalmos may also be present.

Special considerations

Because bruits can signal a life-threatening vascular disorder, frequently check the patient's vital signs and auscultate over the affected arteries. Be especially alert for bruits that become louder or develop a diastolic component.

As needed, administer medications, such as vasodilators, anticoagulants, antiplatelets, or antihypertensives.

Prepare the patient for diagnostic tests, such as blood studies, x-rays, an electrocardiogram, cardiac catheterization, and ultrasonography. Instruct him to report any dizziness or pain, which may indicate a worsening of his condition.

Pediatric pointers

Bruits are common in young children but are usually of little significance; for example, cranial bruits are normal until age 4. However, certain bruits may be significant. Because birthmarks commonly accompany congenital arteriovenous fistulas, carefully auscultate for bruits in a child with port-wine spots or cavernous or diffuse hemangiomas.

BUTTERFLY RASH

Butterfly rash is a sign of systemic lupus erythematosus, but it can also signal dermatologic disorders. Typically, but-

IDENTIFYING BUTTERFLY RASH

In classic butterfly rash, lesions appear on the cheeks and the bridge of the nose, creating a characteristic butterfly pattern. The rash may vary in severity from malar erythema to discoid lesions (plaques).

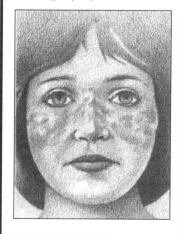

terfly rash appears in a malar distribution across the nose and cheeks. (See *Identifying butterfly rash.*) Similar rashes may appear on the neck, scalp, and other areas. Butterfly rash is sometimes mistaken for sunburn because it can be provoked or aggravated by ultraviolet rays.

History and physical examination

Ask the patient when he first noticed the butterfly rash and if he has been recently exposed to sun. Next, ask about recent weight or hair loss and about the presence of rashes elsewhere on his body. Does he have a family history of lupus erythematosus? Is he taking hydralazine or procainamide (common causes of drug-induced lupus erythematosus)?

BUTTERFLY RASH: COMMON CAUSES AND ASSOCIATED FINDINGS

S&S CAUSES	MAJOR ASSOCIATED SIGNS AND SYMPTOMS											
	Acne	Alopecia	Erythema	Fever	Maculopapular lesions	Malaise	Mucous membrane lesions	Photosensitivity	Plaques	Pruritus	Scaling	Telangiectases
Discoid lupus erythematosus		●	●					●	●	●	●	●
Erysipelas			●	●		●			●	●		
Rosacea			●		●							●
Seborrheic dermatitis	●				●					●	●	
Systemic lupus erythematosus		●	●	●	●	●	●	●			●	●

Inspect the rash, noting any macules, papules, pustules, and scaling. Is the rash edematous? Are areas of hypopigmentation or hyperpigmentation present? Look for blisters or ulcers in the mouth, and note any inflamed lesions. Check for rashes elsewhere on the body.

Common medical causes

● *Discoid lupus erythematosus.* This localized form of lupus erythematosus may produce a unilateral or butterfly rash that consists of mildly scaling, erythematous, raised, sharply demarcated plaques with follicular plugging and central atrophy. Rash may also involve the scalp, ears, chest, or any part of the body exposed to sun. Telangiectases, scarring alopecia, and hypopigmentation or hyperpigmentation may occur later. Other signs include conjunctival redness, dilated capillaries of the nail fold, bilateral parotid gland enlargement, oral lesions, and mottled, reddish blue skin on the legs.

● *Erysipelas.* In this streptococcal infection, butterfly rash appears as warm, indurated, tender, pruritic, edematous, and erythematous plaques, enlarging peripherally with sharply elevated margins; vesicles and bullae may form. Commonly, the rash appears abruptly and covers the bridge of the nose and one or both cheeks, halting at the hairline of the scalp or beard. However, the rash may also appear on the hands and genitals. Associated signs and symptoms include fever, malaise, headache, vomiting, sore throat and, in some patients, cervical lymphadenopathy.

● *Rosacea.* Initially, the butterfly rash may appear as a prominent, nonscaling, intermittent erythema limited to the lower half of the nose or including the chin, cheeks, and central forehead. As rosacea develops, the duration of the rash increases; instead of disappearing after each episode, the rash varies in intensity and is commonly accompanied by telangiectasia. In advanced rosacea, the skin is oily, with papules, pustules, nodules, and telangiectases restricted to the central oval of the face. In men with severe rosacea, butterfly rash may be accompanied by rhinophyma—a thickened, lobulated overgrowth of sebaceous glands and epithelial connective tissue on the lower half of the nose and, possibly, the adjacent cheeks.

• *Seborrheic dermatitis.* The butterfly rash appears as greasy, scaling, slightly yellow macules and papules of varying size; the scalp, beard, eyebrows, portions of the forehead, nasolabial fold, or trunk may also be involved. Associated signs and symptoms may include crusts and fissures (particularly when the external ear and scalp are involved), pruritus, redness, blepharitis, sties, severe acne, and oily skin. Severe seborrheic dermatitis of the face occurs with acquired immunodeficiency syndrome.

• *Systemic lupus erythematosus.* In about 40% of patients with this connective tissue disorder, butterfly rash appears as a red, often scaly, sharply demarcated macular eruption. The rash may be transient in acute lupus or may progress slowly to include the forehead, chin, the area around the ears, and other exposed areas. Common associated skin findings include photosensitivity; scaling, patchy alopecia; mucous membrane lesions; mottled erythema of the palms and fingers; periungual erythema with edema; macular, reddish purple lesions on the volar surfaces of the fingers; telangiectasia of the base of the nails or eyelids; purpura; petechiae; or ecchymoses.

Butterfly rash may also be accompanied by joint pain, stiffness, and deformities—particularly ulnar deviation of the fingers and subluxation of the proximal interphalangeal joints. Related findings include periorbital and facial edema, dyspnea, low-grade fever, malaise, weakness, fatigue, weight loss, anorexia, nausea, vomiting, lymphadenopathy, and hepatosplenomegaly.

Other causes

• *Drugs.* Hydralazine and procainamide can cause a lupus-like syndrome.

Special considerations

Prepare the patient for immunologic studies, complete blood count, and possibly liver studies. Obtain a urine specimen if needed.

Withhold photosensitizing drugs, such as phenothiazines, sulfonamides, sulfonylureas, and thiazide diuretics. Instruct the patient to avoid exposure to the sun or to use a sunscreen. Suggest that he use hypoallergenic makeup to help conceal facial lesions.

Pediatric pointers

Rare in pediatric patients, butterfly rash may occur as part of an infectious disease, such as erythema infectiosum, or "slapped cheek syndrome."

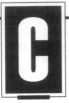

CAPILLARY REFILL TIME, PROLONGED

Capillary refill time is the duration required for color to return to the nail bed of a finger or toe after application of slight pressure, which causes blanching. This duration reflects the quality of peripheral vasomotor function. Normal capillary refill time is less than 3 seconds.

Prolonged refill time isn't diagnostic of any disorder but must be evaluated along with other signs and symptoms. However, it usually signals obstructive peripheral arterial disease or decreased cardiac output.

Capillary refill time is typically tested during a routine cardiovascular assessment. It isn't tested in suspected life-threatening disorders because other, more characteristic signs and symptoms appear earlier.

History and physical examination
If you detect prolonged capillary refill time, take the patient's vital signs and check pulses in the affected limb. Does the limb feel cold or look cyanotic? Does the patient report pain or any unusual sensations in his fingers or toes, especially after exposure to cold?

Take a brief medical history, noting especially previous peripheral vascular disease. Find out which medications the patient is taking.

Common medical causes
• *Aortic aneurysm (dissecting).* Capillary refill time is prolonged in the fingers and toes with a dissecting aneurysm in the thoracic aorta and is prolonged in just the toes with a dissecting aneurysm in the abdominal aorta. Common accompanying signs and symptoms include a pulsating abdominal mass, systolic bruit, and substernal back or abdominal pain.
• *Aortic arch syndrome.* Prolonged capillary refill time in the fingers occurs early in this syndrome. The patient displays absent carotid pulses and possibly unequal radial pulses. Other signs and symptoms usually precede the loss of pulses and include fever, night sweats, arthralgia, weight loss, anorexia, nausea, malaise, skin rash, splenomegaly, and pallor.
• *Arterial occlusion (acute).* Prolonged capillary refill time occurs early in the affected limb. Arterial pulses are usually absent distal to the obstruction; the affected limb appears cool and pale or cyanotic. Intermittent claudication, moderate to severe pain, numbness, and paresthesias or paralysis of the affected limb may occur.
• *Buerger's disease.* Capillary refill time is prolonged in the toes. Exposure to low temperatures turns the feet cold, cyanotic, and numb; later they redden, become hot, and tingle. Other findings include intermittent claudication of the instep, weak peripheral pulses and, in later stages, ulceration, muscle atrophy, and gangrene. If the disease affects the hands, prolonged capillary refill may accompany painful fingertip ulcerations.

- *Cardiac tamponade.* Prolonged capillary refill time is a late sign of decreased cardiac output. Associated signs include tachycardia, cyanosis, dyspnea, neck vein distention, and hypotension.
- *Hypothermia.* Prolonged capillary refill time may appear early as a compensatory response. Associated signs and symptoms depend on the degree of hypothermia and may include some combination of shivering, fatigue, weakness, decreased level of consciousness (LOC), slurred speech, ataxia, muscle stiffness or rigidity, tachycardia or bradycardia, hyporeflexia or areflexia, diuresis, oliguria, bradypnea, decreased blood pressure, and cold, pale skin.
- *Peripheral arterial trauma.* Any trauma to a peripheral artery that reduces distal blood flow also prolongs capillary refill time in the affected extremity. Related findings in that extremity include bruising or pulsating bleeding, weakened pulse, cyanosis, paresthesia, sensory loss, and cool, pale skin.
- *Raynaud's disease.* Capillary refill time is prolonged in the fingers, the usual site of this disease's characteristic episodic arterial vasospasm. Exposure to cold or stress produces blanching in the fingers, then cyanosis, and then erythema before fingers return to normal temperature. Warmth relieves symptoms, which may include paresthesias. Chronic disease may produce trophic changes, such as sclerodactyly, ulcerations, or chronic paronychia.
- *Volkmann's contracture.* Prolonged capillary refill time results from this contracture's characteristic vasospasm. Associated symptoms include loss of mobility and loss of strength in the affected extremity.

Other causes

- *Diagnostic tests.* Cardiac catheterization can cause arterial hematoma or clot formation and prolonged capillary refill time.
- *Drugs.* Drugs that cause vasoconstriction (particularly alpha-adrenergics) prolong capillary refill time.
- *Treatments.* Prolonged capillary refill time can result from an arterial line or umbilical line, which can cause arterial hematoma and obstructed distal blood flow, or an improperly fitting cast, which constricts circulation.

Special considerations

Frequently assess the patient's vital signs, LOC, and affected extremity, and report any changes, such as progressive cyanosis or loss of an existing pulse.

Prepare the patient for diagnostic tests, which may include arteriography or Doppler ultrasonography, to help confirm or rule out arterial occlusion.

Pediatric pointers

Capillary refill time may be prolonged in newborns with acrocyanosis, but this is a normal finding. Typically, prolonged capillary refill time is associated with the same disorders in children as in adults. However, its most common pediatric cause is cardiac surgery such as repair of congenital heart defects.

CARPOPEDAL SPASM

Carpopedal spasm is the violent, painful contraction of the muscles in the hands and feet. It's an important sign of tetany, a potentially life-threatening condition characterized by increased neuromuscular excitation and sustained muscle contraction and commonly associated with hypocalcemia. (See *Identifying carpopedal spasm,* page 112.)

Carpopedal spasm requires prompt evaluation and intervention; untreated, it can cause laryngospasm, seizures, cardiac arrhythmias, and cardiac and respiratory arrest.

IDENTIFYING CARPOPEDAL SPASM

In the hand, carpopedal spasm involves adduction of the thumb over the palm, followed by flexion of the metacarpophalangeal joints, extension of the interphalangeal joints (fingers together), adduction of the hyperextended fingers, and flexion of the wrist and elbow joints. Similar effects occur in the joints of the feet.

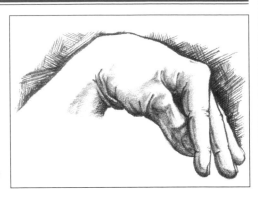

Emergency interventions

 If you detect carpopedal spasm, quickly examine the patient for signs of respiratory distress (laryngospasm, stridor, loud crowing noises, cyanosis) or cardiac arrhythmias, which indicate hypocalcemia. Administer an I.V. calcium preparation, and give emergency respiratory and cardiac support. If calcium infusion doesn't control seizures, administer a sedative, such as chloral hydrate or phenobarbital.

History and physical examination

If the patient isn't in distress, obtain a detailed history. Ask about the onset and duration of the spasms and the degree of pain they produce. Also ask about related signs of hypocalcemia, such as numbness and tingling of the fingertips and feet; other muscle cramps or spasms; and nausea, vomiting, and abdominal pain. Check for previous neck surgery, calcium or magnesium deficiency, tetanus exposure, and hypoparathyroidism.

During the history, form a general impression of the patient's mental status and behavior. If possible, ask family members or friends if they've noticed changes in the patient's behavior. Mental confusion or even personality changes may occur with hypocalcemia.

Inspect the patient's skin and fingernails, noting any dryness or scaling and the presence of ridged, brittle nails.

Common medical causes

• *Hypocalcemia.* Carpopedal spasm is an early sign of hypocalcemia. It's usually accompanied by paresthesia of the fingers, toes, and perioral area; muscle weakness, twitching, and cramping; hyperreflexia; chorea; fatigue; and palpitations. Positive Chvostek's and Trousseau's signs can be elicited. Laryngospasm, stridor, and seizures may appear in severe hypocalcemia.

Chronic hypocalcemia may be accompanied by mental status changes; cramps; dry, scaly skin; brittle nails; and thin, patchy hair and eyebrows.

Other causes

• *Treatments.* Multiple blood transfusions and parathyroidectomy may cause hypocalcemia, resulting in carpopedal spasm. Surgical procedures that impair calcium absorption, such as ileostomy formation and gastric resection with gastrojejunostomy, may also cause hypocalcemia.

Special considerations
Carpopedal spasm can cause severe pain and anxiety, leading to hyperventilation. If this occurs, help the patient slow his breathing through your relaxing touch, reassuring attitude, and clear directions for what he should do. Provide a quiet, dark environment to reduce the patient's anxiety.

Prepare the patient for laboratory tests, such as complete blood count and serum calcium, phosphorus, and parathyroid hormone studies.

Pediatric pointers
Idiopathic hypoparathyroidism is a common cause of hypocalcemia in children. You'll need to carefully monitor children with this condition because carpopedal spasm may herald the onset of epileptiform seizures or generalized tetany followed by prolonged tonic spasms.

CAT CRY

Occurring during infancy, this mewing, kittenlike sound is the primary indicator of cri du chat (or cat cry) syndrome. This syndrome affects 1 in 50,000 neonates, occurs more commonly in females, and causes profound mental retardation and, commonly, death before age 1. The chromosomal defect responsible (deletion of the short arm of chromosome 5) usually appears spontaneously but may be inherited from a carrier parent. The characteristic cry is thought to result from abnormal laryngeal development.

Emergency interventions
 Suspect cri du chat if you detect cat cry in a neonate. Be alert for signs of respiratory distress, such as nasal flaring, cyanosis, a respiratory rate over 60 breaths/minute, and irregular, shallow respirations. Be prepared to suction the infant and to administer warmed oxygen. Keep emergency resuscitation equipment nearby because bradycardia may develop.

History and physical examination
Perform a physical examination and note any abnormalities. If you detect cat cry in an older infant, ask the parents when it developed. Sudden onset of an abnormal cry in an infant with a previously normal, vigorous cry suggests other disorders, not cri du chat. (See "Cry, high-pitched.")

Common medical causes
● *Cri du chat syndrome.* A kittenlike cry begins at birth or shortly thereafter. It's accompanied by profound mental retardation, microcephaly, low birth weight, hypotonia, failure to thrive, and feeding difficulties. Typically, the infant displays a round face with wide-set eyes, strabismus, a broad-based nose with oblique or down-sloping epicanthal folds, an unusually small jaw, and abnormally shaped, low-set ears. He may also have a short neck, webbed fingers, and a simian crease.

Special considerations
Connect the infant to an apnea monitor, and check for signs of respiratory distress. Keep suction equipment and warmed oxygen available. Watch for signs of increased intracranial pressure. Obtain a blood sample for chromosomal analysis. Prepare the infant for a computed tomography scan to rule out other causes of microcephaly. He'll also have an ear, nose, and throat examination to evaluate vocal cords.

Because the infant with cri du chat is usually a poor eater, monitor intake, output, and weight. Instruct the parents to offer small, frequent feedings.

Chest expansion, asymmetrical

Asymmetrical chest expansion is the uneven extension of portions of the chest wall during inspiration. During normal respiration, the thorax uniformly expands upward and outward, then contracts downward and inward. When this process is disrupted, breathing becomes uncoordinated, causing asymmetrical chest expansion.

Asymmetrical chest expansion may develop suddenly or gradually and may affect one or both sides of the chest wall. It may occur as delayed expiration (chest lag), as abnormal movement during inspiration (for example, intercostal retractions, paradoxical movement, or chest-abdomen asynchrony), or as unilateral absence of movement. It usually results from pleural disorders, such as life-threatening hemothorax or tension pneumothorax. (See *Recognizing life-threatening causes of asymmetrical chest expansion.*) However, it can also result from musculoskeletal or neurologic disorders, airway obstruction, or trauma. Regardless of its underlying cause, asymmetrical chest expansion produces rapid and shallow or deep respirations that increase the work of breathing.

Emergency interventions

 If you detect asymmetrical chest expansion, first consider traumatic injury to the patient's ribs or sternum, which can cause flail chest—a life-threatening emergency characterized by paradoxical chest movement. Quickly take the patient's vital signs and look for signs of acute respiratory distress—rapid and shallow respirations, tachycardia, and cyanosis. Use tape or sandbags to temporarily splint the unstable flail segment.

Depending on the severity of respiratory distress, administer oxygen by nasal cannula, mask, or mechanical ventilator. Insert an I.V. line to allow replacement of fluids and administration of pain medication, which helps prevent splinting. Draw a blood sample from the patient for arterial blood gas analysis, and connect him to a cardiac monitor.

Although asymmetrical chest expansion can result from hemothorax, tension pneumothorax, bronchial obstruction, and other life-threatening causes, it's not a cardinal sign of these disorders. Because *any* form of asymmetrical chest expansion can compromise the patient's respiratory status, don't leave the patient unattended. Be alert for signs of respiratory distress.

History and physical examination

Obtain a brief history if you don't suspect flail chest and if the patient isn't experiencing acute respiratory distress. Asymmetrical chest expansion often results from mechanical airflow obstruction, so find out if the patient is experiencing dyspnea or pain during breathing. If so, is he constantly short of breath or does he have intermittent attacks of breathlessness? Does the pain worsen his feeling of breathlessness? Does repositioning, coughing, or any other activity relieve or worsen the dyspnea or pain? Is the pain more noticeable during inspiration or expiration? Can he inhale deeply?

Ask if the patient has a history of pulmonary or systemic illness—frequent upper respiratory infections, asthma, tuberculosis, pneumonia, or cancer. Has he had thoracic surgery? (This typically produces asymmetrical chest expansion on the affected side.) Also ask about blunt or penetrating chest trauma, which may have caused pulmonary injury. And obtain an occupational history to find out if the patient may have inhaled toxic fumes or aspirated a toxic substance on the job.

RECOGNIZING LIFE-THREATENING CAUSES OF ASYMMETRICAL CHEST EXPANSION

Asymmetrical chest expansion can result from several life-threatening disorders. Two common causes—bronchial obstruction and flail chest—produce distinctive chest wall movements that provide important clues about the underlying disorder.

Inspiration

Bronchial obstruction

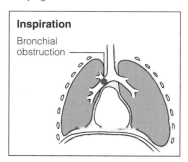

Expiration

Bronchial obstruction

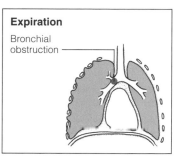

In *bronchial obstruction*, only the unaffected portion of the chest wall expands during inspiration. Intercostal bulging during expiration may indicate that air is trapped in the chest.

Inspiration

Fractured ribs

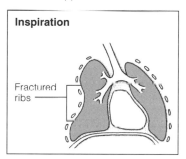

Expiration

Fractured ribs

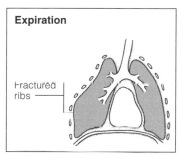

In *flail chest*—a disruption of the thorax due to multiple rib fractures—the unstable portion of the chest wall collapses inward at inspiration and balloons outward at expiration.

Now perform a physical examination. Begin by gently palpating the trachea for midline positioning. Then examine the posterior chest wall for areas of tenderness or deformity. To evaluate the extent of asymmetrical chest expansion, place your hands—fingers together and thumbs abducted toward the spine—flat on both sections of the lower posterior chest wall.

Position your thumbs at the 10th rib, and grasp the lateral rib cage with your hands. As the patient inhales, note the uneven separation of your thumbs and gauge the distance between them. Then repeat this technique on the upper posterior chest wall.

Next, use the ulnar surface of your hand to palpate for vocal or tactile fremitus on both sides of the chest. To check for vocal fremitus, ask the patient to repeat "ninety-nine" as you proceed. Note any asymmetrical vibrations and areas of enhanced, diminished, or absent fremitus. Then percuss and auscultate to detect air and fluid in the lungs and pleural spaces. Finally, auscultate all lung fields for normal and adventitious breath sounds.

Now examine the patient's anterior chest wall, using the same assessment techniques.

Common medical causes
● *Flail chest.* In this life-threatening injury to the ribs or sternum, the unstable portion of the chest wall collapses inward during inspiration and balloons outward during expiration (paradoxical movement). The patient may have ecchymoses, severe localized pain, and other signs of traumatic injury to the chest wall. He may also have tachycardia, cyanosis, and rapid, shallow respirations.
● *Kyphoscoliosis.* Abnormal curvature of the thoracic spine in the anteroposterior direction (kyphosis) and the lateral direction (scoliosis) gradually compresses one lung and distends the other. This produces decreased chest wall movement on the compressed-lung side and expands the intercostal muscles during inspiration on the opposite side. It can also produce ineffective coughing, dyspnea, back pain, and fatigue.
● *Myasthenia gravis.* Progressive loss of ventilatory muscle function produces chest-abdomen asynchrony ("abdominal paradox") that can lead to onset of acute respiratory distress. Typically, the patient's shallow respirations and increased muscle weakness cause severe dyspnea, tachypnea, and possible apnea.
● *Pleural effusion.* Chest lag at end-inspiration occurs gradually in this life-threatening accumulation of fluid, blood, or pus in the pleural space. Usually, some combination of dyspnea, tachypnea, and tachycardia precedes chest lag; the pa-

tient may also have pleuritic pain that worsens with coughing or deep breathing. The area of effusion is delineated by dullness on percussion and by egobronchophony, whispered pectoriloquy, decreased or absent breath sounds, and decreased tactile fremitus. Fever appears if infection causes the effusion.
● *Pneumonia.* Depending on whether consolidation of fluid in the lungs develops unilaterally or bilaterally, asymmetrical chest expansion occurs as inspiratory chest lag or as chest-abdomen asynchrony. The patient will typically have fever, chills, tachycardia, tachypnea, and dyspnea along with crackles, rhonchi, and chest pain that worsens during deep breathing. He may also be fatigued and anorexic and have a productive cough with rust-colored sputum.
● *Pulmonary embolism.* This acute, life-threatening disorder causes chest lag, sudden, stabbing chest pain, and tachycardia. The patient usually has severe dyspnea, blood-tinged sputum, pleural friction rub, and acute anxiety.

Other causes
● *Treatments.* Asymmetrical chest expansion can result from pneumonectomy and surgical removal of several ribs. Chest lag or absence of chest movement may also result from intubation of a mainstem bronchus—a serious complication typically due to incorrect insertion of an endotracheal tube or movement of the tube while it's in the trachea.

Special considerations
If you're caring for an intubated patient, regularly auscultate breath sounds in the lung peripheries to help detect a misplaced tube. If this occurs, prepare the patient for a chest X-ray to allow rapid repositioning of the tube.

Pediatric pointers
Children have a greater risk than adults of mainstem bronchus (especially left bronchus) intubation. But because a

child's breath sounds are commonly referred from one lung to the other because of the small size of the thoracic cage, use chest wall expansion as an indicator of correct tube position.

Congenital abnormalities, such as cerebral palsy and diaphragmatic hernia, can cause asymmetrical chest expansion. In cerebral palsy, asymmetrical facial muscles usually accompany chest-abdomen asynchrony. In life-threatening diaphragmatic hernia, asymmetrical expansion usually occurs on the left side of the chest.

CHEST PAIN

This symptom usually results from disorders that affect thoracic or abdominal organs—the heart, pleurae, lungs, esophagus, rib cage, gallbladder, pancreas, or stomach. It's an important indicator of several acute and life-threatening cardiopulmonary and GI disorders. However, it can also result from musculoskeletal and hematologic disorders, anxiety, and drug therapy.

The cause of chest pain may be difficult to distinguish initially. Chest pain can arise suddenly or gradually and can radiate to the arms, neck, jaw, or back. It can be steady or intermittent, mild or acute. And it can range in character from a sharp shooting sensation to a feeling of heaviness, fullness, or even indigestion. It can be provoked or aggravated by stress, anxiety, exertion, deep breathing, or eating certain foods.

Emergency interventions

 Ask the patient when his chest pain began. Did it arise suddenly or gradually? Is it more severe or frequent now than when it first started? Sudden, severe chest pain requires prompt evaluation and treatment because it may herald a life-threatening disorder.

(See *Managing severe chest pain*, pages 118 and 119.)

History and physical examination
If the chest pain isn't severe, proceed with the history. Ask if the patient feels diffuse pain or can point to the painful area. Sometimes a patient won't perceive the sensation he's feeling as pain, so ask whether he has any discomfort radiating to his neck, jaw, arms, or back. If he does, ask him to describe it. Is it a dull, aching, pressurelike sensation? A sharp, stabbing, knifelike pain? Does he feel it on the surface or deep inside? Find out whether it's constant or intermittent. If it's intermittent, how long does it last? Ask if movement, exertion, breathing, position changes, or eating certain foods worsens or helps relieve the pain. Does anything in particular seem to bring it on?

Review the patient's history for cardiac or pulmonary disease, chest trauma, intestinal disease, or sickle cell anemia. Find out which medications he's taking, if any, and ask about recent dosage or schedule changes.

Take the patient's vital signs, noting tachypnea, fever, tachycardia, hypertension, or hypotension. Look for jugular vein distention and peripheral edema, observe his breathing pattern, and inspect his chest for asymmetrical expansion. Auscultate the lungs for pleural friction rub, crackles, rhonchi, wheezing, or diminished or absent breath sounds. Next, auscultate for murmurs, clicks, gallops, or pericardial friction rub. Palpate for lifts, heaves, thrills, gallops, tactile fremitus, an abdominal mass, and tenderness.

Common medical causes
• *Angina.* In *angina pectoris,* the patient may experience a feeling of tightness or pressure in the chest that he describes as pain or a sensation of indigestion or expansion. Usually, the pain occurs in the retrosternal region over a palm-size or larger area. It may radiate to the neck,

EMERGENCY INTERVENTIONS

MANAGING SEVERE CHEST PAIN

Sudden, severe chest pain may result from several life-threatening disorders. Your evaluation and interventions will depend on the pain's location and character. The flowchart below will help you establish priorities for managing this emergency successfully.

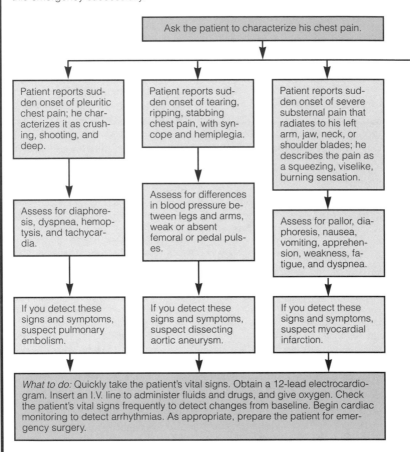

Ask the patient to characterize his chest pain.

Patient reports sudden onset of pleuritic chest pain; he characterizes it as crushing, shooting, and deep.

Patient reports sudden onset of tearing, ripping, stabbing chest pain, with syncope and hemiplegia.

Patient reports sudden onset of severe substernal pain that radiates to his left arm, jaw, neck, or shoulder blades; he describes the pain as a squeezing, viselike, burning sensation.

Assess for diaphoresis, dyspnea, hemoptysis, and tachycardia.

Assess for differences in blood pressure between legs and arms, weak or absent femoral or pedal pulses.

Assess for pallor, diaphoresis, nausea, vomiting, apprehension, weakness, fatigue, and dyspnea.

If you detect these signs and symptoms, suspect pulmonary embolism.

If you detect these signs and symptoms, suspect dissecting aortic aneurysm.

If you detect these signs and symptoms, suspect myocardial infarction.

What to do: Quickly take the patient's vital signs. Obtain a 12-lead electrocardiogram. Insert an I.V. line to administer fluids and drugs, and give oxygen. Check the patient's vital signs frequently to detect changes from baseline. Begin cardiac monitoring to detect arrhythmias. As appropriate, prepare the patient for emergency surgery.

jaw, and arms—classically, to the inner aspect of the left arm. Anginal pain tends to begin gradually, build to its maximum, then slowly subside. Provoked by exertion, emotional stress, or a heavy meal, the pain typically lasts 2 to 10 minutes. Associated findings may include dyspnea, nausea, vomiting, tachycardia, dizziness, diaphoresis, belching, or palpita-

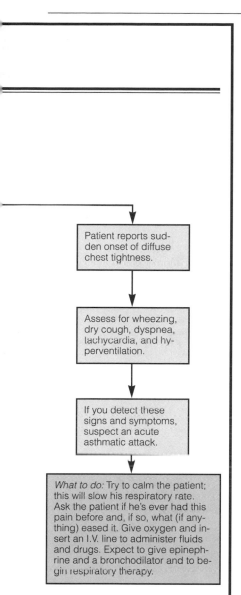

Patient reports sudden onset of diffuse chest tightness.

↓

Assess for wheezing, dry cough, dyspnea, tachycardia, and hyperventilation.

↓

If you detect these signs and symptoms, suspect an acute asthmatic attack.

↓

What to do: Try to calm the patient; this will slow his respiratory rate. Ask the patient if he's ever had this pain before and, if so, what (if anything) eased it. Give oxygen and insert an I.V. line to administer fluids and drugs. Expect to give epinephrine and a bronchodilator and to begin respiratory therapy.

tions. You may hear an atrial gallop (S_4) or murmur during an anginal episode.

In *Prinzmetal's angina,* chest pain occurs when the patient is at rest—or it may awaken him. It may occur with shortness of breath, nausea, vomiting, dizziness, and palpitations. During an attack, you may hear an atrial gallop.

● *Aortic aneurysm (dissecting).* The chest pain associated with this disorder usually begins suddenly and is most severe at its onset. The patient describes an excruciating tearing, ripping, stabbing pain in his chest and neck that radiates to his upper back, abdomen, and lower back. He may also have abdominal tenderness, a palpable abdominal mass, tachycardia, murmurs, syncope, blindness, loss of consciousness, weakness or transient paralysis of the arms or legs, a systolic bruit, systemic hypotension, asymmetrical brachial pulses, lower blood pressure in the legs than in the arms, and weak or absent femoral or pedal pulses. His skin is pale, cool, diaphoretic, and mottled below the waist. Capillary refill time is prolonged in the toes, and palpation reveals decreased pulsation of one or both carotid arteries.

● *Asthma.* In a life-threatening asthmatic attack, diffuse and painful chest tightness arises suddenly along with a dry cough and mild wheezing, which progress to a productive cough, audible wheezing, and severe dyspnea. Related respiratory findings include rhonchi, crackles, prolonged expirations, intercostal and supraclavicular retractions on inspiration, accessory muscle use, flaring nostrils, and tachypnea. Other clinical features include anxiety, tachycardia, diaphoresis, flushing, and cyanosis.

● *Bronchitis.* In its acute form, this disorder produces a burning chest pain or a sensation of substernal tightness. It also produces a cough, initially dry but later productive, that worsens the chest pain. Other findings include low-grade fever, chills, sore throat, tachycardia, muscle and back pain, rhonchi, crackles, and wheezing. Severe bronchitis causes fever of 101° to 102° F (38.3° to 38.9° C) and possibly bronchospasm with worsening wheezing and increased coughing.

CHEST PAIN: COMMON CAUSES AND ASSOCIATED FINDINGS

S&S / CHIEF CAUSES	MAJOR ASSOCIATED SIGNS AND SYMPTOMS												
	Abdominal mass	Abdominal tenderness	Atrial gallop	Breath sounds, decreased	Cough	Crackles	Cyanosis	Diaphoresis	Dizziness	Dyspnea	Fever	Hemoptysis	Murmur
Angina pectoris			●					●	●	●			
Aortic aneurysm (dissecting)	●	●						●					●
Asthma (acute)					●	●	●	●		●			
Bronchitis (acute)					●	●				●			
Cholecystitis	●	●						●		●			
Interstitial lung disease					●	●	●			●			
Lung abscess				●	●	●		●		●	●	●	
Lung cancer					●					●	●	●	
Mitral valve prolapse									●	●			●
Myocardial infarction			●			●		●		●	●		●
Pancreatitis		●				●				●			
Peptic ulcer		●											
Pericarditis										●	●		
Pleurisy				●	●	●				●	●		
Pneumonia				●	●	●	●	●		●	●		
Pneumothorax				●	●		●			●			
Pulmonary embolism					●	●	●	●		●	●	●	

● **Cholecystitis.** This disorder typically produces abrupt epigastric or right upper quadrant pain, which may be sharp or intensely aching. Steady or intermittent pain may radiate to the back. Common associated findings include nausea, vomiting, fever, diaphoresis, and chills. Palpation of the right upper quadrant may detect an abdominal mass, rigidity, distention, and tenderness.

● **Interstitial lung disease.** As this disease advances, it may produce pleuritic

	Nausea or vomiting	Pericardial friction rub	Pleural friction rub	Skin mottling	Syncope	Tachycardia	Tachypnea	Wheezing
		•	•				•	
					•	•	•	
						•	•	•
							•	•
	•							
				•				
								•
						•		
	•							
	•				•	•		
	•							
			•			•		
				•			•	
						•	•	
						•	•	
				•		•	•	•

with a pleural friction rub and a cough that raises copious amounts of purulent, foul-smelling, blood-tinged sputum. The affected side is dull to percussion, and decreased breath sounds and crackles may be heard. The patient will also display diaphoresis, anorexia, weight loss, fever, chills, fatigue, weakness, dyspnea, and clubbing.

• *Lung cancer.* The chest pain associated with lung cancer is commonly described as an intermittent aching felt deep within the chest. If the tumor metastasizes to the ribs or vertebrae, the pain becomes localized, continuous, and gnawing. Associated findings may include a cough (sometimes bloody), wheezing, dyspnea, fatigue, anorexia, weight loss, or fever.

• *Mitral valve prolapse.* Typically, the patient with a prolapsed mitral valve will experience sharp, stabbing precordial chest pain or a precordial ache. The pain can last for seconds or hours and occasionally mimics the pain of ischemic heart disease. The characteristic sign of mitral valve prolapse is a midsystolic click followed by a systolic murmur at the apex. The patient may experience cardiac awareness, migraine headache, dizziness, weakness, episodic severe fatigue, dyspnea, tachycardia, mood swings, or palpitations

• *Myocardial infarction (MI).* The chest pain in MI lasts from 15 minutes to hours. Typically a crushing substernal pain that's unrelieved by rest or nitroglycerin, it may radiate to the patient's left arm, jaw, neck, or shoulder blades. The patient may have pallor, clammy skin, dyspnea, diaphoresis, nausea, vomiting, anxiety, restlessness, and a feeling of impending doom. He may develop hypotension or hypertension, an atrial gallop, murmurs, and crackles. A low-grade fever may arise within 4 days.

• *Pancreatitis.* In its acute form, this disorder usually causes intense pain in the epigastric area that radiates to the back and worsens when the patient is supine.

chest pain along with progressive dyspnea, cellophane-type crackles, nonproductive cough, fatigue, weight loss, clubbing, or cyanosis.

• *Lung abscess.* Pleuritic chest pain develops insidiously in this disorder along

Nausea, vomiting, fever, abdominal tenderness and rigidity, diminished bowel sounds, and crackles at lung bases may also occur. A patient with severe pancreatitis may be extremely restless and have mottled skin, tachycardia, and cold, sweaty extremities. Fulminant pancreatitis causes massive hemorrhage resulting in shock and coma.

• *Peptic ulcer.* In this disorder, sharp, burning pain usually arises in the epigastric region hours after food intake, commonly at night. It lasts longer than anginal pain and is relieved by food or antacids. Other findings may include nausea, vomiting, melena, and epigastric tenderness.

• *Pericarditis.* This disorder produces precordial or retrosternal pain aggravated by deep breathing, coughing, position changes, and occasionally by swallowing. In many cases, the pain is sharp or cutting and radiates to the shoulder and neck. Associated signs and symptoms may include pericardial friction rub, fever, tachycardia, and dyspnea.

• *Pleurisy.* The chest pain of pleurisy arises abruptly and reaches maximum intensity within a few hours. It's sharp—even knifelike—usually unilateral, and located in the lower and lateral aspects of the chest. Deep breathing, coughing, or thoracic movement characteristically aggravates it. Auscultation over the painful area may reveal decreased breath sounds, inspiratory crackles, and a pleural friction rub. Other possible effects are dyspnea, rapid, shallow breathing, cyanosis, fever, or fatigue.

• *Pneumonia.* This disorder produces pleuritic chest pain that increases with deep inspiration and is accompanied by shaking chills and fever. The patient has a dry cough that later becomes productive. Other signs and symptoms may include crackles, rhonchi, tachycardia, tachypnea, myalgias, fatigue, headache, dyspnea, abdominal pain, anorexia, cyanosis, decreased breath sounds, and diaphoresis.

• *Pneumothorax.* Spontaneous pneumothorax, a life-threatening disorder, causes sudden sharp chest pain that's severe, commonly unilateral, and rarely localized; it increases with chest movement. When it's located centrally and radiates to the neck, it may mimic the pain of an MI. After the pain's onset, dyspnea and cyanosis progressively worsen. Breath sounds are decreased or absent on the affected side with hyperresonance or tympany, subcutaneous crepitation, and decreased vocal fremitus. Asymmetrical chest expansion, accessory muscle use, a nonproductive cough, tachypnea, tachycardia, anxiety, and restlessness also occur.

• *Pulmonary embolism.* This disorder produces chest pain or a choking sensation. Typically, the patient first experiences sudden dyspnea with intense angina-like or pleuritic pain aggravated by deep breathing and thoracic movement. Other findings may include tachycardia, tachypnea, cough (nonproductive or producing blood-tinged sputum), a low-grade fever, restlessness, diaphoresis, crackles, a pleural friction rub, diffuse wheezing, dullness to percussion, signs of circulatory collapse (weak, rapid pulse; hypotension), signs of cerebral ischemia (transient unconsciousness, coma, seizures), symptoms of hypoxia (restlessness), and—particularly in the elderly—hemiplegia and other focal neurologic deficits. Less common signs include massive hemoptysis, chest splinting, and leg edema. A patient with a large embolus may have cyanosis and distended neck veins.

• *Sickle cell crisis.* Chest pain associated with sickle cell crisis typically has a bizarre distribution. It may start as a vague pain, commonly located in the back, hands, or feet. As the pain worsens, it becomes generalized or localized to the abdomen or chest, causing severe pleuritic pain. The patient may also have abdominal distention and rigidity, dyspnea, fever, and jaundice.

- **Tuberculosis.** In a patient with this disorder, pleuritic chest pain and fine crackles occur after coughing. Associated signs and symptoms may include night sweats, anorexia, weight loss, fever, malaise, dyspnea, easy fatigability, mild to severe productive cough, occasional hemoptysis, dullness to percussion, increased tactile fremitus, and amphoric breath sounds.

Other causes

- **Chinese restaurant syndrome.** This benign condition—a reaction to excessive ingestion of monosodium glutamate (a common additive in Chinese foods)—mimics the signs of acute MI. The patient may complain of retrosternal burning, ache, or pressure and a burning sensation over his arms, legs, and face; a sensation of facial pressure; shortness of breath; and tachycardia.
- **Drugs.** Abrupt withdrawal of beta blockers can cause rebound angina in patients with coronary heart disease—especially in those who've received high doses for a prolonged period.

Special considerations

As needed, prepare the patient for cardiopulmonary studies, such as an electrocardiogram and a lung scan. Collect a serum sample for cardiac enzyme and other studies.

Explain the purpose and procedure of each diagnostic test to the patient to help alleviate his anxiety. Also explain the purpose of any prescribed medications, and make sure the patient understands the dosage, schedule, and possible adverse effects.

Keep in mind that a patient with chest pain may deny his discomfort, so stress the importance of reporting symptoms to allow adjustment of his treatment.

Pediatric pointers

Even children old enough to talk may have difficulty describing chest pain, so be alert for nonverbal clues, such as restlessness, facial grimaces, or holding the painful area. Ask the child to point to the painful area and then (to find out if it's radiating) to where the pain goes. Determine the pain's severity by asking his parents if the pain interferes with the child's normal activities and behavior. Remember, a child may complain of chest pain in an attempt to get attention or to avoid attending school.

CHEYNE-STOKES RESPIRATIONS

The most common pattern of periodic breathing, Cheyne-Stokes respirations are characterized by a waxing and waning period of hyperpnea that alternates with a shorter period of apnea. This pattern can occur normally in people who live at high altitudes, in the elderly during sleep, and in patients with heart and lung disease. It usually indicates a metabolic disturbance in the brain or increased intracranial pressure (ICP) from a deep cerebral or brain stem lesion.

Cheyne-Stokes respirations may indicate a major change in the patient's condition—usually for the worse. For example, in a patient who's had head trauma or brain surgery, Cheyne-Stokes respirations may signal increasing ICP.

Emergency interventions

 If you detect Cheyne-Stokes respirations in a patient with a history of head trauma, recent brain surgery, or other brain insult, quickly take his vital signs. Keep his head elevated 30 degrees. Perform a rapid neurologic examination to obtain baseline data, and reevaluate neurologic status frequently. If ICP continues to rise, you'll detect changes in the patient's level of consciousness (LOC), pupillary reactions, and ability to move his extremities. ICP monitoring is indicated.

Time the periods of hyperpnea and apnea for 3 to 4 minutes to evaluate respirations and to obtain baseline data. Be alert for prolonged periods of apnea. Frequently check blood pressure; also check skin color to detect signs of hypoxemia. Maintain airway patency and administer oxygen as needed. If the patient's condition worsens, endotracheal intubation is necessary.

History
When the patient's condition permits, obtain a brief history. Ask especially about drug use—large doses of narcotics, hypnotics, or barbiturates can precipitate Cheyne-Stokes respirations.

Common medical causes
• *Heart failure.* In left-sided heart failure, Cheyne-Stokes respirations may occur with exertional dyspnea and orthopnea. Related findings include fatigue, weakness, tachycardia, tachypnea, and crackles. A cough, usually nonproductive but occasionally producing clear or blood-tinged sputum, may also occur.

• *Hypertensive encephalopathy.* In this life-threatening disorder, severe hypertension precedes Cheyne-Stokes respirations. The patient's LOC will be decreased, and he may experience vomiting or seizures, severe headaches, visual disturbances (including transient blindness), and transient paralysis.

• *Increased ICP.* As ICP rises, Cheyne-Stokes is the first irregular respiratory pattern to occur. It's preceded by decreased LOC and accompanied by hypertension, headache, vomiting, impaired or unequal motor movement, and visual disturbances (blurring, diplopia, photophobia, and pupillary changes). In late stages of increased ICP, bradycardia and widened pulse pressure occur.

• *Renal failure.* In end-stage chronic renal failure, Cheyne-Stokes respirations may occur along with bleeding gums, oral lesions, ammonia breath odor, and marked changes in every body system.

• *Stokes-Adams attacks.* Cheyne-Stokes respirations may follow a Stokes-Adams attack—a syncopal episode associated with atrioventricular block. The patient is hypotensive, with a heart rate between 20 and 50 beats/minute. He may also appear pale, shaking, and confused.

Other causes
• *Drugs.* Large doses of hypnotics, narcotics, or barbiturates can precipitate Cheyne-Stokes respirations.

Special considerations
When evaluating Cheyne-Stokes respirations, be careful not to mistake periods of hypoventilation or decreased tidal volume for complete apnea.

Pediatric pointers
Cheyne-Stokes respirations rarely occur in children, except in late heart failure.

CHILLS
[Rigors]

Chills are extreme, involuntary muscle contractions with characteristic paroxysms of violent shivering and teeth-chattering. Commonly accompanied by fever, chills tend to arise suddenly and usually herald the onset of infection. (See *Why chills accompany fever.*) Certain diseases, such as pneumococcal pneumonia, produce only a single, shaking chill. Other diseases, such as malaria, produce intermittent chills with recurring high fever. Still others produce continuous chills for up to 1 hour, precipitating a high fever.

Chills can also result from lymphomas, transfusion reactions, and certain drugs. Chills without fever occur as a normal response to exposure to cold.

WHY CHILLS ACCOMPANY FEVER

Fever usually occurs when exogenous pyrogens activate endogenous pyrogens to reset the body's thermostat to a higher level. At this higher thermostatic set point, the body feels cold and responds through several compensatory mechanisms, including rhythmic muscle contractions, or chills. These muscle contractions in turn generate body heat and help produce fever. This flowchart outlines the events that link chills to fever.

Exogenous pyrogens (infectious organisms, immune complexes, toxins) enter the body.

Phagocytic leukocytes release endogenous pyrogens.

Endogenous pyrogens—possibly with prostaglandins—stimulate temperature-sensitive receptors in the hypothalamus and raise the thermostatic set point to a higher level.

Descending efferent pathways from the hypothalamus innervate effectors such as skeletal muscles and stimulate them to rhythmically contract.

Rhythmic muscle contractions, or chills, generate body heat, which helps produce fever.

History and physical examination

Ask the patient when the chills began and if they're continuous or intermittent. Because fever commonly accompanies chills, take his rectal temperature to obtain a baseline reading. Then check his temperature often to monitor fluctuations and to determine his temperature curve. Typically, a localized infection produces sudden onset of shaking chills, sweats, and high fever. A systemic infection produces intermittent chills with recurring episodes of high fever or continuous chills that may last up to 1 hour and precipitate a high fever.

Ask about related signs and symptoms, such as headache, dysuria, diarrhea, confusion, abdominal pain, cough, sore throat, or nausea. Does the patient have any known allergies or infections or a history of an infectious disorder? Find out which medications he's taking and if any drug has improved or worsened his symptoms. Ask about recent exposure to farm animals, guinea pigs, hamsters, dogs, and birds, such as pigeons, parrots, and parakeets. Also ask about recent insect or animal bites, travel to foreign countries, and contacts with persons who have an active infection.

Common medical causes

• *Acquired immunodeficiency syndrome.* This fatal disorder is caused by infection with human immunodeficiency virus and is transmitted by blood or semen. Most patients develop lymphadenopathy. Other findings may include fatigue, anorexia and weight loss, diarrhea, diaphoresis, skin disorders, and signs of upper respiratory infection.

• *Cholangitis.* Sudden obstruction of the common bile duct is characterized by Charcot's triad—chills with spiking fever, abdominal pain, and jaundice. The patient may have associated pruritus, weakness, and fatigue.

• *Gram-negative bacteremia.* This infection causes sudden chills and fever, nausea, vomiting, diarrhea, and prostration.

• *Hepatic abscess.* This infection most commonly arises abruptly, with chills, fever, nausea, vomiting, diarrhea, anorexia, and severe upper abdominal tenderness and pain that may radiate to the right shoulder.

• *Infective endocarditis.* This infection produces abrupt onset of intermittent, shaking chills with fever. Petechiae commonly develop, and the patient may also have Janeway lesions on his hands and feet and Osler's nodes on his palms and soles. Associated findings include murmur, hematuria, eye hemorrhage, Roth's spots, and signs of cardiac failure (dyspnea, peripheral edema).

• *Influenza.* Initially, this disorder causes abrupt onset of chills, high fever, malaise, headache, myalgias, and nonproductive cough. Some patients may also suddenly develop rhinitis, rhinorrhea, laryngitis, conjunctivitis, hoarseness, and sore throat. Chills generally subside after the first few days, but intermittent fever, weakness, and cough may persist up to 1 week.

• *Malaria.* The malarial paroxysm begins with a period of chills that lasts 1 to 2 hours. A high fever lasting 3 to 4 hours follows, and 2 to 4 hours of profuse diaphoresis complete the paroxysmal cycle. In benign malaria, the paroxysm may be interspersed with periods of well-being. The patient also has a headache, muscle pain, and possibly hepatosplenomegaly.

• *Pelvic inflammatory disease.* This infection causes chills and fever with, typically, lower abdominal pain and tenderness; a profuse, purulent vaginal discharge; and abnormal menstrual bleeding. The patient may also have nausea, vomiting, an abdominal mass, and dysuria.

• *Pneumonia.* A single shaking chill usually heralds the sudden onset of pneumococcal pneumonia; other pneumonias characteristically cause intermittent chills. In any type of pneumonia, related findings may include fever, productive cough with bloody sputum, pleuritic chest pain, dyspnea, tachypnea, and tachycardia. The patient may be cyanotic and diaphoretic, with bronchial breath sounds and crackles, rhonchi, increased tactile fremitus, and grunting respirations. He may also experience achiness, anorexia, fatigue, and headache.

• *Puerperal or postabortal sepsis.* Chills and high fever occur as early as 6 hours or as late as 10 days postpartum or postabortion. The patient may also have a purulent vaginal discharge, an enlarged and tender uterus, abdominal pain, backache, and nausea, vomiting, and diarrhea.

• *Pyelonephritis.* In acute pyelonephritis, the patient develops chills, high fever, and possibly nausea and vomiting over several hours to days. He usually also has anorexia, fatigue, myalgia, flank pain, costovertebral angle tenderness, hematuria or cloudy urine, and urinary frequency, urgency, and burning.

• *Renal abscess.* This disorder initially produces sudden chills and fever. Later effects include flank pain, costovertebral angle tenderness, abdominal muscle spasm, and transient hematuria.

• *Rocky Mountain spotted fever.* This disorder begins with sudden onset of chills, fever, malaise, excruciating headache, and muscle, bone, and joint pain. Typically, the patient's tongue is covered with a thick white coating that gradually turns brown. After 2 to 6 days of fever and occasional chills, a macular or maculopapular rash appears on the hands and feet and then becomes generalized; after a few days, the rash becomes petechial.

• *Septic arthritis.* Chills and fever accompany the characteristic red, swollen, and painful joints this disorder causes.

• *Septic shock.* Initially, septic shock produces chills, fever, and possibly nausea, vomiting, and diarrhea. The patient typically has flushed, warm, and dry skin; normal or slightly low blood pressure; tachycardia; and tachypnea. As septic shock progresses, his arms and legs become cool and cyanotic, and he develops oliguria, thirst, anxiety, restlessness, confusion, and hypotension. Later, his skin becomes cold and clammy, his pulse rapid and thready. He develops severe hypotension, persistent oliguria or anuria, signs of respiratory failure, and coma.

• *Sinusitis.* In acute sinusitis, chills occur along with fever, headache, and pain, tenderness, and swelling over the affected sinuses. Maxillary sinusitis produces pain over the cheeks and upper teeth; ethmoid sinusitis, pain over the eyes; frontal sinusitis, pain over the eyebrows; and sphenoid sinusitis, pain behind the eyes. The primary indicator of sinusitis is nasal discharge, which is commonly bloody for 24 to 48 hours before gradually becoming purulent.

• *Snake bite.* Most pit viper bites that result in envenomation cause chills, typically with fever. Other systemic signs and symptoms may include sweating, weakness, dizziness, fainting, hypotension, nausea, vomiting, diarrhea, and thirst. The area around the snake bite may be marked by immediate swelling and tenderness, pain, ecchymoses, petechiae, blebs, bloody discharge, and local necrosis. The patient may have difficulty speaking, blurred vision, and paralysis. He may also show bleeding tendencies and signs of respiratory distress and shock.

• *Violin spider bite.* This bite produces chills, fever, malaise, weakness, nausea, vomiting, and joint pain within 24 to 48 hours. The patient may also develop skin rash and delirium.

Other causes

• *Drugs.* Amphotericin B heads the list of common drugs associated with chills. However, I.V. bleomycin and intermittent administration of oral antipyretics can also cause chills.

• *I.V. therapy.* Infection at the I.V. insertion site can cause chills, high fever, and local redness, warmth, induration, and tenderness.

• *Transfusion reaction.* A hemolytic reaction may cause chills during the transfusion or immediately afterward. A nonhemolytic febrile reaction may also cause chills.

Special considerations

Check the patient's vital signs often, especially if his chills result from a known or suspected infection. Be alert for such signs of progressive septic shock as hypotension, tachycardia, and tachypnea. If appropriate, obtain samples of blood, sputum, or wound drainage for culture to determine the causative organism. Give antibiotics. Radiographic studies and serum and urine samples may be required.

Because chills are an involuntary response to an increased body temperature set by the hypothalamic thermostat, blankets won't stop a patient's chills or shivering. But keep his room temperature as even as possible. Provide adequate hydration and nutrients, and give antipyretics to help control fever. Irregular use of antipyretics can trigger compensatory chills.

Pediatric pointers
Infants don't get chills because they have poorly developed shivering mechanisms. In addition, most classic febrile childhood infections—such as measles and mumps—don't typically produce chills. But older children and teenagers have chills in mycoplasma pneumonia and acute pyogenic osteomyelitis.

CHVOSTEK'S SIGN

Chvostek's sign is an abnormal spasm of the facial muscles that's elicited by lightly tapping the patient's facial nerve near his lower jaw. This sign usually suggests hypocalcemia but can occur normally in about 25% of people. Typically, it precedes other signs of hypocalcemia and persists until the onset of tetany. It can't be elicited during tetany because of strong muscle contractions. (See *Eliciting Chvostek's sign.*)

Normally, eliciting Chvostek's sign is attempted only in patients with suspected hypocalcemic disorders. But because the parathyroid gland regulates calcium balance, Chvostek's sign may also be tested in patients before neck surgery to provide a baseline.

Emergency interventions
 Test for Trousseau's sign, a reliable indicator of hypocalcemia. (See "Trousseau's sign.") Closely monitor the patient for signs of tetany, such as carpopedal spasms or circumoral and extremity paresthesia.

History
Obtain a brief history. Find out if the patient has had surgery to remove his parathyroid glands or has a history of hypoparathyroidism, hypomagnesemia, or

EXAMINATION TIP

ELICITING CHVOSTEK'S SIGN

Begin by telling the patient to relax his facial muscles. Then stand directly in front of him and tap the facial nerve either just anterior to the earlobe and below the zygomatic arch or between the zygomatic arch and the corner of his mouth. A positive response varies from twitching of the lip at the corner of the mouth to spasm of all facial muscles, depending on the severity of hypocalcemia.

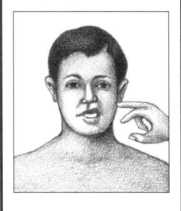

malabsorption disorder. Ask him or his family about mental changes, such as depression or slowed responses, which can accompany chronic hypocalcemia.

Common medical causes
• *Hypocalcemia.* The degree of Chvostek's sign response reflects the patient's serum calcium level. Initially, hypocalcemia produces paresthesia in the fingers, toes, and circumoral area that progresses to muscle tension and carpopedal spasms. The patient may also complain of muscle weakness, fatigue, and palpitations. Muscle twitching, hyperactive deep tendon reflexes, chorei-

form movements, and muscle cramps may also occur. The patient with chronic hypocalcemia may have mental status changes; diplopia; difficulty swallowing; abdominal cramps; dry, scaly skin; brittle nails; and thin, patchy scalp and eyebrow hair.

Other causes
● *Blood transfusion.* A massive transfusion can lower serum calcium levels and allow Chvostek's sign to be elicited.

Special considerations
Collect serum samples for serial calcium studies to evaluate the severity of hypocalcemia and the effectiveness of therapy. Such therapy involves oral or I.V. calcium supplements.

Pediatric pointers
Because Chvostek's sign may be present in healthy infants, it isn't elicited to detect neonatal tetany.

CLUBBING

A nonspecific sign of pulmonary and cyanotic cardiovascular disorders, clubbing is the painless, usually bilateral increase in soft tissue around the terminal phalanges of the fingers or toes. It doesn't involve changes in the underlying bone. In early clubbing, the normal 160-degree angle between the nail and the nail base is about 180 degrees. As clubbing progresses, this angle widens and the base of the nail becomes visibly swollen. In late clubbing, the angle where the nail meets the now-convex nail base extends more than halfway up the nail.

History and physical examination
You'll probably detect clubbing while evaluating other signs of known pulmonary or cardiovascular disease. Therefore, review the patient's current treatment plan because clubbing may resolve with correction of the underlying disorder. Also evaluate the extent of clubbing in both the fingers and toes. (See *Evaluating clubbed fingers,* page 130.)

Common medical causes
● *Bronchiectasis.* Clubbing is a common sign in the late stage of this disorder. You may also see this classic sign: a cough producing copious, foul-smelling, and mucopurulent sputum. Hemoptysis and coarse crackles over the affected area, heard during inspiration, are also characteristic. The patient may complain of weight loss, fatigue, weakness, and dyspnea on exertion. He may also have rhonchi, fever, malaise, and halitosis

● *Bronchitis.* In chronic bronchitis, clubbing may occur as a late sign and is unrelated to the severity of the disease. The patient has a chronic productive cough. He may display barrel chest, dyspnea, wheezing, increased use of accessory muscles, cyanosis, tachypnea, crackles, scattered rhonchi, and prolonged expiration.

● *Emphysema.* Clubbing occurs late in this disease. The patient may have anorexia, malaise, dyspnea, tachypnea, diminished breath sounds, peripheral cyanosis, and pursed-lip breathing. He may also display accessory muscle use, barrel chest, and a productive cough.

● *Endocarditis.* In subacute infective endocarditis, clubbing may be accompanied by fever, anorexia, pallor, weakness, night sweats, fatigue, tachycardia, and weight loss. The patient may also have arthralgia, petechiae, Osler's nodes, splinter hemorrhages, Janeway lesions, splenomegaly, and Roth's spots. Cardiac murmurs are usually present.

● *Heart failure.* Clubbing occurs as a late sign along with wheezing, dyspnea, and fatigue. Other findings may include neck vein distention, hepatomegaly, tachypnea, palpitations, dependent edema, unexplained weight gain, nausea, anorexia, chest tightness, slowed mental

EVALUATING CLUBBED FINGERS

To quickly examine a patient's fingers for early clubbing, gently palpate the bases of his nails. Normally, they'll feel firm—but in early clubbing, nail bases will feel springy when palpated.

To evaluate late clubbing, have the patient place the first phalanges of the forefingers together. Normal nail bases are concave and create a small, diamond-shaped space when the first phalanges are opposed (top). In late clubbing, however, the now-convex nail bases can touch without leaving a space (bottom).

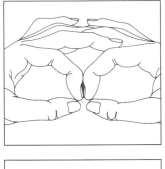

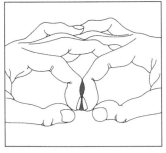

response, hypotension, diaphoresis, narrow pulse pressure, pallor, oliguria, a gallop rhythm (S_3), and crackles on inspiration.

● *Interstitial fibrosis.* Clubbing occurs in almost all patients with advanced interstitial fibrosis. Typically, the patient will also have intermittent chest pain, dyspnea, crackles, fatigue, weight loss, and possible cyanosis.

● *Lung abscess.* Initially, this disorder produces clubbing, which may reverse with resolution of the abscess. It can also produce pleuritic chest pain; dyspnea; crackles; productive cough with a large amount of purulent, foul-smelling, often bloody sputum; and halitosis. The patient may also experience weakness, fatigue, anorexia, headache, malaise, weight loss, and fever with chills. You may hear decreased breath sounds.

● *Lung and pleural cancer.* Clubbing occurs commonly in this cancer. Associated findings may include hemoptysis, dyspnea, wheezing, chest pain, weight loss, anorexia, fatigue, and fever.

Special considerations
Don't mistake curved nails—a normal variation—for clubbing. Always remember that the angle between the nail and its base remains normal in curved nails, but not in clubbing.

Pediatric pointers
In children, clubbing occurs most commonly in cyanotic congenital heart disease and cystic fibrosis. Surgical correction of heart defects may reverse clubbing.

COGWHEEL RIGIDITY

This cardinal sign of Parkinson's disease is marked by muscle rigidity that reacts with superimposed ratchetlike movements when the muscle is passively stretched. This sign can be elicited by stabilizing the patient's forearm and then moving his hand through the range of motion. (Cogwheel rigidity usually appears in the arms but can sometimes be elicited in the ankle.) Both the patient and the examiner can see and feel these characteristic movements, thought to be a combination of rigidity and tremor.

History and physical examination

After you've elicited cogwheel rigidity, take the patient's history to determine when he first noticed associated signs of Parkinson's disease. For example, has he experienced tremors? Did he notice tremors of his hands first? Does he have pill-rolling hand movements? When did he first notice that his movements were becoming slower? How long has he been experiencing stiffness in his arms and legs? Has his handwriting become smaller? While taking the history, observe for signs of pronounced Parkinsonism, such as drooling, a masklike face, dysphagia, monotone speech, and altered gait.

Find out which medications the patient is taking, and ask if they've helped relieve some of his symptoms. If he's taking levodopa and his symptoms have worsened, find out if he's exceeded the prescribed dosage. If you suspect an overdose, withhold the drug.

If the patient has been taking a phenothiazine or another antipsychotic drug and has no history of Parkinson's disease, he may be having an adverse reaction to his medication. Withhold the drug, as appropriate.

Common medical causes

• *Parkinson's disease.* In this disorder, cogwheel rigidity occurs together with an insidious tremor, which usually begins in the fingers (unilateral pill-rolling tremor), increases during stress or anxiety, and decreases with purposeful movement and sleep.

Bradykinesia (slowness of voluntary movements and speech) also occurs. The patient walks with short, shuffling steps; his gait lacks normal parallel motion and may be retropulsive or propulsive. He speaks in a monotone voice and has a masklike facial expression; he may experience drooling; loss of posture control, so that he walks with his body bent forward; dysphagia; or dysarthria. An oculogyric crisis (eyes fixed upward and involuntary tonic movements) or blepharospasm (complete eyelid closure) may also occur.

Other causes

• *Drugs.* Phenothiazines and other antipsychotics—such as haloperidol, thiothixene, and loxapine—can cause cogwheel rigidity. Metoclopramide causes it occasionally.

Special considerations

If the patient has associated muscular dysfunction, assist him with ambulation, feeding, and other activities of daily living, as needed. Provide symptomatic care as appropriate. For example, administer stool softeners if the patient has constipation, or offer a soft diet with small, frequent feedings if he has dysphagia. Refer the patient to the National Parkinson Foundation or the American Parkinson Disease Association, which provide educational materials and support.

Pediatric pointers

Cogwheel rigidity is not common in children.

COLD INTOLERANCE

This increased sensitivity to cold temperatures, which usually develops gradually, reflects damage to the body's temperature-regulating mechanism. The symptom usually results from a tumor or a hormonal deficiency. In elderly patients, onset of cold intolerance reflects normal age-related physiologic changes.

History and physical examination
Find out when the patient first noticed cold intolerance: When did he begin using more blankets or wearing heavier clothing? Ask about associated signs and symptoms, such as changes in vision or in the texture or amount of body hair. If the patient is female, ask her about changes in her normal menstrual pattern.

Before proceeding with the physical examination, obtain a brief history. Does the patient have a history of hypothyroidism or hypothalamic disease? Is he currently taking any medications? If so, is he complying with the prescribed schedule and dosage? Has the regimen been changed recently?

Now perform a physical examination. Begin by taking the patient's vital signs and checking for hypothermia, dry skin, and hair loss. Then ask the patient to straighten and extend his arms. Are his hands shaking? During the examination, note if the patient shivers or complains of chills. Provide a blanket if necessary.

Common medical causes
• *Hypopituitarism.* Clinical features usually develop slowly in this disorder and vary with its severity. Cold intolerance and shivering typically accompany cold, dry, and thin skin with a waxy pallor, and fine wrinkles around the mouth. Other findings may include fatigue, lethargy, menstrual disturbances, impotence, decreased libido, nervousness, irritability, headache, and hunger. If hypopituitarism results from a pituitary tumor, expect neurologic signs and symptoms, such as headache, bilateral temporal hemianopia, loss of visual acuity, and possibly blindness.
• *Hypothalamic lesion.* A patient with hypothalamic damage may show unexplained fluctuations from cold intolerance to heat intolerance. Cold intolerance develops suddenly; the patient typically complains of feeling chilled, shivering, and wearing extra clothes to keep warm. Related findings include amenorrhea, disturbed sleep pattern, increased thirst and urination, vigorous appetite with weight gain, decreased vision, headache, and such personality changes as attacks of rage, laughing, and crying.
• *Hypothyroidism.* Cold intolerance develops early in this disorder and progressively worsens. Other early findings include fatigue, anorexia with weight gain, constipation, and menorrhagia. As hypothyroidism progresses, the patient has loss of libido and slowed intellectual and motor activity. The hair becomes dry and sparse, the nails thick and brittle, and the skin dry, pale, cool, and doughy. Eventually, the patient displays a dull expression with periorbital and facial edema and puffy hands and feet. Relaxation is delayed after deep tendon reflex testing. Bradycardia, abdominal distention, and ataxia may also occur.

Special considerations
Help increase the patient's comfort by regulating his room temperature and by providing extra clothing and blankets. Allow the patient to openly express his concerns about body image changes related to his cold intolerance. Instruct him and his family to adapt the patient's environment to meet his needs.

Prepare the patient for diagnostic tests to determine the cause of cold intolerance. Once the cause is known, explain the disease process to the patient and his family to help alleviate their anxiety. Also explain that, with proper treatment, he can expect relief from his symptoms.

Elder tip
 For elderly patients in the hospital, keep the room temperature around 70° F (21.1° C) or warmer if possible. Also, avoid positioning the patient near drafts, and make sure he has extra blankets as needed. Ad-

vise a patient living at home to follow these same steps. In addition, encourage him to arrange "check-in times" with family and friends, especially during inclement weather, to ensure assistance in times of food shortage or power failure.

Pediatric pointers

In an infant, some degree of cold intolerance is normal, because fat distribution is decreased and the temperature-regulating mechanism is immature at birth. Make sure the parents understand that their infant will quickly lose body heat if he's exposed to cold temperatures. Instruct them to dress the infant warmly for sleep and before going outdoors and to avoid chilling him during his bath.

An infant with cold intolerance due to hypothyroidism may have subtle, nonspecific signs of the underlying disorder—or none at all. He typically shivers and has a subnormal temperature (below 86° F [30° C]), blue lips, and cold, mottled skin, especially on the extremities.

CONFUSION

An umbrella term for puzzling or inappropriate behavior or responses, *confusion* reflects the inability to think quickly and coherently. Depending on its cause, confusion may arise suddenly or gradually and may be temporary or irreversible. Aggravated by stress and sensory deprivation, confusion commonly occurs in hospitalized patients—especially the elderly, in whom it may be mistaken for senility.

When severe confusion arises suddenly and the patient also has hallucinations and psychomotor hyperactivity, his condition is classified as *delirium*. Long-term, progressive confusion with deterioration of all cognitive functions is classified as *dementia*.

Confusion can result from early fluid and electrolyte imbalance or hypoxemia due to pulmonary disorders. It can also have a metabolic, neurologic, cardiovascular, cerebrovascular, or nutritional origin or can result from a severe systemic infection or the effects of toxins, drugs, or alcohol. Confusion may signal worsening of an underlying and perhaps irreversible disease.

History and physical examination

When you take his history, ask the patient to describe what's bothering him. He may not report confusion as his chief complaint but may complain of memory loss, persistent apprehension, or inability to concentrate. He may be unable to respond logically to direct questions. Ask a family member or friend about onset and frequency. Find out, too, if the patient has a history of head trauma or a cardiopulmonary, metabolic, cerebrovascular, or neurologic disorder. Which medications is he taking, if any? Ask about any changes in eating or sleeping habits and in drug or alcohol use.

Now perform a neurologic assessment to establish the patient's level of consciousness.

Common medical causes

● *Brain tumor.* In the early stages of a brain tumor, confusion is usually mild and difficult to detect. As the tumor impinges on cerebral structures, the patient's confusion worsens, and he may display personality changes, bizarre behavior, or sensory and motor deficits. He may also have visual field deficits and aphasia.

● *Dementia.* This group of progressive brain diseases—such as Alzheimer's disease—eventually produces severe and irreversible confusion along with memory loss and intellectual deterioration. (See *Music therapy for Alzheimer's patients,* page 134.) Disorientation, tremors, and gait disturbances may also occur.

● *Fluid and electrolyte imbalance.* The extent of the imbalance determines the

MUSIC THERAPY FOR ALZHEIMER'S PATIENTS

Based on the theory that sound waves affect brain frequencies, muscle tension, breathing, and other body processes, music therapy is currently being used to treat patients with Alzheimer's disease. Music is an external sensory stimulant for Alzheimer's patients, who may not be able to communicate through words or movement. It is thought to tap into remote memories, provide emotional comfort, and improve communication through rhythm.

severity of the patient's confusion. Typically, he'll show signs of dehydration, such as lassitude, poor skin turgor, dry skin and mucous membranes, and oliguria. He may also have hypotension and a low-grade fever.

• *Head trauma.* Concussion, contusion, and brain hemorrhage may produce confusion at the time of injury, shortly afterward, or months or even years afterward. The patient may be delirious, with periodic loss of consciousness. Vomiting, severe headache, pupillary changes, and sensory and motor deficits are also common.

• *Heat stroke.* This disorder causes pronounced confusion that gradually worsens as body temperature rises. Initially, the patient may be irritable and dizzy; later, he may become delirious, have seizures, and lose consciousness.

• *Hypothermia.* Confusion may be an early symptom of this disorder. Typically, the patient displays slurred speech, cold and pale skin, hyperactive deep tendon reflexes, rapid pulse, and decreased

blood pressure and respiratory rate. As his body temperature continues to drop, his confusion progresses to stupor and coma, his muscles develop rigidity, and his respiratory rate decreases further.

• *Hypoxemia.* Acute pulmonary disorders that result in hypoxemia produce confusion that can range from mild disorientation to delirium. Chronic pulmonary disorders produce persistent confusion.

• *Infection.* Severe generalized infections, such as sepsis, commonly produce delirium. Central nervous system (CNS) infections, such as meningitis, cause varying degrees of confusion as well as headache and nuchal rigidity.

• *Low perfusion states.* Mild confusion is an early symptom of decreased cerebral perfusion. Associated findings usually include hypotension, tachycardia or bradycardia, irregular pulse, ventricular gallop, edema, and cyanosis.

• *Nutritional deficiencies.* Inadequate dietary intake of thiamine, niacin, or vitamin B_{12} produces insidious, progressive confusion and possible mental deterioration.

• *Seizure disorders.* Mild to moderate confusion may immediately follow any type of seizure. The confusion usually disappears within several hours.

Other causes

• *Alcohol.* Intoxication causes confusion and stupor, and alcohol withdrawal may cause delirium and seizures.

• *Drugs.* Large doses of CNS depressants produce confusion that can persist for several days after the drug is discontinued. Narcotic and barbiturate withdrawal also causes acute confusion, possibly with delirium. Other drugs that commonly cause confusion include lidocaine, digitalis glycosides, indomethacin, cycloserine, chloroquine, atropine, and cimetidine.

Special considerations

Never leave a confused patient unattended to prevent injury to himself and others. (Apply restraints only if necessary to ensure his safety.) Keep the patient calm and quiet, and plan uninterrupted rest periods. To help him stay oriented, keep a large calendar and a clock visible, and make a list of his activities with specific dates and times. Reintroduce yourself to the patient each time you enter his room.

Pediatric pointers

Confusion can't be determined in infants and very young children. However, older children with acute febrile illnesses commonly experience transient delirium or acute confusion.

CONSTIPATION

Constipation is defined as small, infrequent, or difficult bowel movements. Because normal bowel movements can vary in frequency and from individual to individual, constipation must be determined in light of the patient's normal elimination pattern. Constipation may be a minor annoyance or, rarely, a symptom of a life-threatening disorder such as acute intestinal obstruction. Untreated, constipation can lead to headache, anorexia, and abdominal discomfort and can adversely affect the patient's lifestyle and well-being.

Constipation usually occurs when the urge to defecate is suppressed and the muscles associated with bowel movements remain contracted. Because the autonomic nervous system controls bowel movements—by sensing rectal distention from fecal contents and by stimulating the external sphincter—any factor that influences this system may cause bowel dysfunction. (See *How habits and stress cause constipation,* page 136.)

History and physical examination

Ask the patient to describe the frequency and consistency of his bowel movements and the size of his stools. How long has he had constipation? Acute constipation usually has an organic cause, such as an anal or rectal disorder. In a patient over age 45, recent onset of constipation may be an early symptom of colorectal cancer. Conversely, chronic constipation typically has a functional cause and may be related to stress.

Does the patient have pain related to constipation? If so, when did he first notice it, and where is it located? Cramping abdominal pain and distention suggest obstipation—extreme, persistent constipation due to intestinal tract obstruction. Ask the patient if elimination worsens or helps relieve the pain. Elimination usually worsens pain, but in disorders such as irritable bowel syndrome, it may relieve it.

Ask the patient to describe his typical daily diet. Estimate his daily fiber and fluid intake. Ask about any changes in eating habits, in medication or alcohol use, or in physical activity. Has he experienced recent emotional distress? Has constipation affected his family life or social contacts? Also ask about his job. A sedentary or stressful job can contribute to constipation.

Find out whether the patient has a history of GI, rectoanal, neurologic, or metabolic disorders; abdominal surgery; or radiation therapy. Then ask about the medications he's taking, including over-the-counter preparations, such as laxatives, mineral oil, stool softeners, and enemas.

Inspect the abdomen for distention or scars from previous surgery. Then auscultate for bowel sounds, and characterize their motility. Percuss all four quadrants, and gently palpate for abdominal tenderness, a palpable mass, or hepatomegaly. Next, examine the patient's rectum. Spread his buttocks to expose the anus, and inspect for inflammation,

HOW HABITS AND STRESS CAUSE CONSTIPATION

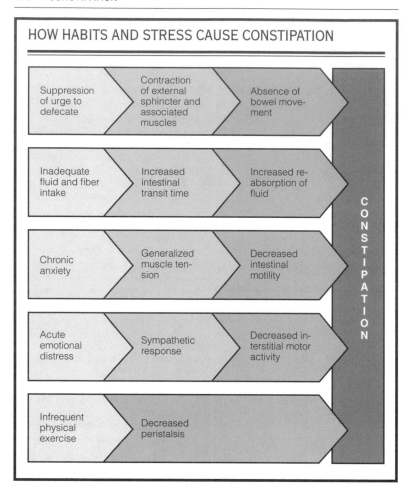

lesions, scars, fissures, and external hemorrhoids. Use a disposable glove and lubricant to palpate the anal sphincter for laxity or stricture. Also palpate for rectal masses and fecal impaction. Finally, obtain a stool sample and test it for occult blood.

As you evaluate the patient, remember that constipation can also result from several life-threatening disorders, such as acute intestinal obstruction and mesenteric artery ischemia—but it doesn't herald these conditions.

Common medical causes

● *Anal fissure.* A crack or laceration in the lining of the anal wall can cause acute constipation—usually due to the patient's fear of the severe tearing or burning pain associated with bowel movements. He may notice a few drops of blood streaking toilet tissue or his underclothes.

● *Anorectal abscess.* In this disorder, constipation occurs together with severe, throbbing, localized pain and tenderness at the abscess site. The patient may also have localized inflammation, swelling, and purulent drainage and complain of fever and malaise.

- *Cirrhosis.* In the early stages of cirrhosis, the patient has constipation along with nausea, vomiting, and a dull pain in the right upper quadrant. Other early findings include indigestion, anorexia, flatulence, hepatomegaly, and possibly splenomegaly and diarrhea.

- *Diabetic neuropathy.* This type of neuropathy produces episodic constipation or diarrhea. Other signs and symptoms may include dysphagia, postural hypotension, syncope, and painless bladder distention with overflow incontinence. A male patient may also experience impotence and retrograde ejaculation.

- *Diverticulitis.* In this disorder, constipation or diarrhea occurs with left lower quadrant pain and tenderness and possibly a palpable abdominal mass. The patient may have mild nausea, flatulence, or a low-grade fever.

- *Hemorrhoids.* Thrombosed hemorrhoids cause constipation as the patient tries to avoid the severe pain of defecation. The hemorrhoids may bleed during defecation.

- *Hepatic porphyria.* Abdominal pain—which may be severe, colicky, localized, or generalized—precedes constipation in hepatic porphyria. The patient may also have fever, sinus tachycardia, labile hypertension, excessive diaphoresis, severe vomiting, photophobia, urine retention, nervousness or restlessness, disorientation, and possibly visual hallucinations. His deep tendon reflexes may be diminished or absent. Some patients have skin lesions causing itching, burning, erythema, altered pigmentation, and edema in areas exposed to light. Severe hepatic porphyria can produce delirium, coma, seizures, paraplegia, or complete flaccid quadriplegia.

- *Hypothyroidism.* This disorder causes early and insidious onset of constipation. Other early signs and symptoms include fatigue, sensitivity to cold, anorexia with weight gain, and menorrhagia.

- *Intestinal obstruction.* Constipation associated with this disorder varies in severity and onset with the location and extent of the obstruction. In partial obstruction, constipation may alternate with leakage of liquid stool. In complete obstruction, obstipation may occur. Constipation can be the earliest symptom of partial colon obstruction, but it usually occurs later if the level of the obstruction is more proximal. Associated findings may include episodes of colicky abdominal pain, abdominal distention, nausea, or vomiting. The patient may also have hyperactive bowel sounds, visible peristaltic waves, a palpable abdominal mass, and abdominal tenderness.

- *Irritable bowel syndrome.* This common syndrome usually produces chronic constipation, although some patients may have intermittent, watery diarrhea and others may complain of alternating constipation and diarrhea. Stress may trigger nausea and abdominal distention and tenderness, but defecation usually relieves these symptoms. Typically, the stools are scybalous and contain visible mucus.

- *Mesenteric artery ischemia.* This life-threatening disorder produces sudden constipation with failure to expel stool or flatus. Initially, it also produces severe abdominal pain, tenderness, vomiting, and anorexia. Later, the patient may develop abdominal guarding, rigidity, and distention; tachycardia; tachypnea; fever; and signs of shock, such as cool, clammy skin and hypotension. A bruit may be heard.

- *Spinal cord lesion.* Constipation may occur in this disorder along with urine retention, sexual dysfunction, pain, and possibly motor weakness, paralysis, or sensory impairment below the level of the lesion.

Other causes

- *Diagnostic tests.* Constipation can result from retention of barium given during certain GI studies.

• **Drugs.** Many patients experience constipation when taking narcotic analgesics, vinca alkaloids, calcium channel blockers, antacids containing aluminum or calcium, anticholinergics, and drugs with anticholinergic effects (such as tricyclic antidepressants). Excessive use of laxatives or enemas can also lead to constipation.

• **Surgery and radiation therapy.** Constipation can result from rectoanal surgery, which may traumatize nerves, and abdominal irradiation, which may cause intestinal stricture.

Special considerations

As indicated, prepare the patient for diagnostic tests, such as proctosigmoidoscopy, colonoscopy, barium enema, plain abdominal X-rays, and an upper GI series.

Stress the importance of a high-fiber diet, and encourage the patient to drink sufficient fluids. (Explain to the patient that he may experience temporary bloating or flatulence after adding fiber to his diet.) Also encourage him to exercise at least 1½ hours each week if possible.

If the patient is on bed rest, reposition him frequently, and help him perform active or passive exercises, as indicated. Teach him abdominal toning exercises if his abdominal muscles are weak, and relaxation techniques to help him reduce stress related to constipation.

Caution the patient not to strain during defecation to prevent injuring rectoanal tissue. Instruct him to avoid using laxatives or enemas. If the patient has been abusing these products, begin weaning him from them. Use a disposable glove and lubricant to remove impacted fecal contents. (Check if an oil-retention enema can be given first to soften the fecal mass.)

Pediatric pointers

The high content of casein and calcium in cow's milk can produce hard stools and possibly constipation in bottle-fed infants. Other causes of constipation in infants include inadequate fluid intake, Hirschsprung's disease, and anal fissures.

In older children, constipation usually results from inadequate fiber intake and excessive intake of milk. However, it may also result from bowel spasm, mechanical obstruction, and hypothyroidism.

CORNEAL REFLEX, ABSENT

The corneal reflex is tested bilaterally by drawing a fine-pointed wisp of sterile cotton from a corner of each eye to the cornea. Normally, even though only one eye is tested at a time, the patient blinks bilaterally each time either cornea is touched. This is the corneal reflex. When this reflex is absent, however, neither eyelid closes when the cornea of one is touched. (See *Eliciting the corneal reflex.*)

The site of the afferent fibers for this reflex is in the ophthalmic branch of the trigeminal nerve (cranial nerve V); the efferent fibers are located in the facial nerve (cranial nerve VII). Unilateral or bilateral absence of the corneal reflex may result from damage to these nerves.

History and physical examination

If you're unable to elicit the corneal reflex, look for other signs of trigeminal nerve dysfunction. To test the three sensory portions of the nerve, touch each side of the patient's face on the brow, cheek, and jaw with a cotton wisp, and ask him to compare the sensations.

If you suspect facial nerve involvement, note if both the upper face (brow and eyes) and lower face (cheek, mouth, and chin) are weak bilaterally. Lower motor neuron facial weakness affects the face on the same side as the lesion, whereas upper motor neuron weakness affects the side opposite the lesion—primarily the lower facial muscles.

Because an absent corneal reflex may signify such progressive neurologic disorders as Guillain-Barré syndrome, ask the patient about associated symptoms, such as facial pain, dysphagia, and limb weakness.

Common medical causes

● *Acoustic neuroma.* This tumor affects the trigeminal nerve, causing a diminished or absent corneal reflex, tinnitus, and unilateral hearing impairment. Facial palsy and anesthesia, palate weakness, and signs of cerebellar dysfunction (ataxia, nystagmus) may result if the tumor impinges on the adjacent cranial nerves, brain stem, and cerebellum.

● *Bell's palsy.* A common cause of a diminished or absent corneal reflex, this disorder causes paralysis of cranial nerve VII. It can also produce complete hemifacial weakness or paralysis, and drooling on the affected side. The affected side also sags and appears masklike. The eye on this side can't be shut and tears constantly.

● *Brain stem infarction or injury.* An absent corneal reflex can occur on the side opposite the lesion when infarction or injury affects cranial nerve V or VII. Associated findings may include decreased level of consciousness, dysphagia, dysarthria, contralateral limb weakness, and early signs and symptoms of increased intracranial pressure, such as headache and vomiting.

In massive brain stem infarction or injury, the patient also displays respiratory changes, such as apneustic breathing or periods of apnea; bilateral pupillary dilation or constriction with decreased responsiveness to light; rising systolic blood pressure; widening pulse pressure; bradycardia; and coma.

● *Guillain-Barré syndrome.* In this polyneuropathic disorder, a diminished or absent corneal reflex accompanies ipsilateral loss of facial muscle control. Dys-

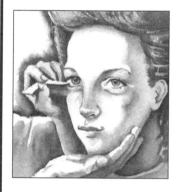
arthria and dysphagia also may occur. Muscle weakness, the primary neurologic symptom of this disorder, typically starts in the legs, then extends to the arms and facial nerves within 72 hours. Other findings include paresthesia, respiratory muscle paralysis, respiratory insufficiency, postural hypotension, incontinence, diaphoresis, and tachycardia.

Special considerations

When the corneal reflex is absent, you'll need to take measures to protect the patient's affected eye from injury. For example, lubricate the eye with artificial tears to prevent drying, cover the cornea with a shield, and avoid excessive corneal reflex testing.

Prepare the patient for cranial X-rays or a computed tomography scan.

Pediatric pointers

Brain stem lesions and injuries are the most common causes of absent corneal reflexes in children; Guillain-Barré syndrome occurs less commonly. Infants, especially those born prematurely, may have an absent corneal reflex due to anoxic damage to the brain stem.

COSTOVERTEBRAL ANGLE TENDERNESS

This elicited symptom indicates sudden distention of the renal capsule. It almost always accompanies unelicited, dull, constant flank pain in the costovertebral angle (CVA) just lateral to the sacrospinal muscle and below the 12th rib. This associated pain typically travels anteriorly in the subcostal region toward the umbilicus.

Percussing the CVA elicits CVA tenderness. (See *Eliciting CVA tenderness.*) A patient who doesn't have this symptom will perceive a thudding, jarring, or pressure-like sensation when tested, but no pain. A patient with a disorder that distends the renal capsule will experience intense pain as the renal capsule stretches and stimulates the afferent nerves, which emanate from the spinal cord at levels T11 through L2 and innervate the kidney.

History and physical examination

After detecting CVA tenderness, determine the possible extent of renal damage. First, find out if the patient has other symptoms of renal or urologic dysfunction. Ask about voiding habits: How frequently does he urinate and in what amounts? Has he noticed any change in intake or output? If so, when did he notice the change? (Ask about fluid intake before judging his output abnormal.) Has he had nocturia, difficulty starting a stream, or pain or burning during urination? Does he strain to urinate without being able to do so (tenesmus)? Ask about urine color; brown or bright red urine may contain blood.

Explore other signs and symptoms. For example, if the patient is experiencing pain in his flank, abdomen, or back, when did he first notice it? How severe is it, and where is it located?

Find out if the patient or a family member has a history of urinary tract infections, congenital anomalies, calculi, or other obstructive nephropathies or uropathies. Ask about a history of renovascular disorders, such as occlusion of the renal arteries or veins.

Perform a brief physical examination. Begin by taking the patient's vital signs. Fever and chills in a patient with CVA tenderness may indicate acute pyelonephritis. If the patient has hypertension and bradycardia, be alert for other autonomic effects of renal pain, such as diaphoresis and pallor. Inspect, auscultate, and gently palpate the abdomen for clues to the underlying cause of CVA tenderness. Be alert for abdominal distention, hypoactive bowel sounds, or palpable masses.

Common medical causes

• *Calculi.* Infundibular and ureteropelvic or ureteral calculi produce CVA tenderness and flank pain. The patient may also have nausea, vomiting, severe abdominal pain, abdominal distention, and decreased bowel sounds.

• *Perirenal abscess.* Causing exquisite CVA tenderness, this disorder may also produce severe unilateral flank pain, dysuria, persistent high fever, chills, erythema of the skin, and sometimes a palpable abdominal mass.

• *Pyelonephritis (acute).* Perhaps the most common cause of CVA tenderness, acute pyelonephritis is accompanied in many cases by a persistent high fever,

EXAMINATION TIP

ELICITING C.V.A. TENDERNESS

To elicit costovertebral angle (CVA) tenderness, have the patient sit upright facing away from you or have him lie prone. Place the palm of your left hand over the left CVA, then strike the back of your left hand with the ulnar surface of your right fist, as shown. Repeat this percussion technique over the right CVA. A patient with CVA tenderness will experience intense pain.

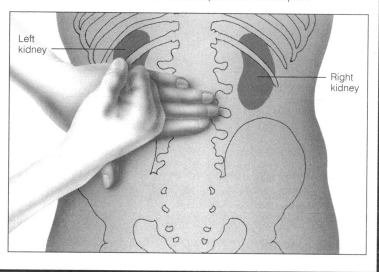

Left kidney

Right kidney

chills, flank pain, weakness, dysuria, hematuria, nocturia, urinary urgency and frequency, and tenesmus.

- **Renal artery occlusion.** In this disorder, the patient experiences flank pain as well as CVA tenderness. Other findings include nausea, vomiting, decreased bowel sounds, high fever after 1 to 2 days, and severe, continuous upper abdominal pain.

- **Renal vein occlusion.** The patient with this disorder has CVA tenderness and flank pain. He also may have fever, hematuria, and sudden, severe back pain.

Special considerations

Administer pain medication and continue to monitor the patient's vital signs and intake and output. Collect serum and urine samples, and then prepare the patient for radiologic studies, such as excretory urography, renal arteriography, and a computed tomography scan.

Pediatric pointers

An infant with a disorder that distends the renal capsule won't have CVA tenderness. Instead, he'll display nonspecific signs, such as vomiting, diarrhea, and fever. In older children, however, CVA tenderness has the same diagnostic significance as in adults.

COUGH, BARKING

Resonant, brassy, and harsh, a barking cough is part of a complex of signs and symptoms that characterize croup syndrome—a group of pediatric disorders marked by varying degrees of respiratory distress. Croup syndrome is most common in boys and most prevalent in fall; it may recur in the same child.

A barking cough indicates edema of the larynx and surrounding tissue and may signal a life-threatening emergency. Infants and children can rapidly develop airway occlusion from edema because their airways are smaller in diameter than adults'.

Emergency interventions

 Quickly evaluate the child's respiratory status; then take his vital signs. Be particularly alert for tachycardia and signs of hypoxemia. Also check for a decreased level of consciousness (LOC). Try to determine if the child had been playing with any small object that he may have aspirated.

Check for cyanosis in the lips and nail beds. Observe for sternal or intercostal retractions or nasal flaring. Next, note the depth and rate of respirations—they may become increasingly shallow as respiratory distress increases. Observe the child's body position: Is he sitting up, leaning forward, struggling to breathe? Observe his activity level, facial expression, and LOC.

With increasing respiratory distress from airway edema, the child will become restless, with a frightened, wide-eyed expression. As air hunger continues, he'll become lethargic and difficult to arouse.

If the child shows signs of severe respiratory distress, maintain airway patency and provide oxygen. Endotracheal intubation or a tracheotomy may be necessary.

History and physical examination

Ask the child's parents when the barking cough began and what other signs and symptoms accompanied it. When did the child first appear to be ill? Has he had previous episodes of croup syndrome? Did his condition improve upon exposure to cold air? Auscultate for breath sounds. No crackles or rhonchi should be heard.

Spasmodic croup and epiglottitis both typically occur in the middle of the night; the child with spasmodic croup has no fever, but the child with epiglottitis does—a high one. An upper respiratory infection typically is followed by laryngotracheobronchitis.

Common medical causes

● *Epiglottitis.* This life-threatening disorder has become less common because of the increasing use of influenza vaccines. It occurs nocturnally, heralded by a barking cough and a high fever. The child is hoarse, dysphagic, dyspneic, and restless and appears extremely ill and panicky. The cough may progress to severe respiratory distress with sternal and intercostal retractions, nasal flaring, cyanosis, and tachycardia. The child will struggle to get sufficient air as epiglottic edema increases.

● *Laryngotracheobronchitis (acute).* Most common in children between the ages of 9 and 18 months, this viral infection initially produces low to moderate fever, runny nose, poor appetite, and infrequent cough. When the infection descends into the laryngotracheal area, barking cough, hoarseness, and inspiratory stridor occur.

As respiratory distress progresses, substernal and intercostal retractions occur along with tachycardia and shallow, rapid respirations. Sleeping in a dry room worsens these signs. The child becomes restless, irritable, pale, and cyanotic.

• *Spasmodic croup.* Acute spasmodic croup usually occurs during sleep with abrupt onset of a barking cough that awakens the child. He typically won't have a fever but may be hoarse, restless, and dyspneic. As his respiratory distress worsens, the child may exhibit sternal and intercostal retractions, nasal flaring, tachycardia, cyanosis, and an anxious, frantic appearance. The symptoms usually subside within a few hours, but attacks tend to recur.

Other causes
• *Aspiration of a foreign body.* Partial obstruction of the upper airway first produces sudden hoarseness, then a barking cough and inspiratory stridor. Other effects of this life-threatening condition include gagging, tachycardia, dyspnea, decreased breath sounds, wheezing, and possibly cyanosis.

Special considerations
If the child is not in severe respiratory distress, a lateral neck X-ray may be done to visualize any epiglottal edema and a chest X-ray may be done to rule out lower respiratory tract infection. Depending on the child's age and his degree of respiratory distress, oxygen may be administered. Rapid-acting epinephrine and steroids should be considered.

Be sure to observe the child frequently, and monitor the oxygen level if used. Provide the child with periods of rest with minimal interruptions. Maintain a calm, quiet environment and offer reassurance. Encourage the child's parents to stay with him to help alleviate stress.

Teach the parents how to evaluate and treat recurrent episodes. For example, creating steam by running hot water in a sink or shower and sitting with the child in the closed bathroom may help relieve subsequent attacks of croup syndrome. The child may also benefit from being brought outside (properly dressed) to breathe cold night air.

COUGH, NONPRODUCTIVE

A nonproductive cough is a noisy, forceful expulsion of air from the lungs that doesn't yield sputum or blood. It's one of the most common complaints of patients with respiratory disorders.

Coughing is a necessary protective mechanism that clears airway passages. However, a nonproductive cough is not only ineffective but can also cause damage—such as airway collapse or rupture of alveoli or blebs. And a nonproductive cough that later becomes productive is a classic sign of progressive respiratory disease.

The cough reflex generally occurs when mechanical, chemical, thermal, inflammatory, or psychogenic stimuli activate cough receptors. (See *Reviewing the cough mechanism,* page 144.) But external pressure—for example, from subdiaphragmatic irritation or a mediastinal tumor—can also induce it. So can voluntary expiration of air, which occasionally occurs as a nervous habit.

A cough may occur once or several times, as in a paroxysm of coughing, and can worsen by becoming more frequent. An acute cough has a sudden onset and may be self-limiting; a cough that persists beyond 1 month is considered chronic and commonly results from cigarette smoking.

A person may disregard a chronic nonproductive cough or may accept it as normal. In fact, he typically won't seek medical attention unless he has other symptoms.

History and physical examination
Ask the patient when his cough began and whether any body position, time of day, or specific activity affects it. How does the cough sound—harsh, brassy, dry, hacking? Try to determine if the

REVIEWING THE COUGH MECHANISM

Cough receptors are thought to be located in the nose, sinuses, auditory canals, nasopharynx, larynx, trachea, bronchi, pleurae, diaphragm, and possibly the pericardium and GI tract. Once a cough receptor is stimulated, the vagus and glossopharyngeal nerves transmit the impulse to the "cough center" in the medulla. From there, it's transmitted to the larynx and to the intercostal and abdominal muscles. Deep inspiration (illustration at top left) is followed by closure of the glottis (illustration at top right), relaxation of the diaphragm, and contraction of the abdominal and intercostal muscles. The resulting increased pressure in the lungs opens the glottis to release the forceful, noisy expiration known as a cough (bottom illustration).

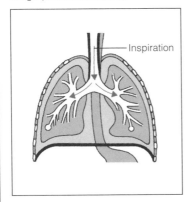

Inspiration

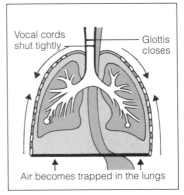

Vocal cords shut tightly

Glottis closes

Air becomes trapped in the lungs

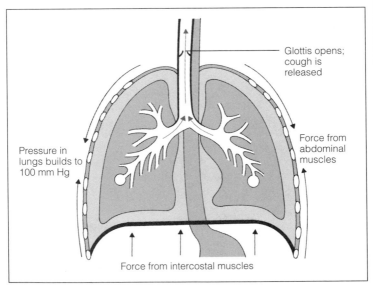

Glottis opens; cough is released

Force from abdominal muscles

Pressure in lungs builds to 100 mm Hg

Force from intercostal muscles

cough is related to smoking or a chemical irritant. If the patient smokes or has smoked, note the number of packs smoked daily multiplied by years (pack-years). Next, ask about the frequency and intensity of coughing. If he has any pain associated with coughing, breathing, or activity, when did it begin? Where is it located?

Ask the patient about recent illness, surgery, or trauma, and find out if he's had any cardiovascular or pulmonary disorders. Also ask about hypersensitivity to drugs, foods, pets, dust, or pollen. Find out which medications the patient takes, if any, and ask about recent changes in schedule or dosages. Also find out about recent changes in his appetite, weight, exercise tolerance, or energy level and recent exposure to irritating fumes, chemicals, or smoke.

As you're taking his history, observe the patient's general appearance and manner: Is he agitated, restless, or lethargic; pale, diaphoretic, or flushed; anxious, confused, or nervous? Also note whether he's cyanotic or has clubbed fingers or peripheral edema.

Now perform a physical examination. Start by taking the patient's vital signs. Next, check the depth and rhythm of his respirations, and note if wheezing or "crowing" noises occur with breathing. Feel the patient's skin: Is it cold or warm, clammy or dry? Check his nose and mouth for congestion, inflammation, drainage, or signs of infection. Inspect his neck for distended veins and tracheal deviation, and palpate for masses or enlarged lymph nodes.

Examine his chest, observing its configuration and looking for abnormal chest wall motion. Do you note any retractions or use of accessory muscles? Percuss for dullness, tympany, or flatness. Auscultate for wheezing, crackles, rhonchi, pleural friction rubs, and decreased or absent breath sounds. Finally, examine the abdomen for distention, tenderness, masses, or abnormal bowel sounds.

Common medical causes

● *Airway occlusion.* Partial occlusion of the upper airway produces sudden onset of dry, paroxysmal coughing. The patient is gagging, wheezing, and hoarse, with stridor, tachycardia, and decreased breath sounds.

● *Aortic aneurysm (thoracic).* This disorder causes a brassy cough with dyspnea, hoarseness, wheezing, and a sudden, sharp substernal pain in the shoulders, lower back, or abdomen. The patient may also have facial or neck edema, neck vein distention, dysphagia, prominent veins over his chest, stridor, and possibly paresthesia or neuralgia.

● *Asthma.* An attack commonly occurs at night and starts with a nonproductive cough and mild wheezing; this progresses to severe dyspnea, audible wheezing, chest tightness, and cough that produces thick mucus. Other signs include apprehension, rhonchi, prolonged expirations, intercostal and supraclavicular retractions on inspiration, accessory muscle use, flaring nostrils, tachypnea, tachycardia, diaphoresis, and flushing or cyanosis.

● *Atelectasis.* As lung tissue deflates, it stimulates cough receptors, causing a nonproductive cough. The patient may also have pleuritic chest pain, anxiety, dyspnea, tachypnea, and tachycardia. His skin may be cyanotic and diaphoretic, his breath sounds may be decreased, his chest may be dull on percussion, and he may exhibit inspiratory lag, substernal or intercostal retractions, decreased vocal fremitus, and tracheal deviation toward the affected side.

● *Bronchitis (chronic).* This disorder starts with a nonproductive, hacking cough that later becomes productive. It also causes prolonged expiration, wheezing, dyspnea, accessory muscle use, barrel chest, cyanosis, tachypnea, crackles, and scattered rhonchi. Clubbing can occur in late stages.

● *Bronchogenic carcinoma.* The earliest indicators of this disorder may be a chronic nonproductive cough, dyspnea, and vague chest pain. The patient may also be wheezing.

● *Common cold.* Colds may start with a nonproductive, hacking cough and progress to some mix of sneezing, headaches, malaise, fatigue, rhinorrhea, myalgia, arthralgia, nasal congestion, and sore throat.

● *Esophageal achalasia.* In this disorder, regurgitation and aspiration produce a dry cough. The patient may also have recurrent pulmonary infections and dysphagia.

● *Esophageal diverticula.* The patient with this disorder has a nocturnal nonproductive cough, regurgitation and aspiration, dyspepsia, and dysphagia. His neck may appear swollen and have a gurgling sound. He may also have halitosis and weight loss.

● *Esophageal occlusion.* This is marked by immediate nonproductive coughing and gagging, with a sensation of something stuck in the throat. Other findings include neck or chest pain, dysphagia, and inability to swallow.

● *Hantavirus pulmonary syndrome.* A nonproductive cough is common in this disorder, which is marked by noncardiogenic pulmonary edema. Other findings include headache, myalgia, fever, nausea, and vomiting.

● *Hypersensitivity pneumonitis.* In this disorder, acute nonproductive coughing, fever, dyspnea, and malaise usually occur 5 to 6 hours after exposure to an antigen.

● *Interstitial lung disease.* A patient with this disorder has a nonproductive cough and progressive dyspnea. He may also be cyanotic and have clubbing, fine crackles, fatigue, variable chest pain, and weight loss.

● *Laryngeal tumor.* A mild, nonproductive cough is an early sign of this disorder, along with minor throat discomfort and hoarseness. Later, dysphagia, dyspnea, cervical lymphadenopathy, stridor, and earache may occur.

● *Laryngitis.* In its acute form, this disorder causes a nonproductive cough with localized pain (especially when the patient is swallowing or speaking) as well as fever and malaise. The hoarseness can range from mild to complete loss of voice.

● *Lung abscess.* This disorder typically begins with a nonproductive cough, weakness, dyspnea, and pleuritic chest pain. The patient may also have diaphoresis, fever, headache, malaise, fatigue, crackles, decreased breath sounds, anorexia, and weight loss. Later, the cough produces large amounts of purulent, foul-smelling, possibly bloody sputum.

● *Pleural effusion.* A nonproductive cough is associated with this disorder along with dyspnea, pleuritic chest pain, and decreased chest motion. The patient also has a pleural friction rub, tachycardia, tachypnea, egophony, flatness on percussion, decreased or absent breath sounds, and decreased tactile fremitus.

● *Pneumonia. Bacterial pneumonia* usually starts with a nonproductive, hacking, painful cough that rapidly becomes productive. Other findings include shaking chills, headache, high fever, dyspnea, pleuritic chest pain, tachypnea, tachycardia, grunting respirations, nasal flaring, decreased breath sounds, fine crackles, rhonchi, and cyanosis. The patient's chest may be dull on percussion.

In *mycoplasmal pneumonia,* a nonproductive cough arises 2 to 3 days after the onset of malaise, headache, and sore throat. The cough can be paroxysmal, causing substernal chest pain. The patient commonly has a fever but won't appear seriously ill.

Viral pneumonia causes a nonproductive, hacking cough and gradual onset of malaise, headache, anorexia, and low-grade fever.

● *Pneumothorax.* This life-threatening disorder causes a dry cough and signs of respiratory distress, such as severe dyspnea, tachycardia, tachypnea, and cyanosis. The patient experiences sudden, sharp chest pain that worsens with chest movement. He also has subcutaneous crepitation, hyperresonance or tympany, decreased vocal fremitus, and decreased or absent breath sounds on the affected side.

• *Pulmonary edema.* Initially, this disorder causes a dry cough, exertional dyspnea, paroxysmal nocturnal dyspnea, orthopnea, tachycardia, tachypnea, dependent crackles, and ventricular gallop. If pulmonary edema is severe, the patient's respirations become more rapid and labored, with diffuse crackles and coughing that produces frothy, bloody sputum.

• *Pulmonary embolism.* Life-threatening pulmonary embolism may produce sudden onset of dry cough along with dyspnea and pleuritic or anginal chest pain. Usually, though, the cough produces blood-tinged sputum. Tachycardia and low-grade fever are also common; less common signs and symptoms include massive hemoptysis, chest splinting, leg edema, and (with a large embolus) cyanosis, syncope, and distended neck veins. The patient may also have a pleural friction rub, diffuse wheezing, dullness on percussion, and decreased breath sounds.

• *Sarcoidosis.* In this disorder, a nonproductive cough is accompanied by dyspnea, substernal pain, and malaise. The patient may also have fatigue, arthralgia, myalgia, weight loss, tachypnea, crackles, lymphadenopathy, hepatosplenomegaly, skin lesions, visual impairment, difficulty swallowing, and arrhythmias.

• *Tracheobronchitis (acute).* Initially, this disorder produces a dry cough that later becomes productive as secretions increase. Chills, sore throat, slight fever, muscle and back pain, and substernal tightness generally precede the cough's onset. Rhonchi and wheezing are usually heard. Severe illness produces a fever of 101° to 102° F (38.3° to 38.9° C) and possibly bronchospasm, with severe wheezing and increased coughing.

Other causes
• *Diagnostic tests.* Pulmonary function tests and bronchoscopy may stimulate cough receptors and trigger coughing.

• *Treatments.* Irritation of the carina during suctioning can trigger a paroxysmal or hacking cough. Intermittent positive pressure breathing or spirometry can also cause nonproductive coughing. Some inhalants, such as pentamidine, may stimulate coughing.

Special considerations
A nonproductive, paroxysmal cough may induce life-threatening bronchospasm. The patient may need a bronchodilator to relieve his bronchospasm and open his airways. Unless he has chronic obstructive pulmonary disease, you may have to give antitussives and sedatives to suppress the cough.

To relieve mucous membrane inflammation and dryness, humidify the air in the patient's room, or instruct him to use a humidifier at home. Tell him to avoid using aerosols, powders, or other respiratory irritants—and to stop smoking, if appropriate. And make sure the patient receives adequate fluids and nutrition.

As indicated, prepare the patient for diagnostic tests, such as X-rays, a lung scan, bronchoscopy, and pulmonary function tests.

Pediatric pointers
A nonproductive cough can be difficult to evaluate in infants and young children because it can't be voluntarily induced and must be observed.

Sudden onset of paroxysmal nonproductive coughing may indicate aspiration of a foreign body—a common danger in children, especially those between 6 months and 4 years old. Nonproductive coughing can also result from several disorders that affect infants and children. In *asthma,* a characteristic nonproductive tight cough can arise suddenly or insidiously as an attack begins. The cough usually becomes productive toward the end of the attack. In *bacterial pneumonia,* a nonproductive, hacking cough arises suddenly and becomes productive in 2 or 3 days. *Acute bronchiolitis* has a peak incidence at age 6, producing paroxysms of nonproductive coughing that become more frequent as the disease progresses.

Acute otitis media commonly occurs in infants and young children because of their short eustachian tubes; it also produces nonproductive coughing. Typically, a child with *measles* has a slight, nonproductive, hacking cough that increases in severity. The earliest sign of *cystic fibrosis* may be a nonproductive, paroxysmal cough from retained secretions. Life-threatening *pertussis* produces a cough that becomes paroxysmal, with an inspiratory "whoop" or crowing sound. *Airway hyperactivity* causes a chronic nonproductive cough that increases with exercise or exposure to cold air. And *psychogenic coughing* may occur when the child is under stress, emotionally stimulated, or seeking attention.

COUGH, PRODUCTIVE

Productive coughing is the body's mechanism for clearing airway passages of accumulated secretions that normal mucociliary action doesn't remove. It's a sudden, forceful, noisy expulsion of air from the lungs that contains sputum or blood (or both). (The sputum's color, consistency, and odor provide important clues about the patient's condition.) It can occur as a single cough or as paroxysmal coughing, and it can be voluntarily induced—although it's usually a reflexive response to stimulation of the airway mucosa.

Productive coughing commonly results from an acute or chronic cardiovascular or respiratory disorder that causes inflammation, edema, and increased mucus production in the airways. It can also result from acquired immunodeficiency syndrome or from inhalation of antigenic or irritating substances or foreign bodies. However, the most common cause of chronic productive coughing is cigarette smoking, which produces mucoid sputum ranging in color from clear to yellow to brown.

Many patients minimize or overlook a chronic productive cough or accept it as normal. Such patients may not seek medical attention until an associated problem—such as dyspnea, hemoptysis, chest pain, weight loss, or recurrent respiratory infections—develops. The delay can have serious consequences because productive coughing is associated with several life-threatening disorders and can also herald airway occlusion from excessive secretions.

Emergency interventions

 A patient with a productive cough can develop acute respiratory distress from thick or excessive secretions, bronchospasm, or fatigue, so examine him before you take his history. Take vital signs and check the rate, depth, and rhythm of respirations. Keep his airway patent, and be prepared to provide supplemental oxygen if he becomes restless or confused or if his respirations become shallow, irregular, rapid, or slow. Look for stridor, wheezing, choking, or gurgling. Be alert for nasal flaring and cyanosis.

A productive cough may signal a severe life-threatening disorder. For example, coughing due to pulmonary edema produces thin, frothy, pink sputum, and coughing due to an asthmatic attack produces thick, mucoid sputum.

History and physical examination

When the patient's condition permits, ask when the cough began, and find out how much sputum he's coughing up each day. (The normal tracheobronchial tree can produce up to 3 oz [90 ml] of sputum per day.) At what time of day does he cough up the most sputum? Does his sputum production seem related to what or when he eats or to his activities or environment? Ask him if he's noticed an increase in sputum production since his coughing began. This may result from external stimuli or from such internal causes as chronic bronchial infection or a lung abscess. Also ask about the color, odor, and consistency of the sputum. Blood-tinged or rust-colored sputum may result from trauma due to coughing or from an underlying condition, such as a pulmonary infection or a tumor. Foul-smelling sputum may result from an anaerobic infection, such as bronchitis or lung abscess.

How does the cough sound? A hacking cough results from laryngeal involvement, whereas a "brassy" cough indicates major airway involvement. Does the patient feel any pain associated with his productive cough? If so, ask about its location and severity and whether it radiates to other areas. Does coughing, changing body position, or inspiration increase or help relieve his pain?

Next, ask the patient about his use of cigarettes, drugs, and alcohol and whether his weight or appetite has changed. Find out if he has a history of asthma, allergies, or respiratory disorders, and ask about recent illnesses, surgery, or trauma. What medications is he taking? Does he work around chemicals or respiratory irritants such as silicone?

Now examine the patient's mouth and nose for congestion, drainage, or inflammation. Note his breath odor: Halitosis can be a sign of pulmonary infection. Inspect his neck for distended veins, and palpate for tenderness and masses or enlarged lymph nodes. Observe his chest for accessory muscle use, retractions, and uneven chest expansion, and percuss for dullness, tympany, or flatness. Finally, auscultate for pleural friction rub and abnormal breath sounds—rhonchi, crackles, or wheezing.

Common medical causes

- **Actinomycosis.** This disorder begins with a cough that produces purulent sputum. Fever, weight loss, fatigue, weakness, dyspnea, night sweats, pleuritic chest pain, and hemoptysis may also occur.

- **Aspiration pneumonitis.** This disorder causes a cough that produces pink, frothy, and possibly purulent sputum. The patient also has marked dyspnea, fever, tachypnea, tachycardia, wheezing, and cyanosis.

- **Bronchiectasis.** The chronic cough of this disorder produces copious, mucopurulent sputum that has characteristic layering (top, frothy; middle, clear; bottom, dense with purulent particles). The patient's sputum may smell foul or sickeningly sweet. Other characteristic findings include hemoptysis, occasional wheezing, rhonchi, exertional dyspnea, weight loss, fatigue, malaise, weakness, recurrent fever, late-stage finger clubbing, and persistent, coarse crackles over the affected lung area.

- **Chemical pneumonitis.** This disorder causes coughing that produces purulent sputum. It can also cause dyspnea, wheezing, orthopnea, fever, malaise, and crackles; mucous membrane irritation of the conjunctivae, throat, and nose; laryngitis; or rhinitis. Signs and symptoms may increase for 24 to 48 hours after exposure, then resolve; if severe, however, they may recur 2 to 5 weeks later.

- **Common cold.** When this disorder causes productive coughing, the sputum is mucoid or mucopurulent. Early indications of the common cold include sneezing, headache, malaise, fatigue, rhinorrhea (watery to tenacious, mucopurulent secretions), nasal congestion, sore throat, myalgia, arthralgia, and a dry, hacking cough.

- **Lung abscess (ruptured).** The cardinal sign of a ruptured lung abscess is coughing that produces copious amounts of purulent, foul-smelling, possibly blood-tinged sputum. A ruptured abscess

PRODUCTIVE COUGH: COMMON CAUSES AND ASSOCIATED FINDINGS

CAUSES	Chest pain	Crackles	Cyanosis	Decreased breath sounds	Dyspnea	Fatigue	Fever	Rhonchi	Sore throat	Tachycardia	Tachypnea	Weight loss	Wheezing
Actinomycosis	●				●	●	●					●	
Aspiration pneumonitis		●	●		●	●	●	●		●	●		●
Bronchiectasis		●			●	●	●	●				●	●
Chemical pneumonitis		●			●		●	●			●		●
Common cold						●	●		●				
Lung abscess	●	●			●	●	●					●	
Lung cancer	●				●	●	●					●	●
Nocardiosis	●			●	●	●						●	
North American blastomycosis	●					●	●					●	
Pneumonia (bacterial)	●	●	●		●	●	●	●		●	●		
Pneumonia (mycoplasma)	●	●				●	●		●				
Psittacosis	●	●					●			●			
Pulmonary edema		●	●		●	●	●			●	●		
Pulmonary embolism	●	●	●		●		●			●	●		●
Pulmonary tuberculosis	●	●			●	●	●	●				●	
Silicosis		●			●	●					●	●	
Tracheobronchitis	●	●					●	●	●				●

MAJOR ASSOCIATED SIGNS AND SYMPTOMS

can also cause diaphoresis, anorexia, clubbing, weight loss, weakness, fatigue, fever with chills, dyspnea, headache, malaise, pleuritic chest pain, halitosis, inspiratory crackles, and tubular or amphoric breath sounds. The patient's chest is dull on percussion on the affected side.

• *Lung cancer.* One of the earliest signs of bronchogenic carcinoma is a chronic cough that produces small amounts of purulent (or mucopurulent), blood-streaked sputum. In a patient with bronchioalveolar cancer, however, coughing produces large amounts of frothy sputum. Other signs and symptoms include dyspnea, anorexia, fatigue, weight loss, chest pain, fever, diaphoresis, wheezing, and clubbing.

• *Nocardiosis.* This disorder causes a productive cough (with purulent, thick, tenacious, and possibly blood-tinged sputum) and fever that may last several months. Other findings include night sweats, pleuritic pain, anorexia, malaise, fatigue, weight loss, and diminished or absent breath sounds. The patient's chest is dull on percussion.

• *North American blastomycosis.* In this chronic disorder, coughing is dry and hacking or produces bloody or purulent sputum. Other findings are pleuritic chest pain, fever, chills, anorexia, weight loss, malaise, fatigue, night sweats, cutaneous lesions (small, painless, nonpruritic macules or papules), and prostration.

• *Pneumonia.* Bacterial pneumonias initially produce a dry cough that becomes productive. Rust-colored sputum occurs in pneumococcal pneumonia; "brick red" or "currant jelly" sputum in *Klebsiella* pneumonia; salmon-colored sputum in staphylococcal pneumonia; and mucopurulent sputum in streptococcal pneumonia. Associated signs and symptoms—shaking chills, high fever, myalgias, headache, tachypnea, tachycardia, dyspnea, cyanosis, diaphoresis, decreased breath sounds, fine crackles, rhonchi, and pleuritic chest pain that increases with chest movement—develop suddenly.

Mycoplasmal pneumonia may cause a cough that produces scant, blood-flecked sputum. Most common, however, is a nonproductive cough that starts 2 to 3 days after the onset of malaise, headache, fever, and sore throat. Paroxysmal coughing causes substernal chest pain. Patients may have crackles but don't usually appear seriously ill.

• *Psittacosis.* The characteristic hacking cough is nonproductive at first but later may produce a small amount of mucoid, blood-streaked sputum. The infection may begin abruptly, with chills, fever, headache, myalgias, and prostration. Other signs and symptoms may include tachypnea, fine crackles, chest pain (rare), epistaxis, photophobia, abdominal distention and tenderness, nausea, vomiting, and a faint macular rash. Severe infection may produce stupor, delirium, and coma.

• *Pulmonary edema.* When severe, this life-threatening disorder causes a cough that produces frothy, bloody sputum. Early signs and symptoms include dyspnea on exertion; paroxysmal nocturnal dyspnea, then orthopnea; and coughing, which may be nonproductive initially. Other clinical features include fever, fatigue, tachycardia, tachypnea, dependent crackles, and ventricular gallop. As the patient's respirations become increasingly rapid and labored, he develops more diffuse crackles and a productive cough, increased tachycardia, and possibly arrhythmias. His skin becomes cold, clammy, and cyanotic; his blood pressure falls; and his pulse becomes thready.

• *Pulmonary embolism.* This life-threatening disorder causes a cough that may be nonproductive or may produce blood-tinged sputum. The first symptom of pulmonary embolism is usually severe dyspnea, which may be accompanied by anginal or pleuritic chest pain. The patient has marked anxiety, a low-grade fever, tachycardia, tachypnea, and diaphoresis. Less common signs include massive hemoptysis, chest splinting, leg edema, and (with a large embolus) cyanosis, syncope, and distended neck veins. The patient may also have a pleural friction rub, diffuse wheezing, crackles, chest dullness on percussion, decreased breath sounds, and signs of circulatory collapse.

• *Pulmonary tuberculosis.* This disorder causes a mild to severe productive cough along with some combination of hemoptysis, malaise, dyspnea, and pleuritic chest pain. Sputum may be scant and mucoid or copious and purulent. Typically, the patient experiences night sweats, easy fatigability, and weight loss. His breath sounds are amphoric. He may have chest dullness on percussion and, after coughing, increased tactile fremitus with crackles.

• *Silicosis.* Productive cough with mucopurulent sputum is the earliest sign of this disorder. The patient also has exertional dyspnea, tachypnea, weight loss, fatigue, general weakness, and recurrent respiratory infections. Auscultation reveals end-inspiratory, fine crackles at the lung bases.

• *Tracheobronchitis.* Inflammation initially causes a nonproductive cough that later—following onset of chills, sore throat, slight fever, muscle and back pain, and substernal tightness—becomes productive as secretions increase. Sputum is mucoid, mucopurulent, or purulent. Rhonchi and wheezing are usually heard. Severe tracheobronchitis may cause a fever of 101° to 102° F (38.3° to 38.9° C) and bronchospasm.

Other causes
• *Diagnostic tests.* Bronchoscopy and pulmonary function tests may increase productive coughing.

• *Drugs.* Expectorants, of course, increase productive coughing. These include ammonium chloride, calcium iodide, guaifenesin, iodinated glycerol, potassium iodide, and terpin hydrate.

• *Respiratory therapy.* Intermittent positive-pressure breathing and incentive spirometry commonly loosen secretions and cause or increase productive cough.

Special considerations
Avoid taking measures to suppress a productive cough because sputum retention

may interfere with alveolar aeration or impair pulmonary resistance to infection. Expect to give mucolytics and expectorants and increase the patient's intake of oral fluids to thin his secretions and increase their flow. In addition, the doctor may order a bronchodilator to relieve bronchospasms and open airways and an antibiotic may be ordered to treat underlying infection.

Humidify the air around the patient; this will relieve mucous membrane inflammation and help loosen dried secretions. Provide chest physiotherapy, such as postural drainage with vibration and percussion to loosen secretions. Aerosol therapy may be necessary.

Provide the patient with uninterrupted rest periods, and don't let him use respiratory irritants. If appropriate, encourage the patient not to smoke because doing so can aggravate his condition.

Teach the patient how to deep-breathe, to cough effectively, and, if appropriate, to splint his incision when he coughs. Tell him to sit or stand upright when coughing, if possible, to facilitate maximum chest expansion. If he's confined to bed rest, change his position often to promote drainage of secretions. Tell the patient to cover his mouth and nose with a tissue when he coughs and to dispose of contaminated tissues properly, to protect himself and others from the cough and secretions. Be sure to provide a container for tissues and sputum.

Prepare the patient for diagnostic tests, such as chest X-rays, bronchoscopy, a lung scan, and pulmonary function tests. And collect sputum samples for culture and sensitivity testing.

Pediatric pointers
Because his airway is narrow, a child with a productive cough can quickly develop airway occlusion and respiratory distress from thick or excessive secretions. Causes of productive cough in children include asthma, bronchiectasis, bronchi-

tis, acute bronchiolitis, cystic fibrosis, and pertussis.

When caring for a child with a productive cough, administer expectorants, but don't expect to give cough suppressants. To soothe inflamed mucous membranes and prevent drying of secretions, provide humidified air or oxygen. Remember, high humidity can induce bronchospasm in a hyperactive child or produce overhydration in an infant.

CRACKLES
[Rales, crepitations]

A common finding in certain cardiovascular and pulmonary disorders, crackles are nonmusical clicking or rattling noises heard during auscultation of breath sounds. They usually occur during inspiration and recur constantly from one respiratory cycle to the next. They can be unilateral or bilateral and moist or dry. They're characterized by their pitch, loudness, occurrence during the respiratory cycle, location, and persistence.

Crackles indicate abnormal movement of air through fluid-filled airways. (See *How crackles develop,* page 154.) They can be irregularly dispersed, as in pneumonia, or localized, as in bronchiectasis. (A few basilar crackles can be heard in normal lungs after prolonged shallow breathing. These normal crackles clear with a few deep breaths.) Usually, though, crackles indicate the degree of an underlying illness. When crackles result from a generalized disorder, they usually occur in the less distended and more dependent areas of the lungs, such as the lung bases when the patient is standing. Crackles due to air passing through inflammatory exudate may not be audible if the involved portion of the lung isn't being ventilated because of shallow respirations.

Emergency interventions

 Quickly take the patient's vital signs and examine for signs of respiratory distress or airway obstruction. Check the depth and rhythm of respirations. Is he struggling to breathe? Check for increased accessory muscle use and chest wall motion, retractions, stridor, or nasal flaring. Provide supplemental oxygen. Endotracheal intubation may be necessary.

History and physical examination

If the patient also has a cough, ask when it began and if it's constant or intermittent. Find out what the cough sounds like and whether he's coughing up sputum or blood. If the cough is productive, determine the sputum's consistency, amount, odor, and color.

Ask the patient if he has any pain. If so, where is it located? When did he first notice it? Does it radiate to other areas? Also ask if movement, coughing, or breathing worsens or helps relieve the pain. Note the patient's position: Is he lying still or moving restlessly?

Obtain a brief medical history. Does the patient have cancer or any known respiratory or cardiovascular problems? Ask about recent surgery, trauma, or illness and whether he has hoarseness or difficulty swallowing. Find out which medications the patient is taking, and ask about tobacco and alcohol use. Also ask about recent weight loss, anorexia, nausea, vomiting, fatigue, weakness, vertigo, and syncope. Has the patient been exposed to irritants, such as vapors, fumes, or smoke?

Now perform a physical examination. Examine the patient's nose and mouth for signs of infection, such as inflammation or increased secretions. Note his breath odor: Halitosis could indicate pulmonary infection. Check his neck for masses, tenderness, swelling, lymphadenopathy, and venous distention.

Inspect the patient's chest for abnormal configuration or uneven expansion.

HOW CRACKLES DEVELOP

Crackles occur when air passes through fluid-filled airways, causing collapsed alveoli to pop open as airway pressure equalizes. They can also occur when membranes lining the chest cavity and the lungs become inflamed. The illustrations below show a normal alveolus and two pathologic alveolar changes, which cause crackles.

Normal alveolus

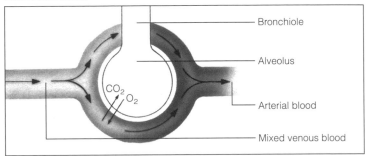

- Bronchiole
- Alveolus
- Arterial blood
- Mixed venous blood

Alveolus in pulmonary edema

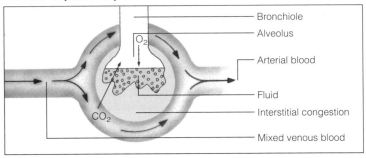

- Bronchiole
- Alveolus
- Arterial blood
- Fluid
- Interstitial congestion
- Mixed venous blood

Alveolus in inflammation

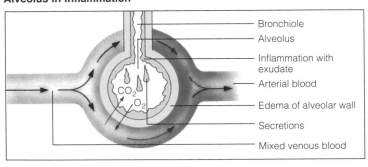

- Bronchiole
- Alveolus
- Inflammation with exudate
- Arterial blood
- Edema of alveolar wall
- Secretions
- Mixed venous blood

Percuss for dullness, tympany, or flatness. Auscultate his lungs for other abnormal, diminished, or absent breath sounds. Listen to his heart for abnormal sounds, and check his hands and feet for edema or clubbing.

Common medical causes

• *Adult respiratory distress syndrome.* This life-threatening disorder causes diffuse, fine to coarse crackles that are usually heard in the dependent portions of the lungs. It also produces cyanosis, nasal flaring, tachypnea, tachycardia, grunting respirations, rhonchi, dyspnea, anxiety, and decreased level of consciousness.

• *Asthma.* A severe attack usually occurs at night or during sleep, causing dry, whistling crackles. An attack typically starts with a dry cough and mild wheezing, then progresses to severe dyspnea, audible wheezing, chest tightness, and productive cough. Other possible findings include apprehension, prolonged expirations, rhonchi, intercostal and supraclavicular retraction on inspiration, accessory muscle use, flaring nostrils, tachypnea, tachycardia, diaphoresis, and flushing or cyanosis.

• *Bronchiectasis.* In this disorder, persistent, coarse crackles are heard over the affected area of the lung. They're accompanied by a chronic cough that produces copious amounts of mucopurulent sputum. Other characteristics include halitosis, occasional wheezing, exertional dyspnea, rhonchi, weight loss, fatigue, malaise, weakness, recurrent fever, and late-stage clubbing.

• *Bronchitis (chronic).* This disorder causes coarse crackles that are usually heard at the lung bases. Prolonged expirations, wheezing, rhonchi, exertional dyspnea, tachypnea, and persistent, productive cough occur because of increased bronchial secretions. Clubbing and cyanosis may occur.

• *Legionnaire's disease.* This disorder produces diffuse moist crackles and cough productive of scant mucoid, nonpurulent, possibly blood-streaked sputum. Usually, prodromal signs and symptoms occur: malaise, fatigue, weakness, anorexia, diffuse myalgias, and possibly diarrhea. Within 12 to 48 hours, the patient develops a dry cough and a sudden high fever with chills. He may also have pleuritic chest pain, headache, tachypnea, tachycardia, nausea, vomiting, dyspnea, mild temporary amnesia, confusion, flushing, mild diaphoresis, and prostration.

• *Lung abscess.* This disorder produces moist, fine to medium inspiratory crackles. Onset is insidious; signs and symptoms including excessive sweating, anorexia, weight loss, fever, fatigue, weakness, dyspnea, clubbing, pleuritic chest pain, pleural friction rub, and cough that produces copious amounts of foul-smelling, purulent sputum that may be blood-tinged. The patient's breath sounds are hollow and tubular or amphoric; the affected side of his chest is dull on percussion.

• *Pneumonia.* *Bacterial pneumonia* produces diffuse fine crackles, sudden onset of shaking chills, high fever, tachypnea, pleuritic chest pain, cyanosis, grunting respirations, nasal flaring, decreased breath sounds, myalgia, headache, tachycardia, dyspnea, cyanosis, diaphoresis, and rhonchi. The patient has a dry cough that later becomes productive.

Mycoplasmal pneumonia produces medium to fine crackles together with a nonproductive cough, malaise, sore throat, headache, and fever. The patient may have blood-flecked sputum.

Viral pneumonia causes diffuse crackles that develop gradually. The patient may also have a nonproductive cough, malaise, headache, anorexia, low-grade fever, and decreased breath sounds.

• *Pulmonary edema.* Moist, bubbling crackles on inspiration are one of the first signs of this life-threatening disorder. Other early findings include dyspnea on exertion; paroxysmal nocturnal dyspnea, then orthopnea; and coughing, which may

CRACKLES: COMMON CAUSES AND ASSOCIATED FINDINGS

CAUSES	MAJOR ASSOCIATED SIGNS AND SYMPTOMS												
	Chest pain	Cough	Cyanosis	Dyspnea	Fatigue	Fever	Hemoptysis	Rhonchi	Tachycardia	Tachypnea	Vomiting	Weakness	Weight loss
Adult respiratory distress syndrome			●	●				●	●	●			
Asthma (acute)	●	●	●	●				●	●	●			
Bronchiectasis		●		●	●	●		●				●	●
Bronchitis (chronic)		●	●	●				●	●				
Legionnaire's disease	●	●		●	●	●	●		●	●	●	●	
Lung abscess	●	●		●	●	●	●					●	●
Pneumonia (bacterial)	●	●	●	●	●	●		●	●	●			
Pneumonia (mycoplasma)		●				●	●		●				
Pneumonia (viral)		●				●			●				
Pulmonary edema		●	●	●				●	●	●			
Pulmonary embolism	●	●	●	●			●	●	●	●			
Pulmonary tuberculosis	●	●		●	●	●	●					●	●
Tracheobronchitis	●	●				●		●					

be nonproductive initially but later produces frothy, bloody sputum. Related clinical effects include tachycardia, tachypnea, and S$_3$ gallop. As the patient's respirations become increasingly rapid and labored, he develops more diffuse crackles, worsening tachycardia, hypotension, a rapid and thready pulse, cyanosis, and cold, clammy skin.

● **Pulmonary embolism.** This life-threatening disorder can cause fine to coarse crackles and a cough that may be dry or that produces blood-tinged sputum. Usually, the first sign of pulmonary embolism is severe dyspnea, which may be accompanied by anginal or pleuritic chest pain. The patient has marked anxiety, a low-grade fever, tachycardia, tachypnea, and diaphoresis. Less common signs include massive hemoptysis, chest splinting, leg edema, and (with a large embolus) cyanosis, syncope, and distended neck veins. The patient may also have a pleural friction rub, diffuse wheezing, chest dullness on percussion, decreased breath sounds, and signs of circulatory collapse.

• *Pulmonary tuberculosis.* In this disorder, fine crackles occur after coughing. The patient has some combination of hemoptysis, malaise, dyspnea, and pleuritic chest pain. Sputum may be scant and mucoid or copious and purulent. Typically, the patient experiences night sweats, easy fatigue, weakness, and weight loss. His breath sounds are amphoric.

• *Tracheobronchitis.* In its acute form, this disorder produces moist or coarse crackles along with a productive cough, chills, sore throat, slight fever, muscle and back pain, and substernal tightness. Rhonchi and wheezing are usually heard. Severe tracheobronchitis may cause a fever of 101° to 102° F (38.3° to 38.9° C) and bronchospasm.

Special considerations

To keep the patient's airway patent, elevate the head of his bed to facilitate his breathing. To liquefy thick secretions and relieve mucous membrane inflammation, administer fluids, humidified air, or oxygen. Diuretics may be needed if crackles result from cardiogenic pulmonary edema. Turn the patient every 1 to 2 hours, and encourage him to breathe deeply. Teach him how to cough effectively and to splint incision areas, if appropriate. Encourage him to avoid smoking and using aerosols, powders, or other products that might irritate his airway. Plan daily uninterrupted rest periods to help him relax and sleep.

Prepare the patient for diagnostic tests, such as chest X-rays, a lung scan, and sputum analysis.

Pediatric pointers

Infants and children can rapidly develop airway occlusion because of their narrow airways. They also develop fatigue from dyspnea sooner than adults and may have more rapid onset and progression of disease.

Crackles in an infant or child may indicate a serious cardiovascular or respiratory disorder. *Pneumonias* produce diffuse, sudden crackles in children. *Esophageal atresia* and *tracheoesophageal fistula* can cause bubbling, moist crackles due to aspiration of food or secretions into the lungs—especially in newborn infants. *Pulmonary edema* causes fine crackles at the bases of the lungs, and *bronchiectasis* produces moist crackles. *Cystic fibrosis* produces widespread, fine to coarse inspiratory crackles and wheezing in infants. And *sickle cell anemia* may produce crackles when it causes pulmonary infarction or infection.

CREPITATION, BONY
[Bony crepitus]

Bony crepitation is a palpable vibration or an audible crunching sound that results when one bone grates against another. It commonly results from a fracture. Or it can happen when bones that have been stripped of their protective articular cartilage grind against each other as they articulate—for example, in advanced arthritic or degenerative joint disorders.

Eliciting bony crepitation can help confirm diagnosis of a fracture, but it can also cause further soft tissue, nerve, or vessel injury. What's more, rubbing fractured bone ends together can convert a closed fracture into an open one if a bone end penetrates the skin. So, after initial detection of crepitation in a patient with a fracture, avoid eliciting this sign.

History and physical examination

If you detect bony crepitation in a patient with a suspected fracture, ask him if he feels any pain and if he can point to the painful area. To prevent lacerating nerves, blood vessels, or other structures, immobilize the affected area by applying a splint that includes the joints above and below the affected area. Elevate the affected area, if possible, and apply cold packs. Inspect for abrasions or lacerations. Find out how and when the injury occurred. Palpate pulses distal to the injury site; check the skin for pallor or coolness. Test motor and sensory function distal to the injury site.

If the patient doesn't have a suspected fracture, ask about a history of osteoarthritis or rheumatoid arthritis. Ask what medications he takes: Has any medication helped ease arthritic discomfort? Take the patient's vital signs and test joint range of motion (ROM).

Common medical causes

• *Fracture.* Besides bony crepitation, a fracture causes acute local pain, hematoma, edema, and decreased ROM. Other findings may include deformity, point tenderness, discoloration of the limb, and loss of limb function. Neurovascular damage may cause prolonged capillary refill time, diminished or absent pulses, mottled cyanosis, paresthesia, and decreased sensation (all distal to the fracture site). An open fracture, of course, produces an obvious skin wound.

• *Osteoarthritis.* In advanced cases of this disorder, joint crepitation may be elicited during ROM testing. The cardinal symptom of osteoarthritis is joint pain, especially during motion and weight bearing. Other findings include joint stiffness that typically occurs after resting and subsides within a few minutes after the patient begins moving.

• *Rheumatoid arthritis.* In advanced cases of this disorder, bony crepitation is heard when the affected joint is rotated. However, rheumatoid arthritis usually de-velops insidiously, producing nonspecific signs and symptoms, such as fatigue, malaise, anorexia, a persistent low-grade fever, weight loss, lymphadenopathy, and vague arthralgias and myalgias. Later, more specific and localized articular signs develop, commonly at the proximal finger joints. These signs usually occur bilaterally and symmetrically and may extend to the wrists, knees, elbows, and ankles. The affected joints stiffen after inactivity. The patient also has limited ROM and increased warmth, swelling, and tenderness of affected joints.

Special considerations

If a fracture is suspected, prepare the patient for X-rays of the affected area, and reexamine his neurovascular status frequently. Keep the affected part immobilized and elevated until treatment begins. Give analgesics to relieve pain.

Pediatric pointers

Bony crepitation in a child usually occurs after a fracture. Obtain an accurate history of the injury, and be alert for the possibility of child abuse. In a teenager, bony crepitation and pain in the patellofemoral joint help diagnose chondromalacia of the patella.

CREPITATION, SUBCUTANEOUS
[Subcutaneous crepitus]

When bubbles of air or other gases (such as carbon dioxide) are trapped in subcutaneous tissue, palpation or stroking of the skin produces a crackling sound called subcutaneous crepitation. The bubbles feel like small, unstable nodules and aren't painful, even though this sign is commonly associated with painful disorders. Usually, the affected tissue is visibly edematous; this can lead to life-

EMERGENCY INTERVENTIONS

MANAGING SUBCUTANEOUS CREPITATION

Subcutaneous crepitation occurs when air or gas bubbles escape into tissues. It may signal life-threatening rupture of an air-filled or gas-producing organ, or may indicate a fulminating anaerobic infection.

Organ rupture
If the patient shows signs of respiratory distress—such as severe dyspnea, tachypnea, accessory muscle use, nasal flaring, air hunger, or tachycardia—quickly test for Hamman's sign to detect trapped air bubbles in the mediastinum.

To test for Hamman's sign, you will need to help the patient assume a left-lateral recumbent position. Then, place your stethoscope over the precordium. If you hear a loud crunching sound that synchronizes with his heartbeat, the patient has a positive Hamman's sign.

Depending on which organ is ruptured, you should be prepared for endotracheal intubation, emergency tracheotomy, or chest tube insertion. Immediately start administering supplemental oxygen. Start an I.V. line to administer fluids and medication, and connect the patient to a cardiac monitor.

Anaerobic infection
If the patient has an open wound with a foul odor and local swelling and discoloration, you must act quickly. Be sure to take the patient's vital signs, checking especially for fever, tachycardia, hypotension, and tachypnea. Next, you should start an I.V. line to administer fluids and medication, and provide supplemental oxygen.

In addition, you should be prepared for emergency surgery to drain and debride the wound. If the patient's condition is life-threatening, you may need to prepare him for transfer to a facility with a hyperbaric chamber.

---

threatening airway occlusion if the edema affects the neck or upper chest.

The air or gas bubbles enter the tissues through open wounds, from the action of anaerobic microorganisms, or from traumatic or spontaneous rupture or perforation of pulmonary or GI organs.

History and physical examination
Because subcutaneous crepitation can indicate a life-threatening disorder, you'll need to perform a rapid initial evaluation. (See *Managing subcutaneous crepitation*.)

When the patient's condition permits, palpate the affected skin to evaluate the location and extent of subcutaneous crepitation and to obtain baseline information.

Repalpate frequently to determine if the subcutaneous crepitation is increasing. Ask the patient if he's experiencing any pain. If he is, find out where the pain is located, how severe it is, and when it began. Ask about recent thoracic surgery, diagnostic tests, respiratory therapy, or a history of trauma or chronic pulmonary disease.

Common medical causes
● *Gas gangrene.* Subcutaneous crepitation is the hallmark of this rare but commonly fatal infection. It's accompanied by local pain, swelling, and discoloration, with formation of bullae and necrosis. The skin over the wound may rupture, revealing dark red or black necrotic mus-

cle and producing foul-smelling watery or frothy discharge. Related findings include tachycardia, tachypnea, moderate fever, cyanosis, and lassitude.

• *Orbital fracture.* This fracture allows air from the nasal sinuses to escape into subcutaneous tissue, causing subcutaneous crepitation of the eyelid and orbit. The most common sign of orbital fracture is periorbital ecchymosis. Visual acuity is usually normal, although a swollen lid may prevent accurate testing. The patient has facial edema, diplopia, a hyphema or, occasionally, a dilated or unreactive pupil on the affected side.

• *Pneumothorax.* Severe pneumothorax produces subcutaneous crepitation in the upper chest and neck. In most cases, the patient has unilateral chest pain that is rarely localized initially and that increases on inspiration. Dyspnea, anxiety, restlessness, tachypnea, cyanosis, tachycardia, accessory muscle use, asymmetrical chest expansion, and a nonproductive cough can also occur. On the affected side, breath sounds are absent or decreased, hyperresonance or tympany may be heard, and decreased vocal fremitus may be present.

• *Rupture of the esophagus.* A ruptured esophagus usually produces subcutaneous crepitation in the neck, chest wall, or supraclavicular fossa. In rupture of the *cervical esophagus,* the patient has excruciating pain in the neck or supraclavicular area, and his neck is resistant to passive motion. He also has local tenderness, soft tissue swelling, dysphagia, odynophagia, and orthostatic vertigo.

Life-threatening rupture of the *intrathoracic esophagus* can produce mediastinal emphysema confirmed by a positive Hamman's sign. The patient has severe retrosternal, epigastric, neck, or scapular pain and edema of the chest wall and neck. He may also display dyspnea, tachypnea, asymmetrical chest expansion, nasal flaring, cyanosis, diaphoresis, tachycardia, hypotension, dysphagia, and fever.

• *Rupture of the trachea or major bronchus.* This life-threatening injury produces abrupt subcutaneous crepitation of the neck and anterior chest wall. The patient has severe dyspnea with nasal flaring, tachycardia, accessory muscle use, hypotension, cyanosis, extreme anxiety, and possibly hemoptysis and mediastinal emphysema, with a positive Hamman's sign.

Other causes

• *Diagnostic tests.* Endoscopic tests such as bronchoscopy can cause rupture or perforation of respiratory or GI organs, producing subcutaneous crepitation.

• *Respiratory treatments.* Mechanical ventilation and intermittent positive pressure breathing can rupture alveoli, producing subcutaneous crepitation.

• *Thoracic surgery.* If air escapes into the tissue in the area of the incision, subcutaneous crepitation can occur.

Special considerations

Monitor the patient's vital signs frequently, especially respirations. Because excessive edema from subcutaneous crepitation in the neck and upper chest can cause airway obstruction, be alert for signs of respiratory distress such as dyspnea. Tell the patient that the affected tissues will eventually absorb the air or gas bubbles, so the subcutaneous crepitation will decrease.

Pediatric pointers

Children may develop subcutaneous crepitation in the neck from ingestion of corrosive substances that perforate the esophagus.

CRY, HIGH-PITCHED
[Cerebral cry]

A high-pitched cry is a brief, sharp, piercing vocal sound produced by a neonate or an infant. Whether acute or chronic, this cry is a late sign of increased intracranial pressure (ICP). However, the acute onset of a high-pitched cry demands emergency treatment to prevent permanent brain damage or death.

Any change in the volume of one of the brain's components—brain tissue, cerebrospinal fluid, and blood—may cause increased ICP. In the neonate, increased ICP may result from intracranial bleeding associated with birth trauma or from congenital malformation, such as craniostenosis and Arnold-Chiari syndrome. In fact, a high-pitched cry may be an early sign of congenital malformation. In an infant, increased ICP may result from meningitis, head trauma, or child abuse.

History and physical examination

Take the infant's vital signs, and then obtain a brief history. Has the infant fallen recently or experienced even minor head trauma? Be sure to ask the mother about any changes in the infant's behavior during the past 24 hours. Has he seemed restless or unlike himself? Has his sucking reflex diminished? Does he cry when moved about? Suspect child abuse if the infant's history is inconsistent.

Next, perform a neurologic examination. Remember that neurologic responses in neonates and young infants are primarily reflex responses. Determine the infant's level of consciousness (LOC). Is he awake, irritable, or lethargic? Does he reach for an attractive object or turn toward the sound of a rattle? Observe the child's posture. Is he in the normal flexed position or in extension or opisthotonos? Examine muscle tone and observe for signs of seizure, such as tremors and twitching.

Now examine the size and shape of the infant's head. Is the anterior fontanel bulging? Measure his head circumference and check pupillary size and response to light. Unilateral or bilateral dilation and sluggish response to light may accompany increased ICP. Finally, test the infant's reflexes; expect Moro's reflex to be diminished.

After completing your examination, elevate the infant's head to promote cerebral venous drainage and decrease ICP. Start an I.V. line, and give diuretics and corticosteroids to decrease ICP. Be sure to keep endotracheal (ET) intubation equipment nearby to secure an airway.

Common medical causes

• *Increased ICP.* A high-pitched cry is a late sign of increased ICP. Typically, the infant also displays bulging fontanels, increased head circumference, and widened sutures. Earlier signs and symptoms of increasing ICP include seizures, bradycardia, possible vomiting, dilated pupils, decreased LOC, increased systolic blood pressure, widened pulse pressure, and altered respiratory pattern.

Special considerations

The infant with increased ICP requires specialized care and monitoring in the intensive care unit. You'll need to monitor his vital signs and neurologic status to detect subtle changes in his condition. Also monitor intake and output. Monitor ICP, restrict fluids, and administer diuretics and corticosteroids.

For an infant with severely increased ICP, ET intubation and mechanical hyperventilation may be needed to decrease partial pressure of arterial carbon dioxide and constrict cerebral blood vessels. Or barbiturate coma or hypothermia therapy may be needed to decrease the infant's metabolic rate.

Remember to avoid jostling the infant, which may aggravate increased ICP. Comfort the infant and maintain a calm, quiet environment because the infant's crying or exposure to environmental stimuli could worsen increased ICP.

CYANOSIS

Cyanosis, a bluish or bluish black discoloration of the skin and mucous membranes, results from excessive concentration of unoxygenated hemoglobin in the blood. This common sign may develop abruptly or gradually. It can be classified as central or peripheral, although the two types may coexist.

Central cyanosis reflects inadequate oxygenation of systemic arterial blood caused by right-to-left cardiac shunting or pulmonary disease or by hematologic disorders. It may occur anywhere on the skin and on the mucous membranes of the mouth, lips, and conjunctiva.

Peripheral cyanosis reflects sluggish peripheral circulation caused by vasoconstriction, reduced cardiac output, or vascular occlusion. It may be widespread or may occur locally in one extremity; however, it doesn't affect mucous membranes. Typically, peripheral cyanosis appears on exposed areas, such as the fingers, nail beds, feet, nose, and ears.

Although cyanosis is an important sign of cardiovascular and pulmonary disorders, it isn't always an accurate gauge of oxygenation. Several factors contribute to its development: hemoglobin level and oxygen saturation, cardiac output, and partial pressure of arterial oxygen (PaO_2). Cyanosis is usually undetectable until the oxygen saturation of hemoglobin falls below 80%. Severe cyanosis is quite obvious, whereas mild cyanosis is more difficult to detect—even in natural, bright light. In dark-skinned patients, cyanosis is most apparent in the mucous membranes and nail beds.

A transient, nonpathologic cyanosis may result from environmental factors. For example, peripheral cyanosis may result from cutaneous vasoconstriction following brief exposure to cold air or water. Central cyanosis may result from reduced PaO_2 at high altitudes.

Emergency interventions

 If the patient displays sudden, localized cyanosis and other signs of arterial occlusion, you'll need to protect the affected limb from injury; however, don't massage the limb. Or, if you see central cyanosis stemming from a pulmonary disorder or shock, perform a rapid evaluation. Take immediate steps to maintain an airway, assist breathing, and monitor circulation.

History and physical examination

If cyanosis accompanies less acute conditions, perform a thorough examination. Begin with a history, focusing on cardiac, pulmonary, and hematologic disorders. Ask about previous surgery. Then begin the physical examination by taking vital signs. Inspect the skin and mucous membranes to determine the extent of cyanosis. Ask the patient when he first noticed the cyanosis. Does it subside and recur? Is it aggravated by cold, smoking, or stress? Alleviated by massage or rewarming? Check for redness, ulceration, and cool, pallid skin. Also note clubbing.

Next, evaluate the patient's level of consciousness. Ask if he has a headache, dizziness, or blurred vision. Then test his motor strength. Ask if he has pain in his arms and legs (especially with walking) or any abnormal sensations (numbness, tingling, or coldness).

Ask about chest pain and its severity. Can the patient identify any aggravating and alleviating factors? Palpate peripheral pulses and test capillary refill time. Also note edema. Auscultate for heart rate and rhythm, noting especially gallops and murmurs. Also auscultate the abdominal aorta and femoral arteries to detect any bruits.

Ask about a cough. Have the patient describe the sputum. Evaluate respiratory rate and rhythm. Check for nasal flaring and use of accessory muscles. Ask about sleep apnea. Does he sleep with his head propped up on pillows? Inspect for asymmetrical chest expansion or barrel chest. Percuss the lungs for dullness or hyperresonance, and auscultate for decreased or adventitious breath sounds.

Inspect the abdomen for ascites, and test for shifting dullness or fluid wave. Percuss and palpate for liver enlargement and tenderness. Also ask about nausea, anorexia, and weight loss.

Common medical causes

• *Arteriosclerotic occlusive disease (chronic).* In this disorder, peripheral cyanosis occurs in the legs whenever they're in a dependent position. Associated signs and symptoms include intermittent claudication and burning pain at rest, paresthesia, pallor, muscle atrophy, weak leg pulses, and impotence. Late signs are leg ulcers and gangrene.

• *Bronchiectasis.* This disorder produces chronic central cyanosis. Its classic sign, though, is a chronic productive cough with copious, foul-smelling, mucopurulent sputum or hemoptysis. Auscultation reveals rhonchi and coarse crackles during inspiration. Other features are dyspnea, recurrent fever and chills, weight loss, malaise, clubbing, and signs of anemia.

• *Buerger's disease.* In this disorder, exposure to cold initially causes the feet to become cold, cyanotic, and numb; later, they redden, become hot, and tingle. Intermittent claudication of the instep is characteristic; it's aggravated by exercise and relieved by rest. Associated clinical features include weak peripheral pulses and, in later stages, ulceration, muscle atrophy, and gangrene.

• *Chronic obstructive pulmonary disease (COPD).* Chronic central cyanosis occurs with this disorder and may be aggravated by exertion. Associated signs and symptoms include exertional dyspnea, productive cough with thick sputum, anorexia, weight loss, pursed-lipped breathing, tachypnea, and use of accessory muscles. Examination reveals wheezing and hyperresonant lung fields. Barrel chest and clubbing are late signs. Tachycardia, diaphoresis, and flushing may also accompany this disorder.

• *Deep vein thrombosis.* In this disorder, acute peripheral cyanosis occurs in the affected extremity along with tenderness, painful movement, edema, warmth, and prominent superficial veins. Also, Homans' sign can be elicited.

• *Heart failure.* Acute or chronic cyanosis may occur in this disorder, typically as a late sign. Cyanosis may be central, peripheral, or both. In left-sided heart failure, central cyanosis occurs with tachycardia, fatigue, dyspnea, cold intolerance, orthopnea, cough, ventricular or atrial gallop, bibasilar crackles, and diffuse apical impulse. In right-sided heart failure, peripheral cyanosis occurs with fatigue, peripheral edema, ascites, jugular vein distention, and hepatomegaly.

• *Lung cancer.* This disorder causes chronic central cyanosis accompanied by fever, weakness, weight loss, anorexia, dyspnea, chest pain, hemoptysis, and wheezing. Atelectasis causes mediastinal shift, decreased diaphragmatic excursion, asymmetrical chest expansion, a dull percussion note, and diminished breath sounds.

• *Peripheral arterial occlusion (acute).* This disorder produces acute cyanosis of one arm or leg or, occasionally, of both legs. Cyanosis is accompanied by paresthesia and sharp or aching pain that worsens when the patient moves. The affected extremity will also be weak, with pale, cool skin. Examination reveals decreased or absent pulse and prolonged capillary refill time.

• *Pneumonia.* In this disorder, acute central cyanosis is usually preceded by fever, shaking chills, cough with purulent sputum, crackles and rhonchi, and pleuritic chest pain that's exacerbated by deep inspiration. Associated signs and symptoms may include tachycardia, dyspnea, tachypnea, diminished breath sounds, diaphoresis, myalgias, fatigue, headache, and anorexia.

● *Pneumothorax.* A cardinal sign of pneumothorax, acute central cyanosis is accompanied by sharp chest pain that's exacerbated by movement, deep breathing, and coughing; asymmetrical chest wall expansion; and shortness of breath. Other possible findings include rapid, shallow respirations; weak, rapid pulse; pallor; neck vein distention; anxiety; and absence of breath sounds over the affected lobe.

● *Polycythemia vera.* A ruddy complexion that can appear cyanotic is characteristic in this chronic myeloproliferative disorder. Other findings are hepatosplenomegaly, headache, dizziness, fatigue, blurred vision, chest pain, intermittent claudication, and coagulation defects.

● *Pulmonary edema.* In this disorder, acute central cyanosis occurs along with dyspnea; orthopnea; frothy, blood-tinged sputum; tachycardia; tachypnea; dependent crackles; ventricular gallop; cold, clammy skin; hypotension; weak, thready pulse; and confusion.

● *Pulmonary embolism.* Acute central cyanosis occurs when a large embolus causes significant obstruction of the pulmonary circulation. Syncope and neck vein distention may also occur. Other common signs and symptoms include dyspnea, chest pain, tachycardia, dry cough or productive cough with blood-tinged sputum, low-grade fever, restlessness, and diaphoresis.

● *Raynaud's disease.* In this disorder, exposure to cold or stress causes the fingers or hands first to blanch and turn cold, then to become cyanotic, and finally to redden with return of normal temperature. Numbness and tingling may also occur.

● *Shock.* In this disorder, acute peripheral cyanosis develops in the hands and feet, which may also be cold, clammy, and pale. Other characteristic clinical features include lethargy, confusion, prolonged capillary refill time, and a rapid, weak pulse. Tachypnea, hyperpnea, and hypotension may also be present.

● *Sleep apnea.* When chronic and severe, sleep apnea causes pulmonary hypertension and cor pulmonale (right-sided heart failure), which can produce chronic cyanosis.

Special considerations

Prepare the patient for such tests as arterial blood gas analysis and complete blood count to determine the cause of cyanosis.

Provide supplemental oxygen to relieve shortness of breath and decrease cyanosis. (Deliver small doses [2 L/minute] in patients with COPD, who may retain carbon dioxide.) Position the patient to ease breathing. As needed, administer diuretics, bronchodilators and antibiotics, or cardiac drugs. Ensure that the patient gets sufficient rest between activities to prevent dyspnea.

Pediatric pointers

Many pulmonary disorders responsible for cyanosis in adults also cause cyanosis in children. In addition, central cyanosis may result from cystic fibrosis, asthma, airway obstruction by a foreign body, acute laryngotracheobronchitis, and epiglottitis. It may also result from congenital heart defects that cause right-to-left intracardiac shunting, such as transposition of the great vessels.

In children, circumoral cyanosis may precede generalized cyanosis. Acrocyanosis (also called "glove and bootee" cyanosis) may occur in infants from excessive crying or exposure to cold. Exercise and agitation enhance cyanosis, so provide comfort and regular rest periods. Also, administer supplemental oxygen during cyanotic episodes.

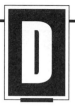

DECEREBRATE POSTURE

[Decerebrate rigidity, abnormal extensor reflex]

Decerebrate posture is usually caused by neurologic deterioration. It's characterized by adduction and extension of the arms, with the wrists pronated and the fingers flexed; stiffly extended legs; plantar flexion of the feet; and, in severe cases, an acutely arched back (opisthotonos). This sign indicates upper brain stem damage, which may result from primary lesions, such as infarction, hemorrhage, or tumor; metabolic encephalopathy; head injury; or brain stem compression associated with increased intracranial pressure (ICP). (See *Comparing decerebrate and decorticate postures,* page 166.)

Decerebrate posture may be elicited by noxious stimuli or may occur spontaneously. It may be unilateral or bilateral. In concurrent brain stem and cerebral damage, decerebrate posture may affect only the arms while the legs remain flaccid. Or decerebrate posture may affect one side of the body and decorticate posture the other. The two postures may also alternate as the patient's neurologic status fluctuates. The duration of each posturing episode usually correlates with the severity of brain stem damage.

Emergency interventions

 As your first priority, ensure a patent airway. Insert an artificial airway, elevate the head of the bed, and turn the patient's head to the side to prevent aspiration (don't disrupt spinal alignment if you suspect spinal cord injury). Suction the patient as necessary.

Next, look for spontaneous respirations. Give supplemental oxygen and ventilate the patient with a handheld resuscitation bag, if necessary. Intubation and mechanical ventilation may be indicated. Keep emergency resuscitation equipment handy. Be sure to check the patient's chart for a no-code order.

History and physical examination

After taking vital signs, determine the patient's level of consciousness (LOC), using the Glasgow Coma Scale as a reference. Then evaluate the pupils for size, equality, and response to light. Test deep tendon reflexes and cranial nerve reflexes, and try to elicit doll's eye sign.

Next, explore the history of the patient's coma. If you're unable to obtain this information, look for clues to the causative disorder, such as hepatomegaly, cyanosis, diabetic skin changes, needle tracks, or obvious trauma. If a family member is available, find out when the patient's LOC began deteriorating. Did it occur abruptly? What did the patient complain of before he lost consciousness? Does he have a history of diabetes, liver disease, cancer, blood clots, or aneurysm? Ask about any accident or trauma that may be responsible for the coma.

COMPARING DECEREBRATE AND DECORTICATE POSTURES

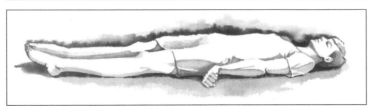

Decerebrate posture results from damage to the upper brain stem. In this posture, the arms are adducted and extended, with the wrists pronated and the fingers flexed. The legs are stiffly extended, with plantar flexion of the feet.

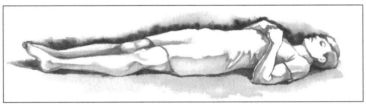

Decorticate posture results from damage to one or both corticospinal tracts. In this posture, the arms are adducted and flexed, with the wrists and fingers flexed on the chest. The legs are stiffly extended and internally rotated, with plantar flexion of the feet.

Common medical causes

● *Brain stem infarction.* When this primary lesion produces a coma, decerebrate posture may also occur. Associated signs and symptoms vary with the severity of the infarct and may include cranial nerve palsies, bilateral cerebellar ataxia, and sensory loss. In a deep coma, all normal reflexes are usually lost, resulting in absent doll's eye sign, a positive Babinski's reflex, and flaccidity.

● *Cerebral lesion.* Whether the etiology is trauma, tumor, abscess, or infarction, any cerebral lesion that increases ICP may also produce decerebrate posture. Typically, this posture is a late sign. Associated findings vary with the lesion's site and extent but commonly include coma, abnormal pupil size and response

to light, and the classic triad of increased ICP—bradycardia, increasing systolic blood pressure, and widening pulse pressure.

● *Hypoglycemic encephalopathy.* Characterized by extremely low blood glucose levels, this disorder may produce decerebrate posture and coma. It also causes dilated pupils, slow respirations, and bradycardia. Muscle spasms, twitching, and seizures eventually progress to flaccidity.

● *Hypoxic encephalopathy.* Severe hypoxia may produce decerebrate posture—the result of brain stem compression associated with anaerobic metabolism and increased ICP. Other findings include coma, a positive Babinski's reflex, absence of doll's eye sign, hypoactive deep tendon reflexes and, possibly, fixed pupils and respiratory arrest.

• ***Pontine hemorrhage.*** Typically, this life-threatening disorder rapidly leads to decerebrate posture with coma. Accompanying signs include total paralysis, absence of doll's eye sign, a positive Babinski's reflex, and small, reactive pupils.

• ***Posterior fossa hemorrhage.*** This subtentorial lesion causes decerebrate posture. Its earlier signs and symptoms include vomiting, headache, vertigo, ataxia, stiff neck, drowsiness, papilledema, and cranial nerve palsies. The patient eventually slips into a coma and, possibly, respiratory arrest.

Other causes

• ***Diagnostic tests.*** Removing spinal fluid during a lumbar puncture to relieve high ICP may precipitate cerebral compression of the brain stem and cause decerebrate posture and coma.

Special considerations

Help prepare the patient for diagnostic tests to determine the cause of his decerebrate posture. In addition to skull X-rays and a computed tomography scan or magnetic resonance imaging, tests may include cerebral angiography, digital subtraction angiography, EEG, brain scan, and ICP monitoring.

Monitor the patient's neurologic status and vital signs every 30 or 60 minutes. In addition, be alert for signs of increased ICP (bradycardia, increasing systolic blood pressure, and widening pulse pressure) and neurologic deterioration (altered respiratory pattern and abnormal temperature).

Inform the patient's family that decerebrate posture is a reflex response—not a voluntary response to pain or a sign of recovery. Offer emotional support.

Pediatric pointers

Children under age 2 may not display decerebrate posture because of nervous system immaturity. However, if they do, it's usually the more severe form with opisthotonos. Opisthotonos is more common in infants and young children than in adults and is usually a terminal sign.

In children, decerebrate posture is usually caused by head injury, but it also occurs in Reye's syndrome—the result of increased ICP causing brain stem compression.

DECORTICATE POSTURE
[Decorticate rigidity, abnormal flexor response]

A sign of corticospinal damage, decorticate posture is characterized by adduction of the arms and flexion of the elbows, wrists and fingers flexed on the chest, extended and internally rotated legs, and plantar flexion of the feet. This posture may occur unilaterally or bilaterally and usually results from cerebrovascular accident (CVA) or head injury. It may be elicited by noxious stimuli or may occur spontaneously. The intensity of the required stimulus, the duration of the posture, and the frequency of spontaneous episodes vary with the severity and location of the cerebral injury.

Although a serious sign, decorticate posture carries a more favorable prognosis than decerebrate posture. However, if the causative disorder extends lower in the brain stem, decorticate posture may progress to decerebrate posture.

Emergency interventions

 Obtain vital signs and evaluate the patient's level of consciousness (LOC). If his LOC is altered, insert an oropharyngeal airway, elevate the head of the bed 30 degrees, and turn the patient's head to the side to prevent aspiration (unless spinal cord injury is suspected). Evaluate his respiratory rate, rhythm, and depth. Prepare to assist respirations with a handheld resuscitation bag or with intubation and mechanical ventilation, if necessary. In addition, institute seizure precautions.

History and physical examination
Test the patient's motor and sensory function. Evaluate pupil size, equality, and response to light. Then test cranial nerve and deep tendon reflexes. Ask about headache, dizziness, nausea, abnormal vision, and numbness or tingling. When did the patient first notice these symptoms? Is his family aware of any behavior changes? Also ask about a history of cerebrovascular disease, cancer, meningitis, encephalitis, upper respiratory infection, or recent trauma.

Common medical causes
• *Brain abscess.* Decorticate posture may occur in this infection. Accompanying findings vary, depending on the size and location of the abscess, but may include aphasia, hemiparesis, headache, dizziness, seizures, nausea, and vomiting. Behavior changes, altered vital signs, and decreased LOC may also occur.
• *Brain tumor.* This disorder may produce decorticate posture that's usually bilateral—the result of increased ICP associated with tumor growth. Related signs and symptoms include headache, behavior changes, memory loss, diplopia, blurred vision or vision loss, seizures, ataxia, dizziness, apraxia, aphasia, paresis, sensory loss, paresthesia, vomiting, papilledema, and signs of hormonal imbalance.
• *Cerebrovascular accident.* Typically, a CVA involving the cerebral cortex produces unilateral decorticate posture, also called spastic hemiplegia. Other clinical features are hemiplegia contralateral to the lesion, dysarthria, dysphagia, unilateral sensory loss, apraxia, agnosia, aphasia, memory loss, decreased LOC, urine retention and incontinence, and constipation. Ocular effects include homonymous hemianopia, diplopia, and blurred vision.

• *Head injury.* Decorticate posture may be a feature of this disorder, depending on the site and severity of head injury. Associated signs and symptoms may include headache, nausea and vomiting, dizziness, irritability, decreased LOC, aphasia, hemiparesis, unilateral numbness, seizures, and pupillary dilation.

Special considerations
Assess the patient frequently to detect subtle signs of neurologic deterioration. Also monitor his neurologic status and vital signs every 30 minutes to 2 hours. Be alert for signs of increased ICP, including bradycardia, increasing systolic blood pressure, and widening pulse pressure.

Pediatric pointers
Decorticate posture is an unreliable sign before age 2 because of nervous system immaturity. In children, this sign usually results from head injury, but it also occurs in Reye's syndrome.

DEEP TENDON REFLEXES, HYPERACTIVE

Hyperactive deep tendon reflexes (DTRs) are abnormally brisk muscle contractions in response to a sudden stretch induced by sharply tapping the muscle's tendon of insertion. This elicited sign may be graded as brisk or pathologically hyperactive. Hyperactive reflexes are commonly accompanied by clonus.

The corticospinal tract and other descending tracts govern the reflex arc—the relay cycle that produces any reflex response. A corticospinal lesion above the level of the reflex arc being tested may result in hyperactive DTRs. Abnormal neuromuscular transmission at the end of the reflex arc may also cause hyperactive DTRs. For example, deficiency of calcium or magnesium may cause hyperactive DTRs because these electrolytes regulate neuromuscular excitability. (See *Tracing the reflex arc in deep tendon reflexes,* pages 170 and 171.)

Although hyperactive DTRs commonly accompany other neurologic findings, they usually lack specific diagnostic value. For example, they're an early, cardinal sign of hypocalcemia.

History and physical examination

After eliciting hyperactive DTRs, begin the neurologic examination with the patient's history. Has he had a spinal cord injury or other trauma? Was he exposed to cold, wind, or water for a prolonged period of time? If the patient is a woman, might she be pregnant? A positive response to any of these questions requires prompt evaluation to rule out life-threatening autonomic hyperreflexia, tetanus, preeclampsia, or hypothermia. Ask about the onset and progression of associated signs and symptoms. Evaluate LOC, and test motor and sensory function in the limbs. Ask about paresthesia. Check for ataxia or tremors and for speech and visual deficits. Test for Chvostek's and Trousseau's signs and for carpopedal spasm. Ask about vomiting or altered bladder habits. Be sure to take vital signs.

Common medical causes

• *Amyotrophic lateral sclerosis.* This disorder produces generalized hyperactive DTRs accompanied by weakness of the hands and forearms and spasticity of the legs. Eventually, the patient develops atrophy of the neck and tongue muscles, fasciculations, occasional weakness of the legs, and possibly bulbar signs (dysphagia, dysphonia, facial weakness, and dyspnea).

• *Brain tumor.* A cerebral tumor causes hyperactive DTRs on the side opposite the lesion. Associated signs and symptoms develop slowly and may include unilateral paresis or paralysis, anesthesia, visual field deficits, spasticity, and a positive Babinski's reflex.

• *Cerebrovascular accident (CVA).* Any CVA that affects the origin of the corticospinal tracts causes sudden onset of hyperactive DTRs on the side opposite the lesion. Unilateral paresis or paralysis, anesthesia, visual field deficits, spasticity, and a positive Babinski's reflex may also occur.

• *Hypocalcemia.* This disorder may produce sudden or gradual onset of generalized hyperactive DTRs with paresthesia, muscle twitching and cramping, positive Chvostek's and Trousseau's signs, carpopedal spasm, and tetany.

• *Hypomagnesemia.* Generalized hyperactive DTRs occur gradually and are accompanied by muscle cramps, hypotension, tachycardia, paresthesia, ataxia, tetany, and possibly seizures.

• *Hypothermia.* Mild hypothermia (90° to 94° F [32.2° to 34.4° C]) produces generalized hyperactive DTRs. Other signs and symptoms include shivering, fatigue, weakness, lethargy, slurred speech, ataxia, muscle stiffness, tachycardia, diuresis, bradypnea, hypotension, and cold, pale skin.

• *Preeclampsia.* Occurring in pregnancy of at least 20 weeks' duration, preeclampsia may cause gradual onset of generalized hyperactive DTRs. Accompanying signs and symptoms include increased blood pressure; abnormal weight gain; edema of the face, fingers, and abdomen after bed rest; oliguria; severe headache; blurred or double vision; epigastric pain; nausea and vomiting; irritability; cyanosis; shortness of breath; and crackles. If preeclampsia progresses to eclampsia, the patient will have seizures.

• *Spinal cord lesion.* Incomplete spinal cord lesions cause hyperactive DTRs below the level of the lesion. In a traumatic lesion, hyperactive DTRs follow resolution of spinal shock. In a neoplastic lesion, hyperactive DTRs gradually replace normal DTRs. Other signs and symptoms are paralysis and sensory loss

(Text continues on page 172.)

TRACING THE REFLEX ARC IN DEEP TENDON REFLEXES

Sharply tapping a tendon initiates a sensory (afferent) impulse that travels along a peripheral nerve to a spinal nerve and then to the spinal cord. The impulse enters the spinal cord through the posterior root, synapses with a motor (efferent)

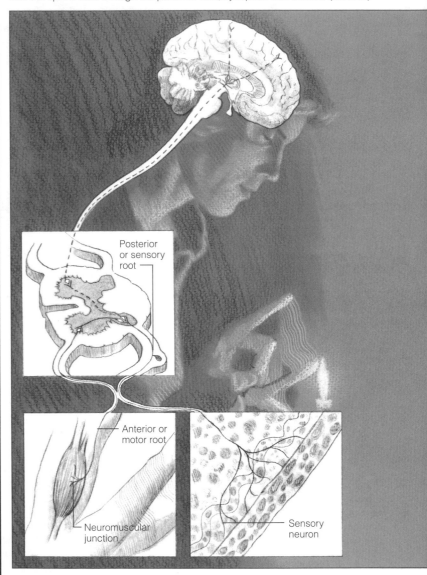

Posterior or sensory root

Anterior or motor root

Neuromuscular junction

Sensory neuron

neuron in the anterior horn on the same side of the spinal cord, and then is transmitted through a motor nerve fiber back to the muscle. When the impulse crosses the neuromuscular junction, the muscle contracts, completing the reflex arc.

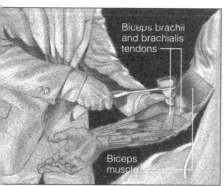

**Biceps reflex
(C5-6 Innervation)**

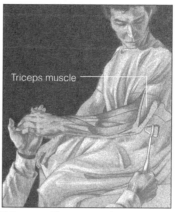

**Triceps reflex
(C7-8 innervation)**

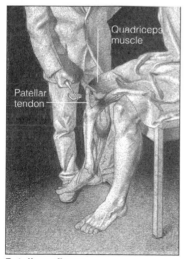

**Patellar reflexes
(L2, 3, 4 innervation)**

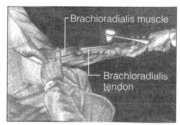

**Brachioradialis reflex
(C5-6 innervation)**

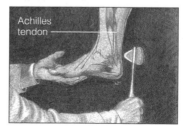

**Achilles tendon reflex
(S1-2 innervation)**

below the level of the lesion, urine retention and overflow incontinence, and alternating constipation and diarrhea. In a lesion above T6, there may also be autonomic hyperreflexia with diaphoresis and flushing above the level of the lesion, headache, nasal congestion, nausea, increased blood pressure, and bradycardia.
• *Tetanus.* In this disorder, sudden onset of generalized hyperactive DTRs accompanies tachycardia, diaphoresis, low-grade fever, painful and involuntary muscle contractions, trismus (lockjaw), and risus sardonicus.

Special considerations

Prepare the patient for diagnostic tests to evaluate hyperactive DTRs. These may include measurement of serum calcium and magnesium levels, spinal X-rays, computed tomography scan, lumbar puncture, and myelography.

If motor weakness accompanies hyperactive DTRs, perform or encourage range-of-motion exercises to preserve muscle integrity. Also, reposition the patient frequently, provide a special mattress, and massage his back to prevent skin breakdown. Administer muscle relaxants and sedatives to relieve severe muscle contractions. Keep emergency resuscitation equipment on hand. Provide a quiet, calm atmosphere to decrease neuromuscular excitability.

Pediatric pointers

Hyperreflexia may be a normal sign in neonates. After age 6, children's reflex responses are similar to those of adults. When testing DTRs in small children, use distraction techniques to elicit reliable results.

Cerebral palsy commonly causes hyperactive DTRs in children. Reye's syndrome causes generalized hyperactive DTRs in stage II and absent DTRs in stage V. Adult causes of hyperactive DTRs may also appear in children.

DEEP TENDON REFLEXES, HYPOACTIVE

Hypoactive deep tendon reflexes (DTRs) are abnormally diminished muscle contractions in response to a sudden stretch induced by sharply tapping the muscle's tendon of insertion. They may be graded as minimal (+) or absent (0). (See *Documenting deep tendon reflexes.*)

The corticospinal tract and other descending tracts govern the reflex arc, the relay cycle that produces any reflex response. Hypoactive DTRs may result from damage to the reflex arc involving the specific muscle, the peripheral nerve, the nerve roots, or the spinal cord at that level. Hypoactive DTRs are an important sign of many disorders, especially when they appear with other neurologic signs and symptoms.

History and physical examination

After eliciting hypoactive DTRs, obtain a thorough history from the patient or a family member. Have him describe current signs and symptoms in detail. Then take a family and drug history.

Next, evaluate the patient's level of consciousness. Test motor function in his limbs, and palpate for muscle atrophy or increased mass. Test sensory function, including pain, touch, temperature, and vibration sense. Ask about paresthesia. To observe gait and coordination, have the patient take several steps. To check for Romberg's sign, ask him to stand with his feet together and eyes closed. Evaluate his speech during conversation. Observe for signs of vision or hearing loss. Abrupt onset of hypoactive DTRs accompanied by muscle weakness may occur in life-threatening Guillain-Barré syndrome, botulism, or spinal cord lesions with spinal shock.

Take vital signs to detect autonomic nervous system effects. Also inspect the skin for pallor, dryness, flushing, or diaphoresis. Auscultate for hypoactive bowel sounds. Ask about nausea, vomiting, constipation, and incontinence. Palpate for bladder distention.

Common medical causes

● *Botulism.* In this disorder, generalized hypoactive DTRs accompany progressive descending muscle weakness. Initially, the patient usually complains of blurred and double vision and, occasionally, of anorexia, nausea, and vomiting. Other early bulbar findings include vertigo, hearing loss, dysarthria, and dysphagia. The patient may have signs of respiratory distress and severe constipation marked by hypoactive bowel sounds.

● *Eaton-Lambert syndrome.* This disorder produces generalized hypoactive DTRs. Early signs include difficulty rising from a chair, climbing stairs, and walking. The patient may complain of achiness, paresthesia, and muscle weakness that's most severe in the morning. Weakness improves with mild exercise and worsens with strenuous exercise.

● *Guillain-Barré syndrome.* This disorder causes bilateral hypoactive DTRs that progress rapidly from hypotonia to areflexia in several days. Typically, this disorder causes muscle weakness that begins in the legs and then extends to the arms and, possibly, to the trunk and neck muscles. Occasionally, weakness may progress to total paralysis. Other clinical features include cranial nerve palsies, pain, paresthesia, and signs of brief autonomic dysfunction, such as sinus tachycardia or bradycardia, flushing, fluctuating blood pressure, and anhidrosis or episodic diaphoresis.

Usually, muscle weakness and hypoactive DTRs peak in severity within 10 to 14 days; then symptoms begin to clear. However, residual hypoactive DTRs and motor weakness may persist in severe cases.

● *Peripheral neuropathy.* A characteristic symptom in end-stage diabetes mellitus, renal failure, and alcoholism, peripheral neuropathy results in progressive hypoactive DTRs. Other effects include motor weakness, sensory loss, paresthesia, tremors, and possibly autonomic dysfunction, such as orthostatic hypotension and incontinence.

● *Polymyositis.* In this disorder, hypoactive DTRs accompany muscle weakness, pain, stiffness, spasms and, possibly, in-

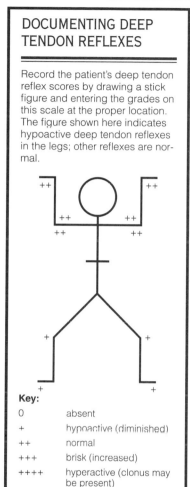

DOCUMENTING DEEP TENDON REFLEXES

Record the patient's deep tendon reflex scores by drawing a stick figure and entering the grades on this scale at the proper location. The figure shown here indicates hypoactive deep tendon reflexes in the legs; other reflexes are normal.

Key:

0	absent
+	hypoactive (diminished)
++	normal
+++	brisk (increased)
++++	hyperactive (clonus may be present)

creased size or atrophy. These effects are usually temporary; affected muscles vary.

• *Spinal cord lesions.* Spinal cord injury or complete transection produces spinal shock, resulting in hypoactive DTRs below the level of the lesion. Associated signs and symptoms may include quadriplegia or paraplegia, flaccidity, loss of sensation below the level of the lesion, and dry, pale skin. Also characteristic are urine retention with overflow incontinence, hypoactive bowel sounds, constipation, and genital reflex loss. Hypoactive DTRs and flaccidity are usually transient; reflex activity may return within several weeks.

• *Syringomyelia.* Permanent bilateral hypoactive DTRs occur early in this slowly progressive disorder. Other clinical features are muscle weakness and atrophy; loss of sensation, usually extending in a capelike fashion over the arms, shoulders, neck, back, and occasionally the legs; deep, boring pain (despite anesthesia) in the limbs; and signs of brain stem involvement (nystagmus, facial numbness, unilateral vocal cord paralysis or weakness, and unilateral tongue atrophy).

Other causes

• *Drugs.* Barbiturates and paralyzing drugs, such as pancuronium and curare, may cause hypoactive DTRs.

Special considerations

Help the patient carry out his daily activities. Try to strike a balance between promoting independence and ensuring his safety. Encourage him to walk with assistance. Make sure personal care articles are within easy reach, and provide an obstacle-free course from his bed to the bathroom. If the patient has sensory deficits, protect him from injury from heat or pressure. Test his bathwater and reposition him frequently, ensuring a soft, smooth bed surface. Keep his skin clean and dry to prevent breakdown. Perform or encourage range-of-motion exercises.

Also encourage a balanced diet with increased protein.

Pediatric pointers

Hypoactive DTRs commonly occur in muscular dystrophy, Friedreich's ataxia, syringomyelia, and spinal cord injury. They also accompany progressive muscular atrophy, which affects preschoolers and adolescents.

Use distraction techniques to test DTRs; assess motor function by watching the infant or child at play.

DEPRESSION

Depression defies easy definition and often eludes diagnosis and treatment. Clinical depression differs from "the blues," periodic bouts of dysphoria that are less persistent and severe than the clinical disorder. Symptoms of depression include depressed mood, loss of interest or pleasure in activities, significant change in appetite or weight, sleep disturbances, restlessness or sluggishness, fatigue or loss of energy, decreased concentration, indecision, feelings of worthlessness or inappropriate guilt, and thoughts of death or suicide. (See *Suicide: Caring for the high-risk patient.*) A diagnosis of depression is likely if a person experiences either of the first two symptoms and four of the remaining eight for at least a 2-week period. A complete psychiatric and physical examination should be conducted to exclude possible medical causes.

Depression is twice as common in women as in men and is especially prevalent among adolescents. It may be caused by psychiatric or organic disorders or the use of certain drugs.

History and physical examination

Try to determine how the patient feels about herself, her family, and her envi-

SUICIDE: CARING FOR THE HIGH-RISK PATIENT

One of the most common factors contributing to suicide is hopelessness—an emotion that a depressed patient frequently experiences. As a result, you'll need to regularly assess depressed patients for suicidal tendencies.

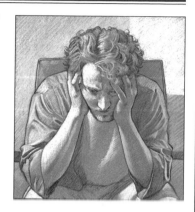

Usually, the patient will provide specific clues to his intentions. For example, you may notice him talking frequently about death or the futility of life, concealing potentially harmful items, giving away personal belongings, or getting legal and financial accounts in order. If you suspect that he's suicidal, follow these care guidelines:

• First, try to determine the patient's suicide potential. Find out how upset he is. Does he have a simple, straightforward suicide plan that's likely to succeed? Does he have a support system—family, friends, a therapist? A patient with low to moderate suicide potential is noticeably depressed but has some form of support system. He may have thoughts of suicide, but no specific plan. A patient with high suicide potential feels profoundly hopeless and has little or no support system. He thinks about suicide frequently and has a plan that's likely to succeed.

• Next, observe precautions. Ensure the patient's safety by removing any objects he could use to harm himself, such as razors, belts, electrical cords, and shoestrings. Know his whereabouts and what he's doing at all times—this may require one-on-one surveillance. Place the patient in a room that's close to your station. Always have someone accompany him off the unit.

• Be alert for in-hospital suicide attempts. Typically, they occur when there's a low staff-to-patient ratio—between shifts, during evening and night shifts, or when a critical event such as a code draws attention away from the patient.

• Finally, arrange for follow-up counseling. Recognize suicidal ideation and behavior as a desperate cry for help. Contact a mental health professional for a referral.

---

ronment. Your goal is to explore the nature of her depression, the extent to which other factors affect it, and her coping mechanisms. Begin by asking what's bothering her. How does her current mood differ from her usual mood? Then ask her to describe the way she feels about herself. What are her plans and dreams? How realistic are they? Is she generally satisfied with what she has accomplished in her work, relationships, and other interests? Observe her body language as she responds. Ask about any changes in her social interactions, sleep patterns, ability to make decisions or concentrate, or normal activities. Explore drug and alcohol use.

Ask the patient about her family—its patterns of interaction and characteristic responses to success and failure. What part does she feel she plays in her family life? Find out if other family members

LIGHT THERAPY FOR DEPRESSION

Because light is associated with maintenance of the body's natural rhythms, it is being used to treat a variety of disorders, including winter depression, also known as seasonal affective disorder (SAD). Although researchers disagree about the exact cause of SAD, many theorize that it results when a person receives insufficient morning light to suppress the hormone melatonin. Too much melatonin can cause depression. Bright light suppresses blood levels of melatonin.

Light therapy is the treatment of choice for patients with this disorder because it is noninvasive and has a high success rate. Therapeutic response is achieved by replacing the light normally found in a long summer day with artificial light. The patient is asked to sit in front of a light box that emits intense bright light. The light enters the eye, hits the retina, and is transmitted by nerve impulses to the pineal gland, which control melatonin secretion.

Intense bright light is the key to this treatment. Full-spectrum light is not required or recommended. Treatment duration varies from 15 minutes to 2 hours daily, and relief typically begins in 3 to 4 days and is completed within 2 weeks. Sessions are usually discontinued when spring arrives, with its longer days.

blue, where does she go and what does she do to feel better? Find out how she feels about her role in the community and the resources that are available to her. Try to determine if she has an adequate support network to help her cope with her depression.

Perform a complete neurologic examination. Test deep tendon reflexes and range of motion. Obtain vital signs and blood for testing, if ordered.

Common medical causes
- *Organic disorders.* Various organic disorders and chronic illnesses produce mild, moderate, or severe depression. Among these are metabolic and endocrine disorders, such as hypothyroidism, hyperthyroidism, and diabetes; infectious diseases, such as influenza, hepatitis, and encephalitis; degenerative diseases, such as Alzheimer's disease, multiple sclerosis, and multi-infarct dementia; and neoplastic disorders such as pancreatic cancer.
- *Psychiatric disorders.* Affective disorders are commonly characterized by abrupt mood swings from depression to elation (mania) or by prolonged episodes of either mood. In fact, severe depression may last for weeks or sometimes longer. More moderate depression occurs in cyclothymic disorders and usually alternates with moderate mania. Moderate depression that is more or less constant over a 2-year period commonly results from dysthymic disorders. In addition, chronic anxiety disorders, such as panic or obsessive-compulsive disorder, may be accompanied by depression.

Other causes
- *Alcohol abuse.* Intoxication or withdrawal commonly produces depression.
- *Drugs.* Various drugs cause depression as an adverse effect. Among the more common are barbiturates, antineoplastic agents such as asparaginase, anticonvulsants such as diazepam, and antiarrhythmics such as disopyramide. Other

have been depressed, and whether anyone important to the patient has been sick or has died in the past year. Finally, ask the patient about her environment. Has her lifestyle changed in the past month? Six months? Year? When she's feeling

depression-inducing drugs include beta-adrenergic blockers such as propranolol, levodopa, indomethacin, cycloserine, corticosteroids, oral contraceptives, and centrally acting antihypertensives, such as reserpine (common in high dosages), methyldopa, and clonidine.

Special considerations

Caring for the depressed patient takes time, tact, and energy. It also requires an awareness of your own vulnerability to feelings of despair that can stem from your interactions with the patient.

Help the patient set realistic goals; encourage her to promote feelings of self-worth by asserting her opinions and making decisions. Because anger typically underlies depression, help the patient acknowledge this emotion and express it safely. To help her overcome feelings of helplessness, plan activities that she can succeed at and teach her to solve problems constructively. Help foster feelings of competence by focusing on past and present experiences in which she was successful. Educate her about the treatments available for depression. (See *Light therapy for depression.*) Try to determine her suicide potential, and take steps to help ensure her safety. The patient may require close surveillance to prevent a suicide attempt.

Make sure the patient receives adequate nourishment and rest, and keep her environment free from stress and excessive stimulation. Assist with diagnostic tests to determine if her depression has an organic cause, and administer drugs as ordered. In addition, arrange for follow-up counseling or contact a mental health professional for a referral.

Elder tip

 When elderly people feel hopeless or powerless, they can become depressed. These feelings may stem from illness, changes in social roles, or the loss of a spouse or friend. Elderly people may be reluctant to discuss their feelings and symptoms. Suicide is a concern in this group. To keep an older person active and promote self-esteem, encourage him to develop hobbies, garden, adopt a pet, or visit with family and friends. If he lives with his family, encourage the family to include him in activities or chores that he would not consider demeaning. Giving an older person choices promotes success.

Pediatric pointers

Because emotional lability is normal in adolescence, depression can be difficult to assess and diagnose in teenagers. Clues to underlying depression may include somatic complaints, sexual promiscuity, low academic achievement, and abuse of alcohol or drugs.

In many cases, use of a family systems model helps determine the cause of depression in adolescents. Once family roles are determined, family therapy or group therapy with peers may help the patient overcome her depression.

DIAPHORESIS

Diaphoresis is profuse sweating—at times, amounting to more than 1 qt (1 L) of sweat per hour. This sign is an autonomic nervous system response to physical or psychogenic stress, fever, or high environmental temperature. When caused by stress, diaphoresis may be generalized or limited to the palms of the hands, soles of the feet, and forehead. When caused by fever or high environmental temperature, it's usually generalized. (See *Understanding diaphoresis,* pages 178 and 179.)

Diaphoresis usually begins abruptly and may be accompanied by other autonomic system signs, such as tachycardia and increased blood pressure. However, it varies with age because sweat glands function immaturely in the infant and are

UNDERSTANDING DIAPHORESIS

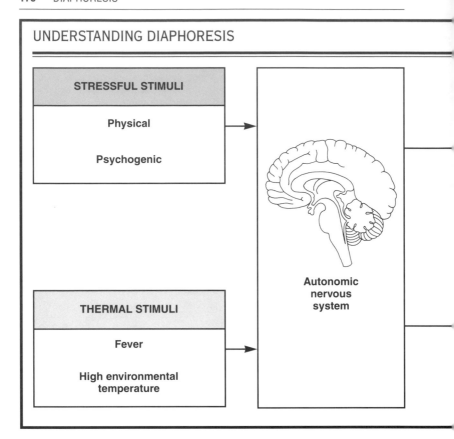

STRESSFUL STIMULI

Physical

Psychogenic

THERMAL STIMULI

Fever

High environmental
temperature

Autonomic
nervous
system

less active in the elderly. As a result, these age-groups may fail to display diaphoresis associated with its common causes.

Intermittent diaphoresis may accompany chronic disorders characterized by recurrent fever; isolated diaphoresis may mark an episode of acute pain or fever. Night sweats may characterize intermittent fever because body temperature tends to return to normal between 2 and 4 a.m. before rising again.

When caused by high external temperature, diaphoresis is a normal response. Acclimatization usually requires several days of exposure to high temperatures; during this process, diaphoresis helps maintain normal body temper-ature. Diaphoresis also commonly occurs during menopause, preceded by a sensation of intense heat (a hot flash). Other causes include exercise or exertion that accelerates metabolism, creating internal heat, and mild to moderate anxiety that helps initiate the fight-or-flight response.

History and physical examination

If the patient is diaphoretic, quickly rule out the possibility of a life-threatening cause. (See *When diaphoresis spells crisis,* page 180.) Begin the history by having the patient describe his chief complaint. Then explore associated signs and symptoms. Note general fatigue and weakness. Does the patient have insom-

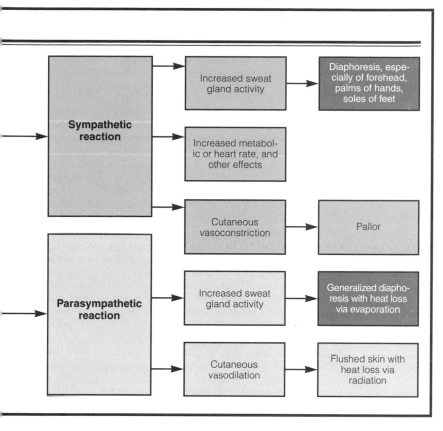

nia, headaches, and changes in vision or hearing? Is he often dizzy? Does he have palpitations? Ask about pleuritic pain, cough, sputum, and difficulty breathing; nausea, vomiting, altered bowel or bladder habits; and abdominal pain. Ask the female patient about amenorrhea. Is she menopausal? Note weight loss or gain. Ask about paresthesia, muscle cramps or stiffness, and joint pain.

Complete the history by asking about travel to tropical countries. Note recent exposure to high environmental temperatures or to pesticides. Was the patient recently bitten by an insect? Check for a history of partial gastrectomy or of drug or alcohol abuse. Finally, obtain a thorough drug history.

Now perform a physical examination. First, determine the extent of diaphoresis by inspecting the patient's trunk and extremities as well as his palms, soles, and forehead. Also check his clothing and bedding for dampness. Note whether diaphoresis occurs during the day or at night. Observe for flushing, abnormal skin texture or lesions, splinter hemorrhages, and increased coarse body hair. Note poor skin turgor and dry mucous membranes.

Then evaluate the patient's mental status and take his vital signs. Observe for fasciculations and flaccid paralysis. Be alert for seizures. Note the patient's facial expression, and examine his eyes for pupillary dilation or constriction, ex-

WHEN DIAPHORESIS SPELLS CRISIS

Diaphoresis is an early sign of certain life-threatening disorders. These guidelines will help you detect such disorders promptly and intervene to minimize patient harm.

If you observe diaphoresis in a patient who complains of blurred vision, be sure to ask him about increased irritability and anxiety. Has he been unusually hungry? Does he have tremors? Take the patient's vital signs, noting hypotension and tachycardia. Then ask about a history of insulin-dependent diabetes. If you suspect *hypoglycemia,* evaluate the patient's blood glucose level using a glucose reagent strip, or send a serum sample to the laboratory. Administer I.V. glucose 50% to return the patient's glucose level to normal. Monitor vital signs and cardiac rhythm. Ensure a patent airway and be prepared to assist breathing and circulation if necessary.

If you observe profuse diaphoresis in a weak, tired, and apprehensive patient, suspect *heat stroke,* which can progress to circulatory collapse. Take vital signs, noting a normal or subnormal temperature. Check for ashen-gray skin and dilated pupils. Was the patient recently exposed to high temperatures and humidity? Was he wearing heavy clothing at the time? Also ask about use of diuretics, which interfere with normal perspiration. Take the patient to a cool room, remove his clothing, and use a fan to direct cool air over his body. Insert an I.V. line and prepare for electrolyte and fluid replacement. Monitor for signs of shock.

If you observe diaphoresis in a patient with a spinal cord injury above T6 or T7, ask about pounding headache, restlessness, blurred vision, and nasal congestion. Take the patient's vital signs, noting bradycardia and extremely elevated blood pressure. If you suspect *autonomic hyperreflexia,* quickly rule out its common complications. Examine the patient for eye pain associated with intraocular hemorrhage and for facial paralysis, slurred speech, or limb weakness associated with intracerebral hemorrhage. Quickly reposition him to remove any pressure stimulus. Also check for a distended bladder or fecal impaction. Remove any kinks from the urinary catheter if necessary. Or administer a suppository or manually remove fecal impaction. If you can't locate and relieve the causative stimulus, start an I.V. line. Prepare to administer hydralazine for hypertension.

If the diaphoretic patient complains of chest pain and dyspnea, suspect *myocardial infarction* or *heart failure.* Connect the patient to a cardiac monitor, ensure a patent airway, and administer supplemental oxygen. Start an I.V. line and administer analgesics. Be prepared to begin emergency resuscitation if cardiac or respiratory arrest occurs.

ophthalmos, and excessive tearing. Test visual fields. Also check for hearing loss and for tooth or gum disease. Percuss the lungs for dullness, and auscultate for crackles, diminished or bronchial breath sounds, and increased vocal fremitus. Look for decreased respiratory excursion. Palpate for lymphadenopathy and hepatosplenomegaly.

Common medical causes

• *Acromegaly.* In this slowly progressive disorder, diaphoresis is a sensitive gauge of disease activity, which involves hypersecretion of growth hormone and increased metabolic rate. The patient has a hulking appearance with an enlarged supraorbital ridge and thickened ears and nose. Other signs and symptoms include warm, oily, thickened skin; enlarged hands, feet, and jaw; joint pain; weight gain; hoarseness; and increased coarse body hair. Increased blood pressure, severe headache, and visual field deficits or blindness may also occur.

• *Anxiety disorders.* Acute anxiety characterizes panic, whereas chronic anxiety characterizes phobias, conversion disorders, obsessions, and compulsions. Whether acute or chronic, anxiety may cause sympathetic stimulation, resulting in diaphoresis. The diaphoresis is most dramatic on the palms, soles, and forehead. It's accompanied by palpitations, tachycardia, tachypnea, tremor, and GI distress. Psychological symptoms—fear, difficulty concentrating, and behavior changes—also occur.

• *Autonomic hyperreflexia.* Occurring after resolution of spinal shock in spinal cord injury above T6, hyperreflexia results in profuse diaphoresis, pounding headache, blurred vision, and dramatically elevated blood pressure. Diaphoresis occurs above the level of the injury, especially on the forehead, and is accompanied by flushing. Other findings may include restlessness, nausea, nasal congestion, and bradycardia.

• *Heart failure.* Typically, diaphoresis follows fatigue, dyspnea, orthopnea, and tachycardia in left-sided heart failure and neck vein distention and dry cough in right-sided heart failure. Other features include tachypnea, cyanosis, dependent edema, crackles, ventricular gallop, and anxiety.

• *Heat exhaustion.* Initially, this condition causes profuse diaphoresis, fatigue, weakness, and anxiety. It may progress to circulatory collapse and shock, marked by confusion, thready pulse, hypotension, tachycardia, and cold, clammy skin. Other features are an ashen-gray appearance, dilated pupils, and normal or subnormal temperature.

• *Hodgkin's disease.* Especially in the elderly, early features of Hodgkin's disease may include night sweats, fever, fatigue, pruritus, and weight loss. Usually, though, Hodgkin's disease initially causes painless swelling of a cervical lymph node. Occasionally, a Pel-Ebstein fever pattern—several days or weeks of fever and chills alternating with afebrile periods with no chills—is present. Systemic symptoms indicate a poor prognosis. Progressive lymphadenopathy eventually causes widespread effects, such as hepatomegaly and dyspnea.

• *Hypoglycemia.* Rapidly induced hypoglycemia may cause diaphoresis accompanied by irritability, tremors, hypotension, blurred vision, tachycardia, hunger, and loss of consciousness.

• *Infective endocarditis (subacute).* Generalized night sweats occur early in this disorder. Accompanying signs and symptoms include intermittent low-grade fever, weakness, fatigue, weight loss, anorexia, and arthralgia. A sudden change in a murmur or the discovery of a new murmur is a classic sign. Petechiae and splinter hemorrhages are also common.

• *Lung abscess.* Drenching night sweats are common in this disorder. Its chief sign, though, is a cough that produces copious purulent, foul-smelling, commonly bloody sputum. Associated findings are fever with chills, pleuritic chest pain, dyspnea, weakness, anorexia, weight loss, headache, malaise, clubbing, tubular or amphoric breath sounds, and dullness on percussion.

• *Myocardial infarction.* Usually, diaphoresis accompanies acute, substernal, radiating chest pain in this life-threatening disorder. Associated signs and symptoms include anxiety, dyspnea, nausea, vomiting, tachycardia, irregular pulse, blood pressure change, fine crackles, pallor, and clammy skin.

● *Pesticide poisoning.* Among the toxic effects of pesticides are diaphoresis, nausea, vomiting, diarrhea, blurred vision, miosis, and excess lacrimation and salivation. The patient may display fasciculations, muscle weakness, and flaccid paralysis. Signs of respiratory depression and coma may also occur.

● *Pheochromocytoma.* This disorder commonly produces diaphoresis. Its cardinal sign, though, is persistent or paroxysmal hypertension. Other effects include headache, palpitations, tachycardia, anxiety, tremors, pallor, flushing, paresthesia, abdominal pain, tachypnea, nausea, vomiting, and orthostatic hypotension.

● *Pneumonia.* Intermittent, generalized diaphoresis accompanies fever and chills in pneumonia. The patient complains of pleuritic chest pain that increases with deep inspiration. Other features are tachypnea, dyspnea, productive cough (with scant and mucoid or copious and purulent sputum), headache, fatigue, myalgia, abdominal pain, anorexia, and cyanosis. Auscultation reveals bronchial breath sounds.

● *Tetanus.* This disorder commonly causes profuse sweating accompanied by low-grade fever, tachycardia, and hyperactive deep tendon reflexes. Early restlessness and pain and stiffness in the jaw, abdomen, and back progress to spasms associated with lockjaw, risus sardonicus, and opisthotonos. Laryngospasm may result in cyanosis or sudden death by asphyxiation.

● *Thyrotoxicosis.* This disorder commonly produces diaphoresis accompanied by heat intolerance, weight loss despite increased appetite, tachycardia, palpitations, an enlarged thyroid, dyspnea, nervousness, diarrhea, tremors, and possibly exophthalmos. Gallops may also occur.

● *Tuberculosis.* Although commonly asymptomatic in primary infection, this disorder may cause night sweats, low-grade fever, fatigue, weakness, anorexia, and weight loss. In reactivation, the patient may have a productive cough with mucopurulent sputum, occasional hemoptysis, and chest pain.

Other causes

● *Drugs.* Sympathomimetics, certain antipsychotics, thyroid hormone, and antipyretics may cause diaphoresis. Aspirin and acetaminophen poisoning also cause this sign.

● *Dumping syndrome.* The result of rapid emptying of gastric contents into the small intestine after partial gastrectomy, this syndrome occurs soon after eating and causes diaphoresis, palpitations, profound weakness, epigastric distress, nausea, and explosive diarrhea.

Special considerations

After an episode of diaphoresis, sponge the patient's face and body and change wet clothes and sheets. Dust skin folds in the groin and axillae and under pendulous breasts with cornstarch or powder to prevent skin irritation. Or tuck gauze or cloth into these folds. Encourage regular bathing.

Replace fluids and electrolytes. Regulate infusions of I.V. saline or lactated Ringer's solution, and monitor urine output. Encourage oral fluids high in electrolytes (such as Gatorade). Enforce bed rest and maintain a quiet environment. Keep the patient's room temperature moderate to prevent additional diaphoresis.

Explain to the patient and his family that diaphoresis signals a return to normal body temperature in an infection and occurs after taking an antipyretic. It may also be a sympathetic reaction to pain or stress.

Prepare the patient for diagnostic tests, including blood tests, cultures, chest X-rays, immunologic studies, biopsy, computed tomography scan, and audiometry.

Pediatric pointers

Diaphoresis commonly results from environmental heat or overdressing an infant or child. Typically, it's most apparent around the head.

Other causes include drug withdrawal associated with maternal addiction, heart failure, thyrotoxicosis, and the effects of drugs, such as antihistamines, ephedrine, haloperidol, and thyroid hormone.

Assess the child's fluid status carefully. Fluid loss through diaphoresis may precipitate hypovolemia more rapidly in a child than in an adult. Monitor input and output, weigh the child daily, and note the duration of each episode of diaphoresis.

DIARRHEA

Usually a sign of intestinal disorders, diarrhea is an increase in the volume of bowel movements compared with the patient's normal bowel habits. It varies in severity and may be acute or chronic. Acute diarrhea may result from acute infection, stress, fecal impaction, or the effects of drugs. Chronic diarrhea may result from chronic infection, obstructive and inflammatory bowel disease, malabsorption syndromes, certain endocrine disorders, and the effects of GI surgery. Periodic diarrhea may result from food intolerance or from ingestion of spicy or high-fiber foods or caffeine.

One or more pathophysiologic mechanisms may contribute to diarrhea. (See *What causes diarrhea,* page 184.) The fluid and electrolyte imbalances it produces may precipitate life-threatening arrhythmias or hypovolemic shock.

Emergency interventions

If the patient's diarrhea is profuse, check for signs of shock: tachycardia, hypotension, and cool, pale, clammy skin.

If you detect these signs, place the patient in the supine position and elevate his legs 20 degrees. Insert an I.V. line for fluid replacement. Monitor for electrolyte imbalances, and look for an irregular pulse, muscle weakness, anorexia, and nausea and vomiting. Keep emergency resuscitation equipment handy.

History and physical examination

If the patient isn't in shock, obtain a history. Explore signs and symptoms associated with diarrhea. Does the patient have abdominal pain and cramps? Difficulty breathing? A rash? Is he weak or fatigued? Find out his drug history. Has he had GI surgery or radiation therapy? Ask the patient to briefly describe his diet. Does he have any known food allergies? Lastly, find out if he's under unusual stress.

Then proceed with the physical examination. Evaluate hydration and check skin turgor. Take blood pressure with the patient lying, sitting, and standing. Inspect the abdomen for distention and palpate for tenderness. Auscultate bowel sounds. Take the patient's temperature and note any chills. Also look for a rash.

Common medical causes

● *Carcinoid syndrome.* In this symptom complex associated with carcinoid tumors, severe diarrhea occurs with severe flushing, abdominal cramps, dyspnea, and palpitations. Associated signs and symptoms include weight loss, anorexia, weakness, and depression.

● *Crohn's disease.* This recurring inflammatory disorder produces diarrhea accompanied by abdominal pain with guarding and tenderness, and nausea. The patient may also display fever, chills, weakness, anorexia, and weight loss.

● *Infections.* Acute viral, bacterial, and protozoal infections (such as cryptosporidiosis) cause the sudden onset of watery diarrhea as well as abdominal pain, cramps, nausea, vomiting, and fever. Significant fluid and electrolyte loss may

WHAT CAUSES DIARRHEA

Ingestion of poorly absorbable material such as bulk-forming laxatives	Local lymphatic or venous obstruction	Stimulation of mucosal intracellular enzymes (cyclic adenosine monophosphate) by bacterial toxins or other factors	Disrupted integrity of small intestinal mucosa	Increased intestinal motility
Excess osmotic load in small intestine	Increased intravascular and intracellular hydrostatic pressure	Active transport of electrolytes into small intestine	Impaired intestinal absorption	Decreased intestinal absorption
Increased fluid drawn into and retained in small intestine	Altered permeability of intestinal mucosa	Excess fluid in small intestine	Excess fluid in small intestine	Excess fluid in small intestine
	Passive secretion of fluid and electrolytes into small intestine			

Diarrhea

cause signs of dehydration and shock. Chronic tuberculosis and fungal and parasitic infections may produce a less severe but more persistent diarrhea, accompanied by epigastric distress, vomiting, weight loss, and possibly passage of blood and mucus.

● *Intestinal obstruction.* Partial intestinal obstruction increases intestinal motility, resulting in diarrhea, abdominal pain with tenderness and guarding, nausea, and possibly distention.

● *Irritable bowel syndrome.* Diarrhea alternates with constipation or normal bowel function. Related findings include dyspepsia, nausea, and abdominal pain, tenderness, and distention.

● *Ischemic bowel disease.* This life-threatening disorder causes bloody diarrhea with abdominal pain. If severe, shock may occur, requiring surgery.

• *Lactose intolerance.* Diarrhea occurs within several hours of ingesting milk or milk products. It's accompanied by cramps, abdominal pain, and flatus.

• *Pseudomembranous enterocolitis.* This potentially life-threatening disorder commonly follows antibiotic administration. It produces copious watery or bloody diarrhea that rapidly precipitates signs of shock. Other features include colicky abdominal pain and distention.

• *Thyrotoxicosis.* In this disorder, diarrhea is accompanied by nervousness, tremor, diaphoresis, weight loss despite increased appetite, dyspnea, palpitations, tachycardia, enlarged thyroid, heat intolerance, and possibly exophthalmos.

• *Ulcerative colitis.* The hallmark of this disorder is recurrent bloody diarrhea with pus or mucus. Other features are tenesmus, hyperactive bowel sounds, cramping lower abdominal pain, low-grade fever, anorexia and, at times, nausea and vomiting. Weight loss, anemia, and weakness are late findings.

Other causes

• *Drugs.* Many antibiotics, such as ampicillin, cephalosporins, tetracyclines, and clindamycin, cause diarrhea. Other drugs that may cause diarrhea include magnesium-containing antacids, colchicine, guanethidine, lactulose, dantrolene, ethacrynic acid, mefenamic acid, methotrexate, metyrosine, and, in high doses, digoxin and quinidine. Laxative abuse can cause acute or chronic diarrhea.

• *Treatments.* Gastrectomy, gastroenterostomy, and pyloroplasty may produce diarrhea. High-dose radiation therapy may produce enteritis associated with diarrhea.

Special considerations

Explain the purpose and procedure of diagnostic tests to the patient. These tests may include blood studies, stool cultures, X-rays, and endoscopy.

Help the patient maintain adequate hydration. Remember that dehydration occurs rapidly in the elderly. Measure liquid stools and weigh the patient daily. Monitor electrolyte levels and hematocrit. Encourage oral fluids and accurately administer I.V. fluid replacements.

Administer analgesics for pain and an opiate to decrease intestinal motility. Ensure the patient's privacy during defecation, and empty bedpans promptly. Clean the perineum thoroughly, and apply ointments to prevent skin breakdown.

Advise the patient to avoid spicy or high-fiber foods (such as fruits), caffeine, and milk. Suggest smaller, more frequent meals if he's had GI surgery or disease. If appropriate, teach the patient stress-reducing exercises, such as guided imagery and deep-breathing techniques, or recommend counseling.

In inflammatory bowel disease (particularly ulcerative colitis), stress the need for medical follow-up. The risk of colon cancer is greater in these patients.

Pediatric pointers

Diarrhea in children commonly results from infection, although chronic diarrhea may result from malabsorption syndrome, anatomic defects, or allergy. Because dehydration and electrolyte imbalance occur rapidly in children, diarrhea can be life-threatening. Diligently monitor all episodes of diarrhea and replace fluids immediately.

DIPLOPIA

Diplopia is double vision—seeing one object as two. This symptom results when extraocular muscles fail to work together, causing images to fall on noncorresponding parts of the retinas. What causes this muscle incoordination? Orbital lesions, the effects of surgery, or impaired function of cranial nerves that supply extraocular muscles (oculomotor, CN III; trochlear, CN IV; abducens, CN VI) may be responsible.

Diplopia usually begins intermittently or affects near or far vision exclusively. It can be classified as monocular or binocular. More common binocular diplopia may result from ocular deviation or displacement, extraocular muscle palsies, or psychoneurosis. It may also follow retinal surgery. Monocular diplopia may result from an early cataract, retinal edema or scarring, iridodialysis, a subluxated lens, a poorly fitting contact lens, or an uncorrected refractive error. Diplopia may also occur in hysteria or malingering.

History and physical examination
If the patient complains of double vision, first check his neurologic status. Evaluate his level of consciousness (LOC), pupil size and response to light, and motor and sensory function. Then take his vital signs. Briefly ask about associated symptoms, especially severe headache. Find out about associated neurologic symptoms first because diplopia can accompany serious disorders.

Now continue with a more detailed examination. Find out when the patient first noticed diplopia. Are the images side-by-side (horizontal), one above the other (vertical), or a combination? Does diplopia affect near or far vision? Does it affect certain directions of gaze? Ask if diplopia has worsened, remained the same, or improved. Does its severity change throughout the day? Worsening of diplopia or its appearance by evening may indicate myasthenia gravis. Find out if the patient can correct diplopia by tilting his head. If so, ask him to show you. (If he has a fourth nerve lesion, tilting of his head toward the opposite shoulder causes compensatory tilting of the unaffected eye. If he has incomplete sixth nerve palsy, tilting of his head toward the

side of the paralyzed muscle may relax the affected lateral rectus muscle.)

Explore associated symptoms such as eye pain. Ask about hypertension, diabetes mellitus, allergies, and thyroid, neurologic, or muscular disorders. Also note a history of extraocular muscle disorders, trauma, or eye surgery.

Observe the patient for ocular deviation, ptosis, proptosis, lid edema, and conjunctival injection. Distinguish between monocular and binocular diplopia by asking the patient to occlude one eye. If he still sees double, he has monocular diplopia. Test visual acuity and extraocular muscles. (See *Testing extraocular muscles.*) Check vital signs.

Common medical causes
- *Alcohol intoxication.* Diplopia is a common symptom of this disorder. It's accompanied by confusion, slurred speech, halitosis, staggering gait, behavior changes, nausea, vomiting, and possible conjunctival injection.
- *Botulism.* Hallmark signs are diplopia, dysarthria, dysphagia, and ptosis. Early findings include dry mouth, sore throat, vomiting, and diarrhea. Later, descending weakness or paralysis of extremity and trunk muscles causes hyporeflexia and dyspnea.
- *Brain tumor.* Diplopia may be an early symptom in this disorder. Accompanying features vary with the tumor's size and location. They may include eye deviation, emotional lability, decreased LOC, headache, vomiting, absence or generalized tonic-clonic seizures, hearing loss, visual field cuts, abnormal pupillary responses, nystagmus, motor weakness, and paralysis.
- *Cavernous sinus thrombosis.* This disorder may produce diplopia and limited eye movement. Associated signs and symptoms include proptosis, orbital and lid edema, diminished or absent pupillary responses, impaired visual acuity, papilledema, and fever.

EXAMINATION TIP

TESTING EXTRAOCULAR MUSCLES

The coordinated action of six muscles controls eyeball movements. To test the function of each muscle and the cranial nerve (CN) that innervates it, ask the patient to look in the direction controlled by that muscle. The six directions you can test make up the *cardinal fields of gaze*. The patient's inability to turn the eye in the designated direction indicates muscle weakness or paralysis.

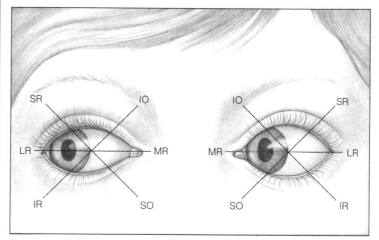

Key:
SR = superior rectus (CN III)
LR = lateral rectus (CN VI)
IR = inferior rectus (CN III)

IO = inferior oblique (CN III)
MR = medial rectus (CN III)
SO = superior oblique (CN IV)

● *Cerebrovascular accident.* Diplopia characterizes this life-threatening disorder when it affects the vertebrobasilar artery. Other clinical features may include unilateral motor weakness or paralysis, ataxia, decreased LOC, dizziness, aphasia, visual field cuts, circumoral numbness, slurred speech, dysphagia, and amnesia.

● *Diabetes mellitus.* Among the long-term effects of this disorder may be diplopia due to isolated third cranial nerve palsy. Diplopia typically begins suddenly and may be accompanied by pain.

● *Encephalitis.* Initially, this disorder may cause a brief episode of diplopia and eye deviation. Usually, though, it begins with sudden onset of high fever, severe headache, and vomiting. As the inflammation progresses, signs of meningeal irritation, decreased LOC, seizures, ataxia, and paralysis may develop.

● *Head injury.* Potentially life-threatening head injuries may cause diplopia, depending on the site and extent of the injury. Associated signs and symptoms may include eye deviation, pupillary changes, headache, decreased LOC, altered vital signs, nausea, vomiting, and motor weakness or paralysis.

• *Intracranial aneurysm.* This life-threatening disorder initially produces diplopia and eye deviation, perhaps accompanied by ptosis and a dilated pupil on the affected side. The patient will complain of a recurrent, severe, unilateral, frontal headache. After rupture of the aneurysm, the headache becomes violent. Associated signs and symptoms include neck and spinal pain and rigidity, decreased LOC, tinnitus, dizziness, nausea, vomiting, and unilateral muscle weakness or paralysis.

• *Multiple sclerosis.* Diplopia is a common early symptom in this disorder. It's usually accompanied by blurred vision and paresthesia. As the disorder progresses, its variable signs and symptoms may include nystagmus, constipation, muscle weakness, paralysis, spasticity, hyperreflexia, intention tremor, gait ataxia, dysphagia, dysarthria, impotence, emotional lability, and urinary frequency, urgency, and incontinence.

• *Myasthenia gravis.* Initially, this disorder produces diplopia and ptosis that worsen throughout the day. It then progressively involves other muscles, resulting in a blank facial expression; a nasal voice; difficulty in chewing, swallowing, and making fine hand movements; and possibly signs of life-threatening respiratory muscle weakness.

• *Ophthalmoplegic migraine.* Occurring mostly in young adults, this disorder results in diplopia that persists for days after the headache. Accompanying signs and symptoms are ptosis, extraocular muscle palsies, and severe, unilateral pain. Irritability, depression, or slight confusion may also occur.

• *Orbital blowout fracture.* This fracture usually causes monocular diplopia affecting the upward gaze, but with marked periorbital edema, diplopia may affect other directions of gaze. In most cases, this fracture causes periorbital ecchymosis. It doesn't usually affect visual acuity, although eyelid edema may prevent accurate testing. Subcutaneous crepitation of the eyelid and orbit is typical. Occasionally, the patient's pupil is dilated and unreactive, and he may have a hyphema.

• *Orbital cellulitis.* Inflammation of the orbital tissues and eyelids causes sudden diplopia. Other findings are eye deviation and pain, purulent drainage, lid edema, chemosis and redness, proptosis, nausea, and fever.

• *Orbital tumors.* Enlarging tumors can cause diplopia. Proptosis and possibly blurred vision may also occur.

• *Thyrotoxicosis.* Diplopia occurs when exophthalmos characterizes the disorder. It's accompanied by impaired eye movement, excessive tearing, lid edema, and possibly inability to close the lids. Other cardinal findings include tachycardia, palpitations, weight loss, diarrhea, tremors, an enlarged thyroid, dyspnea, nervousness, diaphoresis, and heat intolerance.

Other causes

• *Eye surgery.* Fibrosis associated with eye surgery may restrict eye movement, resulting in diplopia.

Special considerations

Continue to monitor vital signs and neurologic status if an acute neurologic disorder is suspected. Prepare the patient for neurologic tests such as a computed tomography scan. Provide a safe environment. In severe diplopia, remove sharp obstacles and assist the patient with ambulation. Also institute seizure precautions, if indicated.

Pediatric pointers

Strabismus, a congenital disorder or one acquired at an early age, produces diplopia; however, in young children, the brain rapidly compensates for double vision by suppressing one image, so diplopia is a rare complaint. School-age children who complain of double vision require a careful examination to rule out serious disorders such as brain tumor.

DIZZINESS

A common symptom, dizziness is a sensation of imbalance or faintness, sometimes associated with giddiness, weakness, confusion, and blurred or double vision. Usually, episodes of dizziness are brief; they may be mild or severe with abrupt or gradual onset. Dizziness aggravated by standing up quickly and alleviated by lying down or by rest suggests hypotension.

Typically, dizziness results from inadequate blood flow and oxygen supply to the cerebrum and spinal cord. It may occur in anxiety, in respiratory and cardiovascular disorders, and in postconcussion syndrome. It's a key symptom in certain serious disorders, such as hypertension and vertebrobasilar artery insufficiency.

Dizziness is commonly confused with vertigo—a sensation of revolving in space or of surroundings revolving about oneself. However, unlike dizziness, vertigo is commonly accompanied by nausea, vomiting, nystagmus, staggering gait, and tinnitus or hearing loss. Dizziness and vertigo may occur together, as in postconcussion syndrome.

Emergency interventions

 If the patient complains of dizziness, first determine its severity and onset. Ask him to describe it. Is the dizziness associated with headache or blurred vision? Next, take the patient's vital signs and ask about a history of high blood pressure. Tell the patient to lie down, and check his vital signs every 15 minutes. Start an I.V. line and prepare to administer medications as ordered.

History and physical examination

Ask about a history of diabetes and cardiovascular disease. Is the patient taking drugs prescribed for high blood pressure? If so, when did he take his last dose?

If the patient's blood pressure is normal, obtain a more complete history. Ask about myocardial infarction, heart failure, or atherosclerosis—which may predispose the patient to cardiac arrhythmias, hypertension, or a transient ischemic attack (TIA). Is there a history of anemia, chronic obstructive pulmonary disease, anxiety disorders, or head injury? Obtain a complete drug history.

Next, explore the patient's dizziness fully. How often does it occur? How long does each episode last? Does his dizziness abate spontaneously or does it lead to loss of consciousness? Find out if dizziness is triggered by sitting up suddenly or stooping over. Does being in a crowd make him feel dizzy? Ask about emotional stress. Has the patient been irritable or anxious? Does he have insomnia or difficulty concentrating? During the interview, look for fidgeting and eyelid twitching. Does the patient startle easily? Also ask about palpitations, chest pain, diaphoresis, shortness of breath, and chronic cough.

Next, perform a physical examination. Begin with a quick neurocheck, assessing level of consciousness (LOC), motor and sensory function, and reflexes. Then inspect for poor skin turgor and dry mucous membranes—signs of dehydration. Auscultate for heart rate and rhythm. Inspect for barrel chest, clubbing, cyanosis, and use of accessory muscles. Also auscultate for breath sounds. Take the patient's blood pressure while he's lying, sitting, and standing to check for orthostatic hypotension. Test capillary refill time in the extremities, and palpate for edema.

Common medical causes

• *Anemia.* Typically, this disorder causes dizziness that's aggravated by postural changes or exertion. Other clinical features include pallor, dyspnea, fatigue, tachycardia, and bounding pulse. Capillary refill time will be prolonged.

• *Cardiac arrhythmias.* Dizziness lasts for several minutes or longer with this disorder and may precede fainting. The patient may experience palpitations; irregular, rapid, or thready pulse; and possibly hypotension. He may also experience weakness, blurred vision, paresthesia, and confusion.

• *Emphysema.* Dizziness may follow exertion or the chronic, productive cough in this disorder. Associated signs and symptoms include dyspnea, anorexia, weight loss, malaise, use of accessory muscles, pursed-lip breathing, tachypnea, peripheral cyanosis, and diminished breath sounds. Barrel chest and clubbing also may be seen.

• *Hypertension.* In this disorder, dizziness may precede fainting. However, it may also be relieved by rest. Other common signs and symptoms include headache and blurred vision. Retinal changes include hemorrhage, sclerosis of retinal blood vessels, exudate, and papilledema.

• *Hyperventilation syndrome.* Episodes of hyperventilation cause dizziness that usually lasts a few minutes; however, if these episodes occur frequently, dizziness may persist between them. Other effects include apprehension, diaphoresis, pallor, dyspnea, chest tightness, palpitations, trembling, fatigue, and peripheral and circumoral paresthesia.

• *Orthostatic hypotension.* This condition produces dizziness that may terminate in fainting or disappear with rest. Related findings include dim vision, spots before the eyes, pallor, diaphoresis, hypotension, tachycardia, and possibly signs of dehydration.

• *Postconcussion syndrome.* Occurring 1 to 3 weeks after a head injury, this syndrome is marked by dizziness, headache (throbbing, aching, bandlike, or stabbing), emotional lability, alcohol intolerance, fatigue, anxiety, and possibly vertigo. Dizziness and other symptoms are intensified by mental or physical stress. The syndrome may persist for years, but symptoms eventually abate.

• *Transient ischemic attack.* Lasting from a few seconds to 24 hours, a TIA commonly signals an impending stroke and may be triggered by turning the head to the side. Dizziness of varying severity occurs during an attack. It's accompanied by unilateral or bilateral diplopia, blindness or visual field deficits, ptosis, tinnitus, hearing loss, paresis, and numbness. Other findings may include dysarthria, dysphagia, vomiting, hiccups, confusion, decreased LOC, and pallor.

Other causes

• *Drugs.* Antianxiety drugs, central nervous system depressants, narcotics, decongestants, antihistamines, antihypertensives, and vasodilators commonly cause dizziness.

Special considerations

Prepare the patient for diagnostic tests, such as blood studies, arteriography, a computed tomography scan, EEG, and magnetic resonance imaging.

Help the patient control dizziness. If he's hyperventilating, have him breathe and rebreathe into his cupped hands or a paper bag. If he experiences dizziness in an upright position, tell him to lie down and rest, then rise slowly. Advise the patient with carotid sinus hypersensitivity to avoid wearing garments that fit tightly at the neck. Instruct the patient who risks a TIA from vertebrobasilar insufficiency to avoid sharply turning his head to one side; have him turn his body.

Elder tip

 Elderly people may lose their sense of equilibrium with age, especially when moving fast.

Encourage a slower pace in walking, climbing steps, and rising from a sitting position. Additional support can come from a railing, cane, or walker. In the home, advise your elderly patient to remove or anchor throw rugs and bath mats and to move electric cords out of high-traffic areas. Also urge him to place non-slip stickers in tubs and shower stalls and to install grab bars on tub and toilet area walls. Tell him to use a bath chair or a raised toilet seat and to rise slowly from each.

Pediatric pointers

Dizziness is less common in children than in adults. Many children have difficulty describing this symptom and will instead complain of tiredness, stomachache, or feeling sick. If you suspect dizziness, assess for vertigo as well. A more common symptom, vertigo may result from vision disorders, ear infections, and the effects of antibiotics.

DOLL'S EYE SIGN, ABSENT
[Negative oculocephalic reflex]

An indicator of brain stem dysfunction, the absence of doll's eye sign is detected by rapid, but gentle, turning of the patient's head from side to side. The eyes remain fixed in midposition, instead of moving laterally toward the side opposite the direction the head is turned. (See *Testing for absent doll's eye sign*, page 192.) Usually, this sign can't be relied upon in a conscious patient because he controls eye movements voluntarily.

The absence of doll's eye sign indicates injury to the midbrain or pons involving cranial nerves III, VI, and VIII. It typically accompanies coma caused by lesions of the cerebellum and brain stem.

Absent doll's eye sign is necessary for a diagnosis of brain death.

A variant of absent doll's eye sign that develops gradually is known as abnormal doll's eye sign: Conjugate eye movement is lost, so one eye may move laterally while the other remains fixed or moves in the opposite direction. Usually, an abnormal doll's eye sign accompanies metabolic coma or increased intracranial pressure (ICP). Associated brain stem dysfunction may be reversible or may progress to deeper coma with absent doll's eye sign.

History and physical examination

Because the patient with an absent doll's eye sign is unresponsive, all questions should be directed to family members or friends. Ask family members if they noticed a sudden change in the patient's affect or mood, speech, or behavior. Did the patient fall or have a seizure before the sign developed? Also, obtain a list of the patient's current medications.

After detecting an absent doll's eye sign, perform a neurologic examination. First evaluate the patient's level of consciousness (LOC) using the Glasgow Coma Scale. Observe for changes in LOC. Note decerebrate or decorticate posture. Examine the pupils for size, equality, and response to light. Check for signs of increased ICP: increased blood pressure, widened pulse pressure, and bradycardia.

Common medical causes

• *Brain stem infarction.* This infarction causes absent doll's eye sign with coma. It also causes limb paralysis, cranial nerve palsies (facial weakness, diplopia, blindness or visual field deficits, nystagmus), bilateral cerebellar ataxia, variable sensory loss, a positive Babinski's reflex, decerebrate posture, and muscle flaccidity.
• *Brain stem tumors.* Absent doll's eye sign accompanies coma in this disorder. This sign may be preceded by hemi-

EXAMINATION TIP

TESTING FOR ABSENT DOLL'S EYE SIGN

To evaluate the patient's oculo-cephalic reflex, hold her upper eyelids open and quickly (but gently) turn her head from side to side, noting eye movements with each head turn.

In absent doll's eye sign, the eyes remain fixed in midposition.

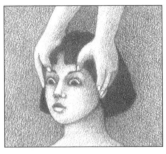

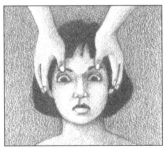

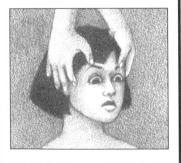

paresis, nystagmus, extraocular nerve palsies, facial pain or sensory loss, facial paralysis, diminished corneal reflex, tinnitus, hearing loss, dysphagia, drooling, vertigo, dizziness, ataxia, and vomiting.

- *Central midbrain infarction.* Accompanying absent doll's eye sign are coma, Weber's syndrome (oculomotor palsy with contralateral hemiplegia), contralateral ataxic tremor, nystagmus, and pupillary abnormalities.
- *Pontine hemorrhage.* Absent doll's eye sign and coma develop within minutes in this life-threatening disorder. Other ominous signs include complete paralysis, decerebrate posture, a positive Babinski's reflex, and small, reactive pupils. The patient may rapidly progress to death.
- *Posterior fossa hematoma.* A subdural hematoma at this location typically causes absent doll's eye sign and coma. These signs may be preceded by characteristic clinical features, such as headache, vomiting, drowsiness, confusion, unequal pupils, dysphagia, cranial nerve palsies, stiff neck, and cerebellar ataxia.

Other causes
- *Drugs.* Barbiturates may produce severe central nervous system depression, resulting in coma and absent doll's eye sign.

Special considerations
Don't try to elicit doll's eye sign in a comatose patient with suspected cervical spine injury; doing so would risk spinal cord damage. Instead, evaluate the oculovestibular reflex with the cold caloric test. Normally, instilling cold water in the ear causes the eyes to move slowly toward the irrigated ear then jerk to the other side. Cold caloric testing may also be done to confirm absent doll's eye sign.

Continue to monitor vital signs and neurologic status in the patient with an absent doll's eye sign.

Pediatric pointers

Normally, doll's eye sign is not present for the first 10 days after birth, and it may be irregular until age 2. After that, it reliably indicates brain stem function.

An absent doll's eye sign in children may accompany coma associated with head injury, near drowning, suffocation, or brain stem astrocytoma.

DYSARTHRIA

Dysarthria, or poorly articulated speech, is characterized by slurring and labored, irregular rhythm. It may be accompanied by a nasal voice tone caused by palate weakness. Whether it occurs abruptly or gradually, dysarthria is usually evident in ordinary conversation. It's confirmed by asking the patient to produce a few simple sounds and words, such as *ba, sh,* and *cat.* However, dysarthria is occasionally confused with aphasia, which involves loss of the ability to produce or comprehend speech.

Dysarthria results from damage to the brain stem that affects cranial nerves IX, X, or XI, usually due to degenerative neurologic disorders. It's a chief sign of olivopontocerebellar degeneration. It may also result from ill-fitting dentures.

Emergency interventions

 If the patient displays dysarthria, ask him about associated difficulty in swallowing. Then determine respiratory rate and depth. Measure vital capacity with a Wright respirometer if available. Obtain blood pressure and heart rate. Tachycardia, slightly increased blood pressure, and shortness of breath are usually early signs of respiratory muscle weakness.

Ensure a patent airway. Place the patient in Fowler's position and suction him if necessary. Administer oxygen and keep emergency resuscitation equipment near-

by. Anticipate intubation and mechanical ventilation in progressive respiratory muscle weakness. Withhold oral fluids if the patient also has dysphagia.

If the patient's dysarthria is not accompanied by respiratory muscle weakness and dysphagia, continue to assess for other neurologic deficits. Compare muscle strength and tone in the limbs. Then evaluate tactile sensation. Ask the patient about numbness or tingling. Test deep tendon reflexes, and note gait ataxia. Next, test visual fields and ask about double vision. Check for signs of facial weakness, such as ptosis. Finally, determine level of consciousness (LOC) and mental status.

History and physical examination

Explore dysarthria fully. When did it begin? Has it gotten better? Speech improves with resolution of a transient ischemic attack, but not in a completed stroke. Ask if dysarthria worsens during the day. Then obtain a drug and alcohol history. Also note a history of seizures.

Perform a complete neurologic examination, including a test of the gag reflex. Assess the patient's cranial nerve integrity. Examine his mouth for ulcerations or cuts that may contribute to poorly articulated speech. If he wears dentures, ensure that they fit properly.

Common medical causes

● *Alcoholic cerebellar degeneration.* This disorder commonly causes chronic, progressive dysarthria along with ataxia, diplopia, ophthalmoplegia, hypotension, and altered mental status.

● *Amyotrophic lateral sclerosis.* Dysarthria occurs when this disorder affects the bulbar nuclei and may worsen as the disease progresses. Other signs and symptoms are dysphagia; difficulty breathing; muscle atrophy and weakness, especially of the hands and feet; fasciculations; spasticity; hyperactive deep tendon reflexes in the legs; and occasionally excessive drooling. Progressive bulbar pal-

DYSARTHRIA: COMMON CAUSES AND ASSOCIATED FINDINGS

CAUSES	Aphasia	Ataxia	Bradykinesia	Diplopia	Drooling	Dysphagia	Dyspnea	Fasciculations	Gait, propulsive	Hyperreflexia	Hypotension	Level of consciousness, decreased	Masklike facies
Alcoholic cerebellar degeneration		●		●							●	●	
Amyotrophic lateral sclerosis					●	●	●	●		●			
Basilar artery insufficiency		●		●									
Botulism				●		●	●						
Cerebrovascular accident (brain stem)				●	●	●	●						
Cerebrovascular accident (cerebral)	●				●	●					●		
Multiple sclerosis		●		●		●				●			
Myasthenia gravis				●	●	●	●						
Olivopontocerebellar degeneration		●											
Parkinson's disease			●		●	●			●				●

Major associated signs and symptoms

sy may cause crying spells or inappropriate laughter.

● **Basilar artery insufficiency.** This disorder causes random, brief episodes of bilateral brain stem dysfunction, resulting in dysarthria. Accompanying it are diplopia, vertigo, facial numbness, ataxia, paresis, and visual field loss, all of which last for minutes to hours.

● **Botulism.** The hallmark of this disorder is acute cranial nerve dysfunction causing dysarthria, dysphagia, diplopia, and ptosis. Early findings include dry mouth, sore throat, weakness, vomiting, and diarrhea. Later, descending weakness or paralysis of muscles in the extremities and trunk causes hyporeflexia and dyspnea.

● **Brain stem cerebrovascular accident (CVA).** This type of CVA is characterized by bulbar palsy, resulting in the triad of dysarthria, dysphonia, and dysphagia. Dysarthria is most severe at onset; it may lessen or disappear with rehabilitation. Other findings may include facial weakness, diplopia, hemiparesis,

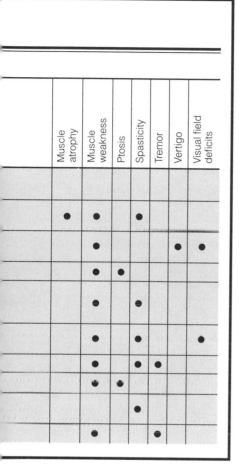

companied by nystagmus, blurred or double vision, dysphagia, ataxia, and intention tremor. These signs and symptoms worsen and subside with exacerbation and remission of the disorder. Other clinical features may include paresthesia, spasticity, hyperreflexia, muscle weakness or paralysis, constipation, and emotional lability. Urinary frequency, urgency, and incontinence may also occur.

• *Myasthenia gravis.* This neuromuscular disorder causes dysarthria associated with nasal voice tone. Typically, the dysarthria worsens during the day. Other findings are dysphagia, drooling, facial weakness, diplopia, ptosis, dyspnea, and muscle weakness.

• *Olivopontocerebellar degeneration.* Dysarthria, a major sign, accompanies cerebellar ataxia and spasticity.

• *Parkinson's disease.* This disorder produces dysarthria and monotone speech. It also produces muscle rigidity, bradykinesia, involuntary tremor usually beginning in the fingers, difficulty in walking, muscle weakness, and a stooped posture. Other features include a masklike facies, dysphagia, and occasionally drooling.

Other causes
• *Drugs.* Large doses of anticonvulsants or barbiturates can cause dysarthria.

Special considerations
Encourage the patient with dysarthria to speak slowly so that he can be understood. Give him time to express himself, and encourage him to use gestures. Dysarthria usually requires consultation with a speech pathologist.

Pediatric pointers
Dysarthria usually results from brain stem glioma, a slow-growing tumor that occurs chiefly in children. It may also result from cerebral palsy.

Dysarthria may be difficult to detect, especially in an infant or a young child who hasn't perfected speech. Be sure to

spasticity, drooling, dyspnea, and decreased LOC.

• *Cerebral CVA.* A massive bilateral CVA causes pseudobulbar palsy. Bilateral weakness produces dysarthria that is most severe at onset. It's accompanied by dysphagia, drooling, dysphonia, bilateral hemianopia, and aphasia. Sensory loss, spasticity, and hyperreflexia may also be present.

• *Multiple sclerosis.* When demyelination affects the brain stem and cerebellum, the patient displays dysarthria ac-

look for other neurologic deficits, too. Encourage a child with dysarthria to speak; his potential for rehabilitation is typically better than an adult's.

DYSMENORRHEA

Dysmenorrhea—painful menstruation—affects over 50% of menstruating women and is the leading cause of lost time from school and work among women of childbearing age. Dysmenorrhea may involve sharp, intermittent pain or dull, aching pain. It's usually characterized by mild to severe cramping or colicky pain in the pelvis or lower abdomen that may radiate to the thighs and lower sacrum. This pain may precede menstruation by several days or may accompany it; it gradually subsides as bleeding tapers off.

Dysmenorrhea may be idiopathic, as in premenstrual syndrome and primary dysmenorrhea, commonly resulting from endometriosis or other pelvic disorders. It may also result from structural abnormalities, such as an imperforate hymen. Stress and poor health may aggravate dysmenorrhea, while rest and mild exercise may relieve it.

History and physical examination

If the patient complains of dysmenorrhea, have her describe the pain fully. Is it intermittent or continuous? Sharp, cramping, or aching? Ask where the pain is located. Is it bilateral? How long has she been experiencing it? Find out when the pain begins and ends and when it's most severe. Does it radiate to the back? Explore associated symptoms, such as nausea and vomiting, altered bowel or urinary habits, bloating, pelvic or rectal pressure, and unusual fatigue, irritability, or depression.

Then obtain a menstrual and sexual history. Ask the patient if her menstrual flow is heavy or scant and whether she has any vaginal discharge between menstrual periods. Does she experience dyspareunia (painful sexual intercourse) and, if so, does it occur with menses? Find out what relieves her cramps. Does she take pain medication? Is it effective? (See *Drug therapy for dysmenorrhea,* opposite, and *Herbal therapy for dysmenorrhea,* page 198.) Note her method of contraception, and check for a history of pelvic infection. Does she have any symptoms of urinary tract obstruction, such as pyuria, incontinence, or urine retention? Ask how she copes with stress.

Next, perform a focused physical examination. Take vital signs, noting fever and any accompanying chills. Inspect the abdomen for distention, and palpate for tenderness and masses. Note costovertebral angle tenderness.

Common medical causes

● *Adenomyosis.* In this disorder, endometrial tissue invades the myometrium, resulting in severe dysmenorrhea with pain radiating to the back or rectum, menorrhagia, and an enlarged, globular uterus.

● *Cervical stenosis.* This structural disorder causes dysmenorrhea and scant or absent menstrual flow.

● *Endometriosis.* Typically, this disorder produces steady, aching pain that begins before menses and peaks at the height of menstrual flow. However, the pain may also occur between menstrual periods. It may arise at the endometrial deposit site or may radiate to the perineum or rectum. Associated symptoms may include premenstrual spotting, dyspareunia, infertility, nausea and vomiting, painful defecation, and rectal bleeding and hematuria with menses.

● *Pelvic inflammatory disease.* Chronic infection produces dysmenorrhea accompanied by fever; malaise; foul-smelling, purulent vaginal discharge; menorrhagia; dyspareunia; severe abdominal pain; nausea and vomiting; and diarrhea.

• **Premenstrual syndrome.** Cramping pain usually begins with menstrual flow and persists for several hours or days, diminishing with decreasing flow. Common associated effects precede menses by several days to 2 weeks and include abdominal bloating, breast tenderness, palpitations, diaphoresis, flushing, depression, and irritability. Other effects may include nausea, vomiting, diarrhea, and headache.

• **Primary (idiopathic) dysmenorrhea.** Increased prostaglandin secretion intensifies uterine contractions, apparently causing mild to severe spasmodic cramping pain in the lower abdomen, which radiates to the sacrum and inner thighs. This pain peaks a few hours before menses.

• **Uterine leiomyomas.** Tumors may cause lower abdominal pain that worsens with menses. The pain may be constant or intermittent. Associated signs and symptoms may include backache, constipation, menorrhagia, and if the tumor is large, signs of ureteral obstruction. Palpation may reveal the tumor mass and an enlarged uterus.

• **Uterine prolapse.** Displacement of the uterus may produce dysmenorrhea and chronic lower back pain, pelvic pressure, fatigue, leukorrhea, dyspareunia, and urinary difficulties.

Other causes

• **Intrauterine devices.** These devices may cause severe cramping and heavy menstrual flow.

Special considerations

In the past, women with dysmenorrhea were considered neurotic. Although current research suggests that prostaglandins contribute to this symptom, old attitudes persist. Encourage the patient to view dysmenorrhea as a medical problem, not as a symptom of maladjustment.

If dysmenorrhea is idiopathic, advise the patient to place a heating pad on her

---

DRUG THERAPY FOR DYSMENORRHEA

To relieve cramping and other symptoms caused by primary dysmenorrhea or the use of an intrauterine device, the patient may receive prostaglandin inhibitors, such as aspirin, ibuprofen, indomethacin, and naproxen. These nonsteroidal anti-inflammatory drugs block prostaglandin synthesis early in the inflammatory reaction, thereby inhibiting prostaglandin action at receptor sites. They also have analgesic and antipyretic effects.

Precautions

Because prostaglandin inhibitors are potentially teratogenic, be sure to rule out the possibility of pregnancy before starting therapy. Advise any patient who suspects she's pregnant to delay therapy until menstruation begins. Administer these drugs cautiously to patients with cardiac decompensation, hypertension, renal dysfunction, or coagulation defects and to those who are receiving ongoing anticoagulant therapy. Because patients who are hypersensitive to aspirin may also be hypersensitive to other prostaglandin inhibitors, watch for signs of gastric ulceration and bleeding.

Adverse effects

Alert the patient to possible adverse effects of prostaglandin inhibitors. Central nervous system effects include dizziness, headache, and visual disturbances. GI effects include nausea, vomiting, heartburn, and diarrhea. Advise the patient to take the drug with milk or after meals to reduce gastric irritation.

HERBAL THERAPY FOR DYSMENORRHEA

Much like conventional drug therapy, herbal therapy uses the "active" chemicals in herbs to treat symptoms of an illness or underlying disturbances in normal physiology.

Herbs are classified according to their taste, which signifies their medicinal action and often their natural affinity to particular body organs. Some herbs are used to treat menstrual problems, including cramps and water retention. Herbal therapy may be used in conjunction with acupuncture, depending on the patient.

Interest in herbal therapy is growing in the United States, possibly because of the increasing number of chronic illnesses that can't be cured by conventional treatments and the debilitating adverse effects that can occur secondary to standard drug therapy. Although herbal therapy is widely accepted and used in Europe and Asia (it's an important part of traditional Chinese medicine), much controversy surrounds its use in the United States for the following reasons:

● There is no licensing body for the practice of herbal medicine.

● The Food and Drug Administration does not regulate the production or marketing of herbs because they're considered food supplements, not medicine.

● Herbs can't be patented because they grow naturally; consequently, pharmaceutical companies have no incentive to study their effectiveness or to develop standardized products.

---

abdomen to relieve pain. Heat reduces abdominal muscle tension and increases blood flow.

Explain the action and adverse effects of oral contraceptives and prostaglandin inhibitors. Rule out the possibility of pregnancy before starting therapy.

Effleurage, a light circular massage with the fingertips, may also provide relief. Other comfort measures include drinking warm beverages, taking a warm shower, performing waist-bending and pelvic-rocking exercises, and walking. Herbal therapy may also be helpful.

Pediatric pointers

Dysmenorrhea is rare during the first year before the menstrual cycle becomes ovulatory. However, the incidence of dysmenorrhea is generally higher among adolescents than older women. Teach the adolescent about dysmenorrhea, and inform her that it's a common medical problem. Encourage good hygiene, nutrition, and exercise.

DYSPEPSIA

Dyspepsia refers to an uncomfortable fullness after meals that's associated with nausea, belching, heartburn, and possibly cramping and abdominal distention. Frequently aggravated by spicy, fatty, or high-fiber foods and by excess caffeine intake, dyspepsia without other symptoms indicates impaired digestive function.

Dyspepsia usually results from GI disorders, apparently when altered gastric secretions lead to excess stomach acidity. It may also stem from cardiac, pulmonary, and renal disorders; the effects of drugs; emotional upset; and overly rapid eating or improper chewing. It usually occurs a few hours after eating and lasts for a variable period of time. Its severity depends on the amount and type of food eaten and on GI motility. Additional food or antacids may relieve the discomfort.

History and physical examination

If the patient complains of dyspepsia, begin by asking him to describe it fully. How often and when does it occur, specifically in relation to meals? Do any drugs or activities relieve or aggravate it? Has the patient had nausea, vomiting, melena, hematemesis, cough, or chest pain? Ask what drugs he's currently taking. Also find out about any recent surgery. Does he have a history of renal, cardiovascular, or pulmonary disease? Has he noticed any change in the amount or color of his urine?

Focus the physical examination on the abdomen. Inspect for distention, ascites, scars, jaundice, uremic frost, or bruising. Then auscultate for bowel sounds and characterize their motility. Palpate and percuss the abdomen, noting any tenderness, pain, organ enlargement, or tympany.

Last, examine other body systems. Ask about behavior changes and evaluate level of consciousness. Auscultate for gallops and crackles. Percuss the lungs to detect consolidation. Note peripheral edema and any swelling of lymph nodes.

Common medical causes

• *Cholelithiasis.* Dyspepsia may occur with gallstones, usually after intake of fatty foods. Biliary colic, a more common symptom of gallstones, causes acute pain that may radiate to the back, shoulders, and chest. The patient may have diaphoresis, tachycardia, chills, low-grade fever, petechiae, and bleeding tendencies. Jaundice with pruritus, dark urine, and clay-colored stools may also occur.

• *Cirrhosis.* Dyspepsia in this chronic disorder varies in intensity and duration and is relieved by antacids. Other GI effects are anorexia, nausea, vomiting, flatulence, diarrhea, constipation, abdominal distention, and epigastric or right upper quadrant pain. Weight loss, jaundice, hepatomegaly, ascites, dependent edema, fever, bleeding tendencies, and muscle weakness are also common. Skin changes include severe pruritus, extreme dryness, easy bruising, and such lesions as telangiectasis and palmar erythema.

• *Duodenal ulcer.* A primary symptom of duodenal ulcer, dyspepsia ranges from a vague feeling of fullness or pressure to a boring or aching sensation in the middle or right epigastrium. It usually occurs 1½ to 3 hours after eating and is relieved by food or antacids. The pain may awaken the patient at night with heartburn and water brash (fluid regurgitation). Abdominal tenderness and weight gain may occur; vomiting and anorexia are rare.

• *Gastric dilation (acute).* Epigastric fullness is an early symptom of this life-threatening disorder. Accompanying dyspepsia are nausea and vomiting, upper abdominal distention, succussion splash, and apathy. The patient may display signs and symptoms of dehydration, such as poor skin turgor and dry mucous membranes, and of electrolyte imbalance, such as irregular pulse and muscle weakness. Gastric bleeding may produce hematemesis and melena.

• *Gastric ulcer.* Typically, dyspepsia and heartburn after eating occur early in this disorder. The cardinal symptom, though, is epigastric pain that may not be relieved by food and may be accompanied by vomiting, fullness, and abdominal distention. Weight loss and GI bleeding are also characteristic.

• *Gastritis (chronic).* In this disorder, dyspepsia is relieved by antacids and aggravated by spicy foods or excessive caffeine. It occurs with anorexia, a feeling

DYSPEPSIA: COMMON CAUSES AND ASSOCIATED FINDINGS

CAUSES	MAJOR ASSOCIATED SIGNS AND SYMPTOMS												
	Abdominal distention	Abdominal pain	Anorexia	Bruising, easy	Chest pain	Cough	Edema	Hepatomegaly	Jaundice	Nausea and vomiting	Oliguria	Tachycardia	Weight loss
Cholelithiasis		●							●	●		●	
Cirrhosis	●	●	●	●			●	●	●	●			●
Duodenal ulcer		●								●			
Gastric dilation (acute)	●									●			
Gastric ulcer	●	●								●			●
Gastritis (chronic)		●	●							●			
Heart failure		●	●		●	●	●	●		●		●	
Hepatitis			●					●	●	●			
Pulmonary embolus					●	●						●	
Pulmonary tuberculosis			●			●							●
Uremia		●	●				●				●	●	

of fullness, vague epigastric pain, belching, nausea, and vomiting.

● **Heart failure.** Common in right-sided heart failure, transient dyspepsia may occur with chest tightness and a constant ache or sharp pain in the right upper quadrant. Typically, this disorder also causes hepatomegaly, anorexia, nausea, vomiting, bloating, ascites, tachycardia, distended neck veins, tachypnea, dyspnea, and orthopnea. Other findings include dependent edema, anxiety, fatigue, diaphoresis, hypotension, cough, crackles, ventricular and atrial gallops, and cool, pale skin.

● **Hepatitis.** Dyspepsia occurs in two of the three stages of hepatitis. The preicteric phase produces moderate to severe dyspepsia, fever, malaise, fatigue, arthralgia, coryza, myalgia, nausea, vomiting, an altered sense of taste or smell, and hepatomegaly. Jaundice marks the onset of the icteric phase, along with continued dyspepsia and anorexia, irritability, and severe pruritus. As jaundice clears, dyspepsia and other GI effects also diminish. In the recovery phase, only fatigue remains.

● **Pulmonary embolus.** Sudden dyspnea characterizes this potentially fatal disorder; however, dyspepsia may occur as a severe substernal discomfort. Other findings include tachycardia, tachypnea, cough, pleuritic chest pain, hemoptysis, syncope, cyanosis, and hypotension.

● *Pulmonary tuberculosis.* Vague dyspepsia may occur in this disorder along with anorexia, malaise, and weight loss. Common associated findings include high fever, night sweats, palpitations on mild exertion, a productive cough, dyspnea, and occasional hemoptysis.

● *Uremia.* Of the many GI complaints associated with uremia, dyspepsia may be the earliest and most important. Others include anorexia, nausea, vomiting, bloating, diarrhea, abdominal cramps, epigastric pain, and weight gain. As the renal system deteriorates, findings may include edema, pruritus, pallor, hyperpigmentation, uremic frost, ecchymoses, sexual dysfunction, poor memory, irritability, headache, drowsiness, muscle twitching, seizures, and oliguria.

Other causes

● *Drugs.* Nonsteroidal anti-inflammatory drugs, especially aspirin, commonly cause dyspepsia. Diuretics, antibiotics, antihypertensives, and many other drugs can cause dyspepsia, depending on the patient's tolerance of the dosage.

● *Surgery.* After GI or other surgery, postoperative gastritis can cause dyspepsia, which usually disappears in a few weeks.

Special considerations

Changing the patient's position usually doesn't relieve dyspepsia, but providing food or antacids may. So have food available at all times and give antacids 30 minutes before a meal or 1 hour after it. Because various drugs can cause dyspepsia, give them after meals if possible. Provide a calm environment to reduce stress, and make sure the patient gets plenty of rest. Discuss other ways to deal with stress, such as deep breathing and guided imagery.

Prepare the patient for endoscopy to determine the cause of dyspepsia.

Pediatric pointers

Dyspepsia may occur in adolescents with peptic ulcer disease, but it isn't relieved by food. It may also occur in congenital pyloric stenosis, but projectile vomiting after meals is a more characteristic sign. Lactose intolerance is another potential cause.

DYSPHAGIA

Dysphagia—swallowing difficulty—is a common symptom that's usually easy to localize. It may be constant or intermittent and is classified by the phase of swallowing it affects. (See *Classifying dysphagia by phases of swallowing,* page 202.) Among the factors that can interfere with swallowing are severe pain, obstruction, abnormal peristalsis, impaired gag reflex, and excessive, scanty, or thick oral secretions.

Dysphagia is the most common—and sometimes the only—symptom of esophageal disorders. However, it may also result from oropharyngeal, respiratory, neurologic, and collagen disorders and from the effects of certain toxins and treatments. Dysphagia increases the risk of choking and aspiration and may lead to malnutrition and dehydration.

Emergency interventions

 If the patient suddenly complains of dysphagia and displays signs of respiratory distress, such as dyspnea and stridor, suspect an airway obstruction and quickly perform abdominal thrusts. Prepare to administer oxygen by mask or nasal cannula or to assist with endotracheal intubation.

History and physical examination

If the patient's dysphagia doesn't suggest airway obstruction, begin a health histo-

CLASSIFYING DYSPHAGIA BY PHASES OF SWALLOWING

Swallowing occurs in three distinct phases, and dysphagia can be classified by the phase that it affects. Each phase suggests a specific pathology for dysphagia.

Phase 1
Swallowing begins in the *transfer phase* with chewing and moistening of food with saliva. The tongue presses against the hard palate to transfer the chewed food to the back of the throat; the fifth cranial nerve (CN V) then stimulates the swallowing reflex. Phase 1 dysphagia typically results from a neuromuscular disorder.

Phase 2
In the *transport phase,* the soft palate closes against the pharyngeal wall to prevent nasal regurgitation. At the same time, the larynx rises and the vocal cords close to keep food out of the lungs; breathing stops momentarily as the throat muscles constrict to move food into the esophagus. Phase 2 dysphagia usually indicates spasm or carcinoma.

Phase 3
Peristalsis and gravity work together in the *entrance phase* to move food through the esophageal sphincter and into the stomach. Phase 3 dysphagia results from lower esophageal narrowing by diverticula, esophagitis, and other disorders.

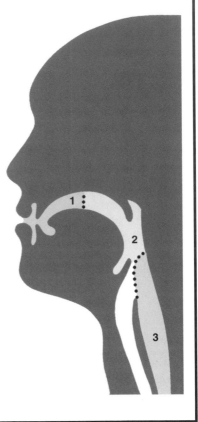

ry. Ask him if it's painful to swallow. If so, is the pain constant or intermittent? Have him point to where the pain is most intense. Does eating alleviate or aggravate it? Is it more difficult for him to swallow solids than liquids? If the patient has difficulty swallowing liquids, ask if hot, cold, and lukewarm fluids affect him differently. Does the symptom disappear after he tries to swallow a few times? Is swallowing easier if he changes position? Ask if he has experienced vomiting, regurgitation, weight loss, anorexia, hoarseness, dyspnea, or cough.

To evaluate the patient's swallowing reflex, place your finger along his thyroid notch and instruct him to swallow. If you feel his larynx rise, the reflex is intact. Next, have him cough to assess his cough reflex. Check his gag reflex if you're sure he has a good swallowing or cough reflex. Listen closely to his speech for signs of muscle weakness. Does he have aphasia or dysarthria? Is his voice nasal, hoarse, or breathy? Assess the patient's mouth carefully, checking for dry mucous membranes and thick, sticky secretions. Observe for tongue and facial weakness. Assess for disorientation, which may make him neglect to swallow.

Common medical causes

● *Achalasia.* Most common in patients ages 20 to 40, this disorder produces phase 3 dysphagia involving solids and liquids. Dysphagia develops gradually and may be precipitated or exacerbated by stress. Occasionally, it's preceded by esophageal colic. Regurgitation of undigested food, especially at night, may cause wheezing, coughing, or choking as well as halitosis. Weight loss, cachexia, hematemesis and, possibly, heartburn are late findings.

● *Airway obstruction.* Life-threatening upper airway obstruction is marked by signs of respiratory distress, such as crowing and stridor. Phase 2 dysphagia occurs with gagging and dysphonia. When hemorrhage obstructs the trachea, dysphagia is usually painless and rapid in onset. When inflammation causes the obstruction, dysphagia may be painful and develop slowly.

● *Amyotrophic lateral sclerosis.* Besides dysphagia, this disease causes muscle weakness and atrophy, fasciculations, dysarthria, dyspnea, shallow respirations, tachypnea, and emotional lability.

● *Bulbar paralysis.* Phase 1 dysphagia occurs along with drooling, difficulty chewing, dysarthria, and nasal regurgitation. Dysphagia is painful and progressive and involves both solids and liquids. Accompanying features may be arm and leg spasticity, hyperreflexia, and emotional lability.

● *Esophageal cancer.* Phase 2 or 3 dysphagia is the earliest and most common symptom of esophageal cancer. Typically, this painless, progressive symptom occurs with rapid weight loss. As the cancer advances, dysphagia becomes painful and constant. The patient will also complain of steady chest pain, cough with hemoptysis, hoarseness, and sore throat. He also may have nausea and vomiting, fever, hiccups, hematemesis, melena, and halitosis.

● *Esophageal compression (external).* Usually caused by a dilated carotid or aortic aneurysm, this rare condition causes phase 3 dysphagia as the primary symptom. Other features depend on the cause of the compression.

● *Esophageal diverticulum.* This disorder causes phase 3 dysphagia when the enlarged diverticulum obstructs the esophagus. Associated findings include food regurgitation, chronic cough, hoarseness, and halitosis.

● *Esophageal obstruction by a foreign body.* Sudden onset of phase 2 or 3 dysphagia, esophageal pain, gagging, and coughing characterize this potentially life-threatening condition. Dyspnea may occur if the obstruction compresses the trachea.

● *Esophageal spasm.* The most striking symptoms of this disorder are phase 2 dysphagia involving solids and liquids and dull or squeezing substernal chest pain that is commonly relieved by drinking a glass of water. The pain may last up to an hour and may radiate to the neck, arm, back, or jaw. Bradycardia may also occur.

● *Esophagitis.* Corrosive esophagitis, resulting from ingestion of alkalies or acids, causes severe phase 3 dysphagia. It occurs with marked salivation, hematemesis, tachypnea, fever, and intense pain in the mouth and anterior chest that is aggravated by swallowing. Signs of shock, such as hypotension and tachycardia, may also occur.

Candidal esophagitis causes phase 2 dysphagia, sore throat, and possibly retrosternal pain on swallowing. In reflux esophagitis, phase 3 dysphagia is a late symptom that usually accompanies stricture development. The patient complains of heartburn that's aggravated by strenuous exercise, bending over, or lying down and relieved by sitting up or taking antacids.

Other features include regurgitation; frequent, effortless vomiting; a dry, nocturnal cough; and substernal chest pain that may mimic angina pectoris. If the esophagus ulcerates, signs of bleeding, such as melena and hematemesis, may occur along with weakness and fatigue.

● *Gastric cancer.* Infiltration of the cardia or esophagus by gastric cancer causes phase 3 dysphagia. It occurs with nausea, vomiting, and pain that may radiate to the neck, back, or retrosternum. In addition, perforation causes massive bleeding with melena.

● *Laryngeal carcinoma (extrinsic).* Phase 2 dysphagia and dyspnea develop late in this disorder. Accompanying features include muffled voice, stridor, pain, halitosis, weight loss, and cachexia. Palpation reveals enlarged cervical nodes.

● *Lead poisoning.* Painless, progressive dysphagia may result from lead poisoning. Related findings include a lead line on the gums, papilledema, ocular palsy, footdrop or wristdrop, and signs of hemolytic anemia, such as abdominal pain and fever. The patient may be depressed and experience severe mental impairment and seizures.

● *Myasthenia gravis.* Fatigue and progressive muscle weakness characterize this disorder and account for painless phase 1 dysphagia and possibly choking. Dysphagia typically follows ptosis and diplopia. Other features include masklike facies, nasal voice, frequent nasal regurgitation, and head bobbing. Shallow respirations and dyspnea may occur with respiratory muscle weakness. Signs and symptoms worsen during menses and with exposure to stress, cold, or infection.

● *Oral cavity tumor.* Painful phase 1 dysphagia develops along with hoarseness and ulcerating lesions.

● *Plummer-Vinson syndrome.* This syndrome causes phase 3 dysphagia involving solids in some women with severe iron deficiency anemia. Related features include upper esophageal pain; atrophy of the oral or pharyngeal mucous membranes; tooth loss; smooth, red, sore tongue; dry mouth; inflamed lips; spoon-shaped nails; pallor; chills; and splenomegaly.

● *Rabies.* Severe phase 2 dysphagia involving liquids results from painful pharyngeal muscle spasms occurring late in this rare, life-threatening disorder. The patient may become dehydrated and possibly apneic. Dysphagia also causes drooling, and in 50% of patients it's responsible for hydrophobia. Eventually, this disorder causes progressive flaccid paralysis that leads to peripheral vascular collapse, coma, and death.

● *Systemic lupus erythematosus.* This disorder may cause progressive phase 2 dysphagia. However, its primary clinical features include nondeforming arthritis, a characteristic butterfly rash, and photosensitivity.

● *Tetanus.* Phase 1 dysphagia usually develops about 1 week after receiving a puncture wound. Other characteristics include marked muscle hypertonicity, hyperactive deep tendon reflexes, tachycardia, diaphoresis, and low-grade fever. Painful, involuntary muscle spasms account for lockjaw (trismus), risus sardonicus, opisthotonos, boardlike abdominal rigidity, and intermittent tonic seizures.

Other causes
● *Radiation therapy.* When used to treat oral cancer, this therapy may cause scant salivation and temporary dysphagia.

● *Surgery.* Recent tracheotomy may cause temporary dysphagia.

Special considerations

At mealtimes, take measures to minimize the patient's risk of choking and aspiration. Place him in an upright position, and have him flex his neck forward slightly and keep his chin at midline.

Stimulate salivation by talking with the patient about food, adding a lemon slice or dill pickle to his tray, and providing mouth care before and after meals. Or administer an anticholinergic or antiemetic to control excess salivation.

Consult with the dietitian to select foods with distinct temperatures and textures. Avoid sticky foods, such as bananas and peanut butter. If the patient has mucus production, avoid uncooked milk products.

During meals, separate solids from liquids, which are harder to swallow. If the patient has decreased saliva production, moisten his food with a little liquid. If he has a weak or absent cough reflex, begin tube feedings or esophageal drips of special formulas.

Prepare the patient for diagnostic tests, such as endoscopy, esophageal manometry, esophagography, and the esophageal acidity test, to pinpoint the cause of dysphagia.

Pediatric pointers

In looking for dysphagia in an infant or a small child, pay close attention to his sucking and swallowing ability. Coughing, choking, or regurgitation during feeding suggests dysphagia.

Corrosive esophagitis and esophageal obstruction by a foreign body are more common causes of dysphagia in children than in adults. However, dysphagia may also result from congenital anomalies, such as annular stenosis, dysphagia lusoria, and esophageal atresia.

DYSPNEA

Commonly a symptom of cardiopulmonary dysfunction, dyspnea is the sensation of difficult or uncomfortable breathing. It's usually reported as shortness of breath. Its severity varies greatly and doesn't always reflect the severity of the underlying cause. Dyspnea may arise suddenly or slowly and may subside rapidly or persist for years.

Most people normally experience dyspnea when they overexert themselves, and its severity depends on their physical condition. In a healthy person, dyspnea is quickly relieved by rest. Pathologic causes of dyspnea include pulmonary, cardiac, neuromuscular, and allergic disorders. Anxiety can cause shortness of breath.

Emergency interventions

 If the patient complains of shortness of breath, quickly look for signs and symptoms of respiratory distress, such as tachypnea, cyanosis, restlessness, and accessory muscle use. Prepare to administer oxygen by nasal cannula, mask, or endotracheal tube. Start an I.V. infusion and begin cardiac monitoring to detect arrhythmias. Expect to insert a chest tube for severe pneumothorax and to apply rotating tourniquets for pulmonary edema.

History and physical examination

If the patient can answer questions without increasing his distress, take a complete history. Ask if the shortness of breath began suddenly or gradually and if it's constant or intermittent. Does it occur with activity or while at rest? If he's had dyspneic attacks before, ask if they're increasing in severity. Can he identify what aggravates or alleviates these attacks? Does he have a productive or nonproductive cough or chest pain? Ask

DYSPNEA: COMMON CAUSES AND ASSOCIATED FINDINGS

CAUSES	MAJOR ASSOCIATED SIGNS AND SYMPTOMS										
	Accessory muscle use	Blood pressure decrease	Breath sounds, decreased	Chest pain	Cough, nonproductive	Cough, productive	Crackles	Cyanosis	Diaphoresis	Edema	Fasciculations
Adult respiratory distress syndrome	●	●					●	●			
Amyotrophic lateral sclerosis											●
Aspiration of a foreign body	●	●	●		●			●	●		
Cor pulmonale	●					●		●		●	
Emphysema	●		●		●						
Flail chest	●	●	●	●				●			
Heart failure	●	●				●	●			●	
Lung cancer				●		●					
Myasthenia gravis											
Myocardial infarction		●		●					●		
Pleural effusion			●		●						
Pneumonia			●	●		●	●	●	●		
Pneumothorax	●	●	●	●	●			●			
Pulmonary edema	●	●				●	●	●	●		
Pulmonary embolism		●	●	●	●	●	●	●	●		
Shock		●									

about recent trauma, and note a history of upper respiratory tract infections, deep vein phlebitis, or other disorders. Ask the patient if he smokes or is exposed to toxic fumes or irritants on the job. Find out if he also has orthopnea, paroxysmal nocturnal dyspnea, or progressive fatigue.

During the physical examination, look for signs of chronic dyspnea such as accessory muscle hypertrophy (especially in the shoulders and neck). Also look for

	Fever	Muscle weakness	Nausea	Neck vein distention	Orthopnea	Stridor	Tachycardia	Tachypnea	Weight loss
							•	•	
		•						•	
							•	•	
					•			•	
								•	•
							•	•	
					•	•	•	•	
	•								•
			•					•	
				•			•		
	•						•	•	
	•						•	•	
							•	•	
					•	•	•	•	
	•					•	•	•	
							•	•	•

oquy. Finally, palpate the abdomen for hepatomegaly.

Common medical causes

• **Adult respiratory distress syndrome (ARDS).** This life-threatening form of noncardiogenic pulmonary edema usually produces acute dyspnea as the first complaint. Progressive respiratory distress then develops with restlessness, anxiety, decreased mental acuity, tachycardia, and crackles and rhonchi in both lung fields. Other findings include cyanosis, tachypnea, motor dysfunction, and intercostal and suprasternal retractions. Severe ARDS can produce signs of shock, such as hypotension and cool, clammy skin.

• **Amyotrophic lateral sclerosis.** Dyspnea develops slowly in this disorder and worsens with time. Other features include dysphagia, dysarthria, muscle weakness and atrophy, fasciculations, shallow respirations, tachypnea, and emotional lability.

• **Aspiration of a foreign body.** Acute dyspnea marks this life-threatening condition, along with paroxysmal intercostal, suprasternal, and substernal retractions. The patient may also display accessory muscle use, inspiratory stridor, tachypnea, decreased or absent breath sounds, asymmetrical chest expansion, anxiety, cyanosis, diaphoresis, and hypotension.

• **Asthma.** Acute dyspneic attacks occur in this chronic disorder, along with audible wheezing, dry cough, accessory muscle use, nasal flaring, intercostal and supraclavicular retractions, tachypnea, tachycardia, diaphoresis, prolonged expiration, flushing or cyanosis, and apprehension.

• **Cor pulmonale.** Chronic dyspnea begins gradually with exertion and progressively worsens until it occurs even at rest. Underlying cardiac or pulmonary disease is usually present. The patient may have a chronic productive cough, wheezing, tachypnea, distended neck veins, dependent edema, and hepatomegaly. He may also experience in-

pursed-lip exhalation, clubbing, peripheral edema, barrel chest, diaphoresis, and distended neck veins. Check blood pressure and auscultate for crackles, abnormal heart sounds or rhythms, egophony, bronchophony, and whispered pectoril-

creasing fatigue, weakness, and light-headedness.

• *Emphysema.* This chronic disorder gradually causes progressive exertional dyspnea. A history of smoking or exposure to an occupational irritant usually accompanies barrel chest, accessory muscle hypertrophy, diminished breath sounds, anorexia, weight loss, malaise, peripheral cyanosis, tachypnea, pursed-lip breathing, prolonged expiration, and possibly a chronic productive cough. Clubbing is a late sign.

• *Flail chest.* Sudden dyspnea results from multiple rib fractures, along with paradoxical chest movement, severe chest pain, hypotension, tachypnea, tachycardia, and cyanosis. Bruising and decreased or absent breath sounds occur over the affected side.

• *Heart failure.* Dyspnea usually develops gradually. Chronic paroxysmal nocturnal dyspnea, orthopnea, tachypnea, tachycardia, palpitations, ventricular gallop, fatigue, dependent peripheral edema, hepatomegaly, dry cough, weight gain, and loss of mental acuity may occur. With acute onset, heart failure may produce distended neck veins, bibasilar crackles, oliguria, and hypotension.

• *Myasthenia gravis.* This neuromuscular disorder causes bouts of dyspnea as the respiratory muscles weaken. In myasthenic crisis, acute respiratory distress may occur, with shallow respiration and tachypnea.

• *Myocardial infarction.* Sudden dyspnea occurs with crushing substernal chest pain that may radiate to the back, neck, jaw, and arms. Other signs and symptoms include nausea, vomiting, diaphoresis, vertigo, hypertension or hypotension, tachycardia, anxiety, and pale, cool, clammy skin.

• *Pleural effusion.* Dyspnea develops slowly and becomes progressively worse in this disorder. A pleural friction rub occurs initially, accompanied by pleuritic pain that worsens with coughing or deep breathing. Other findings include dry cough; dullness on percussion; egophony, bronchophony, or whispered pectoriloquy; tachycardia; tachypnea; weight loss; and decreased chest motion, tactile fremitus, and breath sounds. With infection, fever may occur.

• *Pneumonia.* Dyspnea occurs suddenly, usually accompanied by fever, shaking chills, pleuritic chest pain that worsens with deep inspiration, and a productive cough. Fatigue, headache, myalgia, anorexia, abdominal pain, crackles, rhonchi, tachycardia, tachypnea, cyanosis, decreased breath sounds, and diaphoresis may also occur.

• *Pneumothorax.* This life-threatening disorder causes acute dyspnea unrelated to the severity of pain. Sudden, stabbing chest pain may radiate to the arms, face, back, or abdomen. Other signs include anxiety, restlessness, dry cough, cyanosis, decreased vocal fremitus, tachypnea, tympany, decreased or absent breath sounds on the affected side, asymmetrical chest expansion, splinting, and accessory muscle use. In tension pneumothorax, tracheal deviation accompanies these typical findings. Decreased blood pressure and tachycardia may also occur.

• *Poliomyelitis (bulbar).* Dyspnea develops gradually and progressively worsens. Additional signs and symptoms include fever, facial weakness, dysphasia, hypoactive deep tendon reflexes, decreased mental acuity, dysphagia, nasal regurgitation, and hypopnea.

• *Pulmonary edema.* Commonly preceded by signs of heart failure, such as distended neck veins and orthopnea, this life-threatening disorder causes acute dyspnea. Other features include tachycardia, tachypnea, crackles in both lung fields, S_3 gallop, oliguria, thready pulse, hypotension, diaphoresis, cyanosis, and marked anxiety. The patient's cough may be dry or may produce copious amounts of pink, frothy sputum.

• *Pulmonary embolism.* Acute dyspnea usually accompanied by sudden pleuritic chest pain characterizes this life-threatening disorder. Related findings include tachycardia, low-grade fever, tachypnea, nonproductive or productive cough with blood-tinged sputum, pleural friction rub, crackles, diffuse wheezing, dullness to percussion, decreased breath sounds, diaphoresis, restlessness, and acute anxiety. A massive embolism may cause signs of shock, such as hypotension and cool, clammy skin.

• *Shock.* Dyspnea arises suddenly and worsens progressively in this life-threatening disorder. Related findings include severe hypotension, tachypnea, tachycardia, decreased peripheral pulses, decreased mental acuity, restlessness, anxiety, and cool, clammy skin.

• *Tuberculosis.* Dyspnea commonly occurs with chest pain, crackles, and a productive cough. Other findings include night sweats, fever, anorexia and weight loss, vague dyspepsia, palpitations on mild exertion, and dullness to percussion.

Special considerations

Monitor the dyspneic patient closely. Be as calm and reassuring as possible to reduce his anxiety, and help him into a comfortable position—usually high Fowler's or a forward-leaning position. Support him with pillows, loosen his clothing, and administer oxygen.

Prepare the patient for diagnostic studies, such as arterial blood gas analysis and chest X-rays. As needed, administer bronchodilators, antiarrhythmics, diuretics, and analgesics to dilate bronchioles, correct cardiac arrhythmias, promote fluid excretion, and relieve pain.

Pediatric pointers

Normally, an infant's respirations are abdominal, gradually changing to costal by age 7. Suspect dyspnea in an infant who breathes costally, in an older child who breathes abdominally, or in any child who uses his neck or shoulder muscles to help him breathe.

Both acute epiglottitis and laryngotracheobronchitis (croup) can cause severe dyspnea in a child and may even lead to respiratory or cardiovascular collapse. Expect to administer oxygen, using a hood or cool mist tent.

DYSTONIA

Dystonia is marked by slow involuntary movements of large muscle groups of the limbs, trunk, and neck. This extrapyramidal sign may involve flexion of the foot, hyperextension of the legs, extension and pronation of the arms, arching of the back, and extension and rotation of the neck (spasmodic torticollis). It's typically aggravated by walking and emotional stress and relieved by sleep. It may be intermittent—lasting just a few minutes—or continuous and painful. Occasionally, it causes permanent contractures, resulting in a grotesque posture. Although dystonia may be hereditary or idiopathic, it usually results from extrapyramidal disorders or drugs.

History and physical examination

If possible, include the patient's family in history taking—they may be more aware of behavior changes than the patient is. Begin by asking them when dystonia occurs. Is it aggravated by emotional upset? Does it disappear during sleep? Be sure to ask about a family history of dystonia. Also, obtain a drug history, especially noting the use of phenothiazines and antipsychotics. Dystonia is a common adverse effect of these drugs, and dosage adjustments may be needed to minimize this effect.

Next, examine the patient's coordination and voluntary muscle movement. Observe his gait as he walks across the room; then have him squeeze your fingers to check muscle strength. Check coordination by having him touch your fin-

EXAMINATION TIP

RECOGNIZING DYSTONIA

Dystonia, chorea, and athetosis may occur simultaneously. To differentiate between these three, keep these points in mind:
• *Dystonic* movements are slow and twisting and involve large-muscle groups in the head, neck (as shown below), trunk, and limbs. They may be intermittent or continuous.
• *Choreiform* movements are rapid, highly complex, and jerky.
• *Athetoid* movements are slow, sinuous, and writhing, but *always* continuous; they typically affect the hands and extremities.

Dystonia of the neck (spasmodic torticollis)

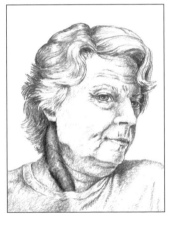

gertip and then his nose repeatedly. Follow this by testing gross motor movement of the leg: Have him place his heel on one knee, slide it down his shin, then return it to his knee. Finally, assess fine motor movement by asking him to touch each finger to his thumb in succession. (See *Recognizing dystonia*.)

Common medical causes

• *Alzheimer's disease.* Dystonia is a late sign of this disorder, which is marked by slowly progressive dementia. The patient typically displays decreased attention span, amnesia, agitation, dysarthria, emotional lability, and an inability to carry out activities of daily living.

• *Dystonia musculorum deformans.* Prolonged, generalized dystonia is the hallmark of this disorder, which usually develops in childhood and worsens with age. It causes foot inversion initially, followed by growth retardation and scoliosis. Late signs include twisted, bizarre postures, limb contractures, and dysarthria.

• *Hallervorden-Spatz disease.* This degenerative disease causes dystonic trunk movements accompanied by choreoathetosis, ataxia, myoclonus, and generalized rigidity. The patient also shows progressive intellectual decline and dysarthria.

• *Huntington's disease.* Dystonic movements mark the preterminal stage of Huntington's disease. Characterized by progressive intellectual decline, this disorder leads to dementia and emotional lability. The patient displays choreoathetosis accompanied by dysarthria, dysphagia, facial grimacing, and wide-based prancing gait.

• *Parkinson's disease.* Dystonic spasms are common in this disease. Other classic features include uniform or jerky rigidity, pill-rolling tremor, bradykinesia, dysarthria, dysphagia, drooling, masklike facies, monotone voice, stooped posture, and propulsive gait.

• *Wilson's disease.* Progressive dystonia and chorea of the arms and legs mark this disorder. Other common signs include hoarseness, bradykinesia, behavior changes, dysphagia, drooling, dysarthria, tremors, and Kayser-Fleischer rings (rusty-brown rings at the periphery of the cornea).

Other causes

- **Drugs.** All types of phenothiazines may cause dystonia. In general, propylamino phenothiazine derivatives are most likely to induce parkinsonian signs and symptoms, and propylpiperazine derivatives are most likely to cause dystonic reactions.

Haloperidol, loxapine, and other antipsychotics usually produce acute facial dystonia. So do antiemetic doses of metoclopramide, excessive doses of levodopa, and metyrosine.

Special considerations

Encourage the patient to obtain adequate sleep and avoid emotional upset. Avoid range-of-motion exercises, which can aggravate dystonia.

If dystonia is severe, protect the patient from injury by raising and padding his bed rails. Provide an uncluttered environment if he's ambulatory.

Pediatric pointers

Children rarely exhibit dystonia before age 10. Common causes include dystonia musculorum deformans, athetoid cerebral palsy, and the residual effects of anoxia at birth.

DYSURIA

Dysuria, painful or difficult urination, is commonly accompanied by urinary frequency, urgency, or hesitancy. This symptom usually reflects lower urinary tract infection (UTI)—a common disorder, especially in women.

Dysuria results from lower UTI or inflammation, which stimulates nerve endings in the bladder and urethra. The pain's onset provides clues to its cause: For example, pain just before voiding usually indicates bladder irritation or distention, whereas pain at the start of urination typically results from bladder outlet irrita-tion. Pain at the end of voiding may signal bladder spasms.

History and physical examination

If the patient complains of dysuria, have him describe its severity and location. When did he first notice it? Did anything precipitate it? Does anything aggravate or alleviate it?

Next, ask about previous urinary or genital tract infections. Has the patient recently undergone invasive procedures, such as cystoscopy or urethral dilatation? Also ask if he has a history of intestinal disease. Ask a female patient about menstrual disorders and use of products that irritate the urinary tract, such as bubble bath salts, feminine deodorants, contraceptive gels, or perineal lotions.

During the physical examination, inspect the urethral meatus for discharge, irritation, or other abnormalities. A pelvic or rectal examination may be necessary.

Common medical causes

- **Appendicitis.** Occasionally, this disorder causes dysuria that persists throughout voiding and is accompanied by bladder tenderness. Appendicitis is characterized by periumbilical abdominal pain that shifts to McBurney's point, anorexia, nausea, vomiting, constipation, slight fever, abdominal rigidity and rebound tenderness, and tachycardia.

- **Bladder tumor.** In this predominantly male disorder, dysuria throughout voiding is a late symptom associated with urinary frequency and urgency, nocturia, hematuria, and perineal, back, or flank pain.

- **Chemical irritants.** Dysuria may result from irritating substances, such as bubble bath salts and feminine deodorants; it's usually most intense at the end of voiding. Other findings may include urinary frequency and urgency, a diminished urine stream and, possibly, hematuria.

- **Cystitis.** Dysuria throughout voiding is common in all types of cystitis, as are

DYSURIA: COMMON CAUSES AND ASSOCIATED FINDINGS

S&S CAUSES	MAJOR ASSOCIATED SIGNS AND SYMPTOMS													
	Abdominal pain	Anorexia	Back pain	Constipation	Costovertebral angle tenderness	Erythema of meatus	Fatigue	Fever	Flank pain	Hematuria	Nausea	Nocturia	Perineal pain	Straining to void
Appendicitis	●	●		●				●			●			
Bladder tumor			●						●	●		●	●	
Chemical irritants										●				
Cystitis (bacterial)			●				●	●		●		●	●	●
Cystitis (chronic interstitial)										●		●		●
Cystitis (tubercular)		●					●		●	●		●		●
Cystitis (viral)								●		●		●		●
Paraurethral gland inflammation										●			●	
Prostatitis (acute)				●			●	●		●	●		●	
Prostatitis (chronic)			●										●	
Pyelonephritis		●			●			●	●	●	●	●		●
Reiter's syndrome		●				●		●		●				
Urinary obstruction														
Vaginitis										●			●	●

urinary frequency, nocturia, straining to void, and hematuria. Bacterial cystitis —the most common cause of dysuria in women—may also produce urinary urgency, perineal and low back pain, suprapubic discomfort, fatigue, and possibly low-grade fever. In chronic interstitial cystitis, dysuria is accentuated at the end of voiding. In tubercular cystitis, dysuria may be accompanied by urinary urgency, flank pain, fatigue, and anorexia. In viral cystitis, severe dysuria occurs with gross hematuria, urinary urgency, and fever.

● *Paraurethral gland inflammation.* Dysuria throughout voiding occurs with urinary frequency and urgency, diminished urine stream, mild perineal pain and, occasionally, hematuria.

● *Prostatitis.* Acute prostatitis commonly causes dysuria throughout or toward the end of voiding. Other findings are diminished urine stream, urinary frequency and urgency, hematuria, suprapubic

Suprapubic pain	Urethral discharge	Urinary frequency	Urine stream, diminished	Urinary urgency	Vaginal discharge	Vomiting	Weakness
							●
		●		●			
		●	●	●			
●		●		●			
		●					
		●		●			
		●		●			
		●	●	●			
		●	●	●		●	
	●	●	●	●			
		●		●		●	●
●	●	●		●			
		●	●	●			
		●		●	●		

clude persistent high fever with chills, costovertebral angle tenderness, flank pain, weakness, urinary urgency and frequency, nocturia, straining on urination, and hematuria. Nausea, vomiting, and anorexia may also occur.

• *Reiter's syndrome.* In this predominantly male disorder, dysuria occurs 1 to 2 weeks after sexual contact. Initially, it occurs with mucopurulent discharge, urinary urgency and frequency, meatal swelling and redness, suprapubic pain, anorexia, weight loss, and low-grade fever. Hematuria, conjunctivitis, arthritic symptoms, a papular skin rash, and penile lesions may follow.

• *Urinary obstruction.* Outflow obstruction by urethral strictures or calculi produces dysuria throughout voiding. (In complete obstruction, bladder distention will develop and dysuria will precede voiding.) Other features are diminished urine stream and urinary frequency and urgency.

• *Vaginitis.* Characteristically, dysuria occurs throughout voiding as urine touches inflamed or ulcerated labia. Other findings include urinary frequency and urgency, nocturia, hematuria, perineal pain, and vaginal discharge.

Other causes

• *Drugs.* Monoamine oxidase inhibitors and metyrosine can cause dysuria.

Special considerations

Monitor vital signs as well as intake and output. Administer prescribed medications, and prepare the patient for such tests as urinalysis and cystoscopy.

Pediatric pointers

If an infant or toddler cries during voiding, use a collection bag to obtain an uncontaminated specimen. Usually, bacterial cystitis causes the dysuria.

fullness, fever, chills, fatigue, myalgia, nausea, vomiting, and constipation. In chronic prostatitis, urethral narrowing causes dysuria throughout voiding. Related effects are urinary frequency and urgency; diminished urine stream; perineal, back, and buttock pain; urethral discharge; and, at times, hematospermia.

• *Pyelonephritis (acute).* More common in females, this disorder causes dysuria throughout voiding. Other features in-

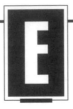

EARACHE
[Otalgia]

Earache usually results from disorders of the external and middle ear associated with infection, obstruction, or trauma. Its severity ranges from a feeling of fullness or blockage to deep, boring pain; at times, it may be difficult to localize precisely. This common symptom may be intermittent or continuous and may develop suddenly or gradually.

History and physical examination
Ask the patient to characterize his earache. How long has he had it? Is it intermittent or continuous? Is it painful or slightly annoying? Can he localize the site of ear pain? Does he have pain in any other areas such as the jaw?

Ask about ear injury or other trauma. Does swimming or showering trigger ear discomfort? Is discomfort associated with itching? If so, find out where itching is most intense and when it began. Ask about ear drainage and, if present, have the patient characterize it. Does he hear ringing or noise in his ears? Ask about dizziness or vertigo. Does it worsen when he changes position? Does he have difficulty swallowing, hoarseness, neck pain, or pain from opening his mouth?

Find out if the patient has recently had a head cold or problems with his eyes, mouth, teeth, jaws, sinuses, or throat. Disorders in these areas may refer pain to the ear along the cranial nerves.

Begin your physical examination by inspecting the external ear for redness, drainage, swelling, or deformity. Then apply pressure to the mastoid process and tragus to elicit any tenderness. Using an otoscope, examine the external auditory canal for lesions, bleeding or discharge, impacted cerumen, foreign bodies, tenderness, or swelling. (See *Using an otoscope correctly*.) Examine the tympanic membrane: Is it intact? Is it pearly gray (normal)? Look for tympanic membrane landmarks: the cone of light, umbo, pars tensa, and the handle and short process of the malleus. Perform the watch tick, whispered voice, Rinne, and Weber's tests to assess for hearing loss.

Common medical causes
• *Barotrauma (acute).* Earache associated with this trauma ranges from mild pressure to severe pain. Tympanic membrane ecchymosis or bleeding into the tympanic cavity may occur, producing a blue drumhead; usually, the eardrum is not perforated.
• *Cerumen impaction.* Impacted cerumen (earwax) may cause a plugged, blocked, or full sensation in the ear. Additional features include partial hearing loss, itching and, possibly, dizziness.
• *Herpes zoster oticus (Ramsay Hunt syndrome).* This disorder causes burning or stabbing ear pain, commonly associated with ear vesicles. The patient also complains of hearing loss and vertigo. Associated signs and symptoms include transitory, ipsilateral, facial paralysis; partial loss of taste; tongue vesicles; and nausea and vomiting.

USING AN OTOSCOPE CORRECTLY

When the patient reports an earache, use an otoscope to inspect ear structures closely. Follow these techniques to obtain the best view and ensure patient safety.

Infant or young child

To inspect an infant's or young child's ear, grasp the *lower* part of the auricle and pull it *down and back* to straighten the upward S curve of the external canal. Then gently insert the speculum into the canal no more than 1.3 cm (½″).

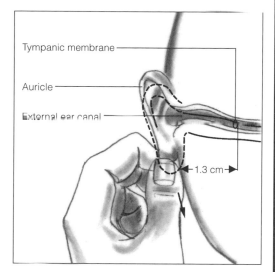

Tympanic membrane

Auricle

External ear canal

←1.3 cm→

Adult

To inspect an adult's ear, grasp the *upper* part of the auricle and pull it *up and back* to straighten the external canal. Then insert the speculum about 2.5 cm (1″). Also use this technique for children over age 3.

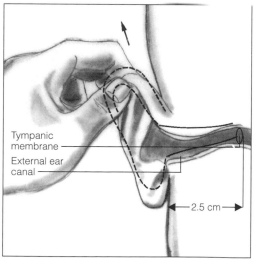

Tympanic membrane

External ear canal

←2.5 cm→

• *Keratosis obturans.* Mild ear pain occurs in this disorder, along with otorrhea and tinnitus. Inspection reveals a white glistening plug obstructing the external meatus.

• *Mastoiditis (acute).* This infection causes a dull ache behind the ear accompanied by low-grade fever (99° to 100° F [37.2° to 37.8° C]). The eardrum appears dull and edematous and may perforate; a purulent discharge is seen in the external canal; and soft tissue near the eardrum may sag.

• *Ménière's disease.* This inner ear disorder can produce a sensation of fullness in the affected ear. Its classic effects, though, include severe vertigo, tinnitus, and sensorineural hearing loss. The patient may also experience nausea and vomiting, diaphoresis, and nystagmus.

• *Otitis externa.* Earache characterizes both types of otitis externa. *Acute otitis externa* begins with mild to moderate ear pain that occurs with tragus manipulation. The pain may be accompanied by low-grade fever, sticky yellow or purulent ear discharge, partial hearing loss, and a feeling of blockage. Later, ear pain intensifies, causing the entire side of the head to ache and throb. Fever may reach 104° F (40° C). Examination reveals eardrum erythema, lymphadenopathy, and swelling of the tragus, external meatus, and external canal. The patient also complains of dizziness and malaise.

Malignant otitis externa abruptly causes ear pain that's aggravated by moving the auricle or tragus. The pain is accompanied by intense itching, purulent ear discharge, fever, parotid gland swelling, and trismus. Examination reveals a swollen external canal with exposed cartilage and temporal bone. Cranial nerve palsy may occur.

• *Otitis media (acute).* This middle ear inflammation may be serous or suppurative. *Acute serous otitis media* may cause a feeling of fullness in the ear, hearing loss, and a vague sensation of top-heaviness. The eardrum may be slightly retracted, amber colored, and marked by air bubbles and a meniscus, or it may be blue-black from hemorrhage.

Hearing loss, a fever that may reach 102° F (38.9° C), and severe, deep, throbbing ear pain characterize *acute suppurative otitis media.* The pain increases steadily over several hours or days and may be aggravated by pressure on the mastoid antrum. Perforated eardrum may occur. Before rupture, the eardrum appears bulging and fiery red. Rupture causes purulent drainage and relieves the pain.

• *Temporomandibular joint infection.* Typically unilateral, this infection produces ear pain that's referred from the jaw joint. The pain is aggravated by pressure on the joint with jaw movement and commonly radiates to the temporal area or the entire side of the head.

Special considerations

Administer analgesics and apply heat to relieve discomfort. Instill eardrops if necessary. Teach the patient how to instill drops if they're prescribed for home use.

Pediatric pointers

Common causes of earache in children are acute otitis media and insertion of foreign bodies that become lodged or infected. In young children, be alert for nonverbal clues to earache, such as crying or ear tugging. To examine the child's ears, place him supine with his arms extended and held securely by his parent. Then hold the otoscope with the handle pointing toward the top of the child's head, and brace it against him with one or two fingers. Because an ear examination may upset the child with an earache, save it for the end of your physical examination.

EDEMA, GENERALIZED

A common sign in severely ill patients, generalized edema is the excessive accumulation of interstitial fluid throughout the body. It varies widely in severity; slight edema may be difficult to detect, especially if the patient is obese, whereas massive edema is immediately apparent.

Generalized edema is typically chronic and progressive. It may result from cardiac, renal, endocrine, or hepatic disorders. However, this sign may also result from severe burns, malnutrition, or the effects of certain drugs and treatments.

Common factors responsible for edema are hypoalbuminemia and excessive sodium ingestion or retention—both of which influence plasma osmotic pressure. (See *Understanding fluid balance,* page 218.) Also, cyclic edema associated with increased aldosterone secretion may occur in premenopausal women.

Emergency interventions

 Quickly determine the edema's severity, including the degree of pitting. (See *Edema: Pitting or nonpitting?* page 219.) If the patient has severe edema, promptly take his vital signs, and check for distended neck veins and cyanotic lips. Auscultate the lungs and heart. Be alert for signs of cardiac failure or pulmonary congestion, such as crackles or ventricular gallop. Place the patient in Fowler's position to promote lung expansion, unless he's hypotensive. Prepare to administer oxygen and I.V. diuretics. Have emergency resuscitation equipment nearby.

History and physical examination

When the patient's condition permits, obtain a complete medical history. First, note when the edema began. Is it affected by position changes? Is it accompanied by shortness of breath or pain in the arms or legs? Find out how much weight the patient has gained. Has his urine output changed?

Next, ask about previous burns or cardiac, renal, hepatic, endocrine, or GI dis-

orders. Also, have the patient describe his diet so you can assess for protein malnutrition. Explore his drug history and note recent I.V. therapy.

Begin the physical examination by comparing the arms and legs for symmetrical edema. Also note ecchymoses and cyanosis. Assess the back, sacrum, and hips of the bedridden patient for dependent edema. Palpate the peripheral pulses, noting whether hands and feet feel cold. Finally, perform a complete cardiac and respiratory assessment.

Common medical causes

● *Angioneurotic edema.* Recurrent attacks of acute, painless, pitting edema affect the skin and mucous membranes, especially those of the respiratory tract. Abdominal pain, nausea, vomiting, and diarrhea accompany visceral edema; dyspnea and stridor accompany life-threatening laryngeal edema.

● *Burns.* Edema and associated tissue damage vary with the severity of the burn. Severe generalized edema (4+) may occur within 2 days of a major burn, whereas localized edema may occur with a less severe burn.

● *Heart failure.* Severe, generalized pitting edema—occasionally anasarca—may follow leg edema late in this disorder. The edema may improve with exercise or elevation of the limbs. Among other classic late findings are hemoptysis, cyanosis, marked hepatomegaly, clubbing, crackles, and a ventricular gallop. Typically, the patient has tachypnea, palpitations, hypotension, weight gain despite anorexia, nausea, slowed mental response, diaphoresis, and pallor. Dyspnea, orthopnea, tachycardia, and fatigue typify left-sided heart failure; distended neck veins typify right-sided heart failure.

● *Myxedema.* In this severe form of hypothyroidism, generalized nonpitting edema is accompanied by dry, waxy, pale skin. Observation also reveals masklike facies, hair loss or coarsening, and psychomotor slowing. Associated findings

UNDERSTANDING FLUID BALANCE

Normally, fluid moves freely between the interstitial and intravascular spaces to maintain homeostasis. Four basic pressures control fluid shifts across the capillary membrane that separates these spaces:

● capillary hydrostatic pressure (the internal fluid pressure on the capillary membrane)
● interstitial fluid pressure (the external fluid pressure on the capillary membrane)
● plasma osmotic pressure (the fluid-attracting pressure from protein concentration within the capillary)
● interstitial osmotic pressure (the fluid-attracting pressure from protein concentration outside the capillary).

Here's how these pressures maintain homeostasis. Normally, capillary hydrostatic pressure is greater than plasma osmotic pressure at the cap-

illary's arterial end, forcing fluid out of the capillary. At the capillary's venous end, the reverse is true: The plasma osmotic pressure is greater than the capillary hydrostatic pressure, drawing fluid into the capillary.

Normally, the lymphatic system transports excess interstitial fluid back to the intravascular space. Edema results when this balance is upset by increased capillary permeability, lymphatic obstruction, persistently increased capillary hydrostatic pressure, decreased plasma osmotic or interstitial fluid pressure, or dilation of precapillary sphincters.

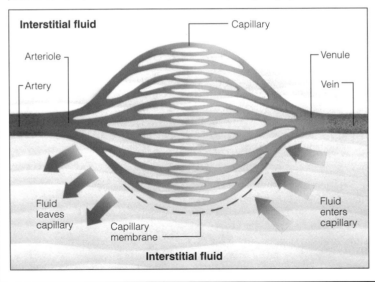

include hoarseness, weight gain, fatigue, cold intolerance, bradycardia, hypoventilation, constipation, abdominal distention, menorrhagia, impotence, and infertility.

● *Nephrotic syndrome.* Generalized pitting edema characterizes this syndrome. In severe cases, anasarca develops, increasing body weight by up to 50%. Other common signs and symptoms are as-

EXAMINATION TIP

 ## EDEMA: PITTING OR NONPITTING?

To differentiate pitting from nonpitting edema, press your finger against a swollen area for five seconds; then remove it quickly. In pitting edema, pressure forces fluid into the underlying tissues, causing an indentation that slowly fills. You can determine the severity of pitting edema by estimating the indentation's depth in centimeters: 1 cm = 1+, 2 cm = 2+, 3 cm = 3+, or 4 cm = 4+.

In nonpitting edema, pressure leaves no indentation because fluid has coagulated in the tissues. Typically, the skin feels unusually firm.

Pitting edema (4+)

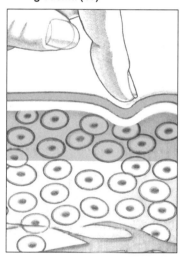

Nonpitting edema

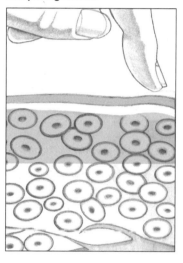

cites, anorexia, fatigue, malaise, depression, and pallor.

● *Pericardial effusion.* Generalized pitting edema may be most prominent in the arms and legs. It may be accompanied by chest pain, dyspnea, orthopnea, nonproductive cough, pericardial friction rub, dysphagia, and fever.

● *Pericarditis (chronic constrictive).* Resembling right-sided heart failure, this disorder usually begins with pitting edema of the arms and legs that may progress to generalized edema. Other signs and symptoms may include ascites, Kussmaul's respirations, dyspnea, fatigue, weakness, abdominal distention, and hepatomegaly.

● *Renal failure.* In acute renal failure, generalized pitting edema occurs as a late sign. In chronic renal failure, generalized edema is less common; its severity depends on the degree of fluid overload. Both forms of renal failure cause oliguria, anorexia, nausea and vomiting, drowsiness, confusion, hypertension, dyspnea, crackles, dizziness, and pallor.

Other causes

• *Drugs.* Any drug that causes sodium retention may aggravate or cause generalized edema. Some examples are antihypertensives, corticosteroids, androgenic and anabolic steroids, estrogens, and nonsteroidal anti-inflammatory drugs, such as phenylbutazone, ibuprofen, and naproxen.

• *I.V. infusions and feedings.* I.V. saline administration or internal feedings may cause sodium and fluid overload, resulting in generalized edema.

Special considerations

Position the patient with his limbs above heart level to promote drainage; reposition him periodically to avoid pressure sores. If the patient develops dyspnea, lower his limbs, elevate the head of the bed, and administer oxygen. Massage reddened areas, especially where dependent edema has formed (back, sacrum, hips, buttocks). Prevent skin breakdown in these areas by placing a pressure mattress, lamb's wool pad, or flotation ring on the patient's bed. Restrict intake of fluids and sodium, and administer diuretics or I.V. albumin. Monitor intake, output, and daily weight.

Monitor serum electrolytes—especially sodium—and albumin levels. Prepare the patient for blood and urine tests, X-rays, echocardiography, or electrocardiography.

Pediatric pointers

Renal failure in children commonly causes generalized edema. Monitor fluid balance closely. Remember that fever or diaphoresis can lead to fluid loss, so promote fluid intake.

Kwashiorkor—protein deficiency malnutrition—is more common in children than in adults and causes anasarca.

EDEMA OF THE ARM

The result of excess interstitial fluid in the arm, this type of edema may be unilateral or bilateral and may develop gradually or abruptly. It may be aggravated by immobility and alleviated by arm elevation and exercise.

Arm edema signals localized fluid imbalance between vascular and interstitial spaces. It commonly results from trauma, venous disorders, toxins, and treatments.

History and physical examination

When taking the patient's history, one of the first questions to ask is how long his arm has been swollen. Then find out if he also has arm pain, numbness, or tingling. Does exercise or arm elevation decrease the edema? Ask about recent arm injury, such as burns or insect stings. Also note recent I.V. therapy, surgery, or radiation therapy for breast cancer.

Determine the edema's severity by comparing the size and symmetry of both arms. Use a tape measure to determine the exact girth. Be sure to note whether the edema is unilateral or bilateral, and test for pitting. Next, examine and compare the color and temperature of both arms. Look for erythema and for ecchymoses or wounds that suggest injury. Palpate and compare radial and brachial pulses. Finally, look for arm tenderness and decreased mobility. If you detect signs of neurovascular compromise, elevate the arm.

Common medical causes

• *Angioneurotic edema.* This common reaction is characterized by sudden onset of painless, nonpruritic edema affecting the hands, feet, eyelids, lips, face, neck, genitalia, or viscera. Although this type of edema usually doesn't itch, it may burn and tingle. If edema spreads to the larynx, signs of respiratory distress may occur.

• *Arm trauma.* Shortly after a crush injury, severe edema may affect the entire arm. Ecchymoses or superficial bleeding, pain or numbness and, possibly, paralysis may occur.

• *Burns.* Two days or less after injury, arm burns may cause mild to severe edema, pain, and tissue damage.

• *Envenomation.* Initially, envenomation by snakes, aquatic animals, or insects may cause edema around the bite or sting that quickly spreads to the entire arm. Pain at the site is common, as are erythema, pruritus and, occasionally, paresthesia. Generalized signs and symptoms, such as nausea, vomiting, weakness, muscle cramps, fever, chills, hypotension, headache and, in severe cases, dyspnea, seizures, and paralysis, may develop later.

• *Superior vena cava syndrome.* Bilateral arm edema usually progresses slowly and is accompanied by facial and neck edema. Dilated veins mark these edematous areas. The patient also complains of headache, vertigo, and visual disturbances.

• *Thrombophlebitis.* This disorder may cause arm edema, pain, and warmth. Deep vein thrombophlebitis can also produce cyanosis, fever, chills, and malaise, whereas superficial thrombophlebitis also causes redness, tenderness, and induration along the vein.

Other causes

• *Treatments.* Localized arm edema may result from infiltration of I.V. fluid into the interstitial tissue. A radical or modified radical mastectomy that disrupts lymphatic drainage may cause edema of the entire arm. Also, radiation therapy for breast cancer may produce arm edema immediately after treatment or months later.

Special considerations

Treatment of the patient with arm edema depends on the underlying cause, but general care measures include elevation of the arm, frequent repositioning, and appropriate use of bandages and dressings to promote drainage and circulation. Make sure you provide meticulous skin care to prevent breakdown and decubiti formation. In addition, administer prescribed analgesics and anticoagulants.

Pediatric pointers

Arm edema rarely occurs in children, except as part of generalized edema. But it may result from arm trauma, such as burns and crush injuries.

EDEMA OF THE FACE

Facial edema refers to localized swelling—around the eyes, for instance—or more generalized facial swelling that may extend to the neck and upper arms. Occasionally painful, this sign may develop gradually or abruptly. At times, it precedes the onset of peripheral or generalized edema. Mild edema may be difficult to detect; the patient or someone who's familiar with his appearance may report it before it's noticed during assessment.

Facial edema results from disruption of the hydrostatic and osmotic pressures that govern fluid movement between the arteries, veins, and lymphatics. It may result from venous, inflammatory, and certain systemic disorders; trauma; allergy; malnutrition; or the effects of drugs, tests, and treatments.

Emergency interventions

 If the patient has facial edema associated with burns or if he reports recent exposure to an allergen, quickly evaluate his respiratory status: Edema may also affect his upper

RECOGNIZING ANGIONEUROTIC EDEMA

Most dramatic in the lips, eyelids, and tongue, angioneurotic edema commonly results from an allergic reaction. It's characterized by rapid onset of painless, nonpitting, subcutaneous swelling that usually resolves in 1 to 2 days. This edema may also involve the hands, feet, genitalia, and viscera; laryngeal edema may cause life-threatening airway obstruction.

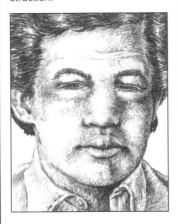

airway, causing life-threatening obstruction. If you detect audible wheezing, inspiratory stridor, or other signs of respiratory distress, administer epinephrine. In severe distress—with absent breath sounds and cyanosis—tracheal intubation, cricothyroidotomy, or tracheotomy may be required. Administer oxygen.

History and physical examination
If the patient isn't in severe distress, take his health history. Ask if facial edema developed suddenly or gradually. Is it more prominent in the early morning, or does it worsen throughout the day? Has the patient noticed any weight gain? If

so, how much and over what length of time? Has he noticed a change in his urine color or output? In his appetite? Take a drug history and ask about recent facial trauma.

Begin the physical examination by characterizing the edema. Is it localized to one part of the face, or does it affect other parts of the body? Determine if it's pitting or nonpitting and grade its severity. Next, take vital signs and assess neurologic status.

Common medical causes
• *Allergic reaction.* Facial edema may characterize both local allergic reactions and anaphylaxis. In life-threatening anaphylaxis, angioneurotic facial edema may occur with urticaria and flushing. (See *Recognizing angioneurotic edema.*) Airway edema causes hoarseness, stridor, and bronchospasm with dyspnea and tachypnea. Signs of shock, such as hypotension and cool, clammy skin, may also occur. A localized reaction produces facial edema, erythema, and urticaria.

• *Cavernous sinus thrombosis.* This rare disorder may begin with unilateral edema that quickly progresses to bilateral edema of the forehead, base of the nose, and eyelids. It may also produce chills, fever, headache, nausea, lethargy, exophthalmos, and eye pain.

• *Chalazion.* A chalazion causes localized swelling and tenderness of the affected eyelid, accompanied by a small red lump on the conjunctival surface.

• *Conjunctivitis.* This inflammation causes eyelid edema, excessive tearing, and itchy, burning eyes. Inspection reveals a thick purulent discharge, crusty eyelids, and conjunctival injection. Corneal involvement causes photophobia and pain.

• *Corneal ulcers (fungal).* Accompanying red, edematous eyelids in this disorder are conjunctival injection, intense pain, photophobia, and severely impaired visual acuity. Copious, purulent eye discharge makes eyelids sticky and crusted. The characteristic dense, central ulcer grows slowly, appears whitish gray, and is surrounded by progressively clearer rings.

- **Dacryoadenitis.** Severe periorbital swelling characterizes this disorder, which may also cause conjunctival injection, purulent discharge, and temporal pain.
- **Dacryocystitis.** Lacrimal sac inflammation causes prominent eyelid edema and constant tearing. In acute cases, pain and tenderness near the tear sac accompany purulent discharge.
- **Facial burns.** Burns may cause extensive edema that impairs respiration. Additional findings may include singed nasal hairs, red mucosa, sooty sputum, and signs of respiratory distress such as inspiratory stridor.
- **Herpes zoster ophthalmicus (shingles).** In this disorder, edematous and red eyelids are usually accompanied by excessive tearing and a serous discharge. Severe unilateral facial pain may occur several days before vesicles erupt.
- **Myxedema.** This disorder eventually causes generalized facial edema, waxy dry skin, hair loss or coarsening, and other signs of hypothyroidism.
- **Nephrotic syndrome.** Commonly the first sign of nephrotic syndrome, periorbital edema precedes dependent and abdominal edema. Associated findings include weight gain, nausea, anorexia, lethargy, fatigue, and pallor.
- **Orbital cellulitis.** Sudden onset of periorbital edema marks this inflammatory disorder, which may be accompanied by a unilateral purulent discharge, hyperemia, exophthalmos, conjunctival injection, fever, and extreme orbital pain.
- **Preeclampsia.** Edema of the face, hands, and ankles is an early sign of this disorder of pregnancy. Other characteristics include excessive weight gain, severe headache, blurred vision, hypertension, and midepigastric pain.
- **Rhinitis (allergic).** In this disorder, red and edematous eyelids are accompanied by paroxysmal sneezing, itchy nose and

eyes, and profuse, watery rhinorrhea. The patient may also have nasal congestion, excessive tearing, headache, sinus pain and, sometimes, malaise and fever.

- **Sinusitis.** *Frontal sinusitis* causes edema of the forehead and eyelids. *Maxillary sinusitis* produces edema in the maxillary area as well as malaise, gingival swelling, and trismus. Both types are also accompanied by facial pain, fever, nasal congestion, purulent nasal discharge, and red, swollen nasal mucosa.
- **Trachoma.** In this disorder, edema affects the eyelid and conjunctiva and is accompanied by eye pain, excessive tearing, photophobia, and eye discharge. Examination reveals an inflamed preauricular node and visible conjunctival follicles.

Other causes

- **Diagnostic tests.** An allergic reaction to contrast media used in radiologic tests may produce facial edema.
- **Drugs.** Long-term use of glucocorticoids may produce facial edema. Any drug that causes an allergic reaction (aspirin, antipyretics, penicillin, and sulfa preparations, for example) may have the same effect.
- **Surgery and transfusion.** Cranial, nasal, or jaw surgery may cause facial edema, as may a blood transfusion that causes an allergic reaction.

Special considerations

Administer analgesics as needed, and apply creams to reduce itching. Unless contraindicated, apply cold compresses to the patient's eyes to decrease edema. Elevate the head of his bed to help drain the accumulated fluid. Urine and blood tests are commonly ordered to help diagnose the cause of facial edema.

Pediatric pointers

Because the pressure in a child's periorbital tissue is lower than an adult's, children are more likely to develop periorbital edema. In fact, periorbital edema is more common than peripheral edema in children with such disorders as heart failure and acute glomerulonephritis. Pertussis may also cause periorbital edema.

EDEMA OF THE LEG

Leg edema results when excess interstitial fluid accumulates in one or both legs. It may affect just the foot and ankle or extend to the thigh. This common sign may be slight or dramatic, and pitting or nonpitting.

Leg edema may result from venous disorders, trauma, and certain bone and cardiac disorders that disturb normal fluid balance. However, several nonpathologic mechanisms may also cause it. For example, prolonged sitting, standing, or immobility may cause bilateral orthostatic edema. Usually, this pitting edema affects the foot and disappears with rest and leg elevation. Increased venous pressure late in pregnancy may cause ankle edema.

History and physical examination
To evaluate the patient, first ask how long he's had the edema. Did it develop suddenly or gradually? Does it decrease if he raises his legs? Is it painful when touched? When he walks? Ask about recent surgery or illness that may have immobilized the patient. Does he have a history of cardiovascular disease? Ask about recent leg injury. Finally, obtain a drug history.

Begin the physical examination by examining each leg for pitting edema. Because leg edema may compromise arterial blood flow, palpate peripheral pulses to detect any insufficiency. Observe leg color and look for unusual vein patterns. Then palpate for warmth, tenderness, or cords, and gently squeeze the calf muscle against the tibia to check for deep pain. If leg edema is unilateral, dorsiflex the foot to look for Homans' sign, which is indicated by calf pain. Finally, note skin ulceration or ulceration in the edematous areas.

Common medical causes
- **Burns.** Two days or less after an injury, leg burns may cause mild to severe edema, pain, and tissue damage.
- **Envenomation.** Mild to severe localized edema may develop suddenly at the site of a bite or sting, along with erythema, pain, urticaria, pruritus, and a burning sensation.
- **Heart failure.** Bilateral leg edema is an early sign in right-sided heart failure. Other effects include weight gain despite anorexia, nausea, chest tightness, hypotension, pallor, tachypnea, palpitations, ventricular gallop, and inspiratory crackles. Pitting ankle edema, hepatomegaly, hemoptysis, and cyanosis signal more advanced heart failure.
- **Leg trauma.** Mild to severe localized edema may form around the trauma site.
- **Osteomyelitis.** When this bone infection affects the lower leg, it usually produces mild to moderate localized edema, which may spread to the adjacent joint. Typically, edema follows fever, localized tenderness, and pain that increases with leg movement.
- **Thrombophlebitis.** Both deep and superficial vein thrombosis may cause unilateral mild to moderate edema. *Deep vein thrombophlebitis* may be asymptomatic or may cause mild to severe pain, warmth, and cyanosis in the affected leg as well as fever, chills, and malaise. *Superficial thrombophlebitis* typically causes pain, warmth, redness, tenderness, and induration along the affected vein.
- **Venous insufficiency (chronic).** Unilateral or bilateral leg edema is moderate to severe in this disorder. Initially, the edema is soft and pitting; later it becomes hard as tissues thicken. Other signs include darkened skin and painless, easily infected stasis ulcers that develop around the ankle.

Other causes
• ***Coronary artery bypass surgery.*** Unilateral venous insufficiency may follow saphenous vein retrieval.
• ***Diagnostic tests.*** Venography is a rare cause of leg edema.

Special considerations
Show the patient with leg edema how to apply antiembolism stockings or bandages to promote venous return. Encourage him to perform leg exercises, and provide analgesics as needed. A compression boot (Unna's boot) may be used to help reduce edema. Have the patient avoid prolonged sitting or standing and elevate his legs as necessary.

Monitor the patient's intake and output, and check his weight and leg circumference daily to detect any change in the edema. Prepare him for diagnostic tests, such as urine studies and X-rays.

Pediatric pointers
Uncommon in children, leg edema may result from osteomyelitis, leg trauma or, rarely, heart failure.

ENURESIS

Enuresis usually refers to nighttime urinary incontinence in a girl over age 5 or a boy over age 6. In rare cases, this sign may continue into adulthood. It's most common in boys and may be classified as primary or secondary. In *primary enuresis,* the child has never achieved bladder control; in *secondary enuresis,* the child achieved bladder control for at least 3 months but has lost it.

Among factors that may contribute to enuresis are delayed development of detrusor muscle control, unusually deep or sound sleep, organic disorders such as urinary tract infection (UTI) or obstruction, and psychological stress. Probably the most important factor, psychological stress commonly results from the birth of a sibling, the death of a parent or loved one, or premature, rigorous toilet training. The child may be too embarrassed or ashamed to discuss his enuresis, which intensifies psychological stress and makes enuresis more likely—thus creating a vicious cycle.

History and physical examination
When taking a history, include the parents as well as the child. First, determine the number of nights each week or month that the child wets the bed. Is there a family history of enuresis? Ask about the child's daily fluid intake. Does he drink much after supper? What are his typical sleep and voiding patterns? Find out if the child has ever had bladder control. If so, try to pinpoint what may have precipitated enuresis, such as an organic disorder or psychological stress. Does the bed-wetting occur at home and away from home? Ask the parents how they've tried to manage the problem, and have them describe the child's toilet training. Observe the child's and parents' attitudes toward bed-wetting. Finally, ask the child if it hurts when he urinates.

Next, perform a physical examination to detect signs of neurologic or urinary tract disorders. Observe the child's gait to assess for motor dysfunction, and test sensory function in the legs. Inspect the urethral meatus for erythema, and obtain a urine specimen. A rectal examination may be required to evaluate sphincter control.

Common medical causes
• ***Detrusor muscle hyperactivity.*** Involuntary detrusor muscle contractions may cause primary or secondary enuresis associated with urinary urgency, frequency, and incontinence. Signs and symptoms of UTI are also common.
• ***Urinary tract infection.*** In children, most UTIs produce secondary enuresis. Associated features include urinary fre-

quency and urgency, dysuria, straining to urinate, and hematuria. Lower back pain, fatigue, and suprapubic discomfort may also occur.

● *Urinary tract obstruction.* Although daytime incontinence is more common, this disorder may produce primary or secondary enuresis. It may also cause flank and lower back pain; upper abdominal distention; urinary frequency, urgency, hesitancy, and dribbling; dysuria; diminished urine stream; hematuria; and variable urine output.

Special considerations

Emotionally support the child and his family. Encourage the parents to accept and support the child. Tell them how to manage enuresis at home.

If the child has detrusor muscle hyperactivity, bladder training may help control enuresis. An alarm device may be useful for the child over age 8. This moisture-sensitive device fits in his mattress and triggers an alarm when wet, waking the child. The alarm conditions him to avoid bed-wetting. This device should be used only in cases where enuresis is having adverse psychological effects on the child.

EPISTAXIS

A common sign, epistaxis can be spontaneous or induced from the front or back of the nose. Most nosebleeds occur in the anterior-inferior nasal septum (Kiesselbach's area), but they may also occur at the point where the inferior turbinates meet the nasopharynx. Usually unilateral, they seem bilateral when blood runs from the bleeding side behind the nasal septum and out the opposite side. Epistaxis ranges from mild oozing to severe—possibly life-threatening—blood loss.

A rich supply of fragile blood vessels makes the nose particularly vulnerable to bleeding. Air moving through the nose can dry and irritate the mucous membranes, forming crusts that bleed when they're removed; dry mucous membranes are also more susceptible to infection, which can produce epistaxis as well. Trauma is another common cause of epistaxis. Additional causes include septal deviations, certain drugs and treatments, and hematologic, coagulation, renal, and GI disorders.

Emergency interventions

 If your patient has severe epistaxis, quickly take his vital signs. Be alert for tachypnea, hypotension, or other signs of hypovolemic shock. Insert a large-gauge I.V. catheter for rapid fluid and blood replacement, and attempt to control bleeding by pinching the nares closed. (However, if you suspect a nasal fracture, *don't* pinch the nares. Instead, place gauze under the patient's nose to absorb the blood.)

Have the hypovolemic patient lie down and turn his head to the side to prevent blood from draining down the back of his throat, which could cause aspiration or vomiting of swallowed blood. If the patient isn't hypovolemic, have him sit upright and tilt his head forward. Constantly check airway patency. If the patient's condition is unstable, begin cardiac monitoring and give supplemental oxygen by mask.

History and physical examination

If your patient isn't in distress, take a health history. Does he have a history of recent trauma? How often has he had nosebleeds in the past? Have the nosebleeds been long or unusually severe? Has the patient recently had surgery in the sinus area? Ask him if he bruises easily and if he has a history of hypertension, bleeding disorders, liver diseases, or other recent illnesses. Find out which drugs he uses, especially anti-inflammatories such as aspirin and anticoagulants such as warfarin.

Continue the physical examination by inspecting the patient's skin for other signs of bleeding, such as ecchymoses and petechiae, and note any jaundice, pallor, or other abnormalities. For a trauma patient, look for associated injuries, such as eye trauma or facial fractures.

Common medical causes

• *Aplastic anemia.* This disorder develops insidiously, eventually producing nosebleeds as well as ecchymoses, retinal hemorrhages, menorrhagia, petechiae, bleeding from the mouth and signs of GI bleeding. Fatigue, dyspnea, headache, tachycardia, and pallor may also occur.

• *Barotrauma.* Commonly seen in airline passengers and scuba divers, barotrauma may cause severe, painful epistaxis when the patient has an upper respiratory infection.

• *Chemical irritants.* Some chemicals, including phosphorus, sulfuric acid, ammonia, printer's ink, and chromates, irritate the nasal mucosa, producing epistaxis.

• *Coagulation disorders.* Such disorders as hemophilia and thrombocytopenic purpura can cause epistaxis along with ecchymoses, petechiae, and bleeding from the gums, mouth, and I.V. puncture sites. Menorrhagia and signs of GI bleeding, such as melena and hematemesis, can occur.

• *Glomerulonephritis (chronic).* This disorder insidiously produces nosebleeds as well as hypertension, proteinuria, hematuria, headache, edema, oliguria, hemoptysis, nausea, vomiting, pruritus, dyspnea, malaise, and fatigue.

• *Hepatitis.* When this disorder interferes with the clotting mechanism, epistaxis and abnormal bleeding tendencies can result. Associated signs and symptoms typically include jaundice, clay-colored stools, pruritus, hepatomegaly, abdominal pain, fever, fatigue, weakness,

dark amber urine, anorexia, nausea, and vomiting.

• *Hypertension.* Hypertension (blood pressure exceeding 140/90 mm Hg) can produce severe epistaxis, usually in the posterior nose, with pulsation above the middle turbinate. Dizziness, a throbbing headache, anxiety, peripheral edema, nocturia, nausea, vomiting, drowsiness, and mental impairment may also occur.

• *Leukemia.* In *acute leukemia,* sudden epistaxis is accompanied by a high fever and other abnormal bleeding, such as bleeding gums, ecchymoses, petechiae, easy bruising, and prolonged menses. These may follow less noticeable signs, such as weakness, lassitude, pallor, chills, recurrent infections, and low-grade fever. In addition, acute leukemia may cause dyspnea, fatigue, malaise, tachycardia, palpitations, a systolic ejection murmur, and abdominal or bone pain.

In *chronic leukemia,* epistaxis is a late sign that may be accompanied by other abnormal bleeding, extreme fatigue, hepatosplenomegaly, weight loss, bone tenderness, edema, macular or nodular skin lesions, pallor, weakness, dyspnea, tachycardia, palpitations, and headache.

• *Nasal fracture.* Unilateral or bilateral epistaxis occurs with nasal swelling, periorbital ecchymoses and edema, pain, nasal deformity, and crepitation of the nasal bones.

• *Polycythemia vera.* A common sign of polycythemia vera, spontaneous epistaxis may be accompanied by bleeding gums; ecchymoses; ruddy cyanosis of the face, nose, ears, and lips; and congestion of the conjunctiva, retina, and oral mucous membranes. Other signs and symptoms depend on the body system affected but may include headache, dizziness, tinnitus, visual disturbances, hypertension, chest pain, intermittent claudication, early satiety and fullness, marked splenomegaly, epigastric pain, pruritus, and dyspnea.

• *Sarcoidosis.* Oozing epistaxis may occur in this disorder, along with a non-

CONTROLLING EPISTAXIS WITH NASAL PACKING

When direct pressure and cautery fail to control epistaxis, nasal packing may be required. *Anterior packing* may be used if the patient has severe bleeding in the anterior nose. Horizontal layers of petroleum gauze strips are inserted into the nostrils near the turbinates.

If the patient has severe bleeding in the posterior nose or if blood from anterior bleeding starts flowing backward, *posterior packing* may be needed. This consists of a gauze pack secured by three strong silk sutures. After the nose is anesthetized, sutures are pulled through the nostrils with a soft catheter and the pack is positioned behind the soft palate. Two of the sutures are tied to a gauze roll under the patient's nose, which keeps the pack in place. The third suture is taped to his cheek. Instead of a gauze pack, a Foley or nasal epistaxis catheter may be inserted through the nose into the area behind the soft palate and inflated with 10 ml of water to compress the bleeding point.

If the patient has nasal packing:
• Watch for signs of respiratory distress such as dyspnea, which may occur if the packing slips and obstructs the airway.
• Keep emergency equipment (flashlights, scissors, and hemostat) at the patient's bedside. Expect to cut the cheek suture (or deflate the catheter) and remove the pack at the first sign of airway obstruction.

• Avoid tension on the cheek suture, which could cause the posterior pack to slip out of place.
• Keep the call bell within easy reach.
• Monitor vital signs frequently. Watch for signs of hypoxia, such as tachycardia and restlessness.
• Elevate the head of the patient's bed, and remind him to breathe through his mouth.
• Administer humidified oxygen, as needed.
• Instruct the patient *not* to blow his nose for 48 hours after the packing is removed

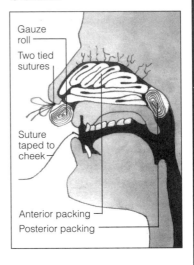

Gauze roll

Two tied sutures

Suture taped to cheek

Anterior packing

Posterior packing

---

productive cough, substernal pain, malaise, and weight loss. Related findings include tachycardia, arrhythmias, parotid gland enlargement, skin lesions, cervical lymphadenopathy, hepatosplenomegaly, and arthritis in the ankles, knees, and wrists.

• *Scleroma.* In this disorder, oozing epistaxis occurs with a watery nasal discharge that becomes foul-smelling and crusty. Progressive anosmia and turbinate atrophy may also occur.

• *Sinusitis (acute).* In this disorder, a bloody or blood-tinged nasal discharge may become purulent and copious after 24 to 48 hours. Associated signs and symptoms may include nasal congestion, pain, tenderness, malaise, headache, low-grade fever, and red, edematous nasal mucosa.

- **Skull fracture.** Depending on the type of fracture, epistaxis can be direct—when blood flows directly down the nares—or indirect—when blood drains through the eustachian tube and into the nose. Abrasions, contusions, lacerations, or avulsions are common. A severe skull fracture may cause decreased level of consciousness, a severe headache, hemiparesis, dizziness, seizures, projectile vomiting, and decreased pulse and respiratory rates.

A *basilar fracture* may also cause bleeding from the pharynx, ears, and conjunctiva along with raccoon eyes and Battle's sign. Cerebrospinal fluid or even brain tissue may leak from the nose or ears. A *sphenoid fracture* may also cause blindness, whereas a *temporal fracture* may also cause unilateral deafness or facial paralysis.

- **Systemic lupus erythematosus.** Commonly affecting women under age 50, this disorder causes oozing epistaxis. However, its more characteristic signs and symptoms include lymphadenopathy, butterfly rash, joint pain and stiffness, anorexia, nausea, vomiting, myalgia, and weight loss.

Other causes

- **Drugs.** Anticoagulants (such as warfarin sodium) and anti-inflammatory drugs (such as aspirin) can cause epistaxis.
- **Surgery and procedures.** Rarely, epistaxis results from facial and nasal surgery, including septoplasty, rhinoplasty, antrostomy, endoscopic sinus procedures, orbital decompression, or dental extraction.

Special considerations

Until the bleeding is completely under control, continue to monitor the patient for signs of hypovolemic shock, such as tachycardia and clammy skin. If external pressure doesn't control the bleeding, insert cotton impregnated with a vasoconstrictor and local anesthetic into the patient's nose.

If bleeding persists, expect to insert anterior or posterior nasal packing. (See *Controlling epistaxis with nasal packing.*) Administer humidified oxygen by face mask to a patient with posterior packing.

A complete blood count may be ordered to evaluate blood loss and detect anemia. Clotting studies, such as prothrombin time and activated partial thromboplastin time, may be required to test coagulation time. Prepare the patient for X-rays if he's recently had a traumatic injury.

Pediatric pointers

In children, nose picking and allergic rhinitis are the most common causes of epistaxis. Biliary atresia, cystic fibrosis, hereditary afibrinogenemia, and nasal trauma from insertion of a foreign body can also cause epistaxis. Rubeola may cause oozing epistaxis along with the characteristic maculopapular rash. Two rare childhood diseases—pertussis and diphtheria—can also cause oozing epistaxis.

Suspect a bleeding disorder if you see excessive umbilical cord bleeding at birth or profuse bleeding during circumcision. Epistaxis commonly begins at puberty in children with hereditary hemorrhagic telangiectasia.

ERYTHEMA
[Erythroderma]

Dilated or congested blood vessels produce red skin, or erythema, the most common sign of skin inflammation or irritation. Erythema may be localized or generalized and may occur suddenly or gradually. Skin color can range from bright red in acute conditions to pale violet or brown in chronic problems. Erythema must be differentiated from purpura, which causes redness from bleeding into the skin. When pressure is applied directly to the skin, erythema blanches momentarily, whereas purpura does not.

Erythema usually results from changes in the arteries, veins, and small vessels that lead to increased small-vessel perfusion. Drugs and neurogenic mechanisms may also allow extra blood to enter the small vessels. In addition, erythema can result from trauma and tissue damage as well as from changes in supporting tissues, which increase vessel visibility.

Emergency interventions

 If your patient has sudden progressive erythema with a rapid pulse rate, dyspnea, hoarseness, and agitation, quickly take his vital signs. These may be signs of anaphylactic shock. Provide emergency respiratory support and give epinephrine.

History and physical examination

If the patient's erythema isn't associated with anaphylaxis, obtain a detailed health history. Find out how long he's had the erythema and where it first began. Ask if he's had any associated pain or itching. Has he recently had a fever, an upper respiratory infection, or joint pain? Does he have a history of skin disease or other illness? Does he or anyone in his family have allergies, asthma, or eczema? Has he been exposed to someone who has had a similar rash or who is now ill?

Obtain a complete drug history, including recent immunizations. Ask about the patient's food intake and any exposure to chemicals.

Begin the physical examination by assessing the extent, distribution, and intensity of erythema. Look for edema and skin lesions, such as urticaria, scales, papules, and purpura. Examine the affected area for warmth, and gently palpate it to check for tenderness or crepitus.

Common medical causes

● *Allergic reactions.* Foods, drugs, chemicals, and other allergens can cause an allergic reaction and erythema. A localized allergic reaction also produces hivelike eruptions and edema.

Anaphylaxis, a life-threatening condition, produces relatively sudden erythema in the form of urticaria. It also produces flushing; facial edema; diaphoresis; weakness; sneezing; possibly airway edema with hoarseness and stridor; bronchospasm with dyspnea and tachypnea; and shock with hypotension and cool, clammy skin.

● *Burns.* In *thermal burns,* erythema and swelling appear first, possibly followed by deep or superficial blisters and other signs of damage that depend on the severity of the burn. *Burns from ultraviolet rays,* such as sunburn, cause delayed erythema and tenderness on exposed areas of the skin.

● *Dermatitis.* Erythema commonly occurs with this family of inflammatory disorders. In *atopic dermatitis,* erythema and intense pruritus precede the development of small papules that may redden, weep, scale, and lichenify.

Contact dermatitis occurs after exposure to an irritant. It quickly produces erythema and vesicles, blisters, or ulcerations on exposed skin.

In *seborrheic dermatitis,* erythema appears with dull red or yellow lesions. Sharply marginated, these lesions are sometimes ring shaped and covered with greasy scales. They usually occur on the scalp, eyebrows, ears, and nasolabial folds but may form a butterfly rash on the face or move to the chest or to skin folds on the trunk.

● *Dermatomyositis.* This disorder, most common in women over age 50, produces a dusky lilac rash on the face, neck, upper torso, and nail beds. Grotton's papules (violet, flat-topped lesions) may appear on finger joints.

• **Erythema annulare centrifugum.** Small pink infiltrated papules appear on the trunk, buttocks, and inner thighs, slowly spreading at the margins and clearing in the center. Itching, scaling, and tissue hardening may occur.

• **Erythema multiforme.** Erythema multiforme major (Stevens-Johnson syndrome) produces sudden hivelike erythema with blisters, and pathognomonic petechial or "iris" lesions that usually appear symmetrically and bilaterally on the face, hands, and feet. Erythema is characteristically preceded by blisters on the lips, tongue, and buccal mucosa; a thick, gray film over the mucous membranes; increased salivation; and an extremely sore throat.

Other early signs include cough, vomiting, diarrhea, corneal ulcers, conjunctival injection with a copious purulent discharge, coryza, epistaxis, and severe inflammation of the urethra, vagina, and anus. The patient may have a fever of 102° to 104° F (38.9° to 40° C). Chest pain, malaise, muscle and joint pain, tachypnea, and a rapid, weak pulse may also occur.

Erythema multiforme minor produces erythematous macules and papules, purpura, and occasional blisters. Characteristic urticarial "iris" lesions may burn or itch slightly; they usually appear in crops and last for 2 to 3 weeks. After 1 week, individual lesions become flat or hyperpigmented. Early signs and symptoms include a mild fever, cough, and sore throat.

• **Erythema nodosum.** Sudden bilateral eruption of tender erythematous nodules characterizes this disorder. These firm, round, protruding lesions usually appear in crops on the shins, knees, and ankles but may occur on the buttocks, arms, calves, and trunk as well. Other effects are mild fever, chills, malaise, muscle and joint pain and, possibly, swollen feet and ankles.

• **Lupus erythematosus.** Both discoid and systemic lupus erythematosus can produce a characteristic butterfly rash. This erythematous eruption may range from a blush with swelling to a scaly, sharply demarcated, macular rash with plaques that may spread to the forehead, chin, ears, chest, and other sun-exposed parts of the body.

In discoid lupus erythematosus, telangiectasia, hyperpigmentation, ear and nose deformity, and mouth, tongue, and eyelid lesions may occur.

In systemic lupus erythematosus, acute onset of erythema may also be accompanied by photosensitivity and mucous membrane ulcers, especially in the nose and mouth. Mottled erythema may occur on the hands, with edema around the nails and macular reddish purple lesions on the fingers. Telangiectasia occurs at the base of the nails or eyelids, along with purpura, petechiae, ecchymoses, and urticaria. Joint pain and stiffness are common. Other findings depend on the body systems affected but typically include low-grade fever, malaise, weakness, headache, depression, lymphadenopathy, fatigue, weight loss, anorexia, nausea, vomiting, diarrhea, and constipation.

• **Psoriasis.** Silvery white scales over a thickened erythematous base usually affect the elbows, knees, chest, scalp, and intergluteal folds. The fingernails may become thick and pitted.

• **Raynaud's disease.** In this disorder, the skin on hands and feet typically blanches and cools after exposure to cold or stress. Later, it becomes warm and purplish red.

• **Rosacea.** Scattered erythema initially develops across the center of the face, followed by superficial telangiectases, papules, pustules, and nodules. Rhinophyma may occur on the lower half of the nose.

• **Rubella.** Typically, flat solitary lesions join to form a blotchy pink erythematous rash that spreads rapidly to the trunk and extremities. Occasionally, small red le-

DRUGS ASSOCIATED WITH ERYTHEMA

Suspect drug-induced erythema in any patient who develops this sign within 1 week of starting a medication. Erythematous lesions can vary in size, shape, type, or amount, but they almost always appear suddenly and symmetrically on the trunk and inner arms. Some drugs that can produce them include:

allopurinol	gentamicin	phenothiazines
anticoagulants	gold	phenylbutazone
antimetabolites	griseofulvin	phenytoin
barbiturates	indomethacin	quinidine
cephalosporins	iodide bromides	salicylates
chlordiazepoxide	isoniazid	sulfonamides
codeine	lithium	sulfonylureas
corticosteroids	nitrofurantoin	tetracyclines
co-trimoxazole	oral contraceptives	thiazides.
diazepam	penicillin	
erythromycin	phenolphthalein	

Some of these drugs—particularly barbiturates, oral contraceptives, phenolphthalein, phenylbutazone, salicylates, sulfonamides, and tetracycline—can cause a "fixed" drug eruption. In this reaction, lesions can appear in any body part and flake off after a few days, leaving a brownish purple pigmentation. Repeated drug administration causes the original lesions to recur and new ones to develop.

sions (Forschheimer's spots) occur on the soft palate. Lesions clear in 4 to 5 days. The rash usually follows a fever (up to 102° F [38.9° C]), headache, malaise, sore throat, lymphadenopathy, a gritty eye sensation, and coryza.

Other causes

• *Drugs.* Many drugs commonly cause erythema. (See *Drugs associated with erythema.*)

• *Radiation and other treatments.* Radiation therapy may produce dull erythema and edema within 24 hours. As the erythema fades, the skin becomes light brown and mildly scaly. Also, any treatment that causes an allergic reaction can cause erythema.

Special considerations

Because erythema can cause fluid loss, closely monitor and replace fluids and electrolytes, especially in patients with burns or widespread erythema. Withhold all medications until the cause of the erythema has been identified; then expect to administer antibiotics and topical or systemic corticosteroids. For the patient with itching skin, expect to give soothing baths or apply open wet dressings containing starch, bran, or sodium bicarbonate. Administer antihistamines and analgesics.

Advise a patient with leg erythema to keep his legs elevated above heart level. For a burn patient with erythema, immerse the affected area in cold water or apply towels soaked in cold water to reduce pain, edema, and erythema.

Prepare the patient for diagnostic tests, such as a skin biopsy to detect cancerous lesions, cultures to identify infectious organisms, and sensitivity studies to confirm allergies.

Pediatric pointers

Erythema neonatorum toxicum, a pink papular rash, normally develops in the first 4 days after birth and spontaneously disappears by the 10th day. Newborns and infants can also develop erythema from infections and other disorders. For instance, candidiasis can produce thick white lesions over an erythematous base on the oral mucosa as well as diaper rash with beefy red erythema.

Roseola, rubeola, scarlet fever, granuloma annulare, and cutis marmorata also cause erythema in pediatric patients.

EXOPHTHALMOS
[Proptosis]

The abnormal protrusion of one or both eyeballs, exophthalmos may result from hemorrhage, edema, or inflammation behind the eye; extraocular muscle relaxation; or space-occupying intraorbital lesions and metastatic tumors. This sign may occur suddenly or gradually, causing mild to dramatic protrusion. Occasionally, the affected eye also pulsates.

In most cases, exophthalmos is easily observed. However, lid retraction may mimic exophthalmos even when protrusion is absent. Similarly, ptosis in one eye may make the other eye appear exophthalmic by comparison. An exophthalmometer can differentiate these signs by measuring ocular protrusion.

History and physical examination

Begin by asking when the patient first noticed exophthalmos. Is it associated with pain in or around the eye? If so, ask him how severe the pain is and how long

he's had it. Then ask about recent sinus infections or vision problems. Take the patient's vital signs, noting fever, which may accompany eye infection. Next, evaluate the severity of exophthalmos with an exophthalmometer. If the eyes bulge severely, look for cloudiness on the cornea, which may indicate ulcer formation. Describe any eye discharge and observe for ptosis. Then check visual acuity, with and without correction, and evaluate extraocular movements.

Common medical causes

- *Cavernous sinus thrombosis.* This disorder usually causes sudden onset of pulsating, unilateral exophthalmos. (See *Detecting unilateral exophthalmos,* page 234.) It may occur with eyelid edema, decreased or absent pupillary reflexes, and impaired extraocular movement and visual acuity. Other features include high fever with chills, papilledema, headache, nausea, vomiting, somnolence and, rarely, seizures.

- *Dacryoadenitis.* Unilateral, slowly progressive exophthalmos is the most common sign of dacryoadenitis. Assessment may also reveal limited extraocular movements (especially on elevation and abduction), ptosis, eyelid edema and erythema, conjunctival injection, eye pain, and diplopia.

- *Foreign body in the eye.* Although rare, exophthalmos may occur with other findings of ocular trauma, such as eye pain, redness, and tearing.

- *Hemangioma.* Most common in young adults, this orbital tumor produces progressive exophthalmos, which may be mild or severe, unilateral or bilateral. Other signs and symptoms may include ptosis, limited extraocular movements, and blurred vision.

- *Lacrimal gland tumor.* Exophthalmos usually develops slowly in one eye, causing its downward displacement toward

EXAMINATION TIP

DETECTING UNILATERAL EXOPHTHALMOS

If one of the patient's eyes seems more prominent than the other, examine them from above the patient's head. Look down across his face, gently draw his lids up, and compare the relationship of the corneas to the lower lids. Abnormal protrusion of one eye suggests unilateral exophthalmos. *Remember:* If you suspect eye trauma, don't do this test.

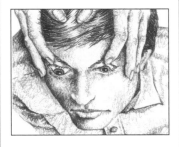

the nose. The patient may also have ptosis and eye deviation and pain.

● *Leiomyosarcoma.* Most common in people over age 45, this tumor is characterized by slowly developing, unilateral exophthalmos. Other effects include diplopia, impaired vision, and intermittent eye pain.

● *Lymphangioma.* Hemorrhage of this congenital tumor causes unilateral or bilateral exophthalmos, among other signs.

● *Optic nerve meningioma.* This tumor commonly produces unilateral exophthalmos and a swollen temple. Impaired visual acuity, visual field deficits, and headache may also occur.

● *Orbital choristoma.* A common sign of this benign tumor, progressive exophthalmos may be associated with diplopia and blurred vision.

● *Orbital emphysema.* Air leaking from the sinus into the orbit usually causes unilateral exophthalmos. Palpation of the globe elicits crepitation.

● *Parasite infestation.* This disorder usually causes painless, progressive exophthalmos in one eye that may spread to the other eye. Associated findings include limited extraocular movements, diplopia, eye pain, and impaired visual acuity.

● *Scleritis (posterior).* Gradual onset of mild to severe unilateral exophthalmos is common in scleritis. Other signs and symptoms include severe eye pain, diplopia, papilledema, limited extraocular movements, and impaired visual acuity.

● *Thyrotoxicosis.* Although a classic sign of this disorder, exophthalmos is absent in many patients. It's usually bilateral, progressive, and severe. Associated ocular features include ptosis, increased tearing, lid lag and edema, photophobia, conjunctival injection, diplopia, and decreased visual acuity. Other findings include an enlarged thyroid, nervousness, heat intolerance, weight loss despite increased appetite, sweating, diarrhea, tremors, palpitations, and tachycardia.

Special considerations

Exophthalmos usually makes the patient self-conscious, so provide privacy and emotional support. Protect the affected eye from trauma, especially drying of the cornea. But *never* place a gauze eye pad or other object over the affected eye; removal could damage the corneal epithelium. If a slit lamp examination is indicated, explain the procedure to the patient. If necessary, refer him to an ophthalmologist for a complete examination.

Pediatric pointers

In children around age 5, a rare tumor—optic nerve glioma—may cause exophthalmos. Rhabdomyosarcoma, a more common tumor, usually affects children between ages 4 and 12 and produces rapid onset of exophthalmos. In Hand-Schüller-Christian syndrome, exophthalmos typically accompanies signs of diabetes insipidus and bone destruction.

EYE DISCHARGE

Usually associated with conjunctivitis, eye discharge refers to the excretion of any substance other than tears. This common sign may occur in one or both eyes, producing scant to copious discharge. The discharge may be purulent, frothy, mucoid, cheesy, or ropey. Sometimes, it can be expressed by applying pressure to the tear sac, punctum, meibomian glands, or canaliculus.

An eye discharge commonly results from inflammatory and infectious eye disorders, but it may also result from certain systemic disorders. (See *Sources of eye discharge,* page 236.) Because this sign may accompany a disorder that threatens vision, it must be assessed and treated immediately.

History and physical examination
Begin your evaluation by finding out when the discharge began. Does it occur at certain times of day or in connection with certain activities? If the patient complains of pain, ask him to show you its exact location and describe its character. Is the pain dull, continuous, sharp, or stabbing? Ask the patient if his eyes itch or burn. Do they tear excessively? Are they sensitive to light? Does he feel like something is in them?

After taking vital signs, carefully inspect the eye discharge, noting its amount and consistency. Then test visual acuity, with and without correction. Examine external eye structures, beginning with the unaffected eye to prevent cross-contamination. Observe for eyelid edema, entropion, crusts, lesions, or trichiasis. Next, ask the patient to blink as you watch for impaired lid movement. If the eyes seem to bulge, measure them with an exophthalmometer. Test the six cardinal fields of gaze. Examine for conjunctival injection and follicles, and for corneal cloudiness or white lesions.

Common medical causes
• *Conjunctivitis.* Four types of conjunctivitis may cause eye discharge with redness and hyperemia. In *allergic conjunctivitis,* a bilateral ropey discharge is accompanied by itching and tearing.

Bacterial conjunctivitis causes a moderate amount of purulent discharge that may form sticky crusts on the eyelids during sleep. Itching, burning, excessive tearing, and the sensation of a foreign body in the eye may also occur. Eye pain indicates corneal involvement.

Fungal conjunctivitis produces copious, thick, purulent discharge that makes eyelids crusty and sticky. Also characteristic are eyelid edema, itching, burning, and tearing. Pain and photophobia occur only with corneal involvement.

Inclusion conjunctivitis causes scant mucoid discharge—especially in the morning—in both eyes, accompanied by pseudoptosis and conjunctival follicles.
• *Corneal ulcers.* Both bacterial and fungal ulcers produce copious, purulent, unilateral eye discharge. Related findings are crusty, sticky eyelids and, possibly, severe pain, photophobia, and impaired visual acuity.

A *bacterial corneal ulcer* is also characterized by an irregular gray-white area on the cornea, blurred vision, unilateral pupil constriction, and conjunctival injection.

A *fungal corneal ulcer* is also characterized by conjunctival injection and eyelid edema and erythema. A painless, dense, whitish gray central ulcer develops slowly and may be surrounded by progressively clearer rings.
• *Erythema multiforme major (Stevens-Johnson syndrome).* A purulent dis-

SOURCES OF EYE DISCHARGE

An eye discharge can come from the tear sac, punctum, meibomian glands, or canaliculi. If the patient reports a discharge that's not immediately apparent, you can express a sample by pressing your fingertip lightly over these structures. Then characterize the discharge and note its source.

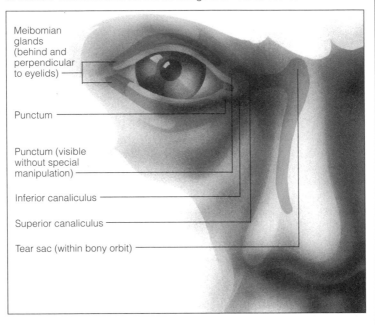

Meibomian glands (behind and perpendicular to eyelids)

Punctum

Punctum (visible without special manipulation)

Inferior canaliculus

Superior canaliculus

Tear sac (within bony orbit)

charge characterizes this disorder. Other ocular effects include severe eye pain, entropion, trichiasis, photophobia, and decreased tear formation. Also typical are erythematous, urticarial, bullous lesions that suddenly erupt over the skin.

● *Herpes zoster ophthalmicus.* This disorder produces moderate to copious serous eye discharge accompanied by excessive tearing. Examination reveals eyelid edema and erythema, conjunctival injection, and a white, cloudy cornea. The patient also complains of eye pain and severe unilateral facial pain that occurs several days before vesicles erupt.

● *Keratoconjunctivitis sicca.* Better known as dry eye syndrome, this disorder typically causes excessive, continuous mucoid discharge and insufficient tearing. Accompanying signs and symptoms include eye pain, itching, burning, a foreign-body sensation, and dramatic conjunctival injection. The patient may also have difficulty closing his eyes.

● *Meibomianitis.* This disorder may produce a continuous frothy eye discharge. The application of pressure on the meibomian glands yields a soft, foul-smelling, cheesy yellow discharge. The eyes also appear chronically red, with inflamed lid margins.

● *Orbital cellulitis.* Although exophthalmos is the most obvious sign of this disorder, a unilateral purulent eye discharge may also be present. Related findings include eyelid edema, conjunctival injection, headache, orbital pain, impaired visual acuity, limited extraocular movement, and fever.

- *Psoriasis vulgaris.* This disorder usually causes a substantial mucus discharge in both eyes, accompanied by redness. The characteristic lesions it produces on the eyelids may extend into the conjunctiva, causing irritation, excessive tearing, and a foreign-body sensation.

- *Trachoma.* A bilateral eye discharge occurs in this disorder, with severe pain, excessive tearing, photophobia, eyelid edema, redness, and visible conjunctival follicles.

Special considerations

Apply warm soaks to soften crusts on eyelids and lashes. Then gently wipe the eyes with a soft gauze pad. Carefully dispose of all used dressings, tissues, and cotton swabs to prevent possible spread of infection. Teach the patient how to avoid contaminating the unaffected eye. Also be sure to sterilize ophthalmic equipment after use.

Explain the diagnostic tests that may be ordered, including culture and sensitivity studies to identify infectious organisms.

Pediatric pointers

In infants, prophylactic eye medication (silver nitrate) commonly causes eye irritation and discharge. However, in children, a discharge usually results from eye trauma and eye or upper respiratory infection.

EYE PAIN
[Ophthalmalgia]

Eye pain may be described as a burning, throbbing, aching, or stabbing sensation in or around the eye. It may also be char-

acterized as a foreign-body sensation. This symptom varies from mild to severe; its duration and exact location provide clues to the causative disorder.

Eye pain usually results from corneal abrasion but may also result from glaucoma and other eye disorders, trauma, and neurologic and systemic disorders. Any of these may stimulate nerve endings in the cornea or external eye, producing pain.

Emergency interventions

 If the patient's eye pain results from a chemical burn, remove contact lenses, if present, and irrigate the eye with at least 1 qt (1 L) of normal saline solution over 10 minutes. Evert the lids and wipe the fornices with a cotton-tipped applicator to remove any particles or chemicals.

History and physical examination

If the patient's eye pain does not result from a chemical burn, take a complete history. Have the patient fully describe the pain. Is it an ache or a sharp pain? How long does it last? Is it accompanied by burning or itching? Find out when it began. Is it worse in the morning or late in the evening? Ask about recent traumatic injury or surgery, especially if the patient complains of sudden, severe pain. Does he have headaches? If so, find out how often and at what time of day they occur.

During the physical examination, *don't* manipulate the patient's eye if you suspect trauma. Carefully assess the lids and conjunctiva for redness, inflammation, and swelling. Then examine the eyes for ptosis or exophthalmos. (See *Examining the external eye*, page 238.) Finally, test visual acuity with and without correction, and assess extraocular movements. Characterize any discharge.

Common medical causes

- *Acute angle-closure glaucoma.* Blurred vision and sudden, excruciating

EXAMINATION TIP

EXAMINING THE EXTERNAL EYE

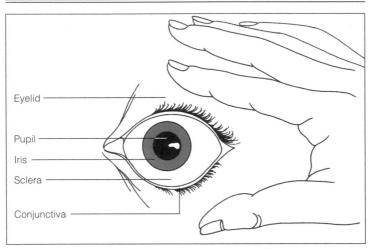

Eyelid

Pupil

Iris

Sclera

Conjunctiva

For the patient with eye pain or other ocular symptoms, examination of the external eye forms an important part of the ocular assessment. Here's how to examine the external eye.

First, inspect the eyelids for ptosis and incomplete closure of the lids. Also observe the lids for edema, erythema, cyanosis, hematoma, and masses. Are the lids everted or inverted? Do the eyelashes turn inward? Have some of them been lost? Do the lashes adhere to one another or contain discharge? Next, examine the lid margins, noting especially any debris, scaling, lesions, or unusual secretions. Also watch for eyelid spasms.

Now gently retract the eyelid with your thumb and forefinger, and assess the conjunctiva for redness, cloudiness, follicles, and blisters or other lesions. Check for chemosis by pressing the lower lid against the eyeball and noting any bulging above this compression point. Observe the sclera, noting any changes from its normal white color.

Next, shine a light across the cornea to detect scars, abrasions, or ulcers. Note any color changes, dots, or opaque or cloudy areas. Also assess the anterior eye chamber, which should be clean, deep, shadow-free, and filled with clear aqueous humor.

Inspect the color, shape, texture, and pattern of the iris. Then assess the pupils' size, shape, and equality. Finally, evaluate their response to light. Are they sluggish, fixed, or unresponsive? Does pupil dilation or constriction occur only on one side?

pain in and around the eye characterize this disorder; the pain may be so severe that it causes nausea and vomiting. Other findings are halo vision, rapidly decreasing visual acuity, and a fixed, nonreactive, moderately dilated pupil.

• *Blepharitis.* Burning pain in both eyelids is accompanied by itching, sticky discharge, and conjunctival injection. Related findings include a foreign-body sensation, lid ulcerations, and loss of eyelashes.

• *Chalazion.* A chalazion causes localized tenderness and swelling on the upper or lower eyelid. Eversion of the lid reveals conjunctival injection and a small red lump.

• *Conjunctivitis.* Some degree of eye pain and excessive tearing occur with four types of conjunctivitis. *Allergic conjunctivitis* causes mild, burning, bilateral pain accompanied by itching, conjunctival injection, and a characteristic ropey discharge. *Bacterial conjunctivitis* causes pain only when it affects the cornea. Otherwise, it produces burning and a foreign body sensation. A purulent discharge and conjunctival injection are also typical.

If it affects the cornea, *fungal conjunctivitis* may cause pain and photophobia. Even without corneal involvement, it produces itchy, burning eyes; a thick, purulent discharge; and conjunctival injection. *Viral conjunctivitis* produces itchy red eyes accompanied by a foreign-body sensation, visible conjunctival follicles, and eyelid edema.

• *Corneal abrasion.* In this type of injury, eye pain is characterized by a foreign-body sensation. Excessive tearing, photophobia, and conjunctival injection are also common.

• *Corneal ulcer.* Both bacterial and fungal corneal ulcers cause severe eye pain. They may also cause a purulent eye discharge, sticky eyelids, photophobia, and impaired visual acuity. In addition, a *bacterial corneal ulcer* produces a grayish white, irregularly shaped ulcer on the cornea, unilateral pupil constriction, and conjunctival injection. A *fungal corneal ulcer* produces conjunctival injection, eyelid edema and erythema, and a dense, cloudy, central ulcer surrounded by progressively clearer rings.

• *Dacryocystitis.* Pain and tenderness near the tear sac characterize acute dacryocystitis. Additional signs include excessive tearing, a purulent discharge, eyelid erythema, and swelling in the lacrimal punctum area.

• *Episcleritis.* Deep eye pain occurs as tissues over the sclera become inflamed. Related effects include photophobia, excessive tearing, conjunctival edema, and a red or purplish sclera.

• *Erythema multiforme major.* This disorder commonly produces severe eye pain, entropion, trichiasis, purulent conjunctivitis, photophobia, and decreased tear formation.

• *Foreign bodies in the cornea and conjunctiva.* Sudden severe pain is common but vision usually remains intact. Other findings include excessive tearing, photophobia, miosis, a foreign-body sensation, a dark speck on the cornea, and dramatic conjunctival injection.

• *Iritis (acute).* Moderate to severe eye pain occurs with severe photophobia, dramatic conjunctival injection, and blurred vision. The constricted pupil may respond poorly to light.

• *Lacrimal gland tumor.* This neoplastic lesion usually produces unilateral eye pain, impaired visual acuity, and some degree of exophthalmos.

• *Ocular laceration and intraocular foreign bodies.* Penetrating eye injuries usually cause mild to severe unilateral eye pain and impaired visual acuity. Eyelid edema, conjunctival injection, and an abnormal pupillary response may also occur.

• *Optic neuritis.* In this disorder, pain in and around the eye occurs with eye movement. Severe vision loss and tunnel vision develop but improve in 2 to 3 weeks. Pupils respond sluggishly to direct light but normally to consensual light.

• *Orbital cellulitis.* This disorder causes dull, aching pain in the affected eye, some degree of exophthalmos, eyelid edema and erythema, purulent discharge, impaired extraocular movement and, occasionally, decreased visual acuity and fever.

• *Scleritis.* This inflammation produces severe eye pain and tenderness, along with conjunctival injection, bluish purple sclera and, possibly, photophobia and excessive tearing.

• *Sclerokeratitis.* Inflammation of the sclera and cornea causes pain, burning, irritation, and photophobia.

• *Subdural hematoma.* Following head trauma, a subdural hematoma commonly causes severe eyeache and headache. Related neurologic signs depend on the hematoma's location and size.

• *Trachoma.* Along with pain in the affected eye, trachoma causes excessive tearing, photophobia, eye discharge, eyelid edema and redness, and visible conjunctival follicles.

• *Uveitis. Anterior uveitis* causes sudden onset of severe pain, dramatic conjunctival injection, photophobia, and a small, nonreactive pupil. Posterior uveitis causes insidious onset of similar features, plus gradual blurring of vision and distorted pupil shape. *Lens-induced uveitis* causes moderate eye pain, conjunctival injection, pupil constriction, and severely impaired visual acuity. The patient usually has only light perception.

Other causes

• *Treatments.* Contact lenses may cause eye pain and a foreign-body sensation. Ocular surgery may also produce eye pain, ranging from a mild ache to a severe pounding or stabbing sensation.

Special considerations

To help ease eye pain, have the patient lie down in a darkened, quiet environment and close his eyes. Prepare him for diagnostic studies, including tonometry and orbital X-rays.

Pediatric pointers

Trauma and infection are the most common causes of eye pain in children. Be alert for nonverbal clues to pain, such as tightly shutting or frequently rubbing the eyes.

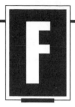

FASCICULATIONS

Fasciculations are local muscle contractions reflecting the spontaneous discharge of a muscle fiber bundle innervated by a single motor nerve filament. These contractions cause visible dimpling or wavelike twitching of the skin but aren't strong enough to produce joint movement. They occur irregularly at frequencies ranging from once every several seconds to two to three times per second; in rare instances, myokymia—continuous, rapid fasciculations that cause a rippling effect—may occur. Because fasciculations are brief and painless, they commonly go undetected or are ignored.

Benign, nonpathologic fasciculations are common and normal. They commonly occur in tense, anxious, or overtired people and typically affect the eyelid, thumb, or calf. However, fasciculations may also indicate a severe neurologic disorder, most notably a diffuse motor neuron disorder that causes loss of control over muscle fiber discharge. They're also an early sign of pesticide poisoning.

Emergency interventions

 Begin by asking the patient about the nature, onset, and duration of his fasciculations. If the onset was sudden, ask about any precipitating events such as exposure to pesticides. *Pesticide poisoning, although uncommon, is a medical emergency requiring prompt and vigorous intervention.* You may need to maintain airway patency, monitor vital signs, give oxygen, and perform gastric lavage or induce vomiting.

History and physical examination

If the patient isn't in severe distress, find out about any sensory changes, such as paresthesia, and any difficulty in speaking, swallowing, breathing, or controlling bowel or bladder function. Ask the patient if he's in pain.

Explore the patient's medical history for neurologic disorders, malignant tumors, and recent infections. Also explore lifestyle, asking especially about stress at home, on the job, or at school.

Perform a physical examination, looking for fasciculations while the affected muscle is at rest. Observe and test for motor and sensory abnormalities, particularly muscle atrophy and weakness, and decreased deep tendon reflexes. If you note these signs, suspect motor neuron disease, and perform a comprehensive neurologic examination.

Common medical causes

- *Amyotrophic lateral sclerosis.* Coarse fasciculations usually begin in the small muscles of the hands and feet, then spread to the forearms and legs. Widespread, symmetrical muscle atrophy and weakness may result in dysarthria; difficulty chewing, swallowing, and breathing; and occasionally choking and drooling.
- *Bulbar palsy.* Fasciculations of the face and tongue commonly appear early. Progressive signs include dysarthria, dysphagia, hoarseness, and drooling. Eventually, weakness spreads to the respiratory muscles.

• *Pesticide poisoning.* Ingestion of organophosphate or carbamate pesticides commonly produces a sudden onset of long, wavelike fasciculations and muscle weakness that rapidly progresses to flaccid paralysis. Other common effects include nausea, vomiting, diarrhea, loss of bowel and bladder control, hyperactive bowel sounds, and abdominal cramping. Cardiopulmonary findings may include bradycardia, dyspnea or bradypnea, and pallor or cyanosis. Other possible signs and symptoms include seizures, visual disturbances (pupillary constriction or blurred vision), and increased secretions (tearing, salivation, pulmonary secretions, or diaphoresis).

• *Poliomyelitis (spinal paralytic).* Coarse fasciculations, usually transient but occasionally persistent, accompany progressive muscle weakness, spasms, and atrophy. The patient may have decreased reflexes, paresthesia, and coldness and cyanosis in the affected limbs. He may also display bladder paralysis, dyspnea, elevated blood pressure, and tachycardia.

• *Spinal cord tumors.* Fasciculations may develop, along with muscle atrophy and cramps, asymmetrically at first and then bilaterally as cord compression progresses. Motor and sensory changes distal to the tumor include weakness or paralysis, areflexia, paresthesia, and a tightening band of pain. Bowel and bladder control may also be lost.

Special considerations

Prepare the patient for diagnostic studies, such as spinal X-rays, myelography, computed tomography scan, magnetic resonance imaging, and electromyography with nerve conduction velocity tests.

Help the patient with progressive neuromuscular degeneration to cope with activities of daily living, and provide appropriate assistive devices.

Teach effective stress management techniques to the patient with stress-induced fasciculations.

Pediatric pointers

Fasciculations, particularly of the tongue, are an important early sign of Werdnig-Hoffmann disease.

FATIGUE

Fatigue is a feeling of excessive tiredness, lack of energy, or exhaustion accompanied by a strong desire to rest or sleep. This common symptom is distinct from weakness, which involves the muscles, but may occur with it.

Fatigue is a normal and important response to physical overexertion, prolonged emotional stress, and sleep deprivation. However, it can also be a nonspecific symptom of a psychological or physiologic disorder—especially viral infections and endocrine, cardiovascular, or neurologic disease.

Fatigue reflects both hypermetabolic and hypometabolic states in which nutrients needed for cellular energy and growth are lacking because of overly rapid depletion, impaired replacement mechanisms, insufficient hormone production, or inadequate nutrient intake or metabolism.

History and physical examination

Obtain a careful history to identify the patient's fatigue pattern. Fatigue that worsens with activity and improves with rest generally indicates a physical disorder; the opposite pattern, a psychological disorder. Also associated with psychological disorders are fatigue lasting longer than 4 months, constant fatigue that's unrelieved by rest, and transient exhaustion that quickly gives way to bursts of energy.

Ask about related symptoms and recent stressful changes in lifestyle. Explore nutritional habits and any appetite or weight changes. Carefully review the patient's medical and psychiatric history for any chronic disorders that commonly produce fatigue. Ask about a family history of such disorders.

Observe the patient's general appearance for overt signs of depression or organic illness. Is he unkempt or expressionless? Does he appear tired or sickly, or have a slumped posture? If warranted, evaluate his mental status, noting especially mental clouding, attention deficits, agitation, or psychomotor retardation.

Common medical causes

• *Acquired immunodeficiency syndrome.* Patients with this disease may report a history of fatigue along with fevers, night sweats, weight loss, diarrhea, and a cough; several concurrent infections may appear soon afterward.

• *Adrenocortical insufficiency.* Mild fatigue, the hallmark of this disorder, initially appears after exertion and stress but later becomes more severe and persistent. Typically, weakness and weight loss accompany GI disturbances, such as nausea, vomiting, anorexia, abdominal pain, and chronic diarrhea; hyperpigmentation; orthostatic hypotension; and a weak, irregular pulse.

• *Anemia.* Fatigue following mild activity is commonly the first symptom of this disorder. Associated findings vary but generally include pallor, tachycardia, and dyspnea.

• *Anxiety.* Chronic, unremitting anxiety invariably produces fatigue, commonly characterized as nervous exhaustion. Other persistent findings include apprehension, indecisiveness, restlessness, insomnia, trembling, and increased muscle tension.

• *Cancer.* In many cases, unexplained fatigue is the earliest sign of cancer. Related findings reflect the type, location, and stage of the cancer and commonly include pain, nausea, vomiting, anorexia, weight loss, abnormal bleeding, and a palpable mass.

• *Chronic fatigue and immune dysfunction syndrome.* This syndrome, whose cause is unknown, is characterized by incapacitating fatigue. Findings also include sore throat, myalgia, and cognitive dysfunction.

• *Chronic obstructive pulmonary disease.* The earliest and most persistent symptoms of this disease are progressive fatigue and dyspnea. The patient may also have a chronic and usually productive cough, weight loss, barrel chest, cyanosis, and slight dependent edema.

• *Diabetes mellitus.* Fatigue, the most common symptom of this disorder, may begin insidiously or abruptly. Related findings include weight loss, polyuria, polydipsia, and polyphagia.

• *Heart failure.* Persistent fatigue and lethargy characterize this disorder. Left-sided heart failure produces exertional and paroxysmal nocturnal dyspnea, orthopnea, and tachycardia. Right-sided heart failure produces distended neck veins and possibly a slight but persistent nonproductive cough. In both types, later signs and symptoms include nausea, anorexia, slowed mental response, unexplained weight gain, and possibly oliguria. Cardiopulmonary findings include tachypnea, inspiratory crackles, palpitations and chest tightness, hypotension, narrowed pulse pressure, ventricular gallop, pallor, diaphoresis, clubbing, and dependent edema.

• *Hypercortisolism.* This disorder typically causes fatigue, related in part to accompanying sleep disturbances. Unmistakable signs include purple striae, acne, hirsutism, increased blood pressure, muscle weakness, truncal obesity with slender extremities, buffalo hump, and moon face.

• *Hypothyroidism.* Fatigue begins early, along with forgetfulness, cold intolerance, weight gain, and constipation.

• *Lyme disease.* Besides fatigue and malaise, symptoms of this tick-borne disease include intermittent headache, fever, chills, expanding red rash, and muscle and joint aches. In later stages, patients may suffer fluctuating meningoencephalitis, arthritis, and cardiac abnormalities such as a brief, fluctuating atrioventricular heart block.

• *Malnutrition.* Easy fatigability commonly occurs in protein-calorie malnutrition, along with lethargy and apathy. The patient may also have weight loss, muscle wasting, sensations of coldness, pallor, edema, and dry, flaky skin.

• *Myasthenia gravis.* The cardinal symptoms of this disorder are easy fatigability and muscle weakness, which worsen with exertion and abate with rest. Related findings depend on the specific muscles affected.

• *Renal failure. Acute renal failure* commonly causes sudden fatigue, drowsiness, and lethargy. Oliguria is an early sign, followed by severe systemic effects: ammonia breath, nausea, vomiting, diarrhea or constipation, and dry skin and mucous membranes. Neurologic signs include muscle twitching and changes in personality and level of consciousness, possibly progressing to seizures and coma.

In *chronic renal failure,* insidious fatigue and lethargy occur with marked changes in all body systems, including GI disturbances, ammonia breath odor, Kussmaul's respirations, bleeding tendencies, poor skin turgor, severe pruritus, paresthesia, visual disturbances, confusion, seizures, and coma.

• *Systemic lupus erythematosus.* Fatigue usually occurs along with generalized aching, malaise, low-grade fever, headache, and irritability. Primary clinical features include joint pain and stiffness, butterfly rash, and photosensitivity. Also common are Raynaud's phenomenon, patchy alopecia, and mucous membrane ulcers.

• *Valvular heart disease.* All types of valvular heart disease commonly produce progressive fatigue and a cardiac murmur. Additional signs and symptoms vary but generally include exertional dyspnea, cough, and hemoptysis.

Other causes

• *Drugs.* Fatigue may result from various drugs, notably antihypertensives and sedatives. In digitalis glycoside therapy, it may indicate toxicity.

• *Surgery.* Most types of surgery cause temporary fatigue, probably due to the combined effects of hunger, anesthesia, and sleep deprivation.

Special considerations

Regardless of the cause of fatigue, you may need to help the patient alter his lifestyle to achieve a balanced diet, a program of regular exercise, and adequate rest. Counsel him about setting priorities, keeping a reasonable schedule, and developing good sleep habits. Teach stress management techniques as appropriate.

If fatigue results from organic illness, help the patient determine which activities he must accomplish, which of these he may need help with, and how to pace himself to ensure sufficient rest. You can help him reduce chronic fatigue by alleviating pain, which may interfere with rest, or nausea, which may lead to malnutrition. The patient may also benefit from a referral to a community health nurse or housekeeping service. If fatigue results from a psychogenic cause, refer him for psychological counseling.

Pediatric pointers

When evaluating a child for fatigue, ask his parents if they've noticed any change in his activity level. Fatigue without an organic cause occurs normally during accelerated growth phases in preschool-age and prepubescent children. However, psychological causes of fatigue must be considered; for instance, a depressed child may try to escape problems at home or school by taking refuge in sleep. In a pubescent child, consider the possibility of drug abuse, particularly of hypnotics and tranquilizers.

FECAL INCONTINENCE

The involuntary passage of feces, fecal incontinence follows any loss or impairment of external anal sphincter control. It can result from the effects of drugs or surgery or from various GI, neurologic, and psychological disorders. In some patients, it may even be a purposeful manipulative behavior.

Fecal incontinence may be temporary or permanent; its onset may be gradual, as in dementia, or sudden, as in spinal cord trauma. Although usually not a sign of severe illness, it can greatly affect the patient's physical and psychological well-being.

History and physical examination
Ask the patient with fecal incontinence about its onset, duration, severity, and any discernible pattern—for instance, at night or with diarrhea. Note the frequency, consistency, and volume of stool passed within the last 24 hours and obtain a stool sample. Focus your history taking on GI, neurologic, and psychological disorders.

Let the history guide your physical examination. If you suspect a brain or spinal cord lesion, perform a complete neurologic examination. If a GI disturbance seems likely, inspect the abdomen for distention, auscultate for bowel sounds, percuss, and palpate for a mass. Inspect the anal area for signs of excoriation or infection. If not contraindicated, check for fecal impaction, which may be associated with incontinence.

Common medical causes
● *Dementias.* Any of these chronic degenerative brain diseases can produce fecal incontinence. Associated signs and symptoms include impaired judgment and abstract thinking, amnesia, emotional lability, hyperactive deep tendon reflexes, aphasia or dysarthria, and possibly diffuse choreoathetoid movements.

● *Head trauma.* Disruption of the neurologic pathways that control defecation can cause fecal incontinence. (See *Neurologic control of defecation,* page 246.) Additional findings depend on the location and severity of the injury and may include decreased level of consciousness, seizures, vomiting, and a wide range of motor and sensory impairments.

● *Inflammatory bowel disease.* Nocturnal fecal incontinence occurs occasionally with diarrhea. Related findings may include abdominal pain, anorexia, weight loss, and hyperactive bowel sounds.

● *Rectovaginal fistula.* Fecal incontinence occurs in tandem with uninhibited passage of flatus.

● *Spinal cord lesion.* Any lesion that causes compression or transection of sensorimotor spinal tracts can lead to fecal incontinence. Incontinence may be permanent, especially with severe lesions of the sacral segments. Other signs and symptoms reflect motor and sensory disturbances below the level of the lesion, such as urinary incontinence, weakness or paralysis, paresthesia, and analgesia and thermoanesthesia.

Other causes
● *Drugs.* Chronic laxative abuse may cause insensitivity to a fecal mass or loss of the colonic defecation reflex.

● *Surgery.* Pelvic, prostate, or rectal surgery occasionally produces temporary fecal incontinence. Colostomy or ileostomy causes permanent or temporary fecal incontinence.

Special considerations
Maintain effective hygienic care, including control of foul odors. Also provide emotional support for the patient because he may feel deep embarrassment. For the patient with intermittent or temporary incontinence, encourage Kegel exercises to strengthen abdominal and perirectal muscles. For the neurologically

NEUROLOGIC CONTROL OF DEFECATION

Three neurologic mechanisms normally regulate defecation: the intrinsic defecation reflex in the colon, the parasympathetic defecation reflex involving sacral segments of the spinal cord, and voluntary control. Here's how they interact:

Fecal distention of the rectum activates the relatively weak intrinsic reflex, causing afferent impulses to spread through the myenteric plexus, initiating peristalsis in the descending and sigmoid colons and in the rectum. Subsequent movement of feces toward the anus causes receptive relaxation of the internal anal sphincter.

To ensure defecation, the parasympathetic reflex magnifies the intrinsic reflex. Stimulation of afferent nerves in the rectal wall circles impulses through the spinal cord and back to the descending and sigmoid colons, rectum, and anus to intensify peristalsis (see illustration).

However, fecal movement and internal sphincter relaxation cause immediate contraction of the external anal sphincter and temporary fecal retention. At this point, conscious control of the external sphincter either prevents or permits defecation. Except in the infant or the neurologically impaired patient, this voluntary mechanism further contracts the sphincter to prevent defecation at inappropriate times, or relaxes it, allowing defecation to occur.

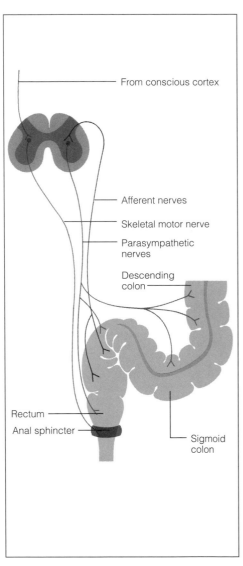

From conscious cortex

Afferent nerves

Skeletal motor nerve

Parasympathetic nerves

Descending colon

Rectum

Anal sphincter

Sigmoid colon

capable patient with chronic incontinence, provide bowel retraining.

Pediatric pointers

Fecal incontinence is normal in an infant and may occur temporarily in a young child who experiences stress-related psychological regression or physical illness with diarrhea. Pediatric fecal incontinence can also result from myclomeningocele.

FETOR HEPATICUS

Fetor hepaticus—a distinctive musty-sweet breath odor—characterizes hepatic encephalopathy, a life-threatening complication of severe liver disease. The odor results from the damaged liver's inability to metabolize and detoxify mercaptans produced by bacterial degradation of methionine, a sulfurous amino acid. As a result, these substances circulate in the blood, are expelled by the lungs, and flavor the breath.

Emergency interventions

 If you detect fetor hepaticus, quickly determine the patient's level of consciousness (LOC). If he's comatose, evaluate his respiratory status. Prepare to intube him and provide ventilatory support if necessary. Start a peripheral I.V. line for fluid administration, begin cardiac monitoring, and insert an indwelling urinary catheter to monitor output. Obtain arterial and venous samples for analysis of blood gas, ammonia, and electrolyte levels.

History and physical examination

If the patient is conscious, closely observe him for signs of impending coma. Evaluate deep tendon reflexes for asterixis, and test for Babinski's sign. Be alert for signs of GI bleeding and shock, common complications of end-stage liver failure. Also watch for increased anxiety, restlessness, tachycardia, tachypnea, hypotension, oliguria, hematemesis, melena, and cool, moist, pale skin. Place the patient in the supine position with his legs elevated 20 degrees, administer oxygen, and increase the infusion rate of I.V. fluids. Draw blood samples for a complete blood count, typing and cross-matching, a clotting profile, and ammonia level. Intubation, ventilation, or cardiopulmonary resuscitation may be necessary.

Continue the physical examination by evaluating the degree of jaundice and abdominal distention and by palpating the liver for degree of enlargement.

Obtain a complete medical history, relying on the patient's family if necessary. Focus on any factors that may have precipitated hepatic disease or coma, such as recent severe infection; overuse of sedatives, analgesics, or diuretics; excessive protein intake; and recent blood transfusion, surgery, or GI bleeding.

Common medical causes

● *Hepatic encephalopathy.* Fetor hepaticus usually occurs in the final stage of this disorder but may occur earlier. Tremors progress to asterixis in the impending stage, along with lethargy, aberrant behavior, and apraxia. Hyperventilation and stupor mark the stuporous stage, and the patient acts agitated when aroused. Seizures and coma herald the final stage, along with decreased pulse and respiratory rates, positive Babinski's sign, hyperactive reflexes, decerebrate posture, and opisthotonos.

Special considerations

Effective treatment of hepatic encephalopathy reduces blood ammonia levels by eliminating ammonia from the GI tract. You may have to administer neomycin or lactulose to suppress bacterial production of ammonia, give sorbitol solution to induce osmotic diarrhea, give potassium supplements to correct alkalosis, provide continuous gastric aspiration of blood, or maintain the patient on a low-protein diet. If these methods aren't successful, hemodialysis or exchange transfusions may be performed.

During treatment, closely monitor the patient's LOC, intake and output, and fluid and electrolyte balance.

Pediatric pointers
A child slipping into a hepatic coma may cry, be disobedient, or become preoccupied with an activity.

FEVER
[Pyrexia]

Because this common sign can arise from disorders affecting virtually every body system, fever alone usually has little diagnostic significance. A persistent high fever, though, is an emergency.

Fever can be classified as low (oral reading of 99° to 100.4° F [37.2° to 38° C]), moderate (100.5° to 104° F [38.1° to 40° C]), or high (above 104° F). A fever over 108° F (42.2° C) causes unconsciousness and, if sustained, leads to permanent brain damage.

Fever may also be classified as remittent, intermittent, sustained, or relapsing. *Remittent fever,* the most common type, is characterized by daily temperature fluctuations above the normal range. *Intermittent fever* is a daily temperature drop into the normal range, then a rise back to above normal. An intermittent fever that fluctuates widely, typically producing chills and sweating, is called a *hectic* or *septic fever. Sustained fever* involves persistent temperature elevation with little fluctuation. *Relapsing fever* consists of alternating feverish and afebrile periods. (See *How fever develops,* pages 250 and 251.)

Further classification involves duration—either brief (less than 3 weeks) or prolonged. Prolonged fevers include fever of unknown origin, a classification used when careful examination fails to detect an underlying cause.

Emergency interventions
 If you detect a fever greater than 106° F (41.1° C), take the patient's other vital signs and determine his level of consciousness (LOC). Administer antipyretic drugs and begin rapid cooling measures: Apply ice packs to the axillae and groin, give tepid sponge baths, or apply a hypothermia blanket. To prevent these measures from evoking a *hypothermic* response, constantly monitor the patient's rectal temperature.

History and physical examination
If the patient's fever is only mild to moderate, ask him when it began and how high it reached. Did the fever disappear and reappear later? Did he experience any other symptoms, such as chills, fatigue, or pain?

Obtain a complete medical history, noting especially immunosuppressive treatments or disorders, infection, trauma, surgery, diagnostic testing, and use of anesthetic or other medications. Ask about recent travel because certain diseases are endemic.

Let the history findings direct your physical examination. Because fever can accompany diverse disorders, this examination may range from a brief evaluation of one body system to a comprehensive review of all systems.

Common medical causes
• *Immune complex dysfunction.* When present, fever usually remains low, although moderate elevations may accompany erythema multiforme. Fever may be remittent or intermittent, as in acquired immunodeficiency syndrome (AIDS) or systemic lupus erythematosus, or sustained, as in polyarteritis. As one of several vague prodromal complaints (such as fatigue, anorexia, and

weight loss), fever produces nocturnal diaphoresis and accompanies such associated signs as diarrhea and persistent cough in AIDS and morning stiffness in rheumatoid arthritis. Other disease-specific findings include headache and possible vision loss (temporal arteritis); pain and stiffness in the neck, shoulders, back, or pelvis (ankylosing spondylitis and polymyalgia rheumatica); skin and mucous membrane lesions (erythema multiforme); and urethritis with urethral discharge and conjunctivitis (Reiter's syndrome).

● *Infectious and inflammatory disorders.* Fever ranges from low (in Crohn's disease and ulcerative colitis) to extremely high (in bacterial pneumonia, necrotizing fasciitis, Ebola virus, and Hantavirus pulmonary syndrome). It may be remittent (as in infectious mononucleosis and otitis media); hectic (as in lung abscess, influenza, and endocarditis); sustained (as in meningitis); or relapsing (as in malaria).

Fever may arise abruptly (as in toxic shock syndrome and Rocky Mountain spotted fever) or insidiously (as in mycoplasmal pneumonia). In hepatitis, fever may represent a disease prodrome; in appendicitis, it follows the acute stage. Its sudden late appearance with tachycardia, tachypnea, and confusion heralds life-threatening septic shock in peritonitis and gram-negative bacteremia.

Associated signs and symptoms involve every system. The cyclic variations of hectic fever typically produce alternating chills and diaphoresis. General systemic complaints include weakness, anorexia, and malaise.

● *Neoplasms.* Primary neoplasms and metastases can produce prolonged fever of varying elevations. For instance, acute leukemia may present insidiously with low fever, pallor, and bleeding tendencies, or more abruptly with high fever, frank bleeding, and prostration. Occasionally, Hodgkin's disease produces Pel-Ebstein fever, an irregularly relapsing fever.

Besides fever and nocturnal diaphoresis, neoplastic disease commonly causes anorexia, fatigue, malaise, and weight loss. Examination may reveal lesions, lymphadenopathy, palpable masses, and hepatosplenomegaly.

● *Thermoregulatory dysfunction.* Sudden onset of fever that rises rapidly and remains as high as 107° F (41.7° C) occurs in life-threatening disorders, such as heatstroke, thyroid storm, and malignant hyperthermia, and in lesions of the central nervous system (CNS). Low or moderate fever appears in dehydration.

Prolonged high fever commonly produces vomiting; anhidrosis; hot, flushed skin; and decreased LOC. Related cardiovascular effects may include tachycardia, tachypnea, or hypotension. Other disease-specific findings may include skin changes—dry skin and mucous membranes and poor skin turgor in dehydration, mottled cyanosis in malignant hyperthermia, diarrhea in thyroid storm, oliguria in dehydration, and ominous signs of increased intracranial pressure (decreased LOC with bradycardia, widened pulse pressure, and increased systolic pressure) in CNS tumor, trauma, or hemorrhage.

Other causes

● *Diagnostic tests.* Immediate or delayed fever infrequently follows radiographic tests that use a contrast medium.

● *Drugs.* Fever and rash commonly result from hypersensitivity to antifungals, sulfonamides, penicillins, cephalosporins, tetracyclines, barbiturates, phenytoin, quinidine, iodides, phenolphthalein, methyldopa, procainamide, and some antitoxins. Fever can also accompany chemotherapy, especially with bleomycin, vincristine, and asparaginase. It can result from drugs that impair sweating, such as anticholinergics, phenothiazines, and monoamine oxidase inhibitors. Fever can also stem from toxic doses of salicylates,

HOW FEVER DEVELOPS

Body temperature is regulated by the hypothalamic thermostat, which has a specific set point under normal conditions. Fever can result from a resetting of this set point or from an abnormality in the thermoregulatory system itself, as shown in this flowchart.

Disruption of hypothalamic thermostat by:
- central nervous system disease
- inherited malignant hyperthermia

Increased production of heat from:
- strenuous exercise or other stress
- chills (skeletal muscle response)
- thyrotoxicosis

Decreased loss of heat from:
- anhidrotic asthenia (heatstroke)
- heart failure
- skin conditions, such as ichthyosis and congenital absence of sweat glands
- drugs that impair sweating

Body invaded by exogenous pyrogens such as bacteria, viruses, or immune complexes

Production of endogenous pyrogens

amphetamines, or tricyclic antidepressants.

Inhalant anesthetics and muscle relaxants can trigger malignant hyperthermia in patients with this inherited trait.
- **Treatments.** After surgery, remittent or intermittent low fever may occur for several days. Transfusion reactions characteristically produce abrupt onset of fever and chills.

Special considerations
Regularly monitor the patient's temperature. Provide increased fluid and nutritional intake. When administering prescribed antipyretic drugs, minimize resultant chills and diaphoresis by following a regular dosage schedule. Promote patient comfort by maintaining a stable room temperature and providing frequent bedding and clothing changes.

with varicella or flulike symptoms because of the risk of precipitating Reye's syndrome.

Common pediatric causes of fever include varicella, croup, dehydration, meningitis, mumps, otitis media, pertussis, roseola infantum, rubella, rubeola, and tonsillitis. Fever can also occur as a reaction to immunizations and antibiotics.

FLANK PAIN

Pain in the flank, the area extending from the ribs to the ilium, is a leading indicator of renal and upper urinary tract disease or trauma. Depending on the cause, this symptom may vary from a dull ache to severe stabbing or throbbing pain, and may be unilateral or bilateral and constant or intermittent. It's aggravated by costovertebral angle (CVA) percussion and, in patients with renal or urinary tract obstruction, by increased fluid intake or ingestion of alcohol, caffeine, and diuretic drugs. Unaffected by position changes, flank pain typically responds only to analgesics or to treatment of the underlying disorder.

Emergency interventions

 If the patient has suffered trauma, quickly look for a visible or palpable flank mass, associated injuries, CVA pain, hematuria, Grey Turner's sign, and signs of shock (such as tachycardia and cool, clammy skin). If any of these is present, insert an I.V. line to allow fluid or drug infusion. Insert an indwelling urinary catheter to monitor urine output and evaluate hematuria. Obtain blood samples for typing and crossmatching, complete blood count, and electrolyte levels.

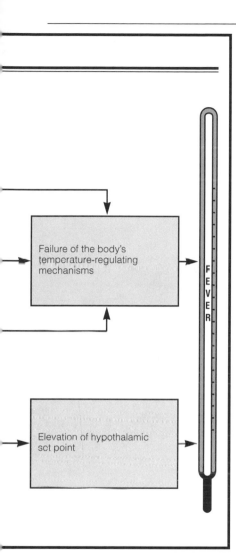

Failure of the body's temperature-regulating mechanisms

FEVER

Elevation of hypothalamic set point

Pediatric pointers

Infants and young children experience higher and more prolonged fevers, more rapid temperature increases, and greater temperature fluctuations than older children and adults.

Keep in mind that seizures commonly accompany extremely high fever, so take appropriate precautions. Also, instruct parents not to give aspirin to a child

FLANK PAIN: COMMON CAUSES AND ASSOCIATED FINDINGS

CAUSES	MAJOR ASSOCIATED SIGNS AND SYMPTOMS										
	Abdominal distention	Abdominal mass	Abdominal pain	Anuria	Back pain	Bladder distention	Blood pressure, decreased	Blood pressure, increased	Bowel sounds, hypoactive	Chills	Costovertebral angle tenderness
Calculi			●		●				●		●
Cortical necrosis (acute)				●							
Obstructive uropathy	●	●	●	●		●			●		●
Papillary necrosis (acute)			●	●					●	●	●
Polycystic kidney disease					●			●			
Pyelonephritis (acute)			●							●	●
Renal infarction			●	●					●		●
Renal neoplasm								●			
Renal trauma	●		●						●		●
Renal vein thrombosis					●						●

History and physical examination

If the patient's condition isn't critical, take a thorough history. Ask about the onset of the flank pain and apparent precipitating events. Have him describe the pain's location, intensity, pattern, and duration. Find out if anything aggravates or alleviates it.

Ask the patient about any changes in his normal pattern of fluid intake and urine output. Explore his history for urinary tract infection (UTI) or obstruction, renal disease, or recent streptococcal infection.

During the physical examination, palpate the patient's flank area and percuss the CVA to determine the extent of pain.

Common medical causes

● *Calculi.* Renal and ureteral calculi produce intense unilateral, colicky flank pain. Typically, initial CVA pain radiates to the flank, suprapubic region, and perhaps the genitalia, with abdominal and low back pain also possible. Nausea and vomiting commonly accompany severe pain. Associated findings include CVA tenderness, hematuria, hypoactive bowel

	Dysuria	Edema, generalized	Fatigue	Fever	Flank mass	Groin pain	Hematuria	Leg pain	Nausea	Nocturia	Oliguria	Perineal pain	Polyuria	Pyuria	Suprapubic pain	Tenesmus	Urinary frequency	Urinary urgency	Urine retention	Vomiting
	●		●	●		●	●		●	●					●	●	●	●		●
				●			●													
							●	●		●			●							●
				●			●				●			●						●
							●				●	●			●	●	●	●		
	●		●	●			●			●					●		●	●		
				●					●		●									●
				●	●		●		●										●	●
					●	●	●		●		●									●
				●			●		●		●									●

sounds, and possibly signs and symptoms of UTI (urinary frequency and urgency, dysuria, nocturia, fatigue, low-grade fever, and tenesmus).

● *Cortical necrosis (acute).* Unilateral flank pain is usually severe. Accompanying findings include gross hematuria, anuria, and fever.

● *Obstructive uropathy.* In acute obstruction, flank pain may be excruciating; in gradual obstruction, it's typically a dull ache. In both, the pain may also localize in the upper abdomen and may radiate to the groin. Nausea and vomiting, abdominal distention, anuria alternating with periods of oliguria and polyuria, and hypoactive bowel sounds may also occur. Additional findings depend on the site and cause of the obstruction; they may include a palpable abdominal mass, CVA tenderness, and bladder distention.

● *Papillary necrosis (acute).* Intense bilateral flank pain occurs along with renal colic, CVA tenderness, and abdominal pain and rigidity. Possible urinary signs include oliguria or anuria, hematuria, and pyuria, with associated high fever, chills, vomiting, and hypoactive bowel sounds.

• *Polycystic kidney disease.* In many patients, dull, aching, bilateral flank pain is the earliest symptom. The pain can become severe and colicky if cysts rupture and clots migrate or cause obstruction. Nonspecific early findings include polyuria, increased blood pressure, and signs of UTI. Later findings include hematuria and perineal, low back, and suprapubic pain.

• *Pyelonephritis (acute).* Intense, constant, unilateral or bilateral flank pain develops over a few hours or days along with typical urinary features: dysuria, nocturia, hematuria, urgency, frequency, and tenesmus. Other common findings include persistent high fever, chills, anorexia, weakness, fatigue, generalized myalgia, abdominal pain, and marked CVA tenderness.

• *Renal infarction.* Unilateral, constant, severe flank pain and tenderness typically accompany persistent, severe upper abdominal pain. The patient may also have CVA tenderness, anorexia, nausea, and vomiting. Fever, hypoactive bowel sounds, hematuria, and oliguria or anuria may also develop.

• *Renal neoplasm.* Unilateral flank pain, gross hematuria, and a palpable flank mass form the classic clinical triad. Flank pain is usually dull and vague, although severe colicky pain can occur during bleeding or passage of clots. Possible associated signs and symptoms include fever, increased blood pressure, and urine retention. Weight loss, leg edema, nausea, and vomiting point to advanced disease.

• *Renal trauma.* Variable bilateral or unilateral flank pain is a common symptom. A visible or palpable flank mass may also exist, along with CVA or abdominal pain—possibly severe and radiating to the groin. Other findings include hematuria, oliguria, abdominal distention, positive Grey Turner's sign, hypoactive bowel sounds, and nausea or vomiting. Severe injury may produce signs of shock, such as tachycardia and cool, clammy skin.

• *Renal vein thrombosis.* Severe unilateral flank and low back pain with CVA and epigastric tenderness typify the rapid onset of venous obstruction. Other features include fever, hematuria, and leg edema. Bilateral flank pain, oliguria, and other uremic signs and symptoms (nausea, vomiting, and uremic fetor) typify bilateral obstruction.

Special considerations
Administer prescribed pain medications. Continue to monitor the patient's vital signs, and maintain precise intake and output records.

Diagnostic evaluation may involve serial urine and serum analysis, excretory urography, flank ultrasonography, computed tomography scan, voiding cystourethrography, cystoscopy, and retrograde ureteropyelography, urethrography, and cystography.

Pediatric pointers
Assessment of flank pain can be difficult if the child can't describe the pain. In such cases, transillumination of the abdomen and flank may help assess bladder distention and identify masses. Common causes of flank pain in children include obstructive uropathy, acute poststreptococcal glomerulonephritis, infantile polycystic kidney disease, and nephroblastoma.

FONTANEL BULGING

In a normal infant, the anterior fontanel, or soft spot, is flat, soft yet firm, and well demarcated against surrounding skull bones. (The posterior fontanel, if not fused at birth, usually closes by age 2 months.) Subtle pulsations may be visible, reflecting the arterial pulse. A bulging

LOCATING FONTANELS

The anterior fontanel lies at the junction of the sagittal, coronal, and frontal sutures. It normally measures about 2.5 cm (1″) by 4 to 5 cm (1½″ to 2″) at birth and usually closes by age 18 to 20 months.

The posterior fontanel lies at the junction of the sagittal and lambdoidal sutures. If it hasn't already fused by the time of birth, it measures 1 to 2 cm (³/₈″ to ³/₄″) and normally closes by age 2 months.

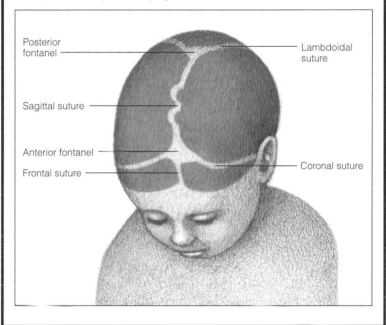

fontanel—widened, tense, and with marked pulsations—is a cardinal sign of meningitis associated with increased intracranial pressure (ICP), a medical emergency. Because prolonged coughing, crying, or lying down can cause transient, physiologic bulging, the infant's head should be observed and palpated while he's upright and relaxed to detect pathologic bulging. (See *Locating fontanels.*)

Emergency interventions

If you detect a bulging fontanel, measure fontanel size and head circumference, and note the overall shape of the head. Take vital signs and determine level of consciousness (LOC) by observing sensory responses, spontaneous activity, and postural reflex activity. Note whether the infant assumes a normal, flexed posture or one of extreme extension, opisthotonos, or hypotonia. Observe movements of his arms and legs—excessive tremulousness or frequent twitching may herald the onset of a seizure. Look for other signs of increased ICP—abnormal respiratory patterns and a distinctive, high-pitched cry.

Ensure airway patency, and have size-appropriate emergency equipment on hand. Provide oxygen, establish I.V. access and, if the infant is having a seizure, stay with him to prevent injury and administer anticonvulsants. Administer antibiotics, antipyretics, and osmotic diuretics to help reduce cerebral edema and ICP, and dexamethasone for edema secondary to head trauma. If these measures fail to reduce ICP, neuromuscular blockage, intubation, mechanical ventilation and, in rare cases, barbiturate coma and total body hypothermia may be necessary.

History
Once the infant's condition is stabilized, you can begin investigating the underlying cause of increased ICP. Obtain his medical history from a parent or caregiver, paying particular attention to any recent infection or trauma, including birth trauma. Has the infant or any family member had a recent rash or fever? Ask about any changes in the infant's behavior, such as frequent vomiting, lethargy, or disinterest in feeding.

Common medical causes
• *Increased ICP.* Besides a bulging fontanel and increased head circumference, other early signs and symptoms are commonly subtle and difficult to discern. They may include behavioral changes, irritability, and fatigue.

As ICP rises, the infant's pupils may dilate and his LOC may decrease to drowsiness and eventual coma. Seizures commonly occur.

Special considerations
Closely monitor the infant's condition, including urine output (by an indwelling catheter if necessary), and continue to observe for seizures. Restrict fluids and

place the infant in the supine position at a 30-degree head-up tilt to enhance cerebral venous drainage and reduce intracranial blood volume.

Explain the purpose and procedure of diagnostic tests to the infant's parents or caregiver. Such tests may include intracranial computed tomography or skull X-ray, cerebral angiography, and a full sepsis workup, including blood and urine cultures.

FONTANEL DEPRESSION

Depression of the anterior fontanel below the surrounding bony ridges of the skull is a sign of dehydration. A common disorder of infancy and early childhood, dehydration can result from insufficient fluid intake but typically reflects excessive fluid loss from severe vomiting or diarrhea. It may also reflect insensible water loss, pyloric stenosis, or tracheoesophageal fistula.

Emergency interventions
 If you detect a markedly depressed fontanel, take vital signs, weigh the infant, and check for signs of shock (tachycardia, tachypnea, and cool, clammy skin). If these signs are present, insert an I.V. line and administer fluids. Have size-appropriate emergency equipment at hand. Anticipate oxygen administration. Monitor urine output by weighing wet diapers.

History
Obtain a thorough patient history from a parent or caretaker, focusing on recent fever, vomiting, diarrhea, and behavioral changes. Monitor the infant's fluid intake and urine output—including the number of wet diapers—over the past 24 hours. Ask about the infant's pre-illness weight, and compare it with his current weight;

weight loss in an infant reflects water loss.

Common medical causes

● *Dehydration.* In *mild dehydration* (5% weight loss), the anterior fontanel appears slightly depressed. The infant has decreased urine output, a normal or slightly elevated pulse rate, possibly a decreased level of activity, and pale, dry skin and mucous membranes.

Moderate dehydration (10% weight loss) causes slightly more pronounced fontanel depression, along with gray skin with poor turgor, dry mucous membranes, and decreased urine output. The infant has normal or decreased blood pressure, an increased pulse rate, and may be lethargic.

Severe dehydration (15% or greater weight loss) may result in a markedly depressed fontanel, along with extremely poor skin turgor, parched mucous membranes, marked oliguria, lethargy, and signs of shock.

Special considerations

Continue to monitor the infant's vital signs and intake and output, and watch for signs of worsening dehydration. Obtain serum electrolyte values to check for increased or decreased sodium, chloride, or potassium levels. In mild dehydration, frequently provide small amounts of clear fluids. If the infant is unable to ingest sufficient fluid, begin I.V. parenteral nutrition.

In moderate or severe dehydration, your first priority is rapid restoration of extracellular fluid volume to treat or prevent shock. Continue to administer I.V. solution with sodium bicarbonate added to combat acidosis. As renal function improves, administer I.V. potassium replacement. Once the infant's fluid status stabilizes, begin to replace depleted fat and protein stores through diet.

Other tests to evaluate dehydration include urinalysis to determine specific gravity and blood tests to determine blood urea nitrogen and serum creatinine levels, osmolality, and acid-base status.

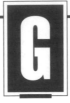

GAG REFLEX ABNORMALITIES
[Pharyngeal reflex abnormalities]

The gag reflex—a protective mechanism that prevents aspiration of food, fluid, and vomitus—normally can be elicited by touching the posterior wall of the oropharynx with a tongue depressor or by suctioning the throat. Prompt elevation of the palate, constriction of the pharyngeal musculature, and a sensation of gagging indicate a normal gag reflex. An abnormal gag reflex—either decreased or absent—interferes with the ability to swallow and, more important, increases susceptibility to life-threatening aspiration.

An impaired gag reflex can result from any lesion affecting its mediators—cranial nerves IX (glossopharyngeal) and X (vagus) or the pons or medulla. It can also occur in a coma or temporarily as a result of anesthesia.

Emergency interventions

 If you detect an abnormal gag reflex, immediately stop the patient's oral intake to prevent aspiration. Quickly evaluate his level of consciousness (LOC). If decreased, place him in a side-lying position to prevent aspiration; if not, place him in Fowler's position. Have suction equipment at hand.

History and physical examination

Ask the patient (or a family member if the patient is unable to communicate) about the onset and duration of swallowing difficulties. Is it more difficult to swallow liquids than solids? Is swallowing more difficult at certain times of the day (as occurs in bulbar palsy associated with myasthenia gravis)? If he also has trouble chewing, suspect more widespread neurologic involvement because chewing involves different cranial nerves.

Explore the patient's medical history for vascular and degenerative disorders. Then assess his respiratory status for evidence of aspiration, and perform a neurologic examination.

Common medical causes

- **Basilar artery occlusion.** This disorder may suddenly diminish or obliterate the gag reflex. It also causes diffuse sensory loss, dysarthria, facial weakness, extraocular muscle palsies, quadriplegia, and decreased LOC.
- **Brain stem glioma.** This lesion causes gradual loss of the gag reflex. Related symptoms reflect bilateral brain stem involvement and include diplopia and facial weakness. Common involvement of the corticospinal pathways causes spasticity and paresis of the arms and legs as well as gait disturbances.
- **Bulbar palsy.** Loss of the gag reflex reflects temporary or permanent paralysis of muscles supplied by cranial nerves IX and X. Other indicators of this paralysis include jaw and facial muscle weakness, dysphagia, loss of sensation at the base of the tongue, increased salivation, possible difficulty articulating and breathing, and fasciculations.
- **Wallenberg's syndrome.** Paresis of the palate and an impaired gag reflex usually develop within hours to days of throm-

bosis. The patient may have analgesia and thermoanesthesia, occurring ipsilaterally on the face and contralaterally on the body, as well as vertigo. He may also display nystagmus, ipsilateral ataxia of the arm and leg, and signs of Horner's syndrome (unilateral ptosis and miosis, and hemifacial anhidrosis).

Other causes
● *Anesthesia.* General and local (throat) anesthesia can produce temporary loss of the gag reflex.

Special considerations
Continually assess the patient's ability to swallow. If his gag reflex is absent, provide tube feedings; if it's merely diminished, try pureed foods. Advise the patient to eat small amounts slowly while in a high Fowler or sitting position. Stay with him while he eats and observe for choking. Remember to keep suction equipment handy in case of aspiration. Keep accurate intake and output records, and assess the patient's nutritional status daily.

Prepare the patient for diagnostic studies, such as computed tomography scan, EEG, lumbar puncture, and arteriography.

Pediatric pointers
Brain stem glioma is a major cause of abnormal gag reflex in children.

GAIT, BIZARRE
[Hysterical gait]

A bizarre gait has no obvious organic basis—rather, it's produced unconsciously by a person with a somatoform disorder (hysterical neurosis) or consciously by a malingerer. The gait has no consistent pattern. It may mimic an organic impairment but characteristically has a more theatrical or bizarre quality with key elements missing—such as a spastic gait without hip circumduction, or leg "paralysis" with normal reflexes and motor strength. Its manifestations may include wild gyrations, exaggerated stepping, leg dragging, or mimicking of unusual walks such as that of a tightrope walker.

History and physical examination
If you suspect that the patient's bizarre gait has no organic cause, begin to investigate other possibilities. Ask the patient when he first developed the unusual gait and whether it coincided with any stressful period or event, such as the death of a loved one or loss of a job. Ask about associated symptoms, and explore any reports of frequent unexplained illnesses and multiple doctor's visits. Subtly try to determine if he'll achieve any gain from malingering, such as added attention or an insurance settlement.

Begin the physical examination by testing the patient's reflexes and sensorimotor function, noting any abnormal response patterns. To quickly check complaints of leg weakness or paralysis, test for Hoover's sign: Place the patient in the supine position and stand at his feet. Cradle a heel in each of your palms, and rest your hands on the table. Ask the patient to raise the affected leg. If he has true motor weakness, the heel of the other leg will press downward; in hysteria or malingering, this movement will be absent. As a further check, observe the patient for normal movements when he's unaware of being watched.

Common medical causes
● *Conversion disorder.* In this rare somatoform disorder, bizarre gait or paralysis may develop after severe stress and is not accompanied by other symptoms. The patient typically seems indifferent toward his impairment.
● *Malingering.* In this rare cause of bizarre gait, the patient may also com-

plain of headache and chest and back pain.

• *Somatization disorder.* Bizarre gait is one of many possible somatic complaints. The patient may exhibit any combination of pseudoneurologic signs and symptoms, such as fainting, weakness, memory loss, dysphagia, visual problems (diplopia, vision loss, blurred vision), loss of voice, seizures, and bladder dysfunction. He may also report pain in the back, joints, and extremities (most commonly the legs) and other complaints in almost any body system. Characteristic GI complaints include pain, bloating, nausea, and vomiting.

The patient's reflexes and motor strength remain normal, but peculiar contractures and arm or leg rigidity may occur. His reputed sensory loss doesn't conform to any known sensory dermatome. In some cases, he won't stand or walk (astasia-abasia), remaining bedridden although still able to move his legs in bed.

Special considerations

A full neurologic workup may be necessary to rule out an organic cause of the patient's abnormal gait.

Remember, even though bizarre gait has no organic basis, it's real to the patient (unless, of course, he's malingering). Avoid expressing judgment about the patient's actions or motives; instead, be supportive and reinforce progress. Because muscle atrophy and bone demineralization can develop in the bedridden patient, encourage the patient to walk and resume his normal activities. Refer him for psychiatric counseling if appropriate.

Pediatric pointers

Bizarre gait is rare before age 8. More common in prepubescence, it usually results from a conversion disorder.

GAIT, PROPULSIVE
[Festinating gait]

Propulsive gait is characterized by a stooped, rigid posture—the patient's head and neck are bent forward, his flexed, stiffened arms are held away from the body, his fingers are extended, and his knees and hips are stiffly bent. During ambulation, this posture results in a forward shifting of the body's center of gravity and consequent impairment of balance, causing increasingly rapid, short, shuffling steps with involuntary acceleration (festination) and lack of control over forward motion (propulsion) or backward motion (retropulsion). (See *Identifying gait abnormalities.*)

Propulsive gait is a cardinal sign of advanced Parkinson's disease, resulting from progressive degeneration of the ganglia, which are primarily responsible for smooth-muscle movement. Because this sign develops gradually and its accompanying effects are often wrongly attributed to aging, propulsive gait often goes unnoticed or unreported until severe disability results.

History and physical examination

Ask the patient when his gait impairment first developed and whether it has recently worsened. Because he may have difficulty remembering, having attributed the gait to "old age," try to obtain information from family members or friends, especially those who see the patient only sporadically.

Also obtain a thorough drug history, including both medication type and dosage. Ask the patient if he has been taking any tranquilizers, especially phenothiazines. If the patient knows he has Parkinson's disease and has been taking levodopa, pay particular attention to the dosage because an overdose can cause

IDENTIFYING GAIT ABNORMALITIES

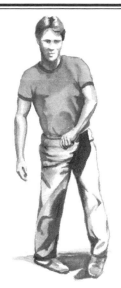

Spastic gait

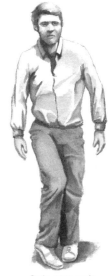

Scissors gait

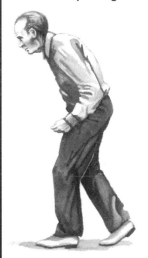

Propulsive gait

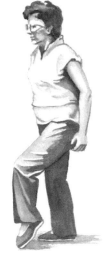

Steppage gait

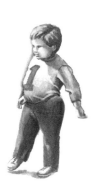

Waddling gait

acute exacerbation of signs and symptoms.

If Parkinson's disease isn't a known or suspected diagnosis, ask the patient if he has been acutely or routinely exposed to carbon monoxide or manganese.

During the physical examination, test and compare strength, range of motion, and sensory function in all extremities.

Common medical causes

• *Carbon monoxide poisoning.* Propulsive gait commonly appears several weeks after acute carbon monoxide intoxication. Earlier effects include muscle rigidity, choreoathetoid movements, generalized seizures, myoclonic jerks, masklike facies, and dementia.

• *Manganese poisoning.* Chronic overexposure to manganese can cause an insidious, usually permanent, propulsive gait. Typical early findings include fatigue, muscle weakness and rigidity, dystonia, resting tremor, choreoathetoid movements, masklike facies, and personality changes.

• *Parkinson's disease.* The characteristic and permanent propulsive gait begins early as a shuffle. As the disease progresses, the gait slows. Cardinal signs of the disease are progressive muscle rigidity, which may be uniform (lead-pipe rigidity) or jerky (cogwheel rigidity); akinesia; and an insidious tremor that begins in the fingers, increases during stress or anxiety, and decreases with purposeful movement and sleep. Besides the gait, akinesia also typically produces a monotone voice, drooling, masklike facies, stooped posture, and dysarthria or dysphagia (or both). Occasionally, it also causes oculogyric crises or blepharospasm.

Other causes

• *Drugs.* Propulsive gait and other extrapyramidal effects can result from use of phenothiazines, other antipsychotics (notably haloperidol, thiothixene, and loxapine) and, infrequently, metoclopramide and metyrosine. Such effects are usually temporary, disappearing within a few weeks after therapy ends.

Special considerations

Because of his gait and associated motor impairment, the patient may have problems performing activities of daily living. Assist him as appropriate, while encouraging his independence and self-reliance. Instruct the patient and his family to allow plenty of time for these activities, especially walking, because he's particularly susceptible to falls resulting from festination and poor balance. Encourage the patient to walk; for safety reasons, remember to stay with him while he's walking, especially if he's on unfamiliar or uneven ground. You may need to refer him to a physical therapist for exercise therapy and gait retraining.

Pediatric pointers

Propulsive gait, usually with severe tremors, typically occurs in juvenile parkinsonism, a rare form. Other rarer causes are Hallervorden-Spatz disease and kernicterus.

GAIT, SCISSORS

Resulting from bilateral spastic paresis (diplegia), scissors gait affects both legs and has little or no effect on the arms. The patient's legs flex slightly at the hips and knees, so he looks like he's crouching. With each step, his thighs adduct and his knees hit or cross in a scissorslike movement. Steps are short, regular, and laborious, as if he were wading through waist-deep water. His feet may be plantar-flexed and turned inward, with a shortened Achilles tendon; as a result, he walks on his toes or the balls of his feet and may scrape his toes on the ground.

History and physical examination

Ask the patient (or a family member, if the patient can't answer) about the onset and duration of the gait. Has it progressively worsened or remained constant? Ask about a history of trauma, including birth trauma, and neurologic disorders. Thoroughly evaluate motor and sensory function and deep tendon reflexes in the legs.

Common medical causes

• *Cerebral palsy.* In the spastic form of this disorder, patients walk on their toes with a scissors gait. Other features include hyperactive deep tendon reflexes, increased stretch reflexes, rapid alternating muscle contraction and relaxation, muscle weakness, underdevelopment of affected limbs, and a tendency toward contractures.

• *Cervical spondylosis with myelopathy.* Scissors gait develops in the late stages of this degenerative disease and steadily worsens. Related findings mimic those of a herniated disk: severe low back pain, which may radiate to the buttocks, legs, and feet; muscle spasms; sensorimotor loss; and muscle weakness and atrophy.

• *Multiple sclerosis.* Progressive scissors gait usually develops gradually, with infrequent remissions. Characteristic muscle weakness, usually in the legs, ranges from minor fatigability to paraparesis with urinary urgency and constipation. Related findings include facial pain, visual disturbances, paresthesia, incoordination, and loss of proprioception and vibration sensation in the ankle and toes.

• *Spinal cord tumor.* Scissors gait can develop gradually from a thoracic or lumbar tumor. Other findings reflect the location of the tumor and may include radicular, subscapular, shoulder, groin, leg, or flank pain; muscle spasms or fasciculations; muscle atrophy; sensory deficits, such as paresthesia and a girdle sensation on the abdomen and chest; hyperactive deep tendon reflexes; bilateral Babinski's reflex; spastic, neurogenic bladder; and sexual dysfunction.

• *Syphilitic meningomyelitis.* Scissors gait appears late in this disorder and may improve with treatment. The patient may also experience sensory ataxia, changes in proprioception and vibration sensation, optic atrophy, and dementia.

• *Syringomyelia.* Scissors gait usually occurs late, along with analgesia and thermoanesthesia, muscle atrophy and weakness, and Charcot's joints. Other effects may include Dupuytren's contracture of the palms, scoliosis, clubfoot, and loss of fingernails, fingers, or toes. Skin in the affected areas is commonly dry, scaly, and grooved.

Special considerations

Because of the sensory loss associated with scissors gait, provide meticulous skin care to prevent skin breakdown and decubitus formation. Also give the patient and his family complete skin care instructions. If appropriate, provide bladder and bowel retraining.

Provide daily active and passive range-of-motion exercises. If appropriate, refer the patient to a physical therapist for gait retraining and for possible in shoe splints or leg braces to maintain proper foot alignment for standing and walking.

Pediatric pointers

The major causes of scissors gait in children are cerebral palsy, hereditary spastic paraplegia, and spinal injury at birth. If spastic paraparesis is present at birth, scissors gait becomes apparent when the child begins to walk, which is usually later than normal.

GAIT, SPASTIC
[Hemiplegic gait]

Spastic gait—sometimes referred to as paretic or weak gait—is a stiff, foot-dragging walk caused by unilateral leg muscle hypertonicity. It indicates focal damage to the corticospinal tract. The affected leg becomes rigid, with a marked decrease in flexion at the hip and knee and possibly plantar flexion and equinovarus deformity of the foot. Because the patient's leg doesn't swing normally at the hip or knee, his foot tends to drag or shuffle, scraping his toes on the ground. To compensate, the pelvis of the affected side tilts upward in an attempt to lift the toes, causing the patient's leg to abduct and circumduct. Also, arm swing is hindered on the same side as the affected leg.

Spastic gait usually develops after a period of flaccidity (hypotonicity) in the affected leg. Whatever the cause, the gait is usually permanent once it develops.

History and physical examination
Find out when the patient first noticed the gait impairment and whether it developed suddenly or gradually. Ask him if it waxes and wanes or if it has worsened progressively. Do fatigue, hot weather, or warm baths or showers worsen the gait? Such exacerbation typically occurs in multiple sclerosis. Focus your medical history questions on neurologic disorders, recent head trauma, and degenerative diseases.

During the physical examination, test and compare strength, range of motion, and sensory function in all limbs. Also observe and palpate for muscle flaccidity or atrophy.

Common medical causes
• *Brain tumor.* Depending on the site and type of tumor, spastic gait usually develops gradually and worsens over time. Accompanying effects may include signs of increased intracranial pressure (headache, nausea, vomiting, and focal or generalized seizures), papilledema, sensory loss on the affected side, dysarthria, ocular palsies, aphasia, and personality changes.

• *Cerebrovascular accident.* Spastic gait usually appears after a period of muscle weakness and hypotonicity on the affected side. Associated effects may include unilateral muscle atrophy, sensory loss, footdrop, aphasia, dysarthria, dysphagia, visual field deficits, diplopia, and ocular palsies.

• *Head trauma.* Spastic gait typically follows the acute stage of head trauma. The patient may also have focal or generalized seizures, personality changes, headache, and focal neurologic signs, such as aphasia and visual field deficits.

• *Multiple sclerosis.* Spastic gait begins insidiously and follows this disorder's characteristic cycle of remission and exacerbation. The gait and other signs and symptoms tend to worsen in warm weather or after a warm bath or shower. Characteristic weakness, usually affecting the legs, ranges from minor fatigability to paraparesis with urinary urgency and constipation. Other effects include facial pain, paresthesia, incoordination, loss of proprioception and vibration sensation in the ankle and toes, and visual disturbances.

Special considerations
Because leg muscle contractures are commonly associated with spastic gait, promote daily exercise—both active and passive. If appropriate, refer the patient to a physical therapist for gait retraining and possible in-shoe splints or leg braces to maintain proper foot alignment for standing and walking.

The patient may have poor balance and a tendency to fall to the paralyzed side, so stay with him while he's walking. Provide a cane or a walker, as indicated.

Pediatric pointers
Causes of spastic gait in children include sickle cell crisis, cerebral palsy, porencephalic cysts, and arteriovenous malformation that causes hemorrhage or ischemia.

GAIT, STEPPAGE

[Equine gait, paretic gait, prancing gait, weak gait]

Steppage gait typically results from footdrop caused by weakness or paralysis of pretibial and peroneal muscles, usually from lower motor neuron lesions. Footdrop causes the foot to hang with the toes pointing down, causing the toes to scrape the ground during ambulation. To compensate, the hip rotates outward and the hip and knee flex in an exaggerated fashion to lift the advancing leg off the ground. The foot is thrown forward and the toes hit the ground first, producing an audible slap. The rhythm of the gait is usually regular, with even steps and normal upper body posture and arm swing. Steppage gait can be unilateral or bilateral and permanent or transient, depending on the site and type of neural damage.

History and physical examination

Begin by asking the patient about the onset of the gait and any recent changes in its character. Find out if any family member has a similar gait. Also find out if the patient has had any traumatic injury to the buttocks, hips, legs, or knees. Ask about a history of chronic disorders that may be associated with polyneuropathy, such as diabetes mellitus, polyarteritis nodosa, or alcoholism. While you're taking the history, observe whether the patient crosses his legs while sitting because this may put pressure on the peroneal nerve.

Inspect and palpate the patient's calves and feet for muscle atrophy and wasting. Using a pin, test for sensory deficits along the entire length of both legs.

Common medical causes

• *Guillain-Barré syndrome.* Typically occurring after recovery from the acute stage of this disorder, steppage gait can be mild or severe, and unilateral or bilateral; it's invariably permanent. In this disorder, muscle weakness usually begins in the legs, extends to the arms and face within 72 hours, and can progress to total motor paralysis and respiratory failure. Other effects include footdrop, transient paresthesia, hypernasality, dysphagia, diaphoresis, tachycardia, orthostatic hypotension, and incontinence.

• *Herniated lumbar disk.* Unilateral steppage gait and footdrop commonly occur with late-stage weakness and atrophy of leg muscles. However, the most pronounced symptom is severe low back pain, which may radiate to the buttocks, legs, and feet, usually unilaterally. Sciatic pain follows, commonly accompanied by muscle spasms and sensorimotor loss. Paresthesia and fasciculations may occur.

• *Multiple sclerosis.* Steppage gait and footdrop typically fluctuate in severity with this disorder's cycle of periodic exacerbations and remissions. Muscle weakness, usually affecting the legs, can range from minor fatigability to paraparesis with urinary urgency and constipation. Related findings include facial pain, visual disturbances, paresthesia, incoordination, and sensory loss in the ankle and toes.

• *Peroneal muscle atrophy.* Bilateral steppage gait and footdrop begin insidiously in this disorder. Foot, peroneal, and ankle dorsiflexor muscles are affected first. Other early signs and symptoms include paresthesia, aching, and cramping in the feet and legs along with coldness, swelling, and cyanosis. As the disorder progresses, all leg muscles become weak and atrophic, with hypoactive or absent deep tendon reflexes. Later, atrophy and sensory losses spread to the hands and arms.

• *Peroneal nerve trauma.* Temporary ipsilateral steppage gait occurs suddenly but resolves with the release of peroneal nerve pressure. It's associated with footdrop and muscle weakness and sensory loss over the lateral surface of the calf and foot.

Special considerations

The patient with steppage gait may tire rapidly when walking because of the extra effort he must expend to lift his feet off the ground. And when he tires, he may stub his toes, causing a fall. To prevent this, help the patient recognize his exercise limits, and encourage him to get adequate rest. Refer him to a physical therapist, if appropriate, for gait retraining and possible application of in-shoe splints or leg braces to maintain correct foot alignment.

Pediatric pointers

Bilateral steppage gait in children may result from Jering-Soppof disease, a rare progressive neuritis.

GAIT, WADDLING

Waddling gait, a distinctive ducklike walk, is an important sign of muscular dystrophy, spinal muscle atrophy or, rarely, congenital hip displacement. It may be present when the child begins to walk or may appear only later in life. The gait results from deterioration of the pelvic girdle muscles—primarily the gluteus medius, hip flexors, and hip extensors. Weakness in these muscles hinders stabilization of the weight-bearing hip during walking, causing the opposite hip to drop and the trunk to lean toward that side in an attempt to maintain balance.

Typically, the legs assume a wide stance and the trunk is thrown back to further improve stability, exaggerating lordosis and abdominal protrusion. In severe cases, leg and foot muscle contractures may cause equinovarus deformity of the foot combined with circumduction or bowing of the legs.

History and physical examination

Ask the patient (or a family member, if the patient is a young child) when the gait first appeared and if it has recently worsened. To determine the extent of pelvic girdle and leg muscle weakness, ask if the patient falls frequently or has difficulty climbing stairs, rising from a chair, or walking. Also find out if the patient was late in learning to walk or holding his head upright. Obtain a family history, focusing on problems of muscle weakness and gait and on congenital motor disorders.

Inspect and palpate the leg muscles, especially in the calves, for size and tone. Check for a positive Gower's sign. Next, assess motor strength and function in the shoulders, arms, and hands, looking for weakness or asymmetrical movements.

Common medical causes

- *Congenital hip dysplasia.* Bilateral hip dislocation produces waddling gait with lordosis and pain.
- *Muscular dystrophy.* In *Duchenne's muscular dystrophy,* waddling gait gradually appears at age 3 to 4 and becomes pronounced by age 6. The gait worsens as the disease progresses, until the child loses the ability to walk and becomes wheelchair-bound—usually by age 12. Early signs are usually subtle: delay in learning to walk, frequent falls, or intermittent calf pain. Common later findings include lordosis with abdominal protrusion, a positive Gower's sign, and equinovarus foot position. As the disease progresses, its effects become more prominent; they commonly include rapid muscle wasting beginning in the legs and spreading to the arms (although calf and upper arm muscles may become hypertrophied, firm, and rubbery), muscle contractures, limited dorsiflexion of the feet and extension of the knees and elbows, obesity, and possibly mild mental retardation.

In *Becker's muscular dystrophy,* waddling gait typically becomes apparent in late adolescence, slowly worsens during the third decade, and culminates in total loss of ambulation. Muscle weakness first appears in the pelvic and upper arm muscles. Progressive wasting with selected muscle hypertrophy produces lordosis with abdominal protrusion, poor balance, a positive Gower's sign, and possibly mental retardation.

In *facioscapulohumeral muscular dystrophy,* waddling gait appears late, after muscle wasting has spread downward from the face and shoulder girdle to the pelvic girdle and legs. Earlier effects include progressive weakness and atrophy of facial, shoulder, and arm muscles, and slight lordosis and pelvic instability.

• ***Spinal muscle atrophy.*** In *Kugelberg-Welander syndrome,* waddling gait occurs early and usually progresses slowly, with loss of ambulation occurring up to 20 years later. Related findings include a positive Gower's sign, ophthalmoplegia, tongue fasciculations, and muscle atrophy in the legs and pelvis, progressing to the shoulders.

In *Werdnig-Hoffmann disease,* waddling gait typically begins when the child learns to walk. The gait progressively worsens, culminating in complete loss of ambulation by adolescence. Associated findings include lordosis with abdominal protrusion and muscle weakness in the hips and thighs.

Special considerations

Perform daily passive and active muscle stretching exercises for both the arms and legs. If possible, have the patient walk at least 3 hours each day (with leg braces if necessary) to maintain muscle strength, reduce contractures, and delay further gait deterioration. Stay near the patient while he's walking, especially if he's on unfamiliar or uneven ground. Caution him against long, unbroken periods of bed rest, which accelerate muscle deterioration. Provide a balanced diet to maintain energy levels and prevent obesity.

Because of the grim prognosis associated with muscular dystrophy and spinal muscle atrophy, provide emotional support for the patient and his family. As indicated, refer him to a local chapter of the Muscular Dystrophy Association. Suggest genetic testing and counseling for the parents if they're considering having another child.

GALLOP, ATRIAL

An atrial, or presystolic, gallop—a fourth heart sound (S_4)—is an extra heart sound that's heard immediately before the first heart sound. This low-pitched sound is best heard with the bell of the stethoscope pressed lightly against the cardiac apex. (See *Locating heart sounds,* page 268.) Some clinicians say an S_4 has the cadence of the "Ten" in Tennessee (Ten = S_4; nes = S_1; see = S_2).

This gallop typically results from hypertension, conduction defects, valvular disorders, and other problems such as ischemia. Occasionally, it helps differentiate angina from other causes of chest pain. An S_4 results from abnormally forceful atrial contraction caused by augmented ventricular filling or by decreased left ventricular compliance. It usually originates from left atrial contraction, is heard at the apex, and doesn't vary with inspiration. It may also originate from right atrial contraction; in that case, it's best heard at the lower left sternal border and intensifies with inspiration. (See *Interpreting heart sounds,* pages 270 and 271.)

An S_4 seldom occurs in normal hearts; however, it may occur in the elderly, in athletes with physiologic hypertrophy of the left ventricle, and in pregnant women because of augmented ventricular filling.

Emergency interventions

 Suspect myocardial ischemia if you auscultate an S_4 in a patient with chest pain. Take the patient's vital signs and quickly look for

EXAMINATION TIP

LOCATING HEART SOUNDS

When auscultating heart sounds, remember that certain sounds are best heard in specific areas. Use these auscultatory points to locate heart sounds quickly and accurately. Then expand your auscultation to nearby areas. Note that the numbers indicate pertinent intercostal spaces.

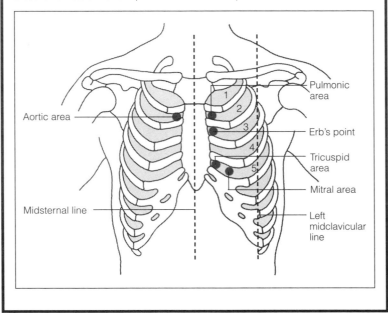

signs of heart failure, such as dyspnea, crackles, and distended neck veins. If you detect these signs, connect the patient to a cardiac monitor and obtain an electrocardiogram. Administer antianginal drugs. If the patient has dyspnea, elevate the head of the bed. Then auscultate for abnormal breath sounds. If you detect coarse crackles, start an I.V. line and give oxygen and diuretics, as needed. If the patient has bradycardia, he may require administration of atropine and pacemaker insertion.

History
When the patient's condition permits, ask about a history of hypertension, angina, valvular stenosis, or cardiomyopathy. If appropriate, have him describe the frequency and severity of anginal attacks.

Common medical causes
● *Angina.* An intermittent S_4 characteristically occurs during an anginal attack and disappears when it subsides. This gallop may be accompanied by a paradoxical S_2 or a new murmur. The patient typically complains of anginal chest pain— a feeling of tightness, pressure, achiness, or burning that usually radiates from the retrosternal area to the neck, jaws, left shoulder, and arm. He may also have dyspnea, tachycardia, palpitations,

increased blood pressure, dizziness, diaphoresis, belching, nausea, and vomiting.

● *Aortic insufficiency (acute).* This disorder causes an S_4 accompanied by a soft, short diastolic murmur along the left sternal border. S_2 may be soft or absent. Sometimes, a soft, short midsystolic murmur may be heard over the second right intercostal space. Related cardiopulmonary findings may include tachycardia, S_3, dyspnea, neck vein distention, and crackles. The patient may have fatigue and cool extremities.

● *Aortic stenosis.* This disorder usually causes an S_4, especially when valvular obstruction is severe. Auscultation reveals a harsh, crescendo-decrescendo, systolic ejection murmur that's loudest at the right sternal border near the second intercostal space. Dyspnea, anginal chest pain, and syncope are cardinal associated findings. Crackles, palpitations, fatigue, and diminished carotid pulses may also occur.

● *Cardiomyopathy.* An atrial gallop is a sign associated with cardiomyopathy, regardless of the type—dilated (most common), hypertrophic, or restrictive (least common). Additional findings include dyspnea, orthopnea, crackles, fatigue, syncope, chest pain, palpitations, edema, neck vein distention, S_3, and transient or sustained bradycardia.

● *Hypertension.* One of the earliest findings in systemic arterial hypertension is an atrial gallop. The patient may be asymptomatic, or he may experience headache, weakness, epistaxis, tinnitus, dizziness, or fatigue.

● *Mitral stenosis.* When associated with a normal sinus rhythm, mitral stenosis commonly causes an S_4. Initially, the patient may report exertional dyspnea, fatigue, and possibly palpitations. As the disorder progresses, he may report paroxysmal nocturnal dyspnea, orthopnea, dyspnea at rest, and weakness. Cardinal findings include a loud apical first sound

and an opening snap with a diastolic murmur heard at the apex.

● *Myocardial infarction (MI).* An S_4 is a classic sign of life-threatening MI that may persist even after the infarction heals. Typically, the patient reports crushing substernal chest pain that may radiate to the back, neck, jaw, shoulder, and left arm. Associated signs and symptoms include dyspnea, restlessness, anxiety, a feeling of impending doom, diaphoresis, pallor, clammy skin, nausea, vomiting, and increased or decreased blood pressure.

● *Pulmonary embolism.* This life-threatening disorder causes a right-sided S_4 that's usually heard along the lower left sternal border with a loud pulmonic closure sound. Other features include tachycardia, tachypnea, fever, chest pain, dyspnea, decreased breath sounds, crackles, a pleural friction rub, apprehension, diaphoresis, syncope, and cyanosis. The patient may have a productive cough with blood-tinged sputum or a nonproductive cough.

● *Thyrotoxicosis.* An S_4 and an S_3 may both be auscultated in thyroid hormone overproduction. Other cardinal features include tachycardia, palpitations, weight loss despite increased appetite, diarrhea, tremors, an enlarged thyroid, dyspnea, nervousness, diaphoresis, and heat intolerance. Exophthalmos may also be present.

Special considerations

Prepare the patient for diagnostic tests, such as electrocardiography, echocardiography, cardiac catheterization, and possibly a lung scan.

Pediatric pointers

An atrial gallop may occur normally in children, especially after exercise. However, it may also result from congenital heart diseases, such as atrial septal defect, ventricular septal defect, patent ductus arteriosus, and severe pulmonic stenosis.

INTERPRETING HEART SOUNDS

Detecting subtle variations in heart sounds requires both concentration and practice. Once you recognize normal heart sounds, the abnormal gallops become more obvious.

HEART SOUND AND ITS CAUSE	TIMING AND CADENCE
First heart sound (S₁) Vibrations associated with mitral and tricuspid valve closure	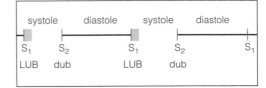
Second heart sound (S₂) Vibrations associated with aortic and pulmonic valve closure	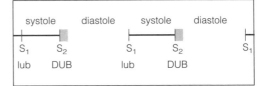
Ventricular gallop (S₃) Vibrations produced by rapid blood flow into the ventricles	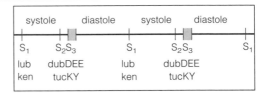
Atrial gallop (S₄) Vibrations produced by an increased resistance to sudden, forceful ejection of atrial blood	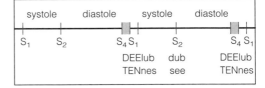
Summation gallop Vibrations produced in middiastole by simultaneous ventricular and atrial gallops, usually caused by tachycardia	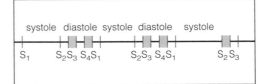

GALLOP, VENTRICULAR

A ventricular gallop is a third heart sound (S_3) associated with rapid ventricular filling in early diastole. Usually palpable, this low-frequency sound occurs about 0.15 second after the second heart sound (S_2). It may originate in either the left or right ventricle. A right-sided gallop usually sounds louder on inspiration and is best heard along the lower left sternal border or over the xiphoid region. A left-sided gallop usually sounds louder on expiration and is best heard at the apex.

Ventricular gallops are easily overlooked because they're usually faint. Fortunately, certain techniques make their detection more likely. These include auscultating in a quiet environment, having the patient cough or raise his legs to augment the sound, and examining the patient in the supine, left lateral, and semi-Fowler positions.

A physiologic ventricular gallop occurs in children and young adults; however, most people lose this third heart sound by age 40. This gallop may also occur during the third trimester of pregnancy. Although the physiologic S_3 has the same timing as the pathologic S_3, its intensity waxes and wanes with respiration. It's also heard more faintly if the patient is sitting or standing.

A pathologic ventricular gallop may be one of the earliest signs of heart failure. It results from one of two mechanisms: rapid deceleration of blood entering a stiff, noncompliant ventricle or rapid acceleration of blood associated with increased flow into the ventricle. The gallop's intensity correlates with the patient's prognosis; a gallop that persists despite therapy indicates a poor prognosis.

A ventricular gallop and an atrial gallop may occur simultaneously. (See *Summation gallop: Two gallops in one*, page 272.)

AUSCULTATION TIPS

Best heard with the diaphragm of the stethoscope at the apex (mitral area).

Best heard with the diaphragm of the stethoscope in the second or third right and left parasternal intercostal spaces with the patient sitting or supine.

Best heard through the bell of the stethoscope at the apex with the patient in the left lateral position. May be visible and palpable during early diastole at the midclavicular line between the fourth and fifth intercostal spaces.

Best heard through the bell of the stethoscope at the apex with the patient in the left semilateral position. May be visible in late diastole at the midclavicular line between the fourth and fifth intercostal spaces. May also be palpable in the midclavicular area with the patient in the left lateral decubitus position.

Best heard through the bell of the stethoscope at the apex with the patient in the left lateral position. May be louder than S_1 or S_2. May be visible and palpable during diastole.

SUMMATION GALLOP: TWO GALLOPS IN ONE

When atrial and ventricular gallops occur simultaneously, they produce a short, low-pitched sound known as a summation gallop. This relatively uncommon gallop occurs during middiastole (between S_2 and S_1) and is best heard with the bell of the stethoscope pressed lightly against the cardiac apex. It may be louder than either S_1 or S_2 and may cause visible apical movement during diastole.

A summation gallop may result from tachycardia or from delayed or blocked atrioventricular (AV) conduction. Tachycardia shortens ventricular filling time during diastole, causing it to coincide with atrial contraction. When the heart rate slows, the summation gallop is replaced by separate atrial and ventricular gallops, producing a quadruple rhythm much like the canter of a horse. Delayed AV conduction also brings atrial contraction closer to ventricular filling, creating a summation gallop.

In most cases, a summation gallop results from heart failure and dilated congestive cardiomyopathy, but it may also accompany other cardiac disorders. Occasionally, it signals further cardiac deterioration. For example, consider the hypertensive patient with a chronic atrial gallop who develops tachycardia and a superimposed ventricular gallop. If this patient abruptly displays a summation gallop, heart failure is the likely cause.

History and physical examination

After auscultating a ventricular gallop, focus your examination on the cardiovascular system. Begin the history by asking the patient if he's had any chest pain. If so, have him describe its character, location, frequency, duration, and any alleviating or aggravating factors. Also ask about palpitations, dizziness, or syncope. Does the patient have difficulty breathing after exertion? While lying down? At rest? Does he have a productive cough? Also ask about a history of cardiac disorders. Is the patient currently receiving any treatment for heart failure? If so, ask which medications he's taking.

During the physical examination, carefully auscultate for murmurs or abnormalities in the first and second heart sounds. Then listen for pulmonary crackles. Next, assess peripheral pulses, noting pulsus alternans—an alternating strong and weak pulse. Finally, palpate the liver to detect enlargement or tenderness, and assess for neck vein distention and peripheral edema.

Common medical causes

● *Aortic insufficiency.* Both acute and chronic aortic insufficiency may produce an S_3. Typically, *acute aortic insufficiency* also causes an S_4 and a soft, short diastolic murmur over the left sternal border. S_2 may be soft or absent. At times, a soft, short midsystolic murmur may be heard over the second right intercostal space. Related findings include tachycardia, dyspnea, neck vein distention, and crackles.

Chronic aortic insufficiency produces an S_3 and a high-pitched, blowing, decrescendo diastolic murmur that's best heard over the second or third right intercostal space or the left sternal border. An Austin Flint murmur—an apical, rumbling, middle to late diastolic murmur—may also occur. Related findings may include palpitations, tachycardia, anginal chest pain, fatigue, dyspnea, orthopnea, and crackles.

● *Cardiomyopathy.* A ventricular gallop is characteristic in this disorder. When accompanied by pulsus alternans and altered S_1 and S_2, this gallop usually signals advanced heart disease. Other effects include fatigue, dyspnea, orthopnea, chest pain, palpitations, syncope, crackles, peripheral edema, neck vein distention, and S_4.

● **Heart failure.** A ventricular gallop is a cardinal sign of heart failure. When it's loud and accompanied by sinus tachycardia, this gallop may indicate severe heart failure. The patient with left-sided heart failure will also have fatigue, exertional dyspnea, paroxysmal nocturnal dyspnea, orthopnea, and possibly a dry cough; with right-sided heart failure, neck vein distention. Other late features include tachypnea, chest tightness, palpitations, anorexia, nausea, dependent edema, weight gain, slowed mental response, diaphoresis, pallor, hypotension, narrowed pulse pressure, and possibly oliguria. In some patients, inspiratory crackles, clubbing, and a tender, palpable liver may be present. As heart failure progresses, hemoptysis, cyanosis, severe pitting edema, and marked hepatomegaly may develop.

● **Mitral insufficiency.** Both acute and chronic mitral insufficiency may produce a ventricular gallop. In *acute mitral insufficiency,* auscultation may also reveal an early or holosystolic decrescendo murmur at the apex, an S_4, and a widely split S_2. Typically, the patient will have sinus tachycardia, tachypnea, orthopnea, dyspnea, crackles, distended neck veins, and fatigue.

In *chronic mitral insufficiency,* a progressively severe ventricular gallop is typical. Auscultation will also reveal a holosystolic, blowing, high-pitched apical murmur. The patient may be asymptomatic or may report fatigue, exertional dyspnea, and palpitations.

● **Thyrotoxicosis.** This disorder may produce ventricular and atrial gallops, but its cardinal features are an enlarged thyroid gland, weight loss despite increased appetite, heat intolerance, diaphoresis, nervousness, tremors, tachycardia, palpitations, diarrhea, and dyspnea.

Special considerations

Monitor the patient with a ventricular gallop; watch for and report tachycardia, dyspnea, crackles, or neck vein distention. Give oxygen, diuretics, and other drugs, such as digoxin and angiotensin-converting enzyme inhibitors, to prevent pulmonary edema.

Prepare the patient for echocardiography, gated blood pool imaging, and cardiac catheterization.

Pediatric pointers

A ventricular gallop is normally heard in children. However, it may accompany congenital abnormalities associated with heart failure, such as large ventricular septal defect and patent ductus arteriosus. It may also result from sickle cell anemia. Clearly, this gallop must be correlated with the patient's associated signs and symptoms to be of diagnostic value.

GENITAL LESIONS IN THE MALE

Among the diverse lesions that may affect the male genitalia are warts, papules, ulcers, scales, and pustules. These common lesions may be painful or painless and occur singly or in multiples. They may be limited to the genitalia or may also occur elsewhere on the body. (See *Recognizing common male genital lesions,* page 274.)

Genital lesions may result from infection, neoplasms, parasites, allergy, or the effects of drugs. In many cases, these lesions profoundly affect the patient's self-image. In fact, the patient may hesitate to seek medical attention because he fears cancer or a sexually transmitted disease (STD).

In addition, genital lesions arising from STDs increase the risk of transmitting human immunodeficiency virus (HIV) between sexual partners. Unfortunately,

RECOGNIZING COMMON MALE GENITAL LESIONS

A wide variety of lesions may affect the male genitalia. Some of the more common ones and their causes appear below.

Penile cancer causes a painless ulcerative lesion on the glans or foreskin, possibly accompanied by a foul-smelling discharge.

Genital herpes begins as a swollen, slightly pruritic wheal and becomes a group of small vesicles or blisters on the foreskin, glans, or penile shaft.

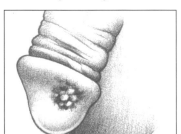

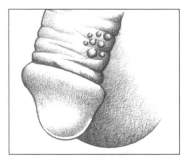

Genital warts are marked by clusters of flesh-colored papillary growths that may be barely visible or several inches in diameter.

Chancroid causes a painful ulcer that's usually less than ¾″ (2 cm) in diameter and bleeds easily. The lesion may be deep and covered by a gray or yellow exudate at its base.

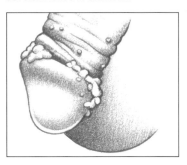

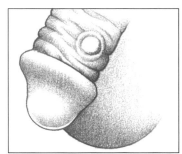

if the patient is treating himself, he may alter the lesions, making differential diagnosis especially difficult.

History and physical examination
Begin by asking the patient when he first noticed the lesion. Did it erupt after he began taking a new drug or after a trip out of the country? Has he had similar lesions before? If so, did he get medical treatment for them? Find out if he's been treating the lesion himself. If so, how? Does he have any itching? If so, is it constant or does it bother him only at night?

Note if the lesion is painful. Next, take a complete sexual history, noting the frequency of relations and the number of sexual partners.

Before you examine the patient, observe his clothing. Do his pants fit properly? Tight pants or underwear, especially in nonabsorbent fabrics, may promote the growth of bacteria and fungi. Examine the skin over his entire body, noting the location, size, color, and pattern of the lesions. Do genital lesions resemble those on other parts of the body? Palpate for nodules, masses, and tenderness. Also look for bleeding, edema, or signs of infection such as erythema. Finally, take the patient's vital signs.

Common medical causes

• *Balanitis and balanoposthitis.* Typically, balanitis (glans infection) and posthitis (prepuce infection) occur together (balanoposthitis), causing painful ulceration on the glans, foreskin, or penile shaft. Ulceration is usually preceded by 2 to 3 days of prepuce irritation and soreness, followed by a foul-smelling discharge and edema. The patient may then develop features of acute infection, such as fever with chills, malaise, and dysuria. Without treatment, the ulcers may deepen and multiply. Eventually, the entire penis and scrotum may become gangrenous, resulting in life-threatening sepsis.

• *Bowen's disease.* This painless, premalignant lesion commonly occurs on the penis or scrotum but may also appear elsewhere. It appears as a brownish red, raised, scaly, indurated plaque, which may ulcerate at its center.

• *Chancroid.* In this STD, one or more lesions erupt, usually on the groin, inner thigh, or penis. Within 24 hours, the lesion changes from a reddened area to a small papule. (A similar papule may erupt on the tongue, lip, breast, or umbilicus.) It then becomes an inflamed pustule that rapidly ulcerates. This painful—usually deep— ulcer bleeds easily and commonly has a purulent gray or yellow exudate covering its base. Rarely more than $^3/_4''$ (2 cm) in diameter, it's typically irregular in shape. The inguinal lymph nodes also enlarge, become very tender, and may drain pus.

• *Folliculitis and furunculosis.* Hair follicle infection may cause red, sharply pointed lesions that are tender and swollen with central pustules. If folliculitis progresses to furunculosis, these lesions become hard, painful nodules that may gradually enlarge and rupture, discharging pus and necrotic material. Rupture relieves the pain, but erythema and edema may persist for days or weeks.

• *Genital herpes.* Caused by herpesvirus Type I or Type II, this STD produces fluid-filled vesicles on the glans penis, foreskin, or penile shaft and, occasionally, on the mouth or anus. Usually painless at first, these vesicles may rupture and become extensive, shallow, painful ulcers accompanied by redness, marked edema, and tender, inguinal lymph nodes. Other findings include fever, malaise, and dysuria. If the vesicles recur in the same area, the patient will usually feel localized numbness and tingling before they erupt. Typically, associated inflammation is less marked.

• *Genital warts.* Most common in sexually active males, genital warts initially develop on the subpreputial sac, urethral meatus, and (less commonly) penile shaft and then spread to the perineum and perianal area. These painless warts start as tiny red or pink swellings that may grow to 4″ (10 cm) and become pedunculated. Multiple swellings are common, giving the warts a cauliflower-like appearance. Infected warts are also malodorous.

• *Leukoplakia.* This precancerous disorder is characterized by white, scaly patches on the glans and prepuce accompanied by skin thickening and occasionally fissures.

• *Pediculosis pubis.* This parasitic infestation is characterized by erythematous, itching papules in the pubic area and around the anus, abdomen, and thigh. Inspection may detect grayish white specks (lice eggs) attached to hair shafts. Skin irritation from scratching in these areas is common.

• **Penile cancer.** This cancer usually produces a painless, ulcerative lesion or enlarging "wart" on the glans or foreskin. However, localized pain may occur if the foreskin becomes unretractable. Examination may reveal a foul-smelling discharge from the prepuce, a firm lump in the glans, and enlarged lymph nodes. Late signs and symptoms may include dysuria, pain, bleeding from the lesion, and urine retention and bladder distention associated with obstruction of the urinary tract.

• **Scabies.** Mites burrow under the skin in this disorder, possibly causing crusted lesions on the glans and shaft of the penis and on the scrotum. Lesions may also occur on the wrists, elbows, axillae, and waist. Usually, they're threadlike and $^3/_8"$ to 4" (1 to 10 cm) long and have a swollen nodule or red papule that contains the mite. Nocturnal itching is typical and commonly causes excoriation.

• **Syphilis.** Two to four weeks after exposure to *Treponema pallidum*, one or more primary lesions, or chancres, may erupt on the genitalia; occasionally, they also erupt elsewhere on the body. The chancre usually starts as a small, red, fluid-filled papule and then erodes to form a painless, firm, indurated, shallow ulcer with a clear base or, less commonly, a hard papule. This lesion gradually involutes and disappears. Painless, unilateral regional lymphadenopathy is also typical.

• **Tinea cruris.** Also called "jock itch," this fungal infection usually causes sharply defined, slightly raised, scaling patches on the inner thigh or groin and, less commonly, on the scrotum and penis. Pruritus may be severe.

• **Urticaria.** This common allergic reaction is characterized by intensely pruritic hives, which may appear on the genitalia, especially on the foreskin or shaft of the penis. These distinct, raised, evanescent wheals are surrounded by an erythematous flare.

Other causes

• **Drugs.** Phenolphthalein, barbiturates, and certain broad-spectrum antibiotics, such as tetracycline and sulfonamides, may cause a fixed drug eruption and a genital lesion.

Special considerations

Many disorders produce penile lesions that resemble those of syphilis. Expect to screen every patient with penile lesions for STD, using the dark-field examination and the Venereal Disease Research Laboratory test. In addition, prepare the patient for a biopsy to confirm or rule out penile cancer. Provide emotional support, especially if cancer is suspected.

Explain to the patient how to use prescribed ointments or creams. Use a heat lamp to dry moist lesions, or advise sitz baths to relieve crusting and itching. Also instruct the patient to report any changes in the lesions.

To prevent cross-contamination, wash your hands before and after every patient contact. Wear gloves when handling urine or performing catheter care. Dispose of all needles carefully, and double-bag all material contaminated by secretions.

Pediatric pointers

Contact dermatitis, or "diaper rash," is common in infants; it may produce minor irritation or bright red, weepy, excoriated lesions. Use of disposable diapers and careful cleaning of the penis and scrotum are two measures that help reduce diaper rash.

In children, impetigo may cause pustules with thick, yellow, weepy crusts. Like adults, children may also develop genital warts, but they'll need more reassurance that the treatment (excision) won't hurt or castrate them.

Adolescents ages 15 to 19 have a high incidence of STDs and related genital lesions. However, syphilis may also be congenital.

GRUNTING RESPIRATIONS

Characterized by a deep, low-pitched grunting sound at the end of each breath, these respirations are a chief sign of respiratory distress in infants and children. They may be soft and heard only on auscultation, or loud and clearly audible without a stethoscope. Typically, the intensity of grunting respirations reflects the severity of respiratory distress. The grunting sound coincides with closure of the glottis—an effort to increase end-expiratory pressure in the lungs and prolong alveolar gas exchange, thereby enhancing ventilation and perfusion.

Grunting respirations indicate intrathoracic disease with lower respiratory involvement. Although they may also occur in adults with severe respiratory distress, they're not as common. Whether they occur in children or adults, grunting respirations demand immediate medical attention.

Emergency interventions

 If the patient has grunting respirations, quickly check for associated signs of respiratory distress: wheezing; tachypnea (60 breaths/minute in infants, 40 breaths/minute in children ages 1 to 5, or 30 breaths/minute in children over age 5); accessory muscle use; substernal, subcostal, or intercostal retractions; nasal flaring; tachycardia (160 beats/minute in infants, 120 to 140 beats/minute in children ages 1 to 5, or 120 beats/minute in children over age 5); cyanotic lips or nail beds; hypotension (blood pressure less than 80/40 mm Hg in infants, less than 80/50 mm Hg in children ages 1 to 5, or less than 90/55 mm Hg in children over age 5); and decreased level of consciousness.

If you detect any of these signs, administer oxygen and medications, such as bronchodilators, as ordered. Also have emergency equipment available, and prepare to intubate the patient if necessary.

History and physical examination

After addressing the child's respiratory status, ask his parents when the grunting respirations began. If the patient is a premature infant, find out his gestational age. Ask the parents if anyone in the home has had an upper respiratory infection (URI) recently. Has the child had signs of a URI, such as a runny nose, cough, low-grade fever, or anorexia? Does he have a history of frequent colds or URIs? Ask the parents to describe changes in the child's activity level. Is he lethargic or less alert than usual?

Begin the physical examination by auscultating the lungs, especially the lower lobes. Note diminished or abnormal breath sounds, such as crackles, wheezing, or sibilant rhonchi, which may indicate mucus or fluid buildup. In addition, characterize the color, amount, and consistency of any discharge or sputum.

Common medical causes

● *Asthma.* Grunting respirations may be seen with a severe asthma attack, usually triggered by a URI or allergic exposure. As the attack progresses, dyspnea, audible wheezing, chest tightness, and cough occur. Patients may have a silent chest if air movement is poor. Immediate bronchodilator therapy is needed.

● *Heart failure.* A late sign of left-sided heart failure, grunting respirations accompany increasing pulmonary edema. Other features include crackles, productive cough, and chest wall retractions. Cyanosis may also be present, depend-

POSITIONING THE INFANT FOR CHEST PHYSICAL THERAPY

The infant with grunting respirations may need chest physical therapy to mobilize and drain excess lung secretions. Auscultate first to locate congested areas and determine the best drainage position. Then review the illustrations here, which show the various drainage positions and where to place your hands for percussion. When you percuss the infant, use the fingers of one hand. You'll also vibrate these fingers and move them toward the infant's head to facilitate drainage.

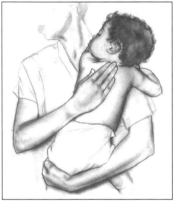

Hold the infant upright and about 30 degrees forward to percuss and drain the apical segments of the upper lobes.

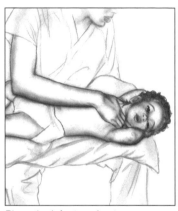

Place the infant supine to percuss and drain the anterior segments of the upper lobes.

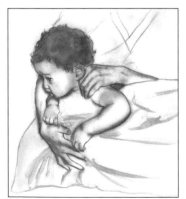

Use this position to percuss and drain the posterior segments of the upper lobes.

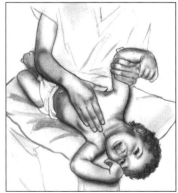

Hold the infant at a 45-degree angle on his side with his head down about 15 degrees to percuss and drain the right middle lobe.

POSITIONING THE INFANT FOR CHEST PHYSICAL THERAPY
(continued)

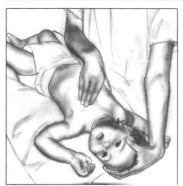

Place the infant in a supine position with his head 30 degrees lower than his feet to percuss and drain the anterior segments of the lower lobes.

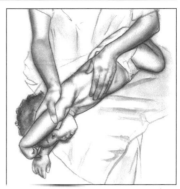

Place the infant on his side with his head down 30 degrees to percuss and drain the lateral basal segments of the lower lobes. Repeat this on the other side.

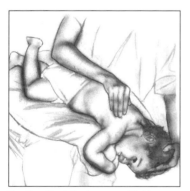

Position the infant prone with his head down 30 degrees to percuss and drain the posterior basal segments of the lower lobes.

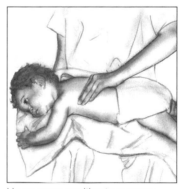

Use a prone position to percuss and drain the superior segments of the lower lobes.

ing on the underlying congenital cardiac defect.

• **Pneumonia.** Life-threatening bacterial pneumonia often follows URIs or colds. *Pneumocystis carinii* pneumonia commonly affects children infected with human immunodeficiency virus. It causes grunting respirations accompanied by high fever, tachypnea, productive cough, anorexia, and lethargy. Auscultation reveals diminished breath sounds, scattered crackles, and sibilant rhonchi over the affected lung. As the disorder progresses, severe dyspnea, substernal and subcostal retractions, nasal flaring, cyanosis, and increasing lethargy may also occur. Some infants display GI signs, such as vomiting, diarrhea, and abdominal distention.

• *Respiratory distress syndrome.* The result of lung immaturity in a premature infant (less than 37 weeks' gestation), this syndrome initially causes audible expiratory grunts along with intercostal, subcostal, or substernal retractions; tachycardia; and tachypnea. Later, as respiratory distress tires the infant, apnea or irregular respirations replace the grunting. Severe respiratory distress is characterized by cyanosis, dramatic nasal flaring, lethargy, bradycardia, and hypotension. Eventually, the infant becomes unresponsive. Auscultation reveals harsh, diminished breath sounds and crackles over the base of the lungs on deep inspiration. Oliguria and peripheral edema may also occur.

Special considerations

Closely monitor the patient's condition. Keep emergency equipment nearby in case respiratory distress worsens. Prepare to administer oxygen using an oxygen hood or tent. Continually monitor arterial blood gas levels and deliver the minimum amount of oxygen possible to avoid retinopathy from excessively high oxygen levels.

Begin inhalation therapy with bronchodilators, and administer I.V. antimicrobials if the patient has pneumonia (or, in some cases, status asthmaticus). Follow these measures with chest physical therapy, as necessary. (See *Positioning the infant for chest physical therapy,* pages 278 and 279.)

Prepare the patient for chest X-rays. Because sedatives are contraindicated in respiratory distress, you'll need to help restrain the restless child during testing, as necessary. To prevent exposure to radiation, wear a lead apron and cover the child's genital area with a lead shield. If a blood culture is ordered, be sure to record any current antibiotic medications on the laboratory request.

Remember to explain all procedures to the patient's parents and to provide emotional support.

GUM BLEEDING
[Gingival bleeding]

Bleeding gums usually result from dental disorders or, less commonly, from blood dyscrasias or the effects of certain drugs. Physiologic causes of this common sign include pregnancy, which can produce gum swelling in the first or second trimester (pregnancy epulis); atmospheric pressure changes, which affect many divers and aviators; and oral trauma. Bleeding, which ranges from slight oozing to life-threatening hemorrhage, may be spontaneous or may follow trauma. Occasionally, direct pressure can control it.

Emergency interventions

 If you detect profuse, spontaneous bleeding in the oral cavity, quickly check the patient's airway and look for signs of cardiovascular collapse, such as tachycardia and hypotension. Suction the patient and apply direct pressure to the bleeding site. Expect to insert an airway, administer I.V. fluids, and collect serum samples for diagnostic evaluation.

History and physical examination

If gum bleeding isn't an emergency, obtain a history. Find out when the bleeding began. Has it been continuous or intermittent? Does it occur spontaneously or when the patient brushes his teeth? Have the patient show you the site of the bleeding if possible.

Determine if the patient or any family members have bleeding tendencies, such as easy bruising or frequent nosebleeds.

How much does the patient bleed after a tooth extraction? Does he have a history of liver or spleen disease? Next, check his dental history. Find out how often he brushes his teeth and goes to the dentist. Has he seen a dentist recently? To evaluate nutritional status, have the patient describe his normal diet and intake of alcohol. Finally, note any prescription and over-the-counter drugs he takes.

Next, perform a complete oral examination. If the patient wears dentures, have him remove them. Examine the gums to determine the site and amount of bleeding. Gums normally appear pink and rippled, with their margins snugly against the teeth. Check for inflammation, pockets around the teeth, swelling, retraction, hypertrophy, discoloration, and gum hyperplasia. Note obvious decay, discoloration, foreign material such as food, and absence of any teeth.

Common medical causes

• *Agranulocytosis.* Spontaneous gum bleeding and other systemic hemorrhages may occur in this hematologic disorder, which typically causes progressive fatigue and weakness, followed by signs of infection, such as fever and chills. Inspection may reveal oral and perianal lesions, which are usually rough-edged with a gray or black membrane.

• *Aplastic anemia.* In this disorder, profuse or scant gum bleeding may follow trauma. Other signs of bleeding, such as epistaxis and ecchymoses, are also characteristic. The patient has progressive weakness and fatigue, shortness of breath, headache, pallor, and possibly fever. Eventually, tachycardia and signs of heart failure, such as neck vein distention and dyspnea, also develop.

• *Ehlers-Danlos syndrome.* In this congenital syndrome, gums bleed easily after toothbrushing. Easy bruising and other signs of abnormal bleeding are also typical. Skin is fragile and hyperelastic; joints are hyperextendible.

• *Gingivitis.* In this disorder, reddened and edematous gums are characteristic. The gingivae between the teeth become bulbous and bleed easily with slight trauma. However, in *acute necrotizing ulcerative gingivitis,* bleeding is spontaneous. The gums also become so painful that the patient may be unable to eat. A characteristic grayish yellow pseudomembrane develops over punched-out gum erosions. Offensive halitosis is typical and may be accompanied by headache, malaise, fever, and cervical adenopathy.

• *Hemophilia.* In hemophilia, hemorrhage occurs from many sites in the oral cavity, especially the gums. *Mild hemophilia* causes easy bruising, hematomas, epistaxis, bleeding gums, and prolonged bleeding during and up to 8 days after even minor surgery. *Moderate hemophilia* produces more frequent episodes of abnormal bleeding and occasional bleeding into the joints, which may cause swelling and pain.

Severe hemophilia causes spontaneous or severe bleeding after minor trauma, possibly resulting in large subcutaneous and intramuscular hematomas. Bleeding into joints and muscles causes pain, swelling, extreme tenderness, and possibly permanent deformity. Bleeding near peripheral nerves causes peripheral neuropathies, pain, paresthesia, and muscle atrophy. Signs of anemia and fever may follow bleeding. Severe blood loss may lead to shock and death.

• *Hereditary hemorrhagic telangiectasia.* This disorder is characterized by red to violet spiderlike hemorrhagic areas on the gums, which blanch on pressure and bleed spontaneously. These telangiectases may also occur on the lips, buccal mucosa, and palate as well as the face, ears, scalp, hands, arms, feet, and under the nails. Epistaxis commonly occurs early and is difficult to control. Hemoptysis and signs of GI bleeding may also occur.

• *Leukemia.* An early sign of acute monocytic, lymphocytic, or myelocytic leukemia, easy gum bleeding is accompanied by gum swelling, necrosis, and petechiae. The soft, tender gums appear glossy and bluish. *Acute leukemia* causes severe prostration marked by high fever and bleeding tendencies, such as epistaxis and prolonged menses. It also may cause dyspnea, tachycardia, palpitations, and abdominal or bone pain. Later effects may include confusion, headaches, vomiting, seizures, papilledema, and nuchal rigidity.

Chronic leukemia usually develops insidiously, producing less severe bleeding tendencies. Other effects may include anorexia, weight loss, low-grade fever, chills, skin eruptions, and enlarged spleen, tonsils, and lymph nodes. Signs of anemia (fatigue and pallor) may occur.

• *Pemphigoid (benign mucosal).* Most common in women between ages 40 and 50, this autoimmune disorder typically causes thick-walled gum lesions that rupture, desquamate, and then bleed easily. Extensive scars form with healing, and the gums remain red for months. Lesions may also develop on other parts of the oral mucosa, conjunctiva and, less commonly, the skin. Secondary fibrous bands may lead to dysphagia, hoarseness, or blindness.

• *Periodontal disease.* Typically, chewing, toothbrushing, or gum probing initiates gum bleeding; however, bleeding may occur spontaneously. As gingivae separate from the bone, pus-filled pockets develop around the teeth and, occasionally, pus can be expressed. Other findings include unpleasant taste with halitosis, facial pain, loose teeth, and dental calculus and plaque.

• *Polycythemia vera.* In this disorder, engorged gums ooze blood following slight trauma. Usually, polycythemia vera turns the oral mucosa—especially the gums and tongue—a deep red-violet. Among associated findings are headache, dyspnea, dizziness, fatigue, paresthesia, tinnitus, double or blurred vision, pruritus, epigastric distress, weight loss, increased blood pressure, ruddy cyanosis, ecchymosis, and hepatosplenomegaly.

• *Thrombocytopenia.* Blood usually oozes between the teeth and gums; however, severe bleeding may follow minor trauma. Associated signs of hemorrhage include large, blood-filled bullae in the mouth, petechiae, ecchymosis, epistaxis, hematuria, and others. Malaise, fatigue, weakness, and lethargy eventually develop.

• *Thrombocytopenic purpura (idiopathic).* Profuse gum bleeding occurs in this disorder. Its classic feature, though, is spontaneous hemorrhagic skin lesions that range from pinpoint petechiae to massive hemorrhages. The patient has a tendency to bruise easily, petechiae on the oral mucosa, and possibly melena, epistaxis, or hematuria.

• *Vitamin K deficiency.* The first sign of this deficiency is usually bleeding gums after toothbrushing. Other signs of abnormal bleeding, such as ecchymosis, epistaxis, and hematuria, may occur. GI bleeding may produce hematemesis and melena; intracranial bleeding may cause decreased level of consciousness and focal neurologic deficits.

Other causes

• *Drugs.* Warfarin and heparin interfere with blood clotting and may cause prolonged gum bleeding. Abuse of aspirin and nonsteroidal anti-inflammatory drugs may alter platelets, producing bleeding gums. Localized gum bleeding may also occur with mucosal "aspirin burn," caused by dissolving aspirin near an aching tooth.

Special considerations

When providing mouth care, avoid using lemon-glycerin swabs, which may burn or dry the gums. Teach the patient about mouth and gum care. Prepare him for diagnostic tests, such as blood tests or facial X-rays.

Pediatric pointers

In newborns, bleeding gums may result from vitamin K deficiency associated with a lack of normal intestinal flora or poor maternal nutrition. In infants who primarily drink cow's milk and don't receive vitamin supplements, bleeding gums can result from vitamin C deficiency.

Encourage parents to instill good oral hygiene habits early. Daily toothbrushing in the morning and before bedtime should begin with eruption of the first tooth. When the child has all of his baby teeth, he should begin receiving regular dental checkups.

GYNECOMASTIA

Occurring only in males, gynecomastia refers to excessive mammary gland development that results in increased breast size. This size change may be barely palpable or immediately obvious. Usually bilateral, gynecomastia may be associated with breast tenderness and milk secretion.

Normally, several hormones regulate breast development. Estrogens, growth hormone, and corticosteroids stimulate ductal growth, while progesterone and prolactin stimulate growth of the alveolar lobules. Although the pathophysiology of gynecomastia isn't fully understood, hormonal imbalance—particularly a change in the estrogen-androgen ratio and an increase in prolactin—is a likely contributing factor. This explains why gynecomastia commonly results from the effects of estrogens and other drugs.

Gynecomastia may also result from hormone-secreting tumors and from endocrine, genetic, hepatic, and adrenal disorders. Physiologic gynecomastia may occur in neonatal, pubertal, and elderly males because of normal fluctuations in hormone levels.

History and physical examination
Begin the history by asking the patient when he first noticed his breast enlargement. How old was he at the time? Since then, have his breasts gotten progressively larger, smaller, or stayed the same? Is gynecomastia accompanied by breast tenderness or discharge? Next, take a thorough drug history, including prescription, over-the-counter, and street drugs. Then explore associated signs and symptoms, such as a testicular mass or pain, loss of libido, decreased potency, or loss of chest, axillary, or facial hair.

Focus the physical examination on the breasts, testicles, and penis. As you examine the breasts, note any asymmetry, dimpling, abnormal pigmentation, or ulceration. Observe the testicles for size and symmetry. Then palpate them to detect nodules, tenderness, or unusual consistency. Look for normal penile development after puberty, and note hypospadias.

Common medical causes
• *Adrenal carcinoma.* Estrogen production by an adrenal tumor may produce a feminizing syndrome in males marked by bilateral gynecomastia, loss of libido, impotence, testicular atrophy, and reduced facial hair growth. Cushingoid signs, such as moon face and purple striae, may occur.
• *Breast cancer.* Painful unilateral gynecomastia develops rapidly in this disorder. Palpation may reveal a hard or stony breast lump suggesting a malignant tumor. Breast examination may also detect changes in breast symmetry; thickening, dimpling, peau d'orange, or ulceration of the skin; and a warm, reddened area. The patient's nipples may produce a watery, bloody, or purulent discharge and may itch or burn. He may also have nipple erosion, deviation, flattening, or retraction.
• *Hepatic carcinoma.* This type of cancer may produce bilateral gynecomastia and other characteristics of feminization, such as testicular atrophy, impotence, and reduced facial hair growth. The patient may have severe epigastric or right upper quadrant pain that's associated with a right upper quadrant mass. A large tumor may

produce a bruit on auscultation. Related findings may include anorexia, weight loss, dependent edema, fever, cachexia, and possibly jaundice or ascites.

● *Hypothyroidism.* This disorder typically produces bilateral gynecomastia along with bradycardia, cold intolerance, weight gain despite anorexia, and mental dullness. The patient may display periorbital edema and puffiness in the face, hands, and feet. His hair appears brittle and sparse and his skin is dry, pale, cool, and doughy.

● *Klinefelter's syndrome.* Painless bilateral gynecomastia first appears during adolescence in this genetic disorder. Before puberty, the patient also has abnormally small testicles and slight mental deficiency; after puberty, he has sparse facial hair, a small penis, decreased libido, and impotence.

● *Pituitary tumor.* This hormone-secreting tumor causes bilateral gynecomastia accompanied by galactorrhea, impotence, and decreased libido. Other effects may include enlarged hands and feet, coarse facial features with prognathism, voice deepening, weight gain, increased blood pressure, diaphoresis, heat intolerance, hyperpigmentation, and thick, oily skin. Paresthesia or sensory loss and muscle weakness commonly affect the limbs. If the tumor expands, it may cause blurred vision, diplopia, headache, or partial bitemporal hemianopia that may progress to blindness.

● *Reifenstein's syndrome.* This genetic disorder produces painless bilateral gynecomastia at puberty. Associated signs may include hypospadias, testicular atrophy, and an underdeveloped penis.

● *Testicular cancer.* Choriocarcinomas, Leydig cell tumors, and other testicular tumors typically cause bilateral gynecomastia, nipple tenderness, and decreased libido. These tumors are usually painless; testicular swelling may be the patient's initial complaint. A firm mass and a heavy sensation in the scrotum may occur.

Other causes

● *Drugs.* Certain drugs produce painful unilateral gynecomastia. Estrogens used to treat prostate cancer, including diethylstilbestrol, estramustine, and chlorotrianisene, directly affect the estrogen-androgen ratio. Drugs that have an estrogen-like effect, such as digitalis glycosides and human chorionic gonadotropin, may do the same. Regular marijuana or heroin use reduces plasma testosterone levels, causing gynecomastia. Other drugs—such as spironolactone, cimetidine, and ketoconazole —produce this sign by interfering with androgen production or action. Some common drugs—phenothiazines, tricyclic antidepressants, and antihypertensives—produce gynecomastia in an unknown way.

● *Treatments.* Gynecomastia may develop within weeks of starting hemodialysis for chronic renal failure. It may also follow major surgery or testicular irradiation.

Special considerations

To make the patient as comfortable as possible, apply cold compresses to his breasts and administer analgesics.

Because gynecomastia may alter the patient's body image, provide emotional support. Reassure the patient that treatment can reduce breast size and that breast tissue can be surgically removed if needed.

Prepare the patient for diagnostic tests, including chest and skull X-rays and blood hormone levels.

Pediatric pointers

In newborns, gynecomastia may be associated with galactorrhea. It usually disappears in a few weeks but may persist until age 2.

Most males have physiologic gynecomastia at some time during adolescence, usually around age 14. This gynecomastia is usually asymmetrical and tender; it commonly resolves within 2 years and rarely persists beyond age 20.

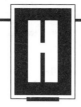

HALO VISION
[Halos]

Halo vision refers to seeing rainbowlike, colored rings around lights or bright objects. The rainbowlike effect can be explained by this physical principle: As light passes through water (in the eye, through tears or the cells of various anteretinal media), it breaks up into spectral colors.

Usually, halo vision develops suddenly; its duration depends on the causative disorder. This symptom may occur in disorders associated with excessive tearing and corneal epithelial edema. The most common and significant of these disorders is acute angle-closure glaucoma, which can lead to blindness. In this ocular emergency, increased intraocular pressure forces fluid into corneal tissues anterior to Bowman's membrane, causing edema. Halos are also an early symptom of cataracts, resulting from dispersion of light by abnormal opacities on the lens.

Nonpathologic causes of excessive tearing associated with halos include poorly fitted or overworn contact lenses, emotional extremes, and exposure to intense light, as in snow blindness.

History and physical examination
One of the first questions to ask the patient is how long he's been seeing halos around lights. When does he usually see them? Patients with glaucoma typically see halos in the morning, when intraocular pressure is most elevated. Ask the patient if light bothers his eyes. Does he have any eye pain? If so, have him describe it. Remember that halos associated with excruciating eye pain or severe headache may point to acute angle-closure glaucoma. Note a history of glaucoma or cataracts.

Next, examine the patient's eyes, noting conjunctival injection, excessive tearing, and lens changes. Examine pupil size, shape, and response to light. Then test visual acuity with an ophthalmoscopic examination.

Common medical causes
● *Cataract.* Halos may be an early symptom of painless, progressive cataract formation. The glare of headlights may blind the patient, making nighttime driving impossible. Other features include blurred vision, impaired visual acuity, and lens opacity, all of which develop gradually.

● *Corneal endothelial dystrophy.* Halos are typically a late symptom in this disorder. Impaired visual acuity may also occur.

● *Glaucoma.* Halos characterize all types of glaucoma. *Acute angle-closure glaucoma* also causes blurred vision followed by severe headache or excruciating pain in and around the affected eye. Examination will reveal a moderately dilated fixed pupil that doesn't respond to light, conjunctival injection, a cloudy cornea, and impaired visual acuity. Nausea and vomiting may also occur. *Chronic angle-closure glaucoma* usually produces no symptoms until pain and blindness occur in advanced disease. Sometimes, halos and blurred vision develop slowly.

COMPENSATING FOR POOR VISION

Halo vision poses a particular safety hazard for elderly people because they have a high incidence of cataracts and glaucoma. Encourage your older patients to have annual eye examinations and to comply with medical therapies, such as wearing glasses and instilling eyedrops. Make sure the patient's room and stairwells are well lit. Place brightly colored tape on the edges of steps.

If the patient drives, discuss his safety with family members. If he needs to take medications, assist him with this daily routine. For instance, draw up a week's worth of insulin in syringes, and label and store them in the refrigerator. Encourage the patient to use a weekly pill container to display the week's supply of pills. If he's an avid reader, tell him local libraries have books in large print. Magnifiers and reading aids are also available.

In *chronic open-angle glaucoma,* halos are a late symptom accompanied by mild eye ache, peripheral vision loss, and impaired visual acuity.

Special considerations

To help minimize halos, remind the patient not to look directly at bright lights.

Halo vision can further complicate poor vision, especially in an elderly patient. (See *Compensating for poor vision.*)

Pediatric pointers

A young child's limited verbal ability may make halos difficult to assess. Usually, halo vision in a child results from congenital cataracts or glaucoma.

HEADACHE

The most common neurologic symptom, a headache may be localized or generalized, producing mild to severe pain. About 90% of all headaches are benign and can be described as muscle-contraction, vascular, or a combination of both. (See *Comparing benign headaches.*) Occasionally, though, this symptom indicates a serious neurologic disorder. Pathologic headaches may result from disorders associated with intracranial inflammation, increased intracranial pressure (ICP), or meningeal irritation. They may also result from ocular or sinus disorders and the effects of drugs, tests, and treatments. Headaches may also be associated with certain metabolic disturbances, such as hypoxemia, hypercapnia, hyperglycemia, and hypoglycemia; however, they're not diagnostically significant in these cases.

Other causes of headaches include fever, eyestrain, dehydration, and systemic febrile illnesses. Some individuals get headaches from coughing, sneezing, heavy lifting, or stooping; others, after seizures.

History and physical examination

If the patient complains of headaches, ask him to describe their character and location. How often does he get a headache? How long does a typical headache last? Try to identify precipitating factors, such as certain foods and exposure to bright lights. Is the patient under stress? Has he been unable to sleep?

Take a drug history and ask about head trauma within the last 4 weeks. Has the patient had nausea, vomiting, photophobia, or any visual changes? Does he feel drowsy, confused, or dizzy? Has he recently developed seizures, or does he have a history of seizures?

COMPARING BENIGN HEADACHES

Of the many patients who report headaches, only about 10% have an underlying medical disorder. The other 90% suffer from benign headaches, which may be classified as muscle-contraction (tension), vascular (migraine and cluster), or a combination of both.

As you review the chart below, you'll see that the two major types—muscle-contraction and vascular headaches—are quite different. In a combined headache, features of both appear. This type of headache may affect the patient with a severe muscle-contraction headache or a late-stage migraine and requires treatment with analgesics and sedatives.

FEATURES	MUSCLE-CONTRACTION HEADACHES	VASCULAR HEADACHES
Incidence	• Most common type, accounting for 80% of all headaches	• More common in women and those with a family history of migraines • Onset after puberty
Precipitating factors	• Stress, anxiety, or tension • Prolonged muscle contraction without structural damage • Eye, ear, and paranasal sinus disorders that produce reflex muscle contractions	• Hormone fluctuations • Alcohol • Emotional upset • Too little or too much sleep • Foods, such as chocolate, cheese, monosodium glutamate, and cured meats; caffeine withdrawal • Weather changes such as shifts in barometric pressure
Intensity and duration	• Produce an aching tightness or a band of pain around the head, especially in the neck, occipital, and temporal areas • Occur frequently and usually last for several hours	• May begin with an awareness of an impending migraine or a 5- to 15-minute prodrome of neurologic deficits, such as visual disturbances; tingling of the face, lips, or hands; dizziness; or unsteady gait • Produce severe, constant, throbbing pain that's typically unilateral and may be incapacitating • Last for 4 to 6 hours
Associated signs and symptoms	• Tense neck and facial muscles	• Anorexia, nausea, and vomiting • Occasionally, photophobia, weakness, fatigue, and sensitivity to loud noises • Depending on the type (classic, common, or hemiplegic mi- *(continued)*

COMPARING BENIGN HEADACHES *(continued)*

FEATURES	MUSCLE-CONTRACTION HEADACHES	VASCULAR HEADACHES
Associated signs and symptoms *(continued)*		graine; or cluster headache), possibly chills, depression, eye pain, ptosis, tearing, rhinorrhea, diaphoresis, and facial flushing
Alleviating factors	• Mild analgesics, muscle relaxants, or other drugs during an attack • Measures to reduce stress, such as biofeedback, relaxation techniques and counseling, and posture correction to prevent attacks	• Methysergide and propranolol to prevent vascular headaches • Ergot or serotonin-receptor drugs at the first sign of a migraine • Rest in a quiet, darkened room • Elimination of irritating foods from diet

Begin the physical examination by evaluating the patient's level of consciousness (LOC). Then check his vital signs. Be alert for signs of increased ICP—widened pulse pressure, bradycardia, altered respiratory pattern, and increased blood pressure. Check pupil size and response to light. Also note any neck stiffness.

Common medical causes
• *Brain abscess.* In this disorder, a headache is localized to the abscess site; it usually intensifies over a few days and is aggravated by straining. Accompanying the headache may be nausea, vomiting, and focal or generalized seizures. The patient's LOC will vary from drowsiness to deep stupor. Depending on the abscess site, associated signs and symptoms may include aphasia, impaired visual acuity, hemiparesis, ataxia, tremors, and personality changes. Signs of infection, such as fever and pallor, usually develop late; however, if the abscess re-

mains encapsulated, these signs may not appear.
• *Brain tumor.* Initially, a tumor causes a localized headache near the tumor site. The headache eventually becomes generalized as the tumor grows. Usually, it's intermittent, deep-seated and dull, and most intense in the morning. It's aggravated by coughing, stooping, Valsalva's maneuver, and changes in head position; it's relieved by sitting and rest. Associated signs and symptoms may include personality changes, altered LOC, motor and sensory dysfunction and, eventually, signs of increased ICP, such as vomiting, increased systolic blood pressure, and widened pulse pressure.
• *Cerebral aneurysm (ruptured).* A sudden, excruciating headache characterizes this life-threatening disorder. The headache may be unilateral and usually peaks within minutes of aneurysmal rupture. The patient may lose consciousness immediately or display a variably altered LOC. Depending on the severity and location of the bleeding, he may also have

nausea and vomiting; signs of meningeal irritation, such as nuchal rigidity and blurred vision; hemiparesis; and other features.

- *Ebola virus.* A headache usually occurs suddenly, commonly on the fifth day of the illness. The patient also has a history of malaise, myalgia, high fever, diarrhea, abdominal pain, dehydration, and lethargy. Pleuritic chest pain, pronounced pharyngitis, and a dry, hacking cough also have been noted. A maculopapular skin rash develops between the fifth and seventh days of the illness. Hematemesis, melena, and bleeding from the nose, gums, and vagina may occur. Death usually occurs in the second week of the illness, preceded by severe blood loss and shock.

- *Encephalitis.* A severe, generalized headache is characteristic in this disorder. Typically, the patient's LOC then deteriorates within 48 hours—perhaps from lethargy to coma. Associated signs and symptoms include fever, nuchal rigidity, irritability, seizures, nausea, vomiting, photophobia, cranial nerve palsies such as ptosis, and focal neurologic deficits, such as hemiparesis and hemiplegia.

- *Hantavirus pulmonary syndrome.* Headache is a common chief complaint in this disorder. Other common complaints include myalgia, fever, nausea, vomiting, and cough. Noncardiogenic pulmonary edema distinguishes this syndrome. Respiratory distress typically follows the onset of a cough. Fever, hypoxia, and (in some patients) serious hypotension typify the hospital course. Other signs and symptoms include an increasing respiratory rate (28 breaths/minute or more) and an increased heart rate (120 beats/minute or more).

- *Hypertension.* This disorder may cause a slightly throbbing occipital headache on awakening that decreases in severity during the day. However, if the patient's diastolic blood pressure exceeds 120 mm Hg, the headache remains constant. Associated signs and symptoms include an

S_4, restlessness, confusion, nausea, vomiting, blurred vision, seizures, and altered LOC.

- *Meningitis.* Sudden onset of a severe, constant, generalized headache that worsens with movement typifies this disorder. Associated signs include nuchal rigidity, positive Kernig's and Brudzinski's signs, hyperreflexia, and possibly opisthotonos. Fever occurs early in meningitis and may be accompanied by chills. As ICP increases, vomiting and, occasionally, papilledema develop. Other features include altered LOC, seizures, ocular palsies, facial weakness, and hearing loss.

- *Subarachnoid hemorrhage.* This hemorrhage commonly produces a sudden, violent headache. Related signs and symptoms include nuchal rigidity, altered LOC that may rapidly progress to coma, nausea, vomiting, seizures, dizziness, and ipsilateral pupil dilation. The patient will also have positive Kernig's and Brudzinski's signs, photophobia, blurred vision, and possibly fever. Focal signs and symptoms, such as hemiparesis, hemiplegia, sensory or vision disturbances, and aphasia, may occur. Signs of elevated intracranial pressure—such as bradycardia and increased blood pressure—may also occur.

- *Subdural hematoma.* Typically associated with head trauma, both acute and chronic subdural hematomas may cause headache and decreased LOC. In *acute subdural hematoma,* head trauma produces headache, drowsiness, confusion, and agitation that may progress to coma. Later findings may include signs of increased ICP and focal neurologic deficits such as hemiparesis.

Chronic subdural hematoma produces a dull, pounding headache that fluctuates in severity and is located over the hematoma. Weeks or months after the initial head trauma, this disorder may cause giddiness, personality changes, confusion, seizures, and altered LOC that progressively worsens. Late signs may

RELIEVING HEADACHE WITH REFLEXOTHERAPY

Also known as reflexology, this bodywork technique is used to treat tension and migraine headaches, among other conditions. It is similar to acupressure, in which hand pressure is applied to specific points on the feet and, less commonly, on the hands or ears.

Reflexotherapy is based on the theory that sensitive nerve endings at reference points on the feet, hands, or ears correspond to all major organs and other parts of the body. Practitioners maintain that applying pressure to these points facilitates movement of life energy along channels in the body to the corresponding body organ or area.

include unilateral pupil dilation, sluggish pupil reaction to light, and ptosis.

● **Temporal arteritis.** A throbbing unilateral headache in the temporal or frontotemporal region is typical in this disorder. It may be accompanied by vision loss, hearing loss, confusion, and fever. The temporal arteries are tender, swollen, nodular, and sometimes erythematous.

Other causes

● **Diagnostic tests.** A lumbar puncture or myelogram may produce a throbbing frontal headache that worsens on standing.

● **Drugs.** A wide variety of drugs may cause headaches. For example, indomethacin produces headaches—usually in the morning—in many patients. Vasodilators and drugs with a vasodilating effect, such as nitrates, typically cause a throbbing headache. This symptom may also follow withdrawal from vasopressors, such as caffeine, ergotamine, or sympathomimetic drugs.

Special considerations

Continue to monitor the patient's vital signs and LOC. Watch for any change in the headache's severity or location.

Prepare the patient for diagnostic tests, such as skull X-rays, computed tomography scan, lumbar puncture, or cerebral arteriography.

To help ease the headache, administer analgesics. Also darken the patient's room and minimize other stimuli. Alternative therapies may also be helpful. (See *Relieving headache with reflexotherapy.*)

Pediatric pointers

If the child is too young to describe his symptom, suspect a headache if you see him banging or holding his head. In an infant, a shrill cry or bulging fontanels may indicate increased ICP and headache. In a school-age child, ask the parents about the child's recent scholastic performance and about any problems at home that may produce a tension headache.

Twice as many boys have migraine headaches as girls. In children over age 3, headache is the most common symptom of a brain tumor.

HEARING LOSS

Affecting nearly 16 million Americans, hearing loss may be temporary or permanent, partial or complete. This common symptom may involve reception of low-, middle-, or high-frequency tones. If the hearing loss doesn't affect speech frequencies, the patient may be unaware of it.

Normally, sound waves enter the external auditory canal, then travel to the middle ear's tympanic membrane and ossicles (incus, malleus, and stapes) and into the inner ear's cochlea. The cochlear division of the eighth cranial (auditory) nerve carries the sound impulse to the brain. This type of sound transmission, called *air conduction,* is normally better than *bone conduction*—sound transmission through bone to the inner ear.

Hearing loss can be classified as conductive, sensorineural, mixed, and functional. *Conductive hearing loss* results from disorders of the external and middle ear that block sound transmission. *Sensorineural hearing loss*—also known as nerve deafness, perceptive deafness, or inner ear deafness—results from disorders of the inner ear, or the eighth cranial nerve. *Mixed hearing loss* combines aspects of both conductive and sensorineural hearing loss. *Functional hearing loss* results from psychological factors; no identifiable organic damage exists.

Hearing loss may result from trauma, infection, allergy, tumors, certain systemic and hereditary disorders, and the effects of ototoxic drugs and treatments. Most commonly, though, it results from presbycusis, a sensorineural hearing loss that usually affects those older than age 50. Other physiologic causes of hearing loss include cerumen (earwax) impaction; barotitis media—unequal pressure on the eardrum—associated with descent in an airplane or elevator, diving, or close proximity to an explosion; and chronic exposure to noise over 90 dB. This noise exposure can occur on the job, at a hobby, or from listening to live or recorded music.

History and physical examination

If the patient reports hearing loss, ask him to describe it fully. Is it unilateral or bilateral? Continuous or intermittent? Ask about a family history of hearing loss. Then obtain the patient's medical history, noting chronic ear infections, ear surgery, and ear or head trauma. Has the patient recently had an upper respiratory infection? After taking a drug history, have the patient describe his occupation and work environment.

Next, explore associated signs and symptoms. Does he have any ear pain? If so, is it unilateral or bilateral? Continuous or intermittent? Ask the patient if he has noticed any discharge from one or both ears. If so, have him describe its color and consistency and note when it began. Does he hear ringing, buzzing, hissing, or other noises in one or both ears? If so, is the noise constant or intermittent? Is he dizzy, too? If so, when did he first notice it?

Begin the physical examination by inspecting the external ear for inflammation, boils, foreign bodies, or discharge. Then apply pressure to the tragus and mastoid to elicit tenderness. If you detect tenderness or external ear abnormalities, ask the doctor whether an otoscopic examination should be done. During the otoscopic examination, note any color change, perforation, bulging, or retraction of the tympanic membrane, which normally looks like a shiny, pearl gray cone.

Next, evaluate the patient's hearing acuity, using the ticking watch and whispered voice tests. Then perform Rinne and Weber's tests to obtain a preliminary evaluation of the type and degree of hearing loss.

Common medical causes

• *Acoustic neuroma.* This eighth cranial nerve tumor causes unilateral, progressive, sensorineural hearing loss. The patient may also have tinnitus, vertigo, and—with cranial nerve compression—facial paralysis.

• *Adenoid hypertrophy.* Eustachian tube dysfunction gradually causes conductive hearing loss accompanied by intermittent ear discharge. The patient also tends to breathe through his mouth and may complain of a sensation of ear fullness.

• *Aural polyps.* If a polyp occludes the external auditory canal, partial hearing loss may occur. The polyp typically bleeds easily and is covered by a purulent discharge.

• *Cholesteatoma.* Gradual hearing loss is characteristic in this disorder. It can be accompanied by vertigo and, at times, facial paralysis. Examination reveals eardrum perforation, pearly white balls in the ear canal, and possible discharge.

• *Cyst.* Ear canal obstruction by a sebaceous or dermoid cyst causes progressive conductive hearing loss. On inspection, the cyst appears like a soft mass.

• *External ear canal tumor (malignant).* A characteristic symptom, progressive conductive hearing loss is accompanied by purulent discharge; deep, boring ear pain; and eventually facial paralysis. Examination may detect the granular bleeding tumor.

• *Glomus jugulare tumor.* This benign tumor initially causes a mild unilateral conductive hearing loss that becomes progressively more severe. The patient may report tinnitus that sounds like his heartbeat. Associated signs and symptoms include gradual congestion in the affected ear, throbbing or pulsating discomfort, bloody otorrhea, facial nerve paralysis, and vertigo. Although the tympanic membrane is normal, a reddened mass appears behind it.

• *Head trauma.* Sudden conductive or sensorineural hearing loss may result from ossicle disruption, ear canal fracture, tympanic membrane perforation, or cochlear fracture associated with head trauma. Typically, the patient will report a headache and have bleeding from his ear. Neurologic features vary and may include impaired vision and altered level of consciousness.

• *Ménière's disease.* Initially, this inner ear disorder produces intermittent, unilateral sensorineural hearing loss that involves only low tones. Later, hearing loss becomes constant and affects other tones. Associated signs and symptoms include intermittent severe vertigo, nausea, vomiting, a feeling of fullness in the ear, a roaring or hollow-seashell tinnitus, diaphoresis, and nystagmus.

• *Nasopharyngeal cancer.* This tumor causes mild unilateral conductive hearing loss when it compresses the eustachian tube. Bone conduction is normal, and inspection reveals a retracted tympanic membrane backed by fluid. When this tumor obstructs the nasal airway, the patient may have bloody nasal and postnasal discharge as well as nasal speech. Cranial nerve involvement produces other findings, such as diplopia and rectus muscle paralysis.

• *Otitis externa.* Conductive hearing loss characterizes both acute and malignant otitis externa and results from debris in the ear canal. In *acute otitis externa,* ear canal inflammation produces pain, itching, and a foul-smelling, sticky yellow discharge. Typically, severe tenderness is elicited by chewing, opening the mouth, and pressing on the tragus or mastoid. The patient may also have a low-grade fever, regional lymphadenopathy, headache on the affected side, and mild to moderate pain around the ear that may later intensify. Examination may reveal greenish white debris or edema in the canal.

In *malignant otitis externa,* debris is also visible in the canal. This life-threatening disorder, which usually strikes diabetics, causes sensorineural hearing loss, pruritus, tinnitus, and severe ear pain.

• *Otitis media.* This middle ear inflammation typically produces unilateral conductive hearing loss. In *acute suppurative otitis media,* the hearing loss develops gradually over a few hours and is usually accompanied by an upper respiratory infection with sore throat, cough, nasal discharge, and headache. Related signs and symptoms may include dizziness, a sensation of fullness in the ear, intermittent or constant ear pain, fever, nausea, and vomiting. Rupture of the bulging, swollen tympanic membrane relieves the pain and produces a brief, bloody, purulent discharge. Hearing will return after the infection subsides.

Hearing loss also develops gradually in *chronic otitis media*. Assessment may reveal a perforated tympanic membrane, purulent ear drainage, earache, nausea, and vertigo.

Commonly associated with an upper respiratory infection or nasopharyngeal carcinoma, *serous otitis media* typically produces a stuffy feeling in the ear and pain that worsens at night. Examination will reveal a retracted—and perhaps discolored—tympanic membrane; air bubbles may be visible behind the membrane.

• *Otosclerosis.* In this hereditary disorder, unilateral conductive hearing loss usually begins in the early twenties and may gradually progress to bilateral mixed loss. The patient may report tinnitus and an ability to hear better in a noisy environment.

• *Skull fracture.* Auditory nerve injury causes sudden unilateral sensorineural hearing loss. Accompanying signs and symptoms may include ringing tinnitus, blood behind the tympanic membrane, and scalp wounds.

• *Temporal bone fracture.* This fracture can cause sudden unilateral sensorineural hearing loss accompanied by hissing tinnitus. The tympanic membrane may be perforated, depending on the fracture's location. Loss of consciousness, Battle's sign, and facial paralysis may also occur.

• *Tympanic membrane perforation.* Commonly caused by trauma from sharp objects or rapid pressure changes, perforation of the tympanic membrane causes abrupt hearing loss. Associated symptoms include ear pain, tinnitus, vertigo, and a sensation of fullness in the ear.

Other causes

• *Drugs.* Typically, ototoxic drugs produce ringing or buzzing tinnitus and a feeling of fullness in the ear. Chloroquine, cisplatin, vancomycin, and aminoglycosides—especially neomycin, kanamycin, and amikacin—may cause irreversible

---

COMPENSATING FOR HEARING LOSS

For an elderly person, hearing loss is not only a safety hazard but also a major impediment to social interaction. Make sure your older patient's regular medical checkups include hearing tests. If he uses a hearing aid, encourage him to wear it. Inform him and his family about devices that can make his life easier, such as amplifiers or light signals for the phone or doorbell, smoke detectors with strobe light or vibrating pod attachments, and communication systems activated by voice or button that alert the person by a pulse sensation.

When speaking to an elderly person, address him in a lower tone. Don't cover your mouth because he may be trying to read your lips. Ask him to repeat what you said, if appropriate, to ensure that he heard you correctly.

---

hearing loss. Loop diuretics, such as furosemide, ethacrynic acid, and bumetanide, usually produce temporary hearing loss. Quinine, quinidine, or high doses of erythromycin or salicylates (such as aspirin) may also cause reversible hearing loss.

• *Radiation therapy.* Irradiation of the middle ear, thyroid, face, skull, or nasopharynx may cause eustachian tube dysfunction, resulting in hearing loss.

• *Surgery.* Myringotomy, myringoplasty, simple or radical mastoidectomy, or fenestrations may cause scarring that interferes with hearing.

Special considerations

When talking with the patient, remember to face him and speak slowly. Don't shout, smoke, eat, or chew gum when talking. (See *Compensating for hearing loss.*)

Prepare the patient for audiometry and auditory evoked-response testing. After testing, the patient may require a hearing aid or cochlear implant to improve his hearing. Instruct him to avoid exposure to loud noise and to use ear protection to arrest loss.

Pediatric pointers
Each year about 3,000 profoundly deaf infants are born in the United States. In about half of these infants, hereditary disorders cause the typically sensorineural hearing loss. Disorders associated with congenital sensorineural hearing loss include albinism, onychodystrophy, cochlear dysplasias, and Pendred's, Waardenburg's, Usher's, and Jervell and Lange-Nielsen syndromes. This type of hearing loss may also result from maternal use of ototoxic drugs, birth trauma, and anoxia during or after birth.

Hereditary disorders associated with sensorineural hearing loss in childhood and adolescence include Paget's disease and Hurler's, Alport's, and Klippel-Feil syndromes. Mumps is the most common pediatric cause of unilateral sensorineural hearing loss. Other causes are meningitis, measles, influenza, and acute febrile illness.

Disorders associated with congenital conductive hearing loss include atresia, ossicle malformation, and other abnormalities. Unlike its effect in adults, serous otitis media commonly causes *bilateral* conductive hearing loss in children. Conductive hearing loss may also occur in children who put foreign objects in their ears.

Because hearing disorders in children may lead to speech, language, and learning problems, early identification and treatment of hearing loss is crucial—before the child is incorrectly labeled as mentally retarded, brain damaged, or a slow learner.

When assessing an infant or young child for hearing loss, remember that you can't use a tuning fork. Instead, test the startle reflex in infants under age 6 months or have an audiologist test brain stem evoked response in neonates, infants, and young children. Also obtain a gestational, perinatal, and family history from the parents.

HEAT INTOLERANCE

Heat intolerance refers to the inability to withstand high temperatures or to maintain a comfortable body temperature. It produces a continuous feeling of being overheated and, at times, profuse diaphoresis. Usually, this symptom develops gradually and is chronic.

Heat intolerance usually results from thyrotoxicosis. In this disorder, excess thyroid hormone stimulates peripheral tissues, increasing basal metabolism and producing excess heat. Although rare, hypothalamic disease may also cause intolerance to heat and cold.

History and physical examination
As you begin the examination, notice how much clothing the patient is wearing. Then ask him when he first noticed his heat intolerance. Did he gradually use fewer blankets at night? Does he have to turn up the air conditioning to keep cool? Is it hard for him to adjust to warm weather? Does he sweat in a hot environment? Find out if the patient's appetite or weight has changed. Also ask about unusual nervousness or other personality changes. Then take a drug history, especially noting use of amphetamines or amphetamine-like drugs. Ask the patient if he takes a prescribed thyroid drug. If so, what is the daily dosage and when did he last take it?

After taking vital signs, inspect the patient's skin for flushing and diaphoresis. Also note tremors and lid lag.

Common medical causes

• *Hypothalamic disease.* In this rare disease, usually caused by pituitary adenoma or hypothalamic or pineal tumors, body temperature fluctuates dramatically, causing alternating heat and cold intolerance. Related features include amenorrhea, disturbed sleep patterns, increased thirst and urination, increased appetite with weight gain, impaired visual acuity, headache, and personality changes, such as bursts of rage or laughter.

• *Thyrotoxicosis.* A classic symptom of thyrotoxicosis, heat intolerance may be accompanied by an enlarged thyroid, nervousness, weight loss despite increased appetite, diaphoresis, diarrhea, tremor, and palpitations. Although exophthalmos is characteristic, many patients don't display this sign. Associated findings may affect virtually every body system. Some common findings include irritability, difficulty concentrating, mood swings, muscle weakness, fatigue, lid lag, tachycardia, full and bounding pulse, widened pulse pressure, dyspnea, and amenorrhea or gynecomastia. Typically, the patient's skin is warm and flushed; premature graying and alopecia occur in both sexes.

Other causes

• *Drugs.* Amphetamines, amphetamine-like appetite suppressants, and excessive doses of thyroid hormone may cause heat intolerance. Anticholinergics may interfere with sweating to cause heat intolerance.

Special considerations

Adjust room temperature to make the patient comfortable. If the patient has diaphoresis, change his clothing and bed linens as necessary, and encourage adequate fluid intake.

Pediatric pointers

Rarely, maternal thyrotoxicosis may be passed to the neonate, resulting in heat intolerance. In most cases, acquired thyrotoxicosis appears between ages 12 and 14, although this, too, is rare. Dehydration can also make a child sensitive to heat.

HEMATEMESIS

Hematemesis, or vomiting of blood, usually indicates GI bleeding above the ligament of Treitz, which suspends the duodenum at its junction with the jejunum. Bright red or blood-streaked vomitus indicates fresh or recent bleeding. Dark red, brown, or black vomitus (the color and consistency of coffee grounds) indicates that blood has been retained in the stomach and partially digested.

Hematemesis usually results from GI disorders but may also result from coagulation disorders or from treatments that irritate the GI tract. Swallowed blood from epistaxis or oropharyngeal erosions may also cause bloody vomitus.

Hematemesis is always an important sign, but its severity depends on the amount, source, and rapidity of the bleeding. Massive hematemesis (vomiting of 500 to 1,000 ml of blood) may rapidly be life-threatening. Hematemesis may be precipitated by straining, emotional stress, use of anti-inflammatory drugs, and alcohol ingestion.

Emergency interventions

 If the patient has massive hematemesis, quickly check his vital signs. If you detect signs of shock, such as tachypnea, hypotension, and tachycardia, place the patient in a supine position and elevate his feet 20 to 30 degrees. Start a large-bore I.V. line for emergency fluid replacement. Also, send a blood sample for typing and crossmatching, and begin oxygen administration. Emergency endoscopy to locate the source of bleeding may be necessary. Prepare to insert a nasogastric (NG) tube for suction or iced lavage. A

Sengstaken-Blakemore tube may be used to compress esophageal varices. (See *Managing hematemesis with intubation.*)

History and physical examination

If the patient's hematemesis isn't immediately life-threatening, begin with a thorough history. First, have the patient describe the amount, color, and consistency of the vomitus. When did he first notice this sign? Has he ever vomited blood before? Find out if he also has bloody or black tarry stools. Note whether hematemesis is usually preceded by nausea, flatulence, diarrhea, or weakness. Has he recently had bouts of retching with or without vomiting?

Next, ask about a history of ulcers or of liver or coagulation disorders. Find out how much alcohol the patient drinks, if any. Is he taking aspirin or another nonsteroidal anti-inflammatory drug (NSAID), such as phenylbutazone or indomethacin? These drugs may cause erosive gastritis or ulcers.

Begin the physical examination by checking for orthostatic hypotension, an early warning sign of hypovolemia. Take blood pressure and pulse with the patient supine, sitting, then standing. A decrease of 10 mm Hg or more in systolic pressure or an increase of 10 beats/minute or more in pulse rate indicates volume depletion. After obtaining other vital signs, inspect the mucous membranes, nasopharynx, and skin for any signs of bleeding or other abnormalities. Finally, palpate the abdomen for tenderness, pain, or masses. Note lymphadenopathy.

Common medical causes

● *Coagulation disorders.* Any disorder that disrupts normal clotting may cause GI bleeding and moderate to severe hematemesis. Bleeding may occur in other body systems as well, resulting in such signs as epistaxis and ecchymosis. Also, each specific coagulation disorder, such as thrombocytopenia or hemophilia, has its own distinct associated effects.

● *Esophageal carcinoma.* A late sign of this disorder, hematemesis may be accompanied by steady chest pain that radiates to the back. Other features include substernal fullness, severe dysphagia, nausea, vomiting with nocturnal regurgitation and aspiration, hemoptysis, fever, hiccups, sore throat, melena, and halitosis.

● *Esophageal rupture.* The severity of hematemesis depends on the cause of the rupture. When instrumentation damages the esophagus, hematemesis is usually slight. However, rupture from Boerhaave's syndrome—increased esophageal pressure from vomiting or retching—or other esophageal disorders typically causes more severe hematemesis. This life-threatening disorder may also produce severe retrosternal, epigastric, neck, or scapular pain accompanied by chest and neck edema. Examination reveals subcutaneous crepitation in the chest wall, supraclavicular fossa, and neck. The patient may also show signs of respiratory distress, such as dyspnea and cyanosis.

● *Esophageal varices (ruptured).* Life-threatening rupture of esophageal varices may produce coffee-ground or massive, bright red vomitus. Signs of shock, such as hypotension or tachycardia, may follow or even precede hematemesis if the stomach fills with blood before vomiting occurs. Melena or painless hematochezia, ranging from slight oozing to massive rectal hemorrhage, may also occur.

● *Gastric carcinoma.* Painless bright red or dark brown vomitus is a late sign of this uncommon cancer. Usually, gastric carcinoma begins insidiously with upper abdominal discomfort. The patient then develops chronic dyspepsia, anorexia, and slight nausea. Later, he may have fatigue, weakness, weight loss, feelings of fullness, melena, altered bowel habits, and signs of malnutrition, such as muscle wasting and dry skin.

● *Gastritis (acute).* Hematemesis and melena are the most common signs of

MANAGING HEMATEMESIS WITH INTUBATION

A patient with hematemesis will need to have a GI tube inserted to allow blood drainage, to aspirate gastric contents, or to perform gastric lavage, if necessary. Here are some of the most common tubes and their uses.

Nasogastric tubes

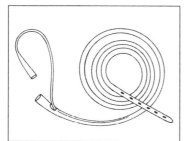

The *Salem-Sump tube* (above), a double-lumen nasogastric (NG) tube, is used to remove stomach fluid and gas or to aspirate gastric contents. It may also be used for gastric lavage, drug administration, or feeding. Its main advantage over the *Levin tube*—a single-lumen NG device—is that it allows atmospheric air to enter the patient's stomach so the tube can float freely instead of risking adhesion and damage to the gastric mucosa.

Wide-bore gastric tubes

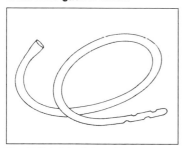

The *Edlich tube* (above) has one wide-bore lumen with four openings near the closed distal tip. A funnel or syringe can be connected at the proximal end. Like the other tubes,

the Edlich can aspirate a large volume of gastric contents quickly.

The *Ewald tube,* a wide-bore tube that allows passage of a large amount of fluid and clots quickly, is especially useful for gastric lavage in patients who have profuse GI bleeding or have ingested poison. Another wide-bore tube, the double-lumen *Levacuator,* has a large lumen for evacuation of gastric contents and a small one for lavage.

Esophageal tubes

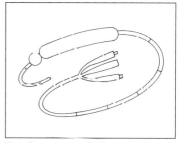

The *Sengstaken-Blakemore tube* (above), a triple-lumen, double-balloon esophageal tube, provides a gastric aspiration port that allows drainage from below the gastric balloon. It can also be used for instilling medication.

A similar tube, the *Linton,* can aspirate esophageal and gastric contents without risking necrosis because it has no esophageal balloon. The *Minnesota esophagogastric tamponade tube,* which has four lumens and two balloons, provides pressure monitoring ports for both balloons without the need for Y-connectors.

acute gastritis. In fact, they may be the only signs, although mild epigastric discomfort, nausea, fever, and malaise may also occur. Massive blood loss will precipitate signs of shock. Typically, the patient has a history of alcohol abuse or has used aspirin or some other NSAID. Gastritis secondary to *Helicobacter pylori* infection is also possible.

• *Mallory-Weiss syndrome.* Characterized by a mucosal tear of the cardia or lower esophagus, this syndrome may produce hematemesis and melena. It's commonly triggered by severe vomiting, retching, or straining (as from coughing). Severe bleeding may precipitate signs of shock, such as tachycardia, hypotension, dyspnea, and cool, clammy skin.

• *Peptic ulcer.* Hematemesis may occur here when a peptic ulcer penetrates an artery, a vein, or highly vascular tissue. Massive—and possibly life-threatening—hematemesis is typical when an artery is penetrated. Other features include melena or hematochezia, chills, fever, and signs of shock and dehydration, such as tachycardia, hypotension, poor skin turgor, and thirst. Usually, the patient will have a history of epigastric pain that's relieved by foods or antacids and of nausea, vomiting, and epigastric tenderness.

Other causes
• *Treatments.* Traumatic NG or endotracheal intubation may cause hematemesis associated with swallowed blood. Nose or throat surgery may also cause this sign in the same way.

Special considerations
Closely monitor the patient's vital signs every 15 minutes, and watch for signs of shock. In addition, keep accurate intake and output records. Place the patient on bed rest in a low or semi-Fowler position to prevent aspiration of vomitus. Keep suctioning equipment nearby and use it as needed. Provide frequent oral hygiene and emotional support—the sight of bloody vomitus can be frightening. Administer histamine-2 blockers I.V.; vasopressin may be required for variceal hemorrhage. As the bleeding tapers off, give hourly doses of antacids by NG tube.

Explain diagnostic tests, such as serum electrolyte studies, endoscopy, and barium swallow. Check the patient's stools regularly for occult blood.

Pediatric pointers
Hematemesis is not nearly as common in children as it is in adults. Occasionally, neonates have hematemesis caused by swallowing maternal blood during delivery or nursing from a cracked nipple. Hemorrhagic disease of the newborn and esophageal erosion may also cause hematemesis in infants, requiring immediate fluid replacement.

HEMATOCHEZIA
[Rectal bleeding]

The passage of bloody stools, hematochezia usually indicates GI bleeding below the ligament of Treitz. In fact, it may be the first sign of lower GI bleeding. However, hematochezia—usually preceded by hematemesis—may also accompany a rapid hemorrhage of 1 L or more from the upper GI tract.

Hematochezia ranges from formed, blood-streaked stools to liquid, bloody stools that may be bright red, dark mahogany, or maroon in color. This sign usually develops abruptly and is heralded by abdominal pain.

Although hematochezia commonly results from GI disorders, it may also result from coagulation disorders, the effects of toxins, and certain diagnostic tests. Always a significant sign, hematochezia may precipitate life-threatening hypovolemia.

Emergency interventions

 If the patient has severe hematochezia, quickly check his vital signs. If you detect signs of shock, such as hypotension and tachycardia, place him in a supine position and elevate his feet 20 to 30 degrees. Prepare to administer oxygen, and start a large-bore I.V. line for emergency fluid replacement. Next, obtain a blood sample for typing and crossmatching. Insert a nasogastric tube. Expect to assist with endoscopy, which may be necessary to detect the source of the bleeding.

History and physical examination

If the patient's hematochezia isn't immediately life threatening, ask him to fully describe the amount, color, and consistency of his bloody stools. (If possible, also inspect and characterize the stools yourself.) How long have his stools been this way? Do they always look the same, or does the amount of blood seem to vary? Ask about associated signs and symptoms.

Next, explore the patient's medical history, focusing on GI and coagulation disorders. Ask about use of GI irritants, such as alcohol, aspirin, and other nonsteroidal anti-inflammatory drugs.

Begin the physical examination by checking for orthostatic hypotension, an early sign of shock. Take the patient's blood pressure and pulse while he's lying down, sitting, and standing. If systolic pressure decreases by 10 mm Hg or more, or pulse rate increases by 10 beats/minute or more when he changes position, suspect volume depletion and impending shock.

Then examine the skin for petechiae or spider angiomas. Palpate the abdomen for tenderness, pain, or masses. Also note lymphadenopathy. Finally, a digital rectal examination must be done to rule out any rectal masses.

Common medical causes

● *Anal fissure.* Slight hematochezia characterizes this disorder; blood may streak the stool or appear on toilet tissue. Accompanying hematochezia is severe rectal pain that may make the patient reluctant to defecate, thereby causing constipation.

● *Angiodysplastic lesions.* Most common in the elderly, these arteriovenous lesions of the ascending colon typically cause chronic, painless, bright red rectal bleeding. Occasionally, this bleeding may result in life-threatening blood loss and signs of shock, such as tachycardia and hypotension.

● *Coagulation disorders.* Moderate to severe hematochezia may occur in these disorders. Bleeding may also occur in other body systems, producing such signs as epistaxis and purpura. Specific coagulation disorders, such as thrombocytopenia and disseminated intravascular coagulation, also produce characteristic associated findings.

● *Colon cancer.* Bright red hematochezia is a telling sign, especially in cancer of the left colon. Early tumor growth in the right colon may cause melena, abdominal aching, pressure, and dull cramps. As the disease progresses, the patient will develop weakness and fatigue. Later, he may also experience pain, diarrhea, anorexia, weight loss, anemia, vomiting, abdominal mass, and signs of obstruction, such as abdominal distention and abnormal bowel sounds.

Cancer of the left colon usually causes early signs of obstruction, including rectal pressure, bleeding, and intermittent fullness or cramping. As the disease progresses, the patient also will develop obstipation, diarrhea, or ribbon-shaped stools. Passage of stool or flatus typically relieves the pain. Stools are grossly bloody.

● *Colorectal polyps.* These polyps are the most common cause of intermittent hematochezia in adults under age 60; however, they sometimes produce no symptoms. When located high in the colon, polyps may cause blood-streaked stools that yield a positive response when tested with guaiac. When the stools are located closer to the rectum, they may bleed freely.

- **Diverticulitis.** Most common in the elderly, this disorder can suddenly cause mild to moderate rectal bleeding after the patient feels the urge to defecate. The bleeding may end abruptly or it may progress to life-threatening blood loss with signs of shock. Associated signs and symptoms may include left lower quadrant pain that's relieved by defecation and alternating episodes of constipation and diarrhea.

- **Esophageal varices (ruptured).** In this life-threatening disorder, hematochezia may range from slight rectal oozing to grossly bloody stools. It may be accompanied by mild to severe hematemesis or melena. This painless—but massive—hemorrhage may precipitate signs of shock, such as tachycardia and hypotension. In fact, signs of shock occasionally precede overt signs of bleeding. Typically, the patient will have a history of chronic liver disease.

- **Food poisoning (staphylococcal).** One to six hours after ingesting food toxins, the patient may have bloody diarrhea. Accompanying signs and symptoms include severe, cramping abdominal pain, nausea and vomiting, and prostration, all of which last a few hours.

- **Hemorrhoids.** Hematochezia may accompany external hemorrhoids, which typically cause painful defecation, resulting in constipation. Less painful internal hemorrhoids usually produce a more chronic hematochezia that may eventually lead to signs of anemia, such as weakness and fatigue.

- **Leptospirosis.** The severe form of this infection—Weil's syndrome—produces hematochezia or melena along with other signs of bleeding, such as epistaxis and hemoptysis. Typically, the bleeding is preceded by a sudden frontal headache and severe thigh and lumbar myalgia that may be accompanied by cutaneous hyperesthesia. Chills and a rapidly rising fever then follow, perhaps with nausea and vomiting. Usually, fever, headache, and myalgia intensify and persist for weeks. Other findings include right upper quadrant tenderness, hepatomegaly, and jaundice.

- **Peptic ulcer.** Upper GI bleeding is a common complication in this disorder. The patient may display hematochezia, hematemesis, or melena, depending on the rapidity and amount of bleeding. If the peptic ulcer penetrates an artery or a vein, massive bleeding may precipitate signs of shock, such as hypotension and tachycardia. Other findings may include chills, fever, and signs and symptoms of dehydration, such as dry mucous membranes, poor skin turgor, and thirst. The patient typically has a history of epigastric pain that's relieved by foods or antacids; he may also complain of nausea and vomiting.

- **Ulcerative proctitis.** Despite an intense urge to defecate, the patient passes only bright red blood, pus, or mucus. Other common signs and symptoms include acute constipation and tenesmus.

Other causes

- **Tests.** Certain procedures, especially colonoscopy, polypectomy, and proctosigmoidoscopy, may cause rectal bleeding. Bowel perforation is rare.

Special considerations

Place the patient on bed rest and check his vital signs every 15 minutes, watching for signs of shock, such as hypotension and tachycardia. Monitor intake and output hourly. Remember to provide emotional support because hematochezia may frighten the patient.

Prepare the patient for blood tests, endoscopy, and GI X-rays. Inspect the patient's stools and test them for occult blood. If necessary, send a stool sample to the laboratory to check for parasites.

Pediatric pointers

Hematochezia is much less common in children than in adults. It may result from structural disorders, such as intussusception and Meckel's diverticulum, or from inflammatory disorders, such as peptic ulcer and ulcerative colitis.

In children, ulcerative colitis typically produces chronic, rather than acute, signs and symptoms and may also cause slow growth and maturation related to malnutrition.

HEMATURIA

A cardinal sign of renal and urinary tract disorders, hematuria is the abnormal presence of blood in the urine. By strict definition, it means three or more red blood cells per high-power microscopic field. Hematuria may be continuous or intermittent, is commonly accompanied by pain, and may be aggravated by prolonged standing or walking. Microscopic hematuria is confirmed by an occult blood indicator, whereas macroscopic hematuria is immediately visible. However, macroscopic hematuria must be distinguished from pseudohematuria.

Hematuria may be classified by the stage of urination it predominantly affects. Bleeding at the start of urination—initial hematuria—usually indicates urethral pathology; bleeding at the end of urination—terminal hematuria—usually indicates pathology of the bladder neck, posterior urethra, or prostate. Bleeding throughout urination—total hematuria—usually indicates pathology above the bladder neck. Another clue to the source of the bleeding is the blood's color. Generally, dark or brownish blood indicates renal or upper urinary tract bleeding, whereas bright red blood indicates lower urinary tract bleeding.

Hematuria may result from one of two mechanisms: rupture or perforation of vessels in the renal system or urinary tract, or impaired glomerular filtration, which allows red blood cells to seep into the urine. Although it usually results from renal and urinary tract disorders, hematuria may also result from certain GI, prostate, vaginal, or coagulation disorders or from the effects of drugs. Invasive therapy or diagnostic tests that involve manipulative instrumentation of the renal and urologic systems may also cause hematuria. Nonpathologic hematuria may result from fever and hypercatabolic states. Transient hematuria may also follow strenuous exercise.

History and physical examination

After detecting hematuria, obtain a pertinent health history. If the patient has macroscopic hematuria, ask him when it began. Does it vary in severity between voidings? Is it worse at the beginning, middle, or end of urination? Is the patient passing any clots? Find out if hematuria has occurred before. To rule out artifactitious hematuria, ask about bleeding hemorrhoids or the onset of menses, if appropriate.

Also ask about recent abdominal or flank trauma. Has the patient been exercising strenuously? Note a history of renal, urinary, prostatic, or coagulation disorders. Then obtain a drug history.

Begin the physical examination by palpating and percussing the abdomen and flanks. Next, percuss the costovertebral angle to elicit tenderness. Check the urinary meatus for bleeding or other abnormalities. Using a chemical reagent strip, test a urine sample for protein. A vaginal or digital rectal examination may be necessary.

Common medical causes

● *Cystitis.* Hematuria is a telling sign in all types of cystitis. Bacterial cystitis usually produces macroscopic hematuria with urinary urgency and frequency, dysuria, nocturia, and tenesmus. The patient complains of perineal and lumbar pain,

(Text continues on page 304.)

HEMATURIA: COMMON CAUSES AND ASSOCIATED FINDINGS

CHIEF CAUSES	Abdominal distention	Abdominal pain	Anuria	Bladder distention	Blood pressure, increased	Bowel sounds, hypoactive	Colicky pain	Costovertebral angle tenderness	Dysuria	Edema, generalized	Edema of the legs	
Cystitis (bacterial)									●			
Cystitis (chronic interstitial)									●			
Cystitis (tubercular)									●			
Cystitis (viral)									●			
Glomerulonephritis (chronic)					●					●		
Obstructive nephropathy		●	●				●	●				
Polycystic kidney disease		●			●		●		●			
Prostatic hyperplasia (benign)				●								
Prostatitis (acute)				●					●			
Prostatitis (chronic)				●					●			
Pyelonephritis (acute)	●						●	●	●			
Renal infarction		●	●		●	●		●				
Renal neoplasm					●		●	●			●	
Renal papillary necrosis (acute)		●	●			●	●	●				
Renal trauma						●						
Renal tuberculosis		●					●		●			
Renal vein thrombosis			●					●			●	
Schistosomiasis							●		●			
Sickle cell anemia												
Vasculitis			●		●							

MAJOR ASSOCIATED SIGNS AND SYMPTOMS

Fever	Flank mass	Flank pain	Lumbar pain	Murmurs	Nausea	Nocturia	Oliguria	Perineal pain	Polyarthralgia	Polyuria	Proteinuria	Purpura	Rash	Urethral discharge	Urinary frequency	Urinary hesitancy	Urinary urgency	Urine stream, diminished	Vomiting
●			●			●		●							●		●		
						●									●				
		●													●		●		
●						●									●		●		
											●								
			●				●			●									
			●	●							●	●			●		●		
						●		●							●	●		●	
●			●		●			●	●						●		●		●
								●						●	●		●		
●		●			●	●									●		●		●
●		●			●		●				●								●
●	●	●			●														●
●		●					●												●
	●	●			●		●						●						●
			●								●				●				
●		●	●				●				●								
				●					●										
●								●				●	●						

suprapubic discomfort, and fatigue and occasionally has a low-grade fever.

More common in women, *chronic interstitial cystitis* occasionally may cause grossly bloody hematuria. Associated features include urinary frequency, dysuria, nocturia, and tenesmus. Both microscopic and macroscopic hematuria may occur in *tubercular cystitis,* which may also cause urinary urgency and frequency, dysuria, tenesmus, flank pain, fatigue, and anorexia. *Viral cystitis* usually produces hematuria, urinary urgency and frequency, dysuria, nocturia, tenesmus, and fever.

• *Chronic glomerulonephritis.* This disorder usually causes microscopic hematuria accompanied by proteinuria, generalized edema, and increased blood pressure. Signs and symptoms of uremia may also occur in advanced disease.

Special considerations

Because hematuria may frighten and upset the patient, be sure to provide emotional support. Check his vital signs at least every 4 hours and monitor intake and output, including the amount and pattern of hematuria. Administer prescribed analgesics and promote bed rest, as indicated.

Prepare the patient for diagnostic tests, such as blood and urine studies, cystoscopy, and renal X-rays or biopsy. Teach the patient how to collect serial urine specimens using the three-glass technique. This technique helps determine whether bleeding occurs at the beginning or end or throughout urination.

HEMIANOPIA

Hemianopia is loss of vision in half the visual field (usually the vertical half) of one or both eyes. It is caused by a lesion affecting the optic chiasm, optic tract, or optic radiation. However, if the visual field defects are identical in both eyes but affect less than half the field of vision in each eye (incomplete homonymous hemianopia), the lesion may be in the occipital lobe; otherwise, it probably involves the parietal or temporal lobe. (See *Recognizing types of hemianopia.*)

Defects in visual perception due to cerebral lesions are usually associated with impaired color vision.

History and physical examination

Suspect a visual field defect if the patient seems startled when you approach him from one side or if he fails to see objects placed directly in front of him. To help determine the type of defect, compare the patient's visual fields to your own (assuming yours are normal). First, ask the patient to cover his right eye while you cover your left eye. Then, move a pen or a similarly shaped object from the periphery of his (and your) uncovered eye into his field of vision. Ask the patient to indicate when he first sees the object. Does he see it at the same time you do? After you do? Repeat this test in each quadrant of both eyes. Then, for each eye, plot the defect by shading the area of a circle that corresponds to the area of vision loss.

Now evaluate the patient's level of consciousness (LOC), take his vital signs, and check his pupillary reaction and motor response. Ask if he has experienced a headache, dysarthria, or seizures. Does he have ptosis, facial or extremity weakness, hallucinations, or loss of color vision? If so, when did the neurologic symptoms start? Obtain a medical history, noting especially eye disorders, hypertension, and diabetes mellitus.

Common medical causes

• *Carotid artery aneurysm.* An aneurysm in the internal carotid artery can cause contralateral or bilateral defects in the visual fields. It can also cause hemiplegia, decreased LOC, headache, aphasia,

RECOGNIZING TYPES OF HEMIANOPIA

Lesions of the optic pathways cause visual field defects. The lesion's site determines the type of defect. For example, a lesion of the optic chiasm involving only those fibers that cross over to the opposite side causes *bitemporal hemianopia*—visual loss in the temporal half of each field. However, a lesion of the optic tract or a complete lesion of the optic radiation produces visual loss in the same half of each field—either left or right *homonymous hemianopia.*

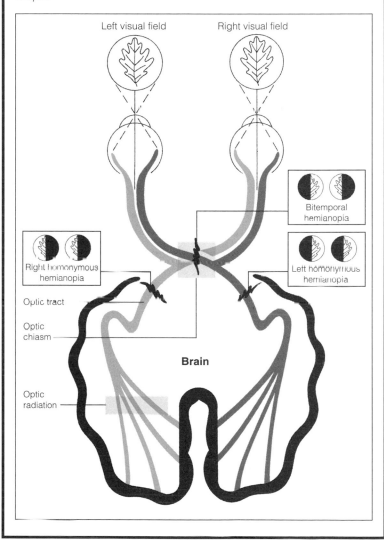

behavior disturbances, and unilateral hypoesthesia.

• *Cerebrovascular accident (CVA).* Hemianopia can result when a hemorrhagic, thrombotic, or embolic CVA affects any part of the optic pathway. Associated signs and symptoms depend on the location and size of the CVA but may include decreased LOC, personality changes, emotional lability, headache, seizures, and intellectual deficits, such as memory loss and poor judgment. The patient may have contralateral hemiplegia, dysarthria, dysphagia, ataxia, unilateral sensory loss, apraxia, agnosia, aphasia, blurred vision, decreased visual acuity, and diplopia. He may also have urine retention or urinary incontinence, constipation, and vomiting.

• *Occipital lobe lesion.* The most common symptoms arising from a lesion of one occipital lobe include incomplete homonymous hemianopia, scotomas, and impaired color vision. The patient may also experience visual hallucinations: flashes of light or color or visions of objects, people, animals, or geometric forms. These may appear in the defective field or may move toward it from the intact field.

• *Parietal lobe lesion.* This lesion produces homonymous hemianopia and sensory deficits, such as an inability to perceive body position or passive movement or to localize tactile, thermal, or vibratory stimuli. It may also cause apraxia and visual or tactile agnosia.

• *Pituitary tumor.* A tumor that compresses nerve fibers supplying the nasal half of both retinas causes complete or partial bitemporal hemianopia that occurs first in the upper visual fields but later can progress to blindness. Related findings include blurred vision, diplopia, headache, and (rarely) somnolence, hypothermia, or seizures.

Special considerations

If the patient's visual field defect is significant, further visual field tests, such as perimetry testing or a tangent screen examination, may be indicated.

Tell the patient the extent of his defect so that he can learn to compensate for it. Advise him to scan his surroundings frequently, turning his head in the direction of the defective visual field so he can directly view objects he'd normally notice peripherally. Also, approach him from the unaffected side. Position his bed so his unaffected side faces the door; if he's ambulatory, remove objects that could cause falls and alert him to other possible hazards. Place his clock and other objects within his field of vision, and avoid putting dangerous objects (such as hot dishes) where he can't see them.

Pediatric pointers

In children, a brain tumor is the most common cause of hemianopia. To help detect this sign, look for nonverbal clues—for example, a child reaching for a toy but missing it. To help the child compensate for hemianopia, place objects within his visual field and teach his parents to do this as well.

HEMOPTYSIS

Frightening to the patient and commonly ominous, hemoptysis is the expectoration of blood or bloody sputum from the lungs or tracheobronchial tree. It's sometimes confused with bleeding from the mouth, throat, nasopharynx, or GI tract. (See *Identifying hemoptysis.*) Expectoration of 200 ml of blood in a single episode suggests severe bleeding; expectoration of 400 ml in 3 hours or more than 600 ml in 16 hours signals a life-threatening crisis.

Hemoptysis usually results from chronic bronchitis, bronchogenic carcinoma, or bronchiectasis. However, it may also result from inflammatory, infectious, cardiovascular, or coagulation disor-

EXAMINATION TIP

 IDENTIFYING HEMOPTYSIS

These guidelines will help you distinguish hemoptysis from epistaxis, hematemesis, and brown, red, or pink sputum.

Hemoptysis
Often frothy because it's mixed with air, blood expectorated in the sputum is typically bright red with an alkaline pH (tested with nitrazine paper). Hemoptysis is strongly suggested by the presence of respiratory signs and symptoms, including a cough, a tickling sensation in the throat, and blood produced from repeated coughing episodes. (You can rule out epistaxis because the patient's nasal passages and posterior pharynx are usually clear.)

Hematemesis
Hematemesis usually originates in the GI tract; the patient vomits or regurgitates coffee-ground material that contains food particles, tests positive for occult blood, and has an acid pH. But he may vomit bright red blood or swallowed blood from the oral cavity and nasopharynx. After an episode of hematemesis, the patient may have stools with traces of blood. Many patients with hematemesis also complain of dyspepsia.

Brown, red, or pink sputum
Brown, red, or pink sputum can result from oxidation of inhaled bronchodilators. Sputum that looks like old blood may result from rupture of an amebic abscess into the bronchus. Red or brown sputum may occur in a patient with pneumonia caused by the enterobacterium *Serratia marcescens.* "Currant jelly" sputum occurs in *Klebsiella* infections.

ders—or, in up to 15% of patients, from unknown causes. Occasionally, it stems from a ruptured aortic aneurysm. (See *What happens in hemoptysis,* page 308.)

The most common causes of *massive hemoptysis* are lung cancer, bronchiectasis, active tuberculosis, and cavitary pulmonary disease from necrotic infections or tuberculosis.

Emergency interventions
 If the patient coughs up copious amounts of blood, endotracheal intubation may be required. Suction frequently to remove blood. Massive hemoptysis can cause airway obstruction and asphyxiation. Insert an I.V. line to allow fluid replacement, drug administration, and blood transfusions if needed. Do an emergency bronchoscopy to iden-

tify the bleeding site. Monitor blood pressure and pulse rate to detect hypotension and tachycardia, and draw an arterial blood sample for laboratory analysis to monitor respiratory status.

History and physical examination
If hemoptysis is mild, ask the patient when the current episode began. Has he ever coughed up blood before? About how much blood is he coughing up now? And how often? Ask about a history of cardiac, pulmonary, or bleeding disorders. If he's receiving anticoagulant therapy, find out the drug, its dosage and schedule, and the duration of therapy. Is he taking other prescription drugs? Does he smoke?

Take the patient's vital signs, and examine his nose, mouth, and pharynx for

WHAT HAPPENS IN HEMOPTYSIS

Hemoptysis results from bleeding into the respiratory tract by bronchial or pulmonary vessels. Bleeding reflects alterations in the vascular walls and in blood-clotting mechanisms. It can reflect any of the following pathophysiologic processes:
• hemorrhage and diapedesis of red blood cells from the pulmonary microvasculature into the alveoli
• necrosis of lung tissue that causes inflammation and rupture of blood vessels or hemorrhage into the alveolar spaces
• rupture of an aortic aneurysm into the tracheobronchial tree
• rupture of distended endobronchial blood vessels from pulmonary hypertension due to mitral stenosis
• rupture of a pulmonary arteriovenous fistula or of bronchial or pulmonary artery or pulmonary venous collateral channels
• sloughing of a caseous lesion into the tracheobronchial tree
• ulceration and erosion of the bronchial epithelium.

sources of bleeding. Inspect the configuration of his chest, and look for abnormal movement during breathing, use of accessory muscles, or retractions. Observe his respiratory rate, depth, and rhythm. Finally, examine his skin for lesions.

Next, palpate the patient's chest for diaphragm level and for tenderness, respiratory excursion, fremitus, and abnormal pulsations; then percuss for flatness, dullness, resonance, hyperresonance, and tympany. Finally, auscultate the lungs, noting especially the quality and intensity of breath sounds. Also auscultate for

heart murmurs, bruits, and pleural friction rubs.

Obtain a sputum sample and examine it for overall quantity, for the amount of blood it contains, and for its color, odor, and consistency.

Common medical causes

• *Aortic aneurysm (ruptured).* An aortic aneurysm occasionally ruptures into the tracheobronchial tree, causing hemoptysis and sudden death.

• *Bronchial adenoma.* This insidious disorder causes recurring hemoptysis in up to 30% of patients, along with a chronic cough and local wheezing.

• *Bronchiectasis.* Inflamed bronchial surfaces and eroded bronchial blood vessels cause hemoptysis, which can vary from blood-tinged sputum to blood (in about 20% of patients). The patient's sputum may also be copious, foul-smelling, and purulent. He may have a chronic cough, coarse crackles, clubbing (a late sign), fever, weight loss, fatigue, weakness, malaise, and dyspnea on exertion.

• *Bronchitis (chronic).* The first sign of this disorder is typically a productive cough that lasts at least 3 months and that eventually leads to production of blood-streaked sputum; massive hemorrhage is unusual. Other respiratory effects include dyspnea, tachypnea, prolonged expirations, wheezing, scattered rhonchi, accessory muscle use, barrel chest, and clubbing (a late sign).

• *Lung abscess.* In about 50% of patients, this disorder produces blood-streaked sputum resulting from bronchial ulceration, necrosis, and granulation tissue. Common associated findings include diaphoresis, anorexia, weight loss, headache, weakness, dyspnea, pleuritic or dull chest pain, clubbing, fever with chills, and a cough with large amounts of purulent, foul-smelling sputum. Auscultation reveals tubular or cavernous breath sounds and crackles. Percussion reveals dullness on the affected side.

• *Lung cancer.* Ulceration of the bronchus commonly causes recurring hemoptysis (an early sign), which can vary from blood-streaked sputum to blood. Related findings include a productive cough, dyspnea, fever, anorexia, weight loss, wheezing, and chest pain (a late symptom).

• *Pneumonia.* In up to 50% of patients, *Klebsiella pneumoniae* produces dark brown or red (currant-jelly) sputum, which is so tenacious the patient has difficulty expelling it from his mouth. Pneumonia begins abruptly with chills, fever, dyspnea, productive cough, and severe pleuritic chest pain. Associated findings may include cyanosis, prostration, tachycardia, decreased breath sounds, and crackles.

Pneumococcal pneumonia produces pinkish or rusty mucoid sputum. It begins with a sudden, shaking chill; a rapidly rising temperature; and, in over 80% of patients, tachycardia and tachypnea. Within a few hours, the patient typically experiences a productive cough along with severe, stabbing, pleuritic pain. The agonizing chest pain leads to rapid, shallow, grunting respirations with splinting. Examination reveals respiratory distress with dyspnea and accessory muscle use, crackles, and dullness on percussion over the affected lung. Malaise, weakness, myalgia, and prostration accompany high fever.

• *Pulmonary edema.* Severe cardiogenic or noncardiogenic pulmonary edema commonly causes frothy, blood-tinged pink sputum, which accompanies severe dyspnea, orthopnea, gasping, anxiety, cyanosis, diffuse crackles, a ventricular gallop, and cold, clammy skin. This life-threatening condition may also cause tachycardia, lethargy, cardiac arrhythmias, tachypnea, hypotension, and a thready pulse.

• *Pulmonary embolism with infarction.* Hemoptysis is a common finding in this life-threatening disorder, although massive hemoptysis is less common. Typical initial symptoms are dyspnea and anginal or pleuritic chest pain. Other common clinical features include tachycardia, tachypnea, low-grade fever, and diaphoresis. Less commonly, splinting of the chest, leg edema, and—with a large embolus—cyanosis, syncope, and distended neck veins may occur. Examination reveals decreased breath sounds, pleural friction rubs, crackles, diffuse wheezing, dullness on percussion, and signs of circulatory collapse (weak, rapid pulse; hypotension), cerebral ischemia (transient loss of consciousness, seizures), and hypoxemia (restlessness and—particularly in the elderly—hemiplegia and other focal neurologic deficits).

• *Pulmonary hypertension (primary).* Features generally develop late and commonly include hemoptysis, exertional dyspnea, and fatigue. Anginalike pain usually occurs with exertion and may radiate to the neck but not to the arms. Other findings include arrhythmias, syncope, cough, and hoarseness.

• *Pulmonary tuberculosis.* Blood-streaked or blood-tinged sputum commonly occurs in this disorder; massive hemoptysis may occur in advanced cavitary tuberculosis. Accompanying respiratory findings include a chronic productive cough, fine crackles after coughing, dyspnea, dullness on percussion, increased tactile fremitus and, possibly, amphoric breath sounds. The patient may also have night sweats, malaise, fatigue, fever, anorexia, weight loss, and pleuritic chest pain.

• *Systemic lupus erythematosus.* In 50% of patients with this disorder, pleuritis and pneumonitis cause hemoptysis, cough, dyspnea, pleuritic chest pain, and crackles. Related findings are a butterfly rash in the acute phase, nondeforming joint pain and stiffness, photosensitivity, Raynaud's phenomenon, seizures or psychosis, anorexia, and lymphadenopathy.

• *Tracheal trauma.* Torn tracheal mucosa may cause hemoptysis, hoarseness, dysphagia, neck pain, airway occlusion, and respiratory distress.

Other causes
● *Diagnostic tests.* Lung or airway injury from bronchoscopy, laryngoscopy, mediastinoscopy, or lung biopsy can cause bleeding and hemoptysis.

Special considerations
Comfort and reassure the patient, who is likely to react to this alarming sign with anxiety and apprehension. Place him in a slight Trendelenburg position to promote drainage of blood from the lung. If necessary to protect the nonbleeding lung, place him in the lateral decubitus position, with the suspected bleeding lung facing down. (Position him cautiously because hypoxemia may worsen with the healthy lung facing up.) Cough suppression may or may not be desirable: Cough suppressants can prevent blood from spreading throughout the lungs, but they can also lead to airway obstruction from accumulated blood.

Prepare the patient for diagnostic tests, such as complete blood count, chest X-rays, sputum culture and smear, coagulation studies, bronchoscopy, lung biopsy, pulmonary arteriography, and lung scan.

Hemoptysis usually stops (but not abruptly) during treatment of the causative disorder, but it may recur in many chronic disorders. Instruct the patient to report recurring episodes and to bring a sputum sample containing blood if he returns for treatment or reevaluation.

Pediatric pointers
Sometimes no cause can be found for pulmonary hemorrhage occurring within the first 2 weeks of life; the prognosis for this condition is poor. Hemoptysis in children may stem from Goodpasture's syndrome, Heiner syndrome, cystic fibrosis, or (rarely) idiopathic primary pulmonary hemosiderosis.

HEPATOMEGALY
[Liver enlargement]

This sign indicates potentially reversible primary or secondary liver disease. It may stem from diverse pathophysiologic mechanisms: dilated hepatic sinusoids (in heart failure), persistently high venous pressure leading to liver congestion (in chronic constrictive pericarditis), dysfunction and engorgement of hepatocytes (in hepatitis), fatty infiltration of parenchymal cells causing fibrous tissue (in cirrhosis), distention of liver cells with glycogen (in diabetes), or infiltration of amyloid (in amyloidosis).

Hepatomegaly may be confirmed by palpation, percussion, or radiologic tests. It may be mistaken for displacement of the liver by the diaphragm in a respiratory disorder, by an abdominal tumor, by a spinal deformity such as kyphosis, by the gallbladder, or by fecal material or a neoplasm in the colon.

History and physical examination
Hepatomegaly is seldom a patient's major complaint. It usually comes to light during palpation and percussion of the abdomen.

If you suspect hepatomegaly, ask the patient about his use of alcohol and exposure to hepatitis. Also ask if he's currently ill or taking any prescribed drugs. If he complains of abdominal pain, ask him to locate and describe it.

Inspect the patient's skin and sclera for jaundice, dilated veins (suggesting generalized congestion), scars from previous surgery, and spider angiomas (common in cirrhosis). Next, inspect the contour of his abdomen. Is it protuberant over the liver or distended (possibly from ascites)? Also, measure his abdominal girth.

Percuss the liver, but be careful to identify structures and conditions that can obscure dull percussion notes, such as the sternum, ribs, breast tissue, pleural effusions, and gas in the colon. (See *Percussing for liver size and position*.) Next, during deep inspiration, palpate the liver's edge (tender and rounded in hepatitis and cardiac decompensation, rocklike in carcinoma, or firm in cirrhosis).

Take the patient's vital signs for baseline data, and assess his nutritional status. An enlarged liver that's functioning poorly will cause muscle wasting, exaggerated skeletal prominences, weight loss, thin hair, and edema.

Evaluate the patient's level of consciousness. When an enlarged liver loses its ability to detoxify waste products, metabolic substances toxic to brain cells accumulate. As a result, watch for personality changes, irritability, agitation, memory loss, inability to concentrate, and—in a severely ill patient—coma.

Common medical causes

• *Amyloidosis.* This rare disorder can cause hepatomegaly and mild jaundice as well as renal, cardiac, and other GI effects.

• *Cirrhosis.* Late in this disorder, the liver becomes enlarged, nodular, and hard. Other late signs and symptoms affect all body systems. *Respiratory findings* include limited thoracic expansion due to abdominal ascites, leading to hypoxia. *Central nervous system findings* include signs and symptoms of hepatic encephalopathy, such as lethargy, slurred speech, asterixis, peripheral neuritis, paranoia, hallucinations, extreme obtundation, and coma.

Hematologic signs include epistaxis, easy bruising, and bleeding gums. *Endocrine findings* include testicular atrophy, gynecomastia, loss of chest and axillary hair, and menstrual irregularities. *Integumentary effects* include abnormal pigmentation, severe pruritus, extreme dryness, poor tissue turgor, spider angiomas, and palmar erythema. The patient may also have fetor hepaticus, en-

PERCUSSING FOR LIVER SIZE AND POSITION

With your patient supine, begin at the right iliac crest to percuss up the right midclavicular line (MCL), as shown below. The percussion note becomes dull when you reach the liver's inferior border— usually at the costal margin but sometimes at a lower point in a patient with liver disease. Mark this point and then percuss down from the right clavicle, again along the right MCL. The liver's superior border usually lies between the fifth and seventh intercostal spaces. Mark the superior border.

The distance between the two marked points represents the approximate span of the liver's right lobe, which normally ranges from 2⅜″ to 4¾″ (6 to 12 cm).

Now assess the liver's left lobe similarly, percussing along the sternal midline. Again, mark the points where you hear dull percussion notes. Also measure the span of the left lobe, which normally ranges from 1½″ to 3⅛″ (4 to 8 cm). Record your findings for use as a baseline.

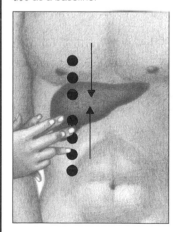

larged superficial abdominal veins, muscle atrophy, right upper quadrant pain that worsens when he sits up or leans forward, and a palpable spleen. Portal hypertension (elevated pressure in the portal vein) causes bleeding from esophageal varices.

• **Diabetes mellitus.** Poorly controlled diabetes in overweight patients commonly produces fatty infiltration of the liver, hepatomegaly, and right upper quadrant tenderness along with polydipsia, polyphagia, and polyuria. These features are more common in type II than in type I diabetes. The chronically enlarged fatty liver typically produces no symptoms except for slight tenderness.

• **Granulomatous disorders.** Sarcoidosis, histoplasmosis, and other such disorders commonly produce a slightly enlarged, firm liver.

• **Hepatic abscess.** Hepatomegaly may accompany fever (a primary sign), nausea, vomiting, chills, weakness, diarrhea, anorexia, and right upper quadrant pain and tenderness.

• **Hepatic neoplasms.** Primary tumors commonly cause hepatomegaly, with pain or tenderness in the right upper quadrant and a friction rub or bruit over the liver. Common related findings are weight loss, anorexia, nausea, and vomiting. Peripheral edema, ascites, jaundice, and a palpable right upper quadrant mass may also be present. Metastatic liver tumors also cause hepatomegaly, but the patient's accompanying signs and symptoms reflect his primary cancer.

• **Hepatitis.** In viral hepatitis, early signs and symptoms include nausea, anorexia, vomiting, fatigue, malaise, photophobia, sore throat, cough, and headache. Hepatomegaly occurs in the icteric phase and continues during the recovery phase. Also, during the icteric phase, the early signs and symptoms diminish and others appear: liver tenderness, slight weight loss, dark urine, clay-colored stools, jaundice, pruritus, right upper quadrant pain, and splenomegaly.

• **Infectious mononucleosis.** Occasionally, this disorder causes hepatomegaly. Prodromal symptoms include headache, malaise, and fatigue. After 3 to 5 days, the patient typically develops sore throat, cervical lymphadenopathy, and temperature fluctuations. He may also develop stomatitis, splenomegaly, exudative tonsillitis, pharyngitis and, possibly, a maculopapular rash.

• **Leukemia and lymphomas.** These proliferative blood cell disorders commonly cause moderate to massive hepatomegaly and splenomegaly as well as abdominal discomfort. General signs and symptoms include malaise, low-grade fever, fatigue, weakness, tachycardia, weight loss, and anorexia.

• **Obesity.** Hepatomegaly can result from fatty infiltration of the liver. Weight reduction reduces liver size.

• **Pancreatic cancer.** In this disorder, hepatomegaly accompanies such classic signs and symptoms as anorexia, weight loss, abdominal or back pain, and jaundice. Other findings include nausea, vomiting, fever, fatigue, weakness, and skin lesions (usually on the legs).

• **Pericarditis.** In chronic constrictive pericarditis, an increase in systemic venous pressure produces marked congestive hepatomegaly. Distended neck veins (more prominent on inspiration) are a common finding. The usual signs of cardiac disease typically are absent; other features include peripheral edema, ascites, and decreased muscle mass.

Special considerations

Prepare the patient for hepatic enzyme, alkaline phosphatase, bilirubin, albumin, and globulin studies to evaluate liver function; also prepare him for X-rays, liver scan, celiac arteriography, computed tomography scan, and ultrasonography to confirm hepatomegaly.

Bed rest, relief from stress, and adequate nutrition are important for the patient with hepatomegaly to help protect liver cells from further damage and to allow the liver to regenerate functioning cells. Hepatotoxic drugs or drugs metabolized by the liver should be given in very small doses, if at all.

Pediatric pointers
Assess hepatomegaly in children the same way you do in adults. Childhood hepatomegaly may stem from Reye's syndrome, biliary atresia, poorly controlled type I diabetes mellitus, or such rare disorders as Wilson's disease, Gaucher's disease, and Niemann-Pick disease.

HOARSENESS

A rough or harsh sound to the voice, hoarseness can result from laryngeal edema, infections, inflammatory lesions, or exudates and from compression or disruption of the vocal cords or recurrent laryngeal nerve. This common sign can also result from thoracic aortic aneurysm, vocal cord paralysis, and systemic disorders, such as Sjögren's syndrome and rheumatoid arthritis. It's characteristically exacerbated by excessive alcohol intake, smoking, inhalation of noxious fumes, excessive talking, and shouting.

Hoarseness can be acute or chronic. For example, chronic hoarseness and laryngitis result when irritating polyps or nodules develop on the vocal cords. Hoarseness may also result from progressive atrophy of the laryngeal muscles and mucosa due to aging, which leads to diminished control of the vocal cords.

History and physical examination
Obtain a patient history. First, consider his age and sex; laryngeal cancer is most common in men ages 50 to 70. Be sure to ask about the onset of hoarseness. Has the patient been overusing his voice? Has he experienced shortness of breath, a sore throat, dry mouth, a cough, or difficulty swallowing dry food? In addition, ask if he's been in or near a fire within the past 48 hours. Be aware that inhalation injury can cause sudden airway obstruction.

Next, explore associated symptoms. Does the patient have a history of cancer, rheumatoid arthritis, or aortic aneurysm? Does he regularly drink alcohol or smoke?

Inspect the oral cavity and pharynx for redness or exudate, which may indicate an upper respiratory infection. Palpate the neck for masses and the cervical lymph nodes and the thyroid for enlargement. Palpate the trachea—is it midline? Ask the patient to stick out his tongue: If he can't, he may have paralysis from cranial nerve involvement. Examine the eyes for corneal ulcers and enlarged lacrimal ducts (signs of Sjögren's syndrome). Dilated neck and chest veins may indicate compression by an aortic aneurysm.

Take the patient's vital signs, noting especially fever and bradycardia. Inspect for asymmetrical chest expansion or signs of respiratory distress (nasal flaring, stridor, and intercostal retractions). Then auscultate for crackles, rhonchi, wheezes, or tubular sounds, and percuss for dullness.

Common medical causes
- *Gastroesophageal reflux.* In this disorder, retrograde flow of gastric juices into the esophagus may spill into the hypopharynx. This, in turn, irritates the larynx, resulting in hoarseness, sore throat, cough, throat clearing, and a sensation of a lump in the throat. The arytenoids and vocal cords may appear red and swollen.
- *Hypothyroidism.* Hoarseness may be an early sign of this disorder. Other findings include fatigue, cold intolerance, weight gain despite anorexia, and menorrhagia.
- *Inhalation injury.* Inhalation injury from a fire or explosion produces hoarseness and coughing, singed nasal hairs,

orofacial burns, and soot-stained sputum. Subsequent signs and symptoms include crackles, rhonchi, and wheezes as well as rapid deterioration to respiratory distress.

● *Laryngeal cancer.* Hoarseness is an early sign of vocal cord cancer but may not occur until later in cancer of other laryngeal areas. The patient usually has a long history of smoking. Other common findings include a mild, dry cough; minor throat discomfort; otalgia; and, sometimes, hemoptysis.

● *Laryngitis.* Persistent hoarseness may be the only sign of *chronic laryngitis.* In *acute laryngitis,* hoarseness or a complete loss of voice develops suddenly. Related findings include pain (especially during swallowing or speaking), cough, fever, profuse diaphoresis, sore throat, and rhinorrhea.

● *Rheumatoid arthritis.* Hoarseness may signal laryngeal involvement. Other findings include pain, dysphagia, a sensation of fullness or tension in the throat, dyspnea on exertion, and stridor.

● *Tracheal trauma.* Torn tracheal mucosa may cause hoarseness, hemoptysis, dysphagia, neck pain, airway occlusion, and respiratory distress.

● *Vocal cord paralysis.* Unilateral vocal cord paralysis causes hoarseness and vocal weakness. Paralysis may accompany signs of trauma, such as pain and swelling of the head and neck.

● *Vocal cord polyps or nodules.* Raspy hoarseness, the chief complaint, accompanies a chronic cough and a crackling voice.

Other causes

● *Treatments.* Surgical trauma to the recurrent laryngeal nerve occasionally results in temporary or permanent unilateral vocal cord paralysis, leading to hoarseness. Prolonged intubation may cause temporary hoarseness.

Special considerations

Carefully observe the patient for stridor, which may indicate bilateral vocal cord paralysis. Advise the patient with laryngitis to use a humidifier. Stress the importance of resting his voice: Talking— even whispering—further traumatizes the vocal cords. Suggest other ways to communicate (such as writing or body language). Urge the patient to avoid alcohol, smoking, and the company of smokers. When hoarseness lasts for more than 2 weeks, indirect or fiber-optic laryngoscopy is indicated to observe the larynx at rest and during phonation.

Pediatric pointers

In children, hoarseness may result from congenital anomalies, such as laryngocele and dysphonia plicae ventricularis. In prepubescent boys, it can stem from juvenile papillomatosis of the upper respiratory tract.

In infants and young children, hoarseness commonly stems from acute laryngotracheobronchitis (croup). Temporary hoarseness commonly results from laryngeal irritation due to aspiration of liquids, foreign bodies, or stomach contents. Hoarseness may also stem from diphtheria, although immunization has made this disease rare.

Help the hoarse child rest his voice. Comfort an infant to minimize crying; play quiet games with him and humidify his environment.

HOMANS' SIGN

Homans' sign is positive when deep calf pain results from strong and abrupt dorsiflexion of the ankle. (See *Eliciting Homans' sign.*) This pain results from venous thrombosis or inflammation of the calf muscles. However, because a positive Homans' sign appears in only 35% of patients with these conditions, it's an

ELICITING HOMANS' SIGN

To elicit this sign, first support the patient's thigh with one hand and his foot with the other. Bend his leg slightly at the knee, then firmly and abruptly dorsiflex the ankle. Resulting deep calf pain indicates a positive Homans' sign. (The patient may also resist ankle dorsiflexion or flex the knee involuntarily if Homans' sign is positive.)

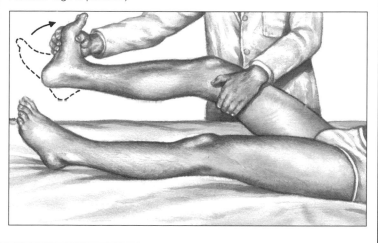

unreliable indicator. Even when accurate, a positive Homans' sign doesn't indicate the extent of the venous disorder.

This elicited sign may be confused with continuous calf pain, which can result from strains, contusions, cellulitis, or arterial occlusion; or with pain in the posterior ankle or Achilles tendon (for example, in a woman with Achilles tendons shortened from wearing high heels).

History and physical examination
When you detect a positive Homans' sign, focus your patient history on signs and symptoms that can accompany deep vein thrombosis (DVT) or thrombophlebitis. These include throbbing, aching, heavy, or tight sensations in the calf and leg pain during or after exercise or routine activity. Further, be sure to ask about predisposing events, such as leg injury, recent surgery, childbirth, and prolonged inactivity.

Next, inspect and palpate the patient's calf for warmth, tenderness, redness, swelling, and the presence of a palpable vein. You'll also need to measure the circumferences of both the patient's calves. The calf with the positive Homans' sign may be larger because of edema and swelling.

Common medical causes
● *Deep vein thrombophlebitis.* A positive Homans' sign and calf tenderness may be the only clinical features of this disorder. But the patient may also have severe pain, heaviness, warmth, and swelling of the affected leg; visible, en-

gorged superficial veins or palpable, cord-like veins; and fever, chills, and malaise.

• *Deep vein thrombosis.* DVT causes a positive Homans' sign along with tenderness over the deep calf veins, slight edema of the calves and thighs, a low-grade fever, and tachycardia. If DVT affects the femoral and iliac veins, you'll notice marked local swelling and tenderness. If DVT is causing venous obstruction, you'll notice cyanosis and, possibly, cool skin in the affected leg.

• *Superficial cellulitis.* This disorder typically affects the legs, but it can also affect the arms. Superficial cellulitis produces pain, redness, tenderness, and edema. Some patients experience fever, chills, tachycardia, headache, and hypotension.

Special considerations

Be sure to place the patient on bed rest with the affected leg elevated above the heart level. Apply warm, moist compresses to the affected area, and administer mild oral analgesics. In addition, prepare the patient to undergo further diagnostic tests, such as Doppler studies and venograms.

Once the patient is ambulatory, advise him to wear elastic support stockings after his discomfort decreases (usually in 5 to 10 days) and to continue wearing them for at least 3 months. Also, instruct the patient to keep the affected leg elevated while sitting and to avoid crossing his legs at the knees because doing so can impair circulation to the popliteal area. (Crossing at the ankles is acceptable.)

If the patient is put on long-term anticoagulant therapy with warfarin, instruct him to report any signs of prolonged clotting time. These include brown or red urine, bleeding gums, bruises, and black, tarry stools. In addition, stress the importance of keeping follow-up appointments so prothrombin time can be monitored.

Pediatric pointers

Homans' sign is seldom assessed in children, who rarely have DVT or thrombophlebitis.

HYPERPNEA

Hyperpnea indicates increased respiratory effort for a sustained period—either a normal rate (at least 12 breaths/minute) with increased depth (a tidal volume greater than 7.5 ml/kg), an increased rate (over 20 breaths/minute) with normal depth, or an increased rate and depth. It may or may not be associated with tachypnea (increased respiratory rate). Hyperpnea differs from sighing (intermittent deep inspirations).

The typical patient with hyperpnea breathes at a normal or an increased rate and inhales deeply, displaying marked chest expansion. He may complain of shortness of breath or stiff lungs if he has a respiratory disorder causing hypoxemia, or he may not be aware of his breathing if he has a metabolic or neurologic disorder causing involuntary hyperpnea. Other causes of hyperpnea include profuse diarrhea or dehydration, ureterosigmoidostomy, and loss of pancreatic juice or bile from GI drainage. All these conditions cause a loss of bicarbonate ions, resulting in metabolic acidosis. Of course, hyperpnea may also accompany strenuous exercise, and voluntary hyperpnea can aid relaxation in patients experiencing stress or pain—as in labor.

Hyperventilation, a consequence of hyperpnea, is characterized by alkalosis (arterial pH above 7.45 and partial pressure of arterial carbon dioxide less than 35 mm Hg). In central neurogenic hyperventilation, brain stem dysfunction (such as a severe cranial injury) increases the rate and depth of respirations. In acute intermittent hyperventilation, the

KUSSMAUL'S RESPIRATIONS: A COMPENSATORY MECHANISM

Kussmaul's respirations—fast, deep breathing without pauses—characteristically sound labored, with deep breaths that resemble sighs. This breathing pattern develops when respiratory centers in the medulla detect decreased blood pH, thereby triggering compensatory fast and deep breathing to remove excess carbon dioxide and restore pH balance.

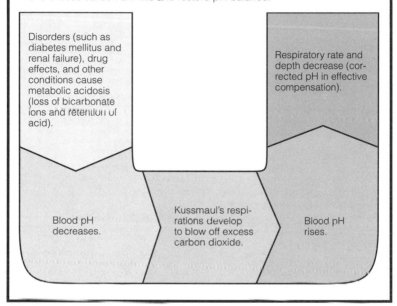

Disorders (such as diabetes mellitus and renal failure), drug effects, and other conditions cause metabolic acidosis (loss of bicarbonate ions and retention of acid).

Respiratory rate and depth decrease (corrected pH in effective compensation).

Blood pH decreases.

Kussmaul's respirations develop to blow off excess carbon dioxide.

Blood pH rises.

respiratory pattern may be a response to hypoxemia, anxiety, fear, pain, or excitement. It may also be a compensatory mechanism for metabolic acidosis, in which case it's known as *Kussmaul's respirations*. (See *Kussmaul's respirations: A compensatory mechanism.*)

History and physical examination
If you observe hyperpnea in a patient whose other signs and symptoms signal a life-threatening emergency, you'll need to intervene quickly and effectively. (See *Managing hyperpnea,* page 318.) However, if the patient's condition isn't grave, first determine his level of consciousness (LOC). If he's alert (and his hyper-

pnea isn't interfering with speaking), ask about any recent illnesses, infections, and ingestion of aspirin or other drugs or chemicals. In addition, find out if the patient has diabetes mellitus or renal disease. Is he excessively thirsty or hungry? Has he recently had severe diarrhea or an upper respiratory infection?

Next, observe the patient for clues to his abnormal breathing pattern. Is he unable to speak, or does he speak only in brief, choppy phrases? Is his breathing abnormally rapid? Examine the patient for cyanosis (especially of the mouth, lips, mucous membranes, and earlobes), restlessness, and anxiety—all signs of decreased tissue oxygenation, as occurs

MANAGING HYPERPNEA

Carefully examine the patient with hyperpnea for related signs of such life-threatening conditions as increased intracranial pressure (ICP), metabolic acidosis, diabetic ketoacidosis, and uremia. Be prepared for rapid intervention.

In increased ICP

If you observe hyperpnea in a patient who has signs of head trauma from a recent accident (soft-tissue injury, edema, or ecchymoses on the face or head) and has lost consciousness, act quickly to prevent further brain stem injury and irreversible deterioration. Then take the patient's vital signs, noting bradycardia, increased systolic blood pressure, or widening pulse pressure—signs of increased ICP. Examine his pupillary reaction.

Elevate the head of the bed 30 degrees (unless you suspect spinal cord injury), and insert an artificial airway. Connect the patient to a cardiac monitor, and continuously observe his respiratory pattern. (Irregular respirations signal deterioration.) Start an I.V. line at a slow infusion rate, and prepare to administer an osmotic diuretic to decrease cerebral edema. Catheterize the patient to measure output, give supplemental oxygen, and keep emergency resuscitation equipment nearby.

In metabolic acidosis

If the patient with hyperpnea doesn't have a head injury, his increased respiratory rate probably indicates metabolic acidosis. If his level of consciousness is decreased, check his history to determine the cause of his metabolic acidosis and appropriate interventions. Suspect shock if the patient has cold, clammy skin. Palpate for a rapid, thready pulse and take his blood pressure, noting hypotension. Elevate his legs 30 degrees, apply pressure dressings to any obvious hemorrhage, start several large-bore I.V. lines, and pre-pare to administer fluids, vasopressors, and blood transfusions.

A patient with hyperpnea who has a history of alcohol abuse, is vomiting profusely, has diarrhea or profuse abdominal drainage, has taken an overdose of aspirin, or is cachectic with a history of starvation may also have metabolic acidosis. Inspect his skin for dryness and poor turgor, indicating dehydration. Take his vital signs, looking for low-grade fever and hypotension. Start an I.V. line for fluid replacement. Draw blood for electrolyte studies, and prepare to give sodium bicarbonate.

In diabetic ketoacidosis

If the patient has a history of diabetes mellitus, is vomiting, and has a fruity breath odor, suspect diabetic ketoacidosis. Catheterize him to monitor output, and infuse saline solution. Perform a finger stick to estimate blood glucose levels with a reagent strip. Obtain a urine specimen to test for glucose and acetone, and draw blood for glucose and ketone tests. You'll need to administer fluids, insulin, potassium, and sodium bicarbonate I.V.

In uremia

If the patient has a history of renal disease, an ammonia odor on his breath, and a fine, white powder on his skin, suspect uremia. Start an I.V. infusion at a slow rate, and prepare to administer sodium bicarbonate. Monitor his electrocardiogram for arrhythmias due to hyperkalemia. Monitor his serum electrolyte, blood urea nitrogen, and creatinine levels, too, until hemodialysis or peritoneal dialysis begins.

in shock. Also observe for intercostal and abdominal retractions, accessory muscle use, and diaphoresis: These signs and symptoms may also indicate deep breathing related to an insufficient supply of oxygen. Next, inspect for draining wounds or signs of infection, and ask about nausea and vomiting. Take the patient's vital signs, noting fever, and be sure to examine his skin and mucous membranes for turgor, possibly indicating dehydration.

Common medical causes

● *Head injury.* Hyperpnea that results from a severe head injury is called central neurogenic hyperventilation. Whether its onset is acute or gradual, this type of hyperpnea indicates damage to the lower midbrain or upper pons. Accompanying signs reflect the site and extent of injury but can include loss of consciousness; soft-tissue injury or bony deformity of the face, head, or neck; facial edema; clear or bloody drainage from the mouth, nose, or ears; raccoon eyes; Battle's sign; absent doll's eye sign; and motor and sensory disturbances.

Signs of increased intracranial pressure include decreased response to painful stimuli, loss of pupillary reaction, bradycardia, increased systolic pressure, and widening pulse pressure.

● *Hyperventilation syndrome.* Acute anxiety triggers episodic hyperpnea, resulting in respiratory alkalosis. Other findings may include agitation, vertigo, syncope, pallor, circumoral and peripheral paresthesia, muscle twitching, carpopedal spasm, weakness, and arrhythmias.

● *Hypoxemia.* Many pulmonary disorders that cause hypoxemia—for example, pneumonia, pulmonary edema, chronic obstructive pulmonary disease, and pneumothorax—may cause hyperpnea and episodes of hyperventilation with chest pain, dizziness, and paresthesia. Other effects include dyspnea, cough,

crackles, rhonchi, wheezes, and decreased breath sounds.

● *Ketoacidosis. Alcoholic ketoacidosis* (usually affecting females with a history of alcohol abuse) typically follows cessation of drinking after a marked increase in alcohol consumption has caused severe vomiting. Kussmaul's respirations begin abruptly; they accompany vomiting for several days, fruity breath odor, slight dehydration, abdominal pain and distention, and absent bowel sounds. The patient is alert and has a normal blood glucose level, unlike the patient with diabetic ketoacidosis.

Diabetic ketoacidosis is potentially life-threatening and typically produces Kussmaul's respirations. The patient usually has polydipsia, polyphagia, and polyuria before the onset of acidosis; he may have a history of diabetes mellitus. Other clinical features include fruity breath odor, orthostatic hypotension, generalized weakness, decreased LOC (lethargy to coma), nausea, vomiting, anorexia, abdominal pain, and rapid, thready pulse.

Starvation ketoacidosis is also potentially life-threatening and can cause Kussmaul's respirations. Its onset is gradual; typical findings include signs of cachexia and dehydration, decreased LOC, bradycardia, and a history of severely limited food intake.

● *Renal failure.* Acute or chronic renal failure can cause life-threatening acidosis with Kussmaul's respirations. Signs and symptoms of severe renal failure include oliguria or anuria, uremic fetor, and dry, scaly yellow skin. Other cutaneous signs are severe pruritus, uremic frost, purpura, and ecchymoses. The patient may complain of nausea and vomiting, weakness, burning pain in the legs and feet, and diarrhea or constipation.

As acidosis progresses, corresponding clinical features include frothy sputum, pleuritic chest pain, and signs of heart failure and pleural or pericardial effusion. Neurologic signs include altered LOC (lethargy to coma), twitching, and seizures. Hyperkalemia and hypertension, if present, require rapid intervention to prevent cardiovascular collapse.

• *Sepsis.* A severe infection may cause lactic acidosis, resulting in Kussmaul's respirations. Other findings may include tachycardia, fever, chills, headache, lethargy, profuse diaphoresis, anorexia, cough, wound drainage, urinary burning, or other signs of local infection.

• *Shock.* Potentially life-threatening metabolic acidosis produces Kussmaul's respirations, hypotension, tachycardia, narrowed pulse pressure, weak pulse, dyspnea, oliguria, anxiety, restlessness, stupor that can progress to coma, and cool, clammy skin. Other clinical features may include external or internal bleeding (in hypovolemic shock); chest pain or arrhythmias and signs of heart failure (in cardiogenic shock); high fever, chills and, rarely, hypothermia (in septic shock); and stridor due to laryngeal edema (in anaphylactic shock). Onset is usually acute in hypovolemic, cardiogenic, or anaphylactic shock, but it may be gradual in septic shock.

Other causes
• *Drugs.* Toxic levels of salicylates, acetazolamide and other carbonic anhydrase inhibitors, and ammonium chloride as well as ingestion of methanol and ethylene glycol, found in antifreeze solutions, can cause Kussmaul's respirations.

Special considerations
Monitor vital signs in all patients with hyperpnea, and observe for increasing respiratory distress or an irregular respiratory pattern signaling deterioration. Prepare for immediate intervention to prevent cardiovascular collapse: Start an I.V. line for administration of fluids, blood transfusions, and vasopressor drugs for hemodynamic stabilization, as ordered, and prepare to give ventilatory support. Prepare the patient for arterial blood gas analysis and blood chemistry studies.

Pediatric pointers
Hyperpnea in children has the same metabolic or neurologic causes as the adult version and requires the same prompt intervention. The most common cause of metabolic acidosis in children is diarrhea, which can cause life-threatening crisis.

In infants, Kussmaul's respirations may accompany acidosis due to inborn errors of metabolism.

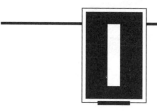

IMPOTENCE

Impotence is the inability to achieve and maintain a penile erection sufficient to complete satisfactory intercourse; ejaculation may or may not be affected. Impotence varies from occasional and minimal to permanent and complete. Occasional impotence occurs in about one-half of adult American men; chronic impotence affects about 10 million American men.

Impotence can also be classified as primary or secondary. A man with *primary impotence* has never been potent with a woman but may achieve normal erections in other situations. This uncommon condition is difficult to treat. *Secondary impotence* carries a more favorable prognosis because, despite present erectile dysfunction, the patient has succeeded in completing intercourse in the past.

Penile erection involves increased arterial blood flow secondary to psychological, tactile, or other sensory stimulation. Trapping of blood within the penis produces increased length, circumference, and rigidity. Impotence results when any component of this process—psychological, vascular, neurologic, or hormonal—malfunctions.

Organic causes of impotence may include vascular disease, diabetes mellitus, hypogonadism, a spinal cord lesion, alcohol and drug abuse, and surgical complications. (The incidence of organic impotence associated with other medical problems increases after age 50.) Psychogenic causes range from performance anxiety and marital discord to moral or religious conflicts.

History and physical examination

If the patient complains of impotence or of a condition that may be causing it, let him describe his problem without interruption. Then begin your assessment in a systematic way, moving from less sensitive to more sensitive matters. Begin with a psychosocial history. Is the patient married, single, or widowed? How long has he been married or had a sexual relationship? What's the age and health status of his sexual partner? Find out about past marriages, if any, and ask him why he thinks they ended. If you can do so discreetly, ask about sexual activity outside marriage or his primary relationship. Also ask about his job history, his typical daily activities, and his living situation. How well does he get along with others in his household?

Focus your medical history on the causes of erectile dysfunction. Does the patient have type II diabetes mellitus, hypertension, or heart disease? If so, ask about its onset and treatment. Also ask about neurologic diseases such as multiple sclerosis (MS). Get a surgical history, emphasizing neurologic, vascular, and urologic surgery. If trauma may be causing the patient's impotence, get information on the date of the injury, its severity, associated effects, and treatment. Ask about intake of alcohol, drug use or abuse, smoking, diet, and exercise. Get a urologic history, including voiding problems and any past injury.

DRUGS THAT MAY CAUSE IMPOTENCE

Many commonly used drugs—especially antihypertensives—can cause impotence. Impotence may be reversible if the drug is discontinued or the dosage reduced. Here are some examples.

amitriptyline	naproxen
atenolol	nortriptyline
cimetidine	perphenazine
clonidine	prazosin
desipramine	propranolol
digoxin	thiazide diuretics
hydralazine	
imipramine	thioridazine
methantheline bromide	tranylcypromine
methyldopa	

Next, ask when the impotence began. How did it progress? What's its current status? Make your questions specific but remember, many men have difficulty discussing sexual problems, and many don't understand the physiology involved. These sample questions may yield helpful data:

When was the first time you remember not being able to initiate or maintain an erection? How often do you wake in the morning or at night with an erection? Do you have wet dreams? Has your sexual drive changed? How often do you try to have intercourse with your partner? How often would you *like* to? Can you ejaculate with or without an erection? Do you experience orgasm with ejaculation?

Ask the patient to rate the quality of a typical erection on a scale of 0 to 10, with 0 being completely flaccid and 10 being completely erect. Using the same scale, also ask him to rate his ability to ejaculate during sexual activity, with 0 being never and 10 being always.

Now perform a brief physical examination. Inspect and palpate the genitalia and prostate gland for structural abnormalities. Assess the patient's sensory function, concentrating on the perineal area. Next, test motor strength and deep tendon reflexes in all extremities, and note other neurologic deficits. Take the patient's vital signs and palpate his pulses for quality. Note any signs of peripheral vascular disease, such as cyanosis and cool extremities. Auscultate for abdominal aortic, femoral, carotid, or iliac bruits, and palpate for thyroid gland enlargement.

Common medical causes

• *Central nervous system disorders.* Spinal cord lesions from trauma produce sudden impotence. A complete lesion above S2 (upper motor neuron lesion) disrupts descending motor tracts to the genital area, causing loss of voluntary erectile control but not the reflexive ability for erection and ejaculation. But a complete lesion in the lumbosacral spinal cord (lower motor neuron lesions) causes loss of reflex ejaculation and reflex erection. Spinal cord tumors and degenerative diseases of the brain and spinal cord (such as MS and amyotrophic lateral sclerosis) cause progressive impotence.

• *Endocrine disorders.* Hypogonadism from testicular or pituitary dysfunction may lead to impotence from deficient secretion of androgens (primarily testosterone). Adrenocortical and thyroid dysfunction and chronic hepatic disease may also cause impotence due to these organs' roles (although minor) in sex hormone regulation.

• *Penile disorders.* Peyronie's disease makes erection painful because the penis is bent, and may make penetration difficult and eventually impossible. Phimosis prevents erection until circumcision releases constricted foreskin. Other inflammatory, infectious, or destructive diseases of the penis may also cause impotence.

• *Psychological distress.* Impotence can result from diverse psychological factors, including depression, performance anxiety, memories of previous traumatic sexual experiences, moral or religious conflicts, and troubled emotional or sexual relationships.

Other causes

• *Alcohol and drugs.* Alcohol and drug abuse are associated with impotence, as are many prescription drugs, especially antihypertensives. (See *Drugs that may cause impotence.*)

• *Surgery.* Surgical injury to the penis, bladder neck, urinary sphincter, rectum, or perineum can cause impotence, as can injury to local nerves or blood vessels.

Special considerations

Care begins by establishing a rapport with the patient. Probably no other medical condition is as potentially frustrating, humiliating, even devastating to a man's self-esteem and significant relationships as impotence. Help the patient feel comfortable about discussing his sexuality. This begins with feeling comfortable about your own sexuality and adopting an accepting attitude about the sexual experiences and preferences of others.

Prepare the patient for screening tests for hormonal irregularities and for Doppler readings of penile blood pressure to rule out vascular insufficiency. Other possible tests include voiding studies, nerve conduction tests, evaluation of nocturnal penile tumescence, and psychological screening.

Treatment for psychogenic impotence may include counseling of both the patient and his sexual partner; treatment for organic impotence focuses on reversing the cause, if possible. Other forms of treatment include surgical revascularization, drug-induced erection, surgical repair of a venous leak, and penile prostheses. Encourage the patient to keep follow-up appointments and to comply with the treatment plan for any underlying medical disorders.

INSOMNIA

Insomnia is the inability to fall asleep, remain asleep, or feel refreshed by sleep. Acute and transient during periods of stress, insomnia may become chronic and cause constant fatigue, extreme anxiety as bedtime approaches, or even psychiatric disorders. A common complaint, it's experienced occasionally by about 25% of Americans and chronically by another 10%.

Physiologic causes of insomnia include jet lag, arguing, and lack of exercise. Its pathophysiologic causes range from medical and psychiatric disorders to pain, drug adverse effects, and idiopathic factors. Complaints of insomnia are subjective and require close investigation; the patient may mistakenly attribute to insomnia his fatigue from an organic cause such as anemia.

History and physical examination

Take a thorough sleep and health history. Find out when the patient's insomnia began and the attending circumstances. Is the patient trying to stop using sedatives? Does he use stimulants, such as amphetamines or pseudoephedrine? What about caffeine-containing drugs and beverages?

Find out if the patient has any chronic or acute conditions whose effects may be disturbing his sleep, particularly cardiac or respiratory disease, or painful or pruritic conditions. What about endocrine or neurologic disorders, or a history of drug or alcohol abuse? Is he a frequent traveler who suffers from jet lag? Does he use his legs a lot during the day, then feel restless at night? Ask about daytime fatigue and regular exercise. Also ask about periods of gasping for air, periods of apnea, and frequent body repositioning. If possible, consult the patient's spouse or sleep partner because the patient may not be aware of his behavior.

Assess the patient's emotional status, and try to estimate his level of self-esteem. Ask about personal and professional problems and psychological stress. Also ask about hallucinations, and note behavior that may indicate alcohol withdrawal.

After reviewing any complaints that suggest an undiagnosed disorder, perform a physical examination.

Common medical causes

• *Alcohol withdrawal syndrome.* Abrupt cessation of alcohol after long-term use causes insomnia that may persist for up to 2 years. Other early effects of this acute syndrome include excessive diaphoresis, tachycardia, increased blood pressure, tremor, restlessness, irritability, headache, nausea, flushing, and nightmares. Progression to delirium tremens produces confusion, disorientation, paranoia, delusions, hallucinations, and seizures.

• *Generalized anxiety disorder.* Hyperattentiveness due to anxiety can cause chronic insomnia. Related findings include signs and symptoms of tension, such as fatigue and restlessness; of autonomic hyperactivity, such as diaphoresis, dyspepsia, and high resting pulse and respiratory rates; and of apprehension.

• *Mood (affective) disorders. Depression* commonly causes chronic insomnia with difficulty falling asleep, waking and being unable to fall back to sleep, or waking early in the morning. Typical adjuncts include dysphoria (a primary symptom), decreased appetite with weight loss or increased appetite with weight gain, and psychomotor agitation or retardation. The patient experiences loss of interest in his usual activities, feelings of worthlessness and guilt, fatigue, difficulty in concentrating, indecisiveness, and recurrent thoughts of death.

Episodes of *mania* produce a decreased need for sleep with an elevated mood and irritability. Related findings include increased energy and activity, fast speech, speeding thoughts, inflated self-esteem, easy distractibility, and involvement in high-risk activities such as reckless driving.

• *Nocturnal myoclonus.* In this seizure disorder, involuntary and fleeting muscle jerks of the legs occur every 20 to 40 seconds, disturbing sleep.

• *Sleep apnea syndrome.* Apneic periods begin with the onset of sleep, continue for 10 to 90 seconds, then end with a series of gasps and arousal. In *central sleep apnea,* respiratory movement ceases for the apneic period; in *obstructive sleep apnea,* upper airway obstruction blocks incoming air, although breathing movements continue. Some patients display both types of apnea. Repeated possibly hundreds of times during the night, this cycle alternates with bradycardia and tachycardia. Associated findings include morning headache, daytime fatigue, hypertension, ankle edema, and such personality changes as hostility, paranoia, and agitated depression.

Other causes

• *Drugs.* Use or abuse of, or withdrawal from, sedatives or hypnotics may produce insomnia. Central nervous system stimulants—including amphetamines, theophylline derivatives, ephedrine, phenylpropanolamine, cocaine, and caffeine-containing beverages—may also produce insomnia.

Special considerations

Prepare the patient for tests to evaluate his insomnia, such as blood and urine studies for 17-hydroxycorticosteroids and catecholamines; sleep EEG; or polysomnography (including electro-oculography, EEG, and electrocardiography).

Teach the patient comfort and relaxation techniques to promote natural sleep. Advise him to awaken and retire at the

TIPS FOR RELIEVING INSOMNIA

COMMON PROBLEMS	CAUSES	INTERVENTIONS
Acropares-thesia	Improper positioning may compress superficial (ulnar, radial, peroneal) nerves, disrupting circulation to the compressed nerve. This causes numbness and tingling in an arm or leg.	Teach the patient to assume a comfortable position in bed, with his limbs unrestricted. If he tends to awaken with a numb leg or arm, teach him to massage and move it until sensation completely returns and then to assume an unrestricted position.
Anxiety	Physical and emotional stress produce anxiety, which causes autonomic stimulation.	Encourage the patient to discuss his fears and concerns, and teach him such relaxation techniques as guided imagery and deep breathing. If ordered, administer a mild sedative such as diazepam before bedtime.
Dyspnea	In many cardiac and pulmonary disorders, a recumbent position and inactivity cause restricted chest expansion, secretion pooling, and pulmonary vascular congestion, leading to coughing and shortness of breath.	Elevate the head of the bed, or provide at least two pillows or a reclining chair to help the patient sleep. Suction him when he awakes, and encourage deep breathing every 2 to 4 hours. Also provide supplementary oxygen via nasal cannula.
Restless leg movement	Excessive exercise during the day may cause tired, aching legs at night, requiring movement for relief.	Help the patient exercise his legs gently by slowly walking with him around the room and down the hall. Administer a muscle relaxant such as diazepam, if ordered.

same time each day and to exercise regularly. Suggest that when he can't sleep, he should get up but remain inactive. Urge him to use his bed only for sleeping, not for relaxing. (See *Tips for relieving insomnia.*)

Advise him to use tranquilizers or sedatives for acute insomnia only when relaxation techniques fail. If appropriate, refer the patient for counseling or to a sleep disorder clinic for biofeedback training or other interventions.

Pediatric pointers
Insomnia may develop with separation anxiety at age 2 or 3, after a stressful or tiring day, or during illness or teething. In children ages 6 to 11, insomnia usually reflects residual excitement from the day's activities; a few children continue

to have bedtime fears. Many foster children display sleep problems.

INTERMITTENT CLAUDICATION

Most common in the legs, intermittent claudication is cramping limb pain brought on by exercise and relieved by 1 to 2 minutes of rest. This pain may be acute or chronic; when acute, it may signal acute arterial occlusion. Intermittent claudication usually occurs in men between ages 50 and 60 with a history of diabetes mellitus, hyperlipidemia, hypertension, or tobacco use. Without treatment, it may progress to pain at rest. In chronic arterial occlusion, limb loss is uncommon because collateral circulation usually develops.

In occlusive artery disease, intermittent claudication results from an inadequate blood supply. Pain in the calf (the most common area) or foot indicates disease of the femoral or popliteal arteries; pain in the buttocks and upper thigh, disease of the aortoiliac arteries. During exercise, the pain typically results from the release of lactic acid due to anaerobic metabolism in the ischemic segment, secondary to obstruction. When exercise stops, the lactic acid clears and the pain subsides.

Intermittent claudication may also have a neurologic cause: narrowing of the vertebral column at the level of the cauda equina. This creates pressure on the nerve roots to the lower extremities. Walking stimulates circulation to the cauda equina, causing increased pressure on those nerves and pain.

Emergency interventions

 If the patient has *sudden intermittent claudication* with severe or aching leg pain at rest, check the leg's temperature and color and palpate pulses. Ask about numbness and tingling. Suspect acute arterial occlusion if pulses are absent; the leg feels cold and looks pale, cyanotic, or mottled; and paresthesia and pain are present.

Don't elevate the leg. Protect it and let nothing press on it. Prepare the patient for preoperative blood tests, urinalysis, electrocardiography, and chest X-rays. Start an I.V. line and administer an anticoagulant and pain medication, as ordered.

History and physical examination

If the patient has *chronic intermittent claudication,* gather history data first. Ask how far the patient can walk before the pain occurs and how long he must rest before it subsides. Can he walk less far now than before, or does he need to rest longer? Is the pain-rest pattern variable? Has this symptom affected his lifestyle?

Get a history of risk factors for atherosclerosis, such as smoking, diabetes, hypertension, or hyperlipidemia. Next, ask about associated signs and symptoms, such as paresthesia in the affected limb and visible changes in the color of the patient's fingers when he's smoking (white to blue to pink), exposed to cold, or under stress. If the patient is male, does he complain of impotence?

Focus the physical examination on the cardiovascular system. Palpate for femoral, popliteal, dorsalis pedis, and posterior tibial pulses. Note their character, amplitude, and bilateral equality. Diminished or absent popliteal and pedal pulses with the femoral pulse present may indicate atherosclerotic disease of the femoral artery. Diminished femoral and distal pulses may indicate disease of the terminal aorta or iliac branches. Absent pedal pulses with normal femoral and popliteal pulses may indicate Buerger's disease.

Listen for bruits over the major arteries. Note color and temperature differences between the legs and between the arms and the legs; also note the leg level where changes in temperature and color occur. Elevate the affected leg for 2 minutes; if it becomes pale or white, blood flow is severely decreased. When the leg hangs down, how long does it take for color to return? (Thirty seconds or longer indicates severe disease.) Check the patient's deep tendon reflexes after exercise; note if they're diminished in his lower extremities.

Examine the feet, toes, and fingers for ulceration, and inspect the hands and lower legs for small, tender nodules and erythema along blood vessels.

In the patient with arm pain, inspect the arms for color change (to white on elevation). Next, palpate for changes in temperature, for muscle wasting, and for a pulsating mass in the subclavian area. Palpate and compare the radial, ulnar, brachial, axillary, and subclavian pulses to identify obstructed areas.

Common medical causes

• *Acute arterial occlusion.* This disorder produces intense intermittent claudication. A saddle embolus may affect both legs. Associated findings include paresthesia, paresis, and sensations of cold in the affected limb. The limb is cool, pale, and cyanotic (mottled) with absent pulses below the occlusion. Capillary refill time is prolonged.

• *Aortic arteriosclerotic occlusive disease.* In this disorder, intermittent claudication occurs in the buttock, hip, thigh, and calf, along with absent or diminished femoral pulses. Bruits can be auscultated over the femoral and iliac arteries. Examination reveals pallor of the affected limb on elevation and profound limb weakness. The leg may be cool to the touch.

• *Arteriosclerosis obliterans.* This disorder usually affects the femoral and popliteal arteries, causing intermittent claudication (the most common symptom) in the calf. Typical associated findings include diminished or absent popliteal and pedal pulses, coolness in the affected limb, pallor on elevation, and profound limb weakness with continuing exercise. Other possible findings include numbness, paresthesia, and—in severe disease—pain at rest in the toes or foot, ulceration, and gangrene.

• *Buerger's disease.* Typically, this disorder produces intermittent claudication of the instep. Early signs include migratory superficial nodules and erythema along extremity blood vessels (nodular phlebitis) and a migratory venous phlebitis. With exposure to cold, the feet initially become cold, cyanotic, and numb; later, they redden, become hot, and tingle. Occasionally, Buerger's disease also affects the hands and can cause painful fingertip ulcerations. Other characteristic findings include impaired peripheral pulses, paresthesia of the hands and feet, and migratory superficial thrombophlebitis.

• *Neurogenic claudication.* Neurospinal disease causes pain from intermittent claudication that requires a longer rest time than the 2 to 3 minutes needed in vascular claudication. Associated findings include paresthesia, weakness and clumsiness when walking, and hypoactive deep tendon reflexes after walking. However, in this disorder, pulses are not affected.

Special considerations

Counsel the patient with intermittent claudication about risk factors. Encourage him to stop smoking, and refer him to a support group, if appropriate.

Promote exercise to improve collateral circulation and increase venous return. (See *Improving circulation in the legs,* page 328.) Advise the patient to avoid prolonged sitting or standing as well as crossing his legs at the knees.

Teach him to inspect his legs and feet for ulcers; to keep his extremities warm, clean, and dry; and to avoid injury.

Urge the patient to immediately report skin breakdown that doesn't heal. Also urge him to report any chest discomfort. Why? Because, when circulation is re-

IMPROVING CIRCULATION IN THE LEGS

To help stimulate circulation in the legs, have your patient perform these exercises (called Berger's exercises) as part of her regular exercise program. Advise doing them four times each day or as often as the doctor specifies, and provide these instructions.

Begin by lying flat on your back; then raise your legs straight up and hold this position for 2 minutes.

Now sit on the edge of a table or any flat surface that's high enough so your legs don't touch the floor. Dangle your legs and swirl them in circles for 2 minutes.

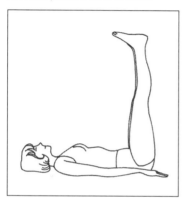

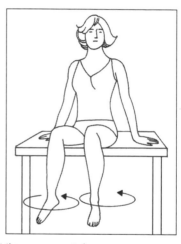

Finally, lie flat for 2 minutes; then repeat the sequence twice.

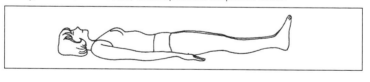

stored to his legs, increased exercise tolerance may lead to angina if he has coronary artery disease that was previously asymptomatic as a result of exercise limitations.

If intermittent claudication interferes with the patient's lifestyle, he may undergo diagnostic tests (Doppler flow studies, arteriography, and digital subtraction angiography) to determine the location and degree of occlusion.

Pediatric pointers
Intermittent claudication rarely occurs in children. Although it sometimes develops in coarctation of the aorta, extensive compensatory collateral circulation typically occurs and prevents manifestation of this sign.

Muscle cramps from exercise and growing pains may be mistaken for intermittent claudication.

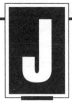

JAUNDICE
[Icterus]

Jaundice is the yellow discoloration of the skin or mucous membranes, indicating excessive levels of conjugated or unconjugated bilirubin in the blood. In fair-skinned patients, it's most noticeable on the face, trunk, and sclera. In dark-skinned patients, it's most noticeable on the hard palate, sclera, and conjunctiva.

Jaundice is most apparent in natural sunlight and may be undetectable in artificial or poor light. It's commonly accompanied by pruritus (because bile pigment damages sensory nerves), dark urine, and clay-colored stools.

Jaundice may result from any of three pathophysiologic processes. (See *Jaundice: Impaired bilirubin metabolism,* page 330.) It may be the only sign of certain disorders such as pancreatic cancer.

History and physical examination

A history of the patient's jaundice is critical in determining its cause. Begin the history by asking the patient when he first noted the jaundice. Does he also have pruritus, clay-colored stools, or dark urine? Ask about past episodes or a family history of jaundice. Does he have any nonspecific signs or symptoms, such as fatigue, fever, or chills; GI signs or symptoms, such as anorexia, abdominal pain, nausea, or vomiting; or cardiopulmonary symptoms, such as shortness of breath or palpitations? Ask about alcohol use and any history of cancer, or liver or gall-

bladder disease. Has the patient lost weight? Obtain a medication history.

Perform the physical examination in a room with natural light. Inspect the skin for texture and dryness and for hyperpigmentation and xanthomas. Look for spider angiomas or petechiae, clubbed fingers, or gynecomastia. If the patient has heart failure, auscultate for arrhythmias, murmurs, and gallops. For all patients, auscultate for crackles and abnormal bowel sounds.

Palpate the lymph nodes for swelling and the abdomen for tenderness, pain, or swelling. Palpate and percuss the liver and spleen for enlargement, and test for ascites with the shifting dullness and fluid wave techniques. Obtain baseline data on the patient's mental status: Slight changes in sensorium may be early signs of deteriorating hepatic function.

Common medical causes

● *Cancer.* Carcinoma of the ampulla of Vater initially produces fluctuating jaundice, mild abdominal pain, recurrent fever, and chills. Occult bleeding may be its first sign. Other findings include weight loss, pruritus, and back pain.

Hepatic cancer may cause jaundice by involving the liver or by metastasizing to cause obstruction of the bile duct. Even advanced cancer causes nonspecific signs and symptoms, such as right upper quadrant discomfort and tenderness, nausea, and slight fever. Examination may reveal hepatomegaly, ascites, peripheral edema, a bruit heard over the liver, and a right upper quadrant mass.

In *pancreatic cancer,* progressive jaundice, possibly with pruritus, may be the

JAUNDICE: IMPAIRED BILIRUBIN METABOLISM

Jaundice occurs in three forms: prehepatic, hepatic, and posthepatic. In all three, bilirubin levels in the blood increase.

In *prehepatic jaundice,* certain conditions and disorders—such as transfusion reactions and sickle cell anemia—cause massive hemolysis. Red blood cells rupture faster than the liver can conjugate bilirubin, so large amounts of unconjugated bilirubin pass into the blood, causing increased intestinal conversion of this bilirubin to water-soluble urobilinogen for excretion in urine and stools. (Unconjugated bilirubin is insoluble in water, so it can't be directly excreted in urine.)

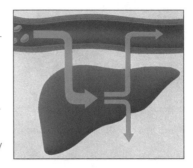

In *hepatic jaundice,* the liver's inability to conjugate or excrete bilirubin leads to increased blood levels of conjugated and unconjugated bilirubin. This occurs in such disorders as hepatitis, cirrhosis, and metastatic cancer and during prolonged use of drugs metabolized by the liver.

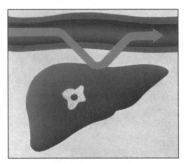

In *posthepatic jaundice,* occurring in biliary and pancreatic disorders, bilirubin forms at its normal rate; however, inflammation, scar tissue, a tumor, or gallstones block the flow of bile into the intestine. This causes an accumulation of conjugated bilirubin in the blood. Water-soluble, the bilirubin is excreted in the urine.

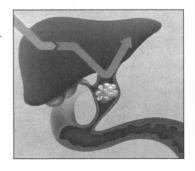

only sign. Related early findings are nonspecific, such as weight loss and back or abdominal pain. Other clinical features include anorexia, nausea, vomiting, fever, steatorrhea, fatigue, weakness, diarrhea, and skin lesions (usually on the legs).

● *Cholangitis.* Obstruction and infection in the common bile duct cause Charcot's triad: jaundice, right upper quadrant pain, and high fever with chills.

• *Cholecystitis.* This disorder produces nonobstructive jaundice in about 25% of patients. Typically, biliary colic occurs and peaks abruptly, persisting for 2 to 4 hours. The pain then localizes to the right upper quadrant and becomes constant. Local inflammation or passage of stones to the common bile duct causes jaundice. Other findings include nausea, vomiting (usually indicating the presence of a stone), fever, profuse diaphoresis, chills, tenderness on palpation, and possibly abdominal distention and rigidity.

• *Cholelithiasis.* This disorder commonly causes jaundice and biliary colic—the primary symptom. It's characterized by severe, steady pain in the right upper quadrant or epigastrium radiating to the right scapula or shoulder and intensifying over several hours. Accompanying signs and symptoms include nausea, vomiting, tachycardia, and restlessness. Occlusion of the common bile duct causes fever, chills, jaundice, clay-colored stools, and abdominal tenderness. After consuming a fatty meal, the patient may experience vague epigastric fullness and dyspepsia.

• *Cirrhosis.* In *Laënnec's cirrhosis,* mild to moderate jaundice with pruritus usually signals hepatocellular necrosis or progressive hepatic insufficiency. Common early findings include ascites, weakness, leg edema, nausea, vomiting, diarrhea or constipation, anorexia, weight loss, and right upper quadrant pain. Massive hematemesis and other bleeding tendencies may occur. Gynecomastia, scanty chest and axillary hair, and testicular atrophy occur in the male patient, whereas menstrual irregularities affect the female patient. The liver and parotid gland may be enlarged, the fingers clubbed, and Dupuytren's contracture present. Other findings include mental changes, asterixis, fetor hepaticus, spider angiomas, and palmar erythema.

In *primary biliary cirrhosis,* fluctuating jaundice may appear years after the onset of other signs and symptoms, such as pruritus that worsens at bedtime (often the first sign), weakness, fatigue, weight loss, and poorly defined abdominal pain. Chronic itching commonly leads to skin excoriation. Associated findings may include hyperpigmentation; indications of malabsorption, including nocturnal diarrhea, steatorrhea, purpura, and osteomalacia; hematemesis from esophageal varices; ascites; edema; xanthelasmas; xanthomas on the palms, soles, and elbows; and hepatomegaly.

• *Dubin-Johnson syndrome.* In this inherited syndrome, fluctuating jaundice—increasing with stress—is the major sign, appearing as late as age 40. Related findings include slight hepatic enlargement and tenderness, upper abdominal pain, nausea, and vomiting.

• *Heart failure.* Jaundice due to liver dysfunction occurs in severe right-sided heart failure. Other effects include jugular vein distention, cyanosis, dependent edema of the legs and sacrum, steady weight gain, confusion, hepatomegaly, nausea, vomiting, abdominal discomfort, and anorexia due to visceral edema. Ascites is a late sign. Oliguria and marked weakness and anxiety may also occur. If left-sided heart failure develops first, other findings may include fatigue, dyspnea, orthopnea, paroxysmal nocturnal dyspnea, tachypnea, arrhythmias, and tachycardia.

• *Hepatic abscess.* Multiple abscesses may cause jaundice, but the primary effects are persistent fever with chills and sweating. Other, but possibly misleading, findings include steady, severe pain in the right upper quadrant or midepigastrium that may be referred to the shoulder; vomiting, nausea, and anorexia; hepatomegaly; and ascites.

• *Hepatitis.* Dark urine and clay-colored stools usually develop before jaundice in the late stages of acute viral hepatitis. Early systemic signs and symptoms vary and include fatigue, nausea, vomiting, malaise, arthralgias, myalgias, headache, anorexia, photophobia, pharyngitis, cough, diarrhea or constipation, and a low-grade fever associated with liver and lymph node enlargement. During the icteric phase (which subsides in 2 to 3 weeks unless complications occur), systemic signs subside, but an enlarged, palpable liver may be present along with weight loss, anorexia, and right upper quadrant pain and tenderness.

● *Pancreatitis (acute).* Edema of the head of the pancreas and obstruction of the common bile duct can cause jaundice. Usually, this disorder's primary symptom is severe epigastric pain that commonly radiates to the back. Lying with the knees flexed on the chest or sitting up and leaning forward brings relief. Early associated signs and symptoms include nausea, persistent vomiting, and abdominal distention. Other findings include fever, tachycardia, abdominal rigidity and tenderness, hypoactive bowel sounds, and crackles.

Severe pancreatitis produces extreme restlessness; mottled skin; cold, diaphoretic extremities; and paresthesia and tetany—signs and symptoms of hypocalcemia. Fulminant pancreatitis causes massive hemorrhage.

● *Sickle cell anemia.* Hemolysis produces jaundice in this disorder. Other findings include impaired growth and development and increased susceptibility to infection; life-threatening thrombotic complications; and, commonly, leg ulcers and painful, swollen joints with fever and chills. Bone aches and chest pain may also occur. Severe hemolysis may cause hematuria and pallor, chronic fatigue, dyspnea (or dyspnea on exertion), and tachycardia. During sickle cell crisis, the patient may have severe bone, abdominal, thoracic, and muscular pain; low-grade fever; and increased weakness, jaundice, and dyspnea.

Other causes

● *Drugs.* Many drugs may cause hepatic injury and resultant jaundice. Some examples include phenylbutazone, I.V. tetracycline, isoniazid, oral contraceptives, sulfonamides, mercaptopurine, ery-thromycin estolate, niacin, troleandomycin, androgenic steroids, and phenothiazines.

● *Treatments.* Upper abdominal surgery may cause postoperative jaundice. It occurs secondary to hepatocellular damage from manipulation of organs, leading to edema and obstructed bile flow; from administration of tetracyclines or halothane; or from prolonged surgery with shock, blood loss, or blood transfusion.

A surgical shunt used to reduce portal hypertension (such as a portacaval shunt) may also produce jaundice.

Special considerations

Encourage the patient with a hepatic disorder to decrease protein intake sharply and increase intake of carbohydrates. If he has obstructive jaundice, encourage a balanced, nutritious diet (avoiding high-fat foods) and frequent small meals. To help decrease the itching of pruritus, bathe the patient frequently, and apply an antipruritic lotion such as calamine.

Prepare the patient for diagnostic tests to evaluate biliary and hepatic function. Laboratory studies may include urine and fecal urobilinogen, serum bilirubin, hepatic enzymes and cholesterol, prothrombin time, and a complete blood count. Other tests may include ultrasonography, cholangiography, liver biopsy, and exploratory laparotomy.

Pediatric pointers

Physiologic jaundice is common in newborns, developing 3 to 5 days after birth. In infants, obstructive jaundice usually results from congenital biliary atresia. Choledochal cyst—a congenital cystic dilation of the common bile duct—may also cause jaundice in children, particularly those of Japanese descent.

Other causes of jaundice include Crigler-Najjar syndrome, Gilbert's syndrome, Rotor's syndrome, thalassemia major, hereditary spherocytosis, erythroblastosis fetalis, Hodgkin's disease, and infectious mononucleosis.

JAW PAIN

Jaw pain may arise from either or both of the bones that hold the teeth in the jaw—the maxilla, or upper jaw, and the mandible, or lower jaw. Jaw pain also includes pain in the temporomandibular joint (TMJ), where the mandible meets the temporal bone.

Jaw pain may develop gradually or abruptly and may range from barely noticeable to excruciating, depending on its cause. It usually results from disorders of the teeth, soft tissue, or glands of the mouth or throat, or from local trauma or infections. Systemic causes include musculoskeletal, neurologic, cardiovascular, endocrine, immunologic, metabolic, or infectious disorders. Myocardial infarction (MI) and tetany also produce jaw pain, as do drugs (especially phenothiazines) and dental or surgical procedures.

Jaw pain is seldom a primary indicator of any one disorder—but some of its causes represent medical emergencies.

History and physical examination

Begin your examination by asking the patient to describe the pain's character, intensity, and frequency. When did he first notice the jaw pain? Where on the jaw does he feel pain? Does the pain radiate to other areas? Sharp or burning pain arises from the skin or subcutaneous tissues. Causalgia, an intense burning sensation, usually results from damage to the fifth cranial or trigeminal nerve. This type of superficial pain is easily localized, unlike dull, aching, boring, or throbbing pain, which originates in muscle, bone, or joints. Also ask about aggravating or alleviating factors.

Explore associated signs and symptoms. Ask about joint or chest pain, fatigue, headache, malaise, anorexia, weight loss, intermittent claudication, diplopia, and hearing loss. (Keep in mind that jaw pain may accompany more characteristic signs and symptoms of life-threatening disorders, such as chest pain in MI.)

Focus your physical examination on the jaw. Inspect the painful area for redness, and palpate for edema or warmth. Facing the patient directly, look for facial asymmetry indicating swelling. Check the TMJs by placing your fingertips just anterior to the external auditory meatus and asking the patient to open and close and to thrust out and retract his jaw. Note the presence of crepitus, an abnormal scraping or grinding sensation in the joint. (Clicks heard when the jaw is widely spread apart are normal.) How wide can the patient open his mouth? Less than $1^1/4''$ (3 cm) or more than $2^1/4''$ (6 cm) between upper and lower teeth is abnormal. Next, palpate the parotid area for pain and swelling, and inspect and palpate the oral cavity for lesions, tongue elevation, or masses.

Common medical causes

● *Angina pectoris.* Angina may produce jaw pain (usually radiating from the substernal area) and left arm pain. Unlike the pain associated with an MI, anginal pain is less severe and is commonly triggered by exertion, emotional stress, or eating a heavy meal. It usually subsides with rest and administration of nitroglycerin. Other signs and symptoms may include shortness of breath, nausea and vomiting, tachycardia, dizziness, diaphoresis, belching, and palpitations.

● *Arthritis.* In *osteoarthritis,* which usually affects the small hand joints, aching jaw pain increases with activity (talking, eating) and subsides with rest. Other features are crepitus heard and felt over the TMJ, enlarged joints with a restricted range of motion (ROM), and stiffness on awakening that improves with activity. Redness and warmth are usually absent.

Rheumatoid arthritis causes symmetrical pain in all the joints, including the jaw (it generally affects proximal finger joints first). Joints display limited ROM and are tender, warm, swollen, and stiff after inactivity, especially in the morning. Myalgia is common. Systemic signs and symptoms include fatigue, weight loss, malaise, anorexia, lymphadenopathy, and mild fever. Painless, movable rheumatoid nodules may appear on the elbows, knees, and knuckles. Progressive disease causes deformities, crepitation with joint rotation, muscle weakness and atrophy around the involved joint, and multiple systemic complications.

● *Head and neck cancer.* Many types of head and neck cancer, especially those of the oral cavity and nasopharynx, produce aching jaw pain of insidious onset. Other findings include a history of leukoplakia ulcers of the mucous membranes; palpable masses in the jaw, mouth, and neck; dysphagia; bloody discharges; drooling; lymphadenopathy; and trismus.

● *Hypocalcemic tetany.* Besides painful muscle contractions of the jaw and mouth, this life-threatening disorder produces paresthesia and carpopedal spasms. The patient may complain of weakness, fatigue, and palpitations. Examination reveals hyperreflexia and positive Chvostek's and Trousseau's signs. Muscle twitching, choreiform movements, and muscle cramps may also occur. In severe hypocalcemia, laryngeal spasm may occur with stridor, cyanosis, seizures, and cardiac arrhythmias.

● *Myocardial infarction.* Initially, this life-threatening disorder causes intense, crushing substernal pain that is unrelieved by rest or nitroglycerin. The pain may radiate to the lower jaw, left arm, neck, back, or shoulder blades. (Rarely, jaw pain occurs without chest pain.) The patient may have pallor, clammy skin, dyspnea, profuse diaphoresis, nausea and vomiting, anxiety, restlessness, and a feeling of impending doom. Associated findings may include low-grade fever, blood pressure changes, arrhythmias, atrial gallop, new murmurs (usually from mitral insufficiency), and crackles.

● *Sinusitis.* Maxillary sinusitis produces intense boring pain in the maxilla and cheek that may radiate to the eye. This type of sinusitis also causes a feeling of fullness, increased pain on percussion of the first and second molars, and—in nasal obstruction—loss of the sense of smell. Sphenoid sinusitis causes chronic pain at the mandibular ramus, vertex of the head, and temporal area and a scanty nasal discharge. Other signs and symptoms of both types of sinusitis include fever, halitosis, headache, malaise, cough, sore throat, and fever.

● *Suppurative parotitis.* Bacterial infection of the parotid gland by *Staphylococcus aureus* tends to develop in debilitated patients with dry mouth or poor oral hygiene. Besides abrupt onset of jaw pain, high fever, and chills, findings include redness and edema of the overlying skin; a tender, swollen gland; and pus at the second top molar (Stensen's ducts). Infection may lead to disorientation, shock, and death.

● *Temporal arteritis.* Common in patients over age 60, this disorder produces sharp jaw pain after chewing or talking. Nonspecific signs and symptoms include low-grade fever, generalized muscle pain, malaise, fatigue, anorexia, and weight loss. Vascular lesions produce jaw pain; throbbing, unilateral headache in the frontotemporal region; swollen, nodular, tender temporal arteries; and, at times, erythema of the overlying skin.

● *Temporomandibular joint syndrome.* This common syndrome produces jaw pain at the TMJ; spasm and pain of the masticating muscle; clicking, popping, or crepitus of the TMJ; and restricted jaw movement. Unilateral, localized pain may radiate to other head and neck areas. The patient typically reports teeth clenching, bruxism, and emotional stress. He may also experience ear pain, headache, deviation of the jaw to the affected side upon opening the mouth, and jaw subluxation or dislocation, especially after yawning.

● **Tetanus.** A rare, life-threatening disorder caused by a bacterial toxin, tetanus produces stiffness and pain in the jaw and difficulty opening the mouth. Early nonspecific signs and symptoms (commonly unnoticed or mistaken for influenza) include headache, irritability, restlessness, low-grade fever, and chills. Examination reveals tachycardia, profuse diaphoresis, and hyperreflexia. Progressive disease leads to painful, involuntary muscle spasms that spread to the abdomen, back, or face. The slightest stimulus may produce reflex spasms of any muscle group. Ultimately, laryngospasms, respiratory distress, and seizures may occur.

● **Trigeminal neuralgia.** This disorder causes paroxysmal attacks of intense unilateral jaw pain (stopping at the facial midline) or rapid-fire shooting sensations in one of the divisions of the trigeminal nerve (usually the mandibular or maxillary division). This superficial pain, felt mainly over the lips and chin and in the teeth, lasts from 1 to 15 minutes. Mouth and nose areas may be hypersensitive. Involvement of the ophthalmic branch of the trigeminal nerve causes a diminished or absent corneal reflex on the same side. Stimulating the nerve—for example, by lightly touching the cheeks—triggers an attack. Exposure to heat or cold and consumption of hot or cold foods or beverages can also spur an attack.

Other causes

● **Drugs.** Some drugs, such as phenothiazines, affect the extrapyramidal tract, causing dyskinesias; others cause tetany of the jaw secondary to hypocalcemia.

Special considerations

If the patient is in severe pain, withhold food, liquids, and normally taken drugs until the diagnosis is confirmed. Administer pain medications. Prepare the patient for diagnostic tests such as jaw X-rays. Apply an ice pack if the jaw is swollen, and discourage the patient from talking or moving his jaws.

Pediatric pointers

Be alert for nonverbal signs of jaw pain, such as rubbing the affected area or wincing while talking or swallowing. Jaw pain in children sometimes stems from disorders not common in adults. Mumps, for example, causes unilateral or bilateral swelling from the lower mandible to the zygomatic arch. Parotiditis due to cystic fibrosis also causes jaw pain. Always consider the possibility of abuse when jaw pain is due to trauma.

JUGULAR VEIN DISTENTION

Jugular vein distention is the abnormal fullness and height of the pulse waves in the internal or external jugular veins. When the supine patient's head is elevated 45 degrees, a pulse wave height greater than 1 1/2" (4 cm) above the angle of Louis indicates distention. Engorged, distended veins reflect increased venous pressure in the right side of the heart. This common sign characteristically occurs in heart failure and other cardiovascular disorders.

Emergency interventions

 Evaluating jugular vein distention involves visualizing and evaluating venous pulsations. (See *Evaluating jugular vein distention,* page 336.) If you detect jugular vein distention in a patient with pale, clammy skin who suddenly appears anxious and dyspneic, take his blood pressure. If you note hypotension and pulsus paradoxus, suspect cardiac tamponade. Elevate the foot of the bed 20 to 30 degrees, give supplemental oxygen, and monitor cardiac status. Start an I.V. line for fluid administration, and keep cardiopulmonary resuscitation equipment close by. Assemble equipment for emergency pericardiocentesis to relieve pressure on the

EVALUATING JUGULAR VEIN DISTENTION

First, position the supine patient so that you can visualize pulsations reflected from the right atrium. Elevate the head of the bed from 45 to 90 degrees. (In the normal patient, veins distend only when the patient lies flat.) Next, locate the angle of Louis, or sternal notch—the reference point for measuring venous pressure. To do so, palpate the clavicles where they join the sternum (the suprasternal notch). Place your first two fingers on the suprasternal notch. Then, without lifting them from the skin, slide them down the sternum until you feel a bony protuberance—the angle of Louis.

Now find the internal jugular vein. (This indicates venous pressure more reliably than the external jugular vein.) Shine a flashlight across the patient's neck to create shadows that highlight his venous pulse. Be sure to distinguish jugular venous pulsations from carotid arterial pulsations. One way to do this is to palpate the vessel: Arterial pulsations continue, whereas venous pulsations disappear with light finger pressure. Also, with changes in body position, venous pulsations increase or decrease, but arterial pulsations remain constant.

Next, locate the highest point along the vein where you can see pulsations. Using a centimeter ruler, measure the distance between that high point and the sternal notch. Record this finding as well as the angle at which the patient is lying. A finding greater than 4 cm above the sternal notch, with the head of the bed at a 45-degree angle, indicates jugular vein distention.

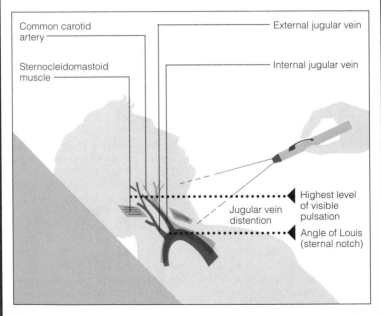

Common carotid artery

Sternocleidomastoid muscle

External jugular vein

Internal jugular vein

Jugular vein distention

Highest level of visible pulsation

Angle of Louis (sternal notch)

heart. Throughout the procedure, monitor the patient's blood pressure, heart rhythm, and respirations.

History and physical examination

If the patient isn't in severe distress, obtain a personal history. Has he gained weight recently? Does he have difficulty putting on shoes? Ask about chest pain, shortness of breath, paroxysmal nocturnal dyspnea, swollen ankles, anorexia, nausea, vomiting, and history of cancer or heart, pulmonary, or renal disease.

Next, perform a physical examination. Take vital signs. Tachycardia, tachypnea, and increased blood pressure indicate fluid overload that's stressing the heart. Inspect and palpate the extremities and face for edema. Then weigh the patient.

Now auscultate the lungs for crackles and the heart for gallops and a pericardial friction rub. Inspect the abdomen for distention, and palpate and percuss for an enlarged liver. Finally, monitor urine output and note any decrease.

Common medical causes

● *Cardiac tamponade.* This life-threatening condition produces jugular vein distention along with anxiety, restlessness, cyanosis, chest pain, dyspnea, hypotension, tachycardia, tachypnea, pulsus paradoxus, muffled heart sounds, and clammy skin.

● *Heart failure.* Sudden or gradual development of right-sided heart failure commonly causes jugular vein distention along with possible weakness and anxiety, cyanosis, dependent edema of the legs and sacrum, steady weight gain, confusion, and hepatomegaly. Other findings may include nausea, vomiting, abdominal discomfort, and anorexia due to visceral edema. Ascites is a late sign. Massive right-sided heart failure may produce anasarca and oliguria.

If left-sided heart failure precedes right-sided failure, jugular vein distention is a late sign. Other features include fatigue, dyspnea, orthopnea, paroxysmal nocturnal dyspnea, tachypnea, tachycardia, and arrhythmias. Auscultation reveals crackles and a ventricular gallop.

● *Hypervolemia.* Markedly increased intravascular fluid volume causes jugular vein distention along with rapid weight gain, elevated blood pressure, bounding pulse, peripheral edema, dyspnea, and crackles.

● *Pericarditis (chronic constrictive).* Progressive signs and symptoms of restricted heart filling cause jugular vein distention that's more prominent on inspiration (Kussmaul's sign). The patient usually complains of chest pain. Other clinical features typically include fluid retention with dependent edema, hepatomegaly, ascites, and pericardial friction rub.

● *Superior vena cava obstruction.* A tumor or, rarely, thrombosis may gradually lead to jugular vein distention when the veins of the head, neck, and arms fail to empty effectively, causing facial, neck, and upper-arm edema. Metastasis to the mediastinum may cause dyspnea, cough, substernal chest pain, and hoarseness.

Special considerations

If the patient has cardiac tamponade, prepare him for pericardiocentesis. If he has heart failure, administer diuretics. If the patient doesn't have cardiac tamponade, restrict fluids and monitor intake and output. Routinely change his position to avoid skin breakdown from peripheral edema. Teach him about treatments, such as a low-sodium diet.

Pediatric pointers

Jugular vein distention is difficult to evaluate in most infants and toddlers because of their short, thick necks. Even in school-age children, measurement of jugular vein distention can be unreliable because the sternal angle may not be the same distance above the right atrium as in adults (2" to 2¾" [5 to 7 cm]).

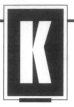

KEHR'S SIGN

A cardinal sign of hemorrhage within the peritoneal cavity, Kehr's sign is referred left shoulder pain due to diaphragmatic irritation by intraperitoneal blood. Usually, the pain arises when the patient assumes the supine position or lowers his head. Such positioning increases the contact of free blood or clots with the left diaphragm, involving the phrenic nerve.

Kehr's sign usually develops right after the hemorrhage, although onset is sometimes delayed up to 48 hours. It's a classic sign of a ruptured spleen, and also occurs with a ruptured ectopic pregnancy.

Emergency interventions

 After you detect Kehr's sign, quickly take the patient's vital signs. If the patient shows signs of hypovolemia, elevate his feet 30 degrees. In addition, you'll need to insert a large-bore I.V. for fluid and blood replacement and an indwelling urinary catheter. Begin monitoring intake and output. Draw blood to determine hematocrit and give supplemental oxygen.

Inspect the patient's abdomen for bruises and distention, and palpate for tenderness. Percuss for Ballance's sign— an indicator of massive perisplenic clotting and free blood in the peritoneal cavity from a ruptured spleen.

Common medical causes
• *Intra-abdominal hemorrhage.* Kehr's sign usually accompanies intense ab-dominal pain, abdominal rigidity, and muscle spasm. Other findings vary with the cause of bleeding.

Special considerations
In anticipation of surgery, withhold oral intake and prepare the patient for abdominal X-rays, computed tomography and ultrasound scans, and possibly paracentesis, peritoneal lavage, and culdocentesis. Give analgesics as needed.

Pediatric pointers
Because a child may have difficulty describing pain, watch for nonverbal clues such as rubbing the shoulder.

KERNIG'S SIGN

A reliable early indicator of meningeal irritation, Kernig's sign elicits both resistance and hamstring muscle pain when the examiner attempts to extend the knee while the hip and knee are both flexed 90 degrees. (See *Eliciting Kernig's sign.*) This sign is usually elicited in meningitis or subarachnoid hemorrhage. In these potentially life-threatening disorders, hamstring muscle resistance results from stretching the blood- or exudate-irritated meninges surrounding spinal nerve roots.

Kernig's sign can also indicate herniated disk and spinal tumor. In these disorders, sciatic pain results from disk or tumor pressure on spinal nerve roots.

EXAMINATION TIP

ELICITING KERNIG'S SIGN

To elicit Kernig's sign, place the patient in a supine position. Flex her leg at the hip and knee, as shown here. Then try to extend the leg while you keep the hip flexed. Pain and possibly spasm in the hamstring muscle with resistance to further extension indicate meningeal irritation.

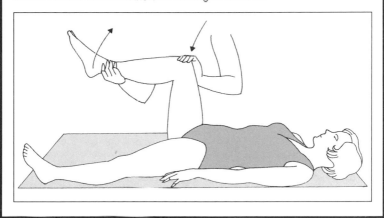

History and physical examination

If you elicit a positive Kernig's sign and suspect life-threatening meningitis or subarachnoid hemorrhage, prepare at once for emergency intervention. (See *When Kernig's sign signals CNS crisis,* page 340.)

If meningeal irritation isn't suspected, ask the patient if he feels any back pain that radiates down one or both legs. Does he also feel leg numbness, tingling, or weakness? Ask about other signs and symptoms, and find out if he has a history of cancer or back injury. Then perform a physical examination, concentrating on motor and sensory function.

Common medical causes

● *Lumbosacral herniated disk.* A positive Kernig's sign may be elicited in this disorder, but the cardinal and earliest feature is sciatic pain on the affected side or on both sides. Associated findings include postural deformity (lumbar lordosis or scoliosis), paresthesia, hypoactive deep tendon reflexes in the involved leg, and dorsiflexor muscle weakness.
● *Meningitis.* Usually, Kernig's sign is positive early in meningitis. Fever also occurs early, possibly with chills. Other signs and symptoms of meningeal irritation may include nuchal rigidity, hyperreflexia, Brudzinski's sign, and opisthotonos. As intracranial pressure (ICP) increases, headache and vomiting may occur. In severe meningitis, the patient may experience stupor, coma, and seizures. Cranial nerve involvement may produce ocular palsies, facial weakness, deafness, and photophobia. An erythematous maculopapular rash may occur in viral meningitis; a purpuric rash may be seen in meningococcal meningitis.
● *Spinal cord tumor.* Kernig's sign can be elicited occasionally, but the earliest symptom is usually pain felt locally or

EMERGENCY INTERVENTIONS

WHEN KERNIG'S SIGN SIGNALS C.N.S. CRISIS

Kernig's sign may signal a life-threatening central nervous system (CNS) disorder: meningitis or subarachnoid hemorrhage. If you elicit this sign, take the patient's vital signs to obtain baseline information. Then test for Brudzinski's sign to obtain further evidence of meningeal irritation. (See *Testing for Brudzinski's sign,* page 104.) Next, ask the patient or his family to describe the onset of illness. Typically, progressive onset of headache, fever, nuchal rigidity, and confusion suggests meningitis. Conversely, sudden onset of severe headache, nuchal rigidity, photophobia, and possibly loss of consciousness usually indicates subarachnoid hemorrhage.

Meningitis

If you suspect meningitis, ask about recent infections—especially tooth abscesses. Ask about exposure to infected persons or places where meningitis is endemic. Usually, meningitis is a complication of another bacterial infection. Draw blood for culture to determine the causative organism. Also find out if the patient has a history of I.V. drug abuse, open-head injury, or endocarditis. Insert an I.V. line and administer antibiotics immediately.

Subarachnoid hemorrhage

If you suspect subarachnoid hemorrhage, ask about a history of hypertension, cerebral aneurysm, head trauma, or arteriovenous malformations. Also ask about sudden withdrawal of antihypertensive drugs.

Check the patient's pupils for dilation, and assess for signs of increasing intracranial pressure, such as bradycardia, increased systolic blood pressure, and widened pulse pressure. Insert an I.V. line and administer supplemental oxygen.

---

along the spinal nerve, commonly in the leg. Associated findings may include weakness or paralysis distal to the tumor, paresthesia, urine retention or incontinence, fecal incontinence, and sexual dysfunction.

• *Subarachnoid hemorrhage.* Kernig's sign and Brudzinski's sign can both be elicited within minutes after the initial bleed. The patient experiences sudden onset of severe headache, nuchal rigidity, and decreased level of consciousness. Photophobia, fever, nausea, vomiting, dizziness, and seizures are possible. Focal signs may include hemiparesis or hemiplegia, aphasia, and sensory or visual disturbances. Increasing ICP may produce bradycardia, increased blood pressure, respiratory pattern change, and rapid progression to coma.

Special considerations

Prepare the patient for diagnostic tests, such as computed tomography, magnetic resonance imaging, spinal X-rays, and myelography. Closely monitor his vital signs, ICP, and cardiopulmonary and neurologic status. Ensure bed rest, quiet, and minimal stress.

If the patient has subarachnoid hemorrhage, darken the room and elevate the head of the bed at least 30 degrees to reduce ICP. If he has a herniated disk or spinal tumor, he may require pelvic traction.

Pediatric pointers

Kernig's sign is considered ominous in children because of their greater potential for rapid deterioration.

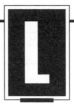

LEG PAIN

Although leg pain commonly signifies a musculoskeletal disorder, it can also result from more serious vascular or neurologic disorders. (See *Common causes of local leg pain,* page 342.) The pain may arise suddenly or gradually and may be localized or affect the entire leg. Constant or intermittent, it may feel dull, burning, sharp, shooting, or tingling. Leg pain commonly affects locomotion, limiting weight bearing. Severe leg pain that follows cast application for a fracture may signal limb-threatening compartment syndrome. Sudden onset of severe leg pain in a patient with underlying vascular insufficiency may signal acute deterioration, possibly requiring an arterial graft or amputation.

Emergency interventions

 If the patient has acute leg pain and a history of trauma, quickly take his vital signs and determine the leg's neurovascular status. Observe the patient's leg position and check for swelling, gross deformities, or abnormal rotation. Also, be sure to check distal pulses and note skin color and temperature. Impaired circulation may be indicated if the affected leg is pale, cool, and pulseless. Emergency surgery may be required.

History and physical examination

When the patient's condition permits, ask him when the pain began and have him describe its intensity, character, and pattern. Is the pain worse in the morning, at night, or with movement? If it doesn't prevent him from walking, must he rely on a crutch or other assistive device? Also ask him about the presence of other signs and symptoms.

Find out if the patient has a history of leg injury or surgery and if he or a family member has a history of joint, vascular, or back problems. Also ask what medications the patient is taking and whether they've helped to relieve his leg pain.

Begin the physical examination by watching the patient walk, if his condition permits. Observe how he holds his leg while standing and sitting. Palpate the legs, buttocks, and lower back to determine the extent of pain and tenderness. If fracture has been ruled out, test range of motion (ROM) in the hip and knee. Also check reflexes with the patient's leg straightened and raised, noting any action that causes pain. Then compare both legs for symmetry, movement, and active ROM. If the patient wears a leg cast, splint, or restrictive dressing, carefully check distal circulation, sensation, and mobility, and stretch his toes to elicit any associated pain.

Common medical causes

• *Bone neoplasm.* Continuous deep or boring pain, generally worse at night, may be the first symptom. Later, skin breakdown and impaired circulation may occur, along with cachexia, fever, and impaired mobility.

• *Compartment syndrome.* Progressive, intense, lower leg pain that increases with passive muscle stretching is a cardinal sign of this limb-threatening disorder.

COMMON CAUSES OF LOCAL LEG PAIN

Various disorders—such as those listed below—cause hip, knee, ankle, or foot pain, which may radiate to surrounding tissues and be reported as leg pain. Local pain is commonly accompanied by tenderness, swelling, and deformity in the affected area.

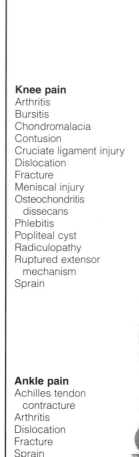

Hip pain
Arthritis
Avascular necrosis
Bursitis
Dislocation
Fracture
Sepsis
Tumor

Knee pain
Arthritis
Bursitis
Chondromalacia
Contusion
Cruciate ligament injury
Dislocation
Fracture
Meniscal injury
Osteochondritis
  dissecans
Phlebitis
Popliteal cyst
Radiculopathy
Ruptured extensor
  mechanism
Sprain

Foot pain
Arthritis
Bunion
Callus or corn
Dislocation
Flat foot
Fracture
Gout
Hallux rigidus
Hammer toe
Ingrown toenail
Köhler's disease
Morton's neuroma
Occlusive vascular
  disease
Plantar fasciitis
Plantar wart
Radiculopathy
Tabes dorsalis
Tarsal tunnel syndrome

Ankle pain
Achilles tendon
  contracture
Arthritis
Dislocation
Fracture
Sprain
Tenosynovitis

Restrictive dressings or traction may aggravate the pain, which typically worsens despite analgesia. Other findings may include muscle weakness and paresthesia, but apparently normal distal circulation. With irreversible muscle ischemia, you'll also find paralysis and absent pulse.

• *Fracture.* Severe, acute pain accompanies swelling and ecchymosis in the affected leg. Movement produces extreme pain, and the leg may be unable to bear weight. Neurovascular status distal to the fracture may be impaired, causing paresthesia, absent pulse, mottled cyanosis, and cool skin. Deformity, muscle spasms, and bony crepitation may occur.

• *Infection.* Local leg pain, erythema, swelling, and warmth characterize both soft tissue and bone infections. Fever and tachycardia may be present with other systemic signs.

• *Occlusive vascular disease.* Continuous cramping pain in the legs and feet may worsen with walking, inducing claudication. The patient may report increased pain at night and complain of cold feet and cold intolerance. Examination may reveal ankle and lower leg edema, decreased or absent pulses, and decreased capillary refill time. (See the entry "Intermittent claudication.")

• *Sciatica.* In this disorder, pain that's described as shooting, aching, or tingling radiates down the back of the leg along the sciatic nerve. Typically, activity exacerbates the pain and rest relieves it. The patient may limp to avoid aggravating the leg pain and may have difficulty moving from a sitting to a standing position.

• *Strain or sprain.* Acute strain causes sharp, transient pain and rapid swelling, followed by leg tenderness and ecchymosis. Chronic strain produces stiffness, soreness, and generalized leg tenderness several hours after the injury; active and passive motion may be painful or impossible. A sprain causes local pain, especially during joint movement; ecchymosis and possibly local swelling and loss of mobility develop.

• *Thrombophlebitis.* Discomfort may range from calf tenderness to severe pain accompanied by swelling, warmth, and a feeling of heaviness in the affected leg. The patient may also have fever, chills, malaise, muscle cramps, and a positive Homans' sign. Assessment may reveal visibly engorged, palpable superficial veins.

• *Varicose veins.* Mild to severe leg symptoms may develop, including nocturnal cramping; a feeling of heaviness; diffuse, dull aching after prolonged standing or walking; and aching during menses. Assessment may reveal palpable nodules, orthostatic edema, and stasis pigmentation of the calves and ankles.

• *Venous stasis ulcers.* Localized pain and bleeding arise from infected ulcerations on the calves. Mottled, bluish pigmentation is characteristic, and local edema may also occur.

Special considerations

If the patient has acute leg pain, closely monitor his neurovascular status by frequently checking distal pulses and evaluating the temperature and color of both legs. Also monitor thigh and calf circumference to evaluate bleeding into tissues from a possible fracture site. Prepare him for X-rays. Use sandbags to immobilize the leg; apply ice and possibly skeletal traction. If a fracture isn't suspected, prepare the patient for laboratory tests to detect an infectious agent or for such tests as venography, Doppler ultrasonography, or plethysmography to determine vascular competency. Withhold food and fluids until the need for surgery has been eliminated, and withhold analgesics until a preliminary diagnosis is made.

If the patient has chronic leg pain, instruct him in using anti-inflammatory drugs and performing ROM exercises. If necessary, teach him how to use a cane, walker, or other assistive device. Discuss with the patient and his family any lifestyle changes that may be necessary until leg pain resolves. If physical therapy is necessary, stress the importance of establishing a daily exercise regimen.

Pediatric pointers
Common pediatric causes of leg pain include fracture, osteomyelitis, and bone neoplasms. If parents fail to give an adequate explanation for a leg fracture, consider the possibility of child abuse.

LEVEL OF CONSCIOUSNESS, DECREASED

A decrease in level of consciousness (LOC)—from lethargy to stupor to coma—usually results from neurologic disorders and commonly signals life-threatening complications of hemorrhage, trauma, or cerebral edema. However, this sign can also result from metabolic, GI, musculoskeletal, urologic, and cardiopulmonary disorders; severe nutritional deficiency; the effects of toxins; and use of certain drugs. LOC can deteriorate suddenly or gradually and can remain altered temporarily or permanently.

Consciousness is affected by the reticular activating system (RAS), an intricate network of neurons whose axons extend from the brain stem, thalamus, and hypothalamus to the cerebral cortex. Disturbance in any part of this integrated system prevents the intercommunication that makes consciousness possible. Loss of consciousness results from a bilateral cerebral disturbance, a reticular activating system disturbance, or both. Cerebral dysfunction characteristically produces the least dramatic decrease in a patient's LOC. In contrast, dysfunction of the RAS produces the most dramatic decrease in a patient's LOC—coma.

The most sensitive indicator of decreased LOC is a change in the patient's mental status. The Glasgow Coma Scale can also be used to quickly evaluate a patient's LOC, based on his ability to respond to verbal, sensory, and motor stimulation.

Emergency interventions
 After evaluating the patient's airway, breathing, and circulation, use the Glasgow Coma Scale to quickly determine LOC and to obtain baseline data. (See *Glasgow Coma Scale.*) If the patient's score is 13 or less, emergency surgery may be necessary. Insert an artificial airway, elevate the head of the bed 30 degrees and, if spinal cord injury has been ruled out, turn the patient's head to the side. Prepare to suction the patient, if necessary. Remember to hyperventilate him first to reduce carbon dioxide levels. Then, determine the rate, rhythm, and depth of spontaneous respirations. Support his breathing with a handheld resuscitation bag, if necessary. If the patient's Glasgow Coma Scale score is 7 or less, intubation and resuscitation may be necessary.

Continue to monitor the patient's vital signs, being alert for signs of increasing intracranial pressure (ICP), such as bradycardia and widening pulse pressure. When his airway, breathing, and circulation are stabilized, perform a neurologic examination.

History
Try to obtain history information from the patient, if he's lucid, and from his family. Did the patient complain of headache, dizziness, nausea, visual or hearing disturbances, weakness, fatigue, or any other problems before his LOC decreased? Has his family noticed any changes in the patient's behavior, personality, memory, or temperament? Also ask about a history of neurologic disease, cancer, or recent trauma; drug and alcohol use; and the development of other signs and symptoms.

Because decreased LOC can result from disorders that affect virtually every

EXAMINATION TIP

GLASGOW COMA SCALE

You've probably heard the terms lethargic, obtunded, or stuporous used to describe progressive decreases in a patient's level of consciousness (LOC). However, the Glasgow Coma Scale provides a more accurate, less subjective method of recording such changes, grading consciousness in relation to eye opening and motor and verbal responses.

For this test, you'll assess the patient's ability to respond to verbal, motor, and sensory stimulation. The scoring system doesn't determine the exact LOC, but it does provide an easy way to describe the patient's basic status and helps to detect and interpret changes from baseline findings.

A decreased reaction score in one or more categories may signal an impending neurologic crisis. A patient scoring 7 or less on the scale manifests severe neurologic damage.

TEST	REACTION	SCORE
Best eye response		
	Open spontaneously	4
	Open to verbal command	3
	Open to pain	2
	No response	1
Best motor response		
	Obeys verbal command	6
	Localizes painful stimulus	5
	Flexion—withdrawal	4
	Flexion—abnormal (docorticate rigidity)	3
	Extension (decerebrate rigidity)	2
	No response	1
Best verbal response		
	Oriented and converses	5
	Disoriented and converses	4
	Inappropriate words	3
	Incomprehensible sounds	2
	No response	1
Total		3 to 15

body system, tailor the remainder of your evaluation according to the patient's associated symptoms.

Common medical causes

● *Adrenal crisis.* Decreased LOC, ranging from lethargy to coma, may develop within 8 to 12 hours of onset. Early associated findings include progressive weakness, irritability, anorexia, headache, nausea and vomiting, diarrhea, abdominal pain, and fever. Later signs include hypotension; rapid, thready pulse; oliguria; cool, clammy skin; and flaccid extremities. The patient with chronic adrenocortical hypofunction may have hyperpigmented skin and mucous membranes.

● *Brain abscess.* Decreased LOC varies from drowsiness to deep stupor, depending on abscess size and site. Early signs reflect increasing ICP: constant intractable headache, nausea, vomiting, and seizures. Typical later features include ocular disturbances, such as nystagmus, vision loss, pupillary inequality, and signs of infection such as fever. Other findings may include personality changes, confusion, abnormal behavior, dizziness, facial weakness, aphasia, ataxia, tremor, and hemiparesis.

● *Brain tumor.* LOC decreases slowly, from lethargy to coma. The patient may also experience apathy, behavior changes, memory loss, and decreased attention span; he may complain of morning headache, dizziness, vision loss, ataxia, or sensorimotor disturbances. Aphasia and seizures are possible, along with signs of hormonal imbalance, such as fluid retention or amenorrhea. In later stages, papilledema, vomiting, bradycardia, and widening pulse pressure also appear. The patient may exhibit a decorticate or decerebrate posture.

● *Cerebral aneurysm (ruptured).* Somnolence, confusion and, at times, stupor characterize a moderate bleed; deep coma occurs in often-fatal severe bleeding. Usually, onset is abrupt, with sudden, severe headache, nausea, and vomiting. Nuchal rigidity, back and leg pain, fever, restlessness, irritability, occasional seizures, and blurred vision reflect meningeal irritation. The type and severity of other findings depend on the site and severity of the hemorrhage, and include hemiparesis, hemisensory defects, dysphagia, and visual defects.

● *Cerebrovascular accident (CVA).* LOC changes vary in degree and onset, depending on a lesion's size and location and the presence of edema. *Thrombotic CVA* usually follows multiple transient ischemic attacks. Onset may be abrupt or take several minutes, hours, or days. *Embolic CVA* occurs suddenly, and deficits reach their peak almost at once. *Hemorrhagic CVA* deficits usually develop over minutes or hours.

Associated findings vary with CVA type and severity and may include disorientation; intellectual deficits, such as memory loss and poor judgment; personality changes; and emotional lability. Other possible findings include dysarthria, dysphagia, ataxia, aphasia, apraxia, agnosia, unilateral sensorimotor loss, and visual disturbances. In addition, urine retention or incontinence, constipation, headache, vomiting, and seizures may occur.

● *Diabetic ketoacidosis.* This life-threatening disorder produces a fairly rapid decrease in LOC, ranging from lethargy to coma. It's commonly preceded by polydipsia, polyphagia, and polyuria. The patient may complain of weakness, anorexia, abdominal pain, nausea, and vomiting. He may also exhibit orthostatic hypotension; fruity breath odor; Kussmaul's respirations; warm, dry skin; and a rapid, thready pulse.

● *Encephalitis.* Within 24 to 48 hours after onset, the patient may develop LOC changes ranging from lethargy to coma. He may also have abrupt onset of fever, headache, nuchal rigidity, vomiting, irritability, seizures, aphasia, ataxia, hemiparesis, nystagmus, photophobia, myoclonus, and cranial nerve palsies.

● *Encephalopathy.* In *hepatic encephalopathy,* signs and symptoms develop in four stages. *Prodromal stage*: slight personality changes (disorientation, forgetfulness, slurred speech) and a slight tremor. *Impending stage*: tremor progressing to asterixis (the hallmark of hepatic encephalopathy), lethargy, aberrant behavior, and apraxia. *Stuporous stage*: stupor and hyperventilation, with the patient noisy and abusive when aroused. *Comatose stage*: coma with decerebrate posture, hyperactive reflexes, positive Babinski's reflex, and fetor hepaticus.

In life-threatening *hypertensive encephalopathy*, LOC progressively decreases from lethargy to stupor to coma. In addition to markedly elevated blood pressure, the patient may experience severe headache, vomiting, seizures, visual disturbances, transient paralysis, and eventually Cheyne-Stokes respirations.

In *hypoglycemic encephalopathy,* LOC rapidly deteriorates from lethargy to coma. Early signs and symptoms include nervousness, restlessness, and confusion; hunger; alternate flushing and cold sweats; and headache, trembling, and palpitations. Blurred vision progresses to motor weakness, hemiplegia, dilated pupils, pallor, decreased pulse, shallow respirations, and seizures. Flaccidity and decerebrate posture appear late.

Depending on its severity, *hypoxic encephalopathy* produces a sudden or gradual decrease in LOC, leading to coma and brain death. Early, the patient appears confused and restless, even combative, with cyanosis and increased heart and respiratory rates and blood pressure. Later, his respiratory pattern becomes abnormal, and assessment reveals decreased pulse, blood pressure, and deep tendon reflexes (DTRs); Babinski's reflex; absent doll's eye sign; and fixed pupils.

In *uremic encephalopathy*, LOC decreases gradually from lethargy to coma.

Early, the patient may appear apathetic, inattentive, confused, and irritable and may complain of headache, nausea, fatigue, and anorexia. Other findings may include vomiting, tremors, edema, papilledema, hypertension, cardiac arrhythmias, dyspnea, crackles, Kussmaul's and Cheyne-Stokes respirations, and oliguria.

● *Heatstroke.* As body temperature increases, LOC gradually decreases from lethargy to coma. Early signs and symptoms include malaise, tachycardia, tachypnea, orthostatic hypotension, muscle cramps, and syncope. The patient may be irritable, anxious, and dizzy and may report a severe headache. His skin will be hot, flushed, and diaphoretic; later, when fever exceeds 105° F (40.5° C), the skin becomes hot, flushed, and anhidrotic. Pulse and respiratory rates increase markedly, while blood pressure drops precipitously. Other findings include vomiting, diarrhea, dilated pupils, and Cheyne-Stokes respirations.

● *Hypernatremia.* This disorder, life-threatening if acute, causes LOC to deteriorate from lethargy to coma. The patient will be irritable and exhibit twitches progressing to seizures. Other signs and symptoms may include dry mucous membranes, nausea, malaise, fever, thirst, flushed skin, and a weak, thready pulse.

● *Hyperosmolar hyperglycemic nonketotic syndrome.* LOC decreases rapidly from lethargy to coma. Early findings include polyuria, polydipsia, weight loss, and weakness. Later, the patient may develop hypotension, poor skin turgor, dry skin and mucous membranes, tachycardia, tachypnea, oliguria, and seizures.

● *Hypokalemia.* LOC gradually decreases to lethargy; coma is rare. Other findings include confusion, nausea, vomiting, diarrhea, and polyuria; weakness, decreased reflexes, and malaise; and dizziness, hypotension, and arrhythmias.

● *Hyponatremia.* This disorder, life-threatening if acute, produces decreased LOC in late stages. Early nausea and malaise may progress to behavior changes, incoordination, and eventually seizures and coma.

● *Hypothermia.* In *severe hypothermia* (temperature below 90° F [32.2° C]), LOC decreases from lethargy to coma. DTRs disappear, and ventricular fibrillation occurs—possibly followed by cardiopulmonary arrest. In *mild to moderate hypothermia,* the patient may experience memory loss and slurred speech in addition to shivering, weakness, fatigue, and apathy. Other early signs include ataxia, muscle stiffness, and hyperactive DTRs; diuresis; tachycardia and decreased respiratory rate and blood pressure; and cold, pale skin. Later, muscle rigidity and decreased reflexes may develop, along with peripheral cyanosis, bradycardia, arrhythmias, severe hypotension, decreased respirations, and oliguria.

● *Intracerebral hemorrhage.* This life-threatening disorder produces rapid, steady loss of consciousness within hours, commonly accompanied by severe headache, dizziness, nausea, and vomiting. Associated signs and symptoms vary and may include increased blood pressure, irregular respirations, Babinski's reflex, seizures, aphasia, decreased sensations, hemiplegia, decorticate or decerebrate posture, and dilated pupils.

● *Meningitis.* Confusion and irritability are expected, although stupor, coma, and seizures may occur in severe meningitis. Fever develops early, possibly accompanied by chills. Associated findings include severe headache, nuchal rigidity, hyperreflexia, and possibly opisthotonos. The patient exhibits Kernig's and Brudzinski's signs and possibly ocular palsies, photophobia, facial weakness, and hearing loss.

● *Seizure disorders. Complex partial seizures* produce decreased LOC, manifested as a blank stare, purposeless behavior (picking at clothing, wandering, lip smacking or chewing motions), and unintelligible speech. They may be heralded by an aura and followed by several minutes of mental confusion.

Absence seizures usually involve a brief change in LOC, indicated by blinking or eye rolling, blank stare, and slight mouth movements.

Generalized tonic-clonic seizures typically begin with a loud cry and sudden loss of consciousness. Muscle spasm alternates with relaxation. Tongue biting, incontinence, labored breathing, apnea, and cyanosis may also occur. Consciousness returns after the seizure, but the patient remains confused and may have difficulty talking. He may complain of drowsiness, fatigue, headache, muscle aching, and weakness and may fall into deep sleep.

Atonic seizures produce sudden unconsciousness for a few seconds.

Status epilepticus, rapidly recurring seizures without intervening periods of physiologic recovery and return of consciousness, can be life-threatening.

● *Shock.* Decreased LOC—lethargy progressing to stupor and coma—occurs late. Associated findings include confusion, anxiety, and restlessness; hypotension; tachycardia; weak pulse with narrowing pulse pressure; dyspnea; oliguria; and cool, clammy skin. *Hypovolemic shock* also produces massive or insidious bleeding, either internally or externally.

Cardiogenic shock may produce chest pain or arrhythmias and signs of heart failure, such as dyspnea, cough, edema, neck vein distention, or weight gain. *Septic shock* may be accompanied by high fever and chills. *Anaphylactic shock* usually involves stridor.

● *Subdural hemorrhage (acute).* In this potentially life-threatening disorder, consciousness progressively decreases from somnolence to coma, preceded by agitation and confusion. The patient may also experience headache, fever, unilateral pupil dilation, decreased pulse and respirations, widening pulse pressure, seizures, hemiparesis, and Babinski's reflex.

• ***Thyroid storm.*** LOC decreases suddenly and can progress to coma. Irritability, restlessness, confusion, and psychotic behavior precede the deterioration. Associated signs and symptoms include tremors and weakness; visual disturbances; tachycardia, arrhythmias, and angina; warm, moist, flushed skin; and vomiting, diarrhea, and fever to 105° F (40.5° C).

• ***Transient ischemic attack.*** Abrupt decrease in LOC varies in severity and disappears gradually within 24 hours. Site-specific findings may include vision loss, nystagmus, aphasia, dizziness, dysarthria, unilateral hemiparesis or hemiplegia, tinnitus, paresthesia, dysphagia, or staggering or uncoordinated gait.

Other causes
• ***Alcohol.*** Use of alcohol causes varying degrees of sedation, irritability, and incoordination; intoxication commonly causes stupor.

• ***Drugs.*** Sedation and other degrees of decreased LOC can result from an overdose of aspirin or central nervous system depressants, such as barbiturates.

Special considerations
Reassess the patient's LOC and neurologic status at least hourly. Carefully monitor ICP, intake, and output. Ensure airway patency and proper nutrition. Take precautions to help ensure the patient's safety. Keep him on bed rest with the side rails up. Apply restraints only if absolutely necessary because their use may increase his agitation and confusion. Talk to the patient even if he appears comatose; your voice may help reorient him to reality.

Pediatric pointers
The primary cause of decreased LOC in children is head trauma, which usually results from physical abuse or motor vehicle accident. Other causes include accidental poisoning, hydrocephalus, and meningitis or brain abscess following ear or respiratory infection. To reduce the parents' anxiety, include them in the child's care. Offer them support and realistic explanations of their child's condition.

LIGHT FLASHES

A cardinal symptom of vision-threatening retinal detachment, light flashes can occur locally or throughout the visual field. Usually, the patient reports seeing spots, stars, or lightning streaks. Light flashes can arise suddenly or gradually and can indicate temporary or permanent vision impairment. They usually signal the splitting of the posterior vitreous membrane into two layers; the inner layer detaches from the retina while the outer layer remains fixed to it. The sensation of light flashes may result from vitreous traction on the retina, hemorrhage caused by a tear in the retinal capillary, or strands of solid vitreous floating in a local pool of liquid vitreous.

Emergency interventions
 Until retinal detachment is ruled out, restrict the patient's eye and body movement.

History and physical examination
Ask the patient when the light flashes began. Can he pinpoint their location, or do they occur throughout the visual field? If the patient is experiencing eye pain or a headache, have him describe it. Also ask if he wears or has ever worn corrective lenses and if he or a family member has a history of eye or vision problems. Ask if he has any other medical problems— especially hypertension or diabetes mellitus, which can cause retinopathy. Also, obtain an occupational history because the patient's light flashes may be related to job stress or to eye strain.

Perform a complete eye and vision examination, especially if trauma is apparent or suspected. Begin by inspecting the external eye, lids, lashes, and tear puncta for abnormalities and the iris and sclera for signs of bleeding. Check pupils for size and shape, reaction to light, accommodation, and consensual light response. Next, test visual acuity in each eye, then visual fields. Document any light flashes the patient reports during this test.

Common medical causes
● *Head trauma.* A patient who has sustained minor head trauma may report "seeing stars" when the injury occurs. He may also complain of localized pain at the injury site, along with generalized headache and dizziness. Later, he may develop nausea, vomiting, and decreased level of consciousness.
● *Migraine headache.* Light flashes—possibly accompanied by an aura—may herald a classic migraine headache. As these symptoms subside, the patient typically experiences a severe, throbbing, unilateral headache that usually lasts 1 to 12 hours and may be accompanied by numbness and tingling of the lips, face, or hands; slight confusion; dizziness; photophobia; nausea; and vomiting.
● *Retinal detachment.* Light flashes described as floaters or spots are localized in the portion of the visual field where the retina is detaching. With macular involvement, the patient may experience painless visual impairment resembling a curtain covering the visual field.
● *Vitreous detachment.* Sudden onset of light flashes may be accompanied by visual floaters. Both eyes may be affected, but usually one at a time.

Special considerations
If the patient has retinal detachment, prepare him for reattachment surgery. Explain that after surgery, he may need to continue wearing bilateral eye patches and may have activity and position restrictions until the retina heals completely.

If the patient doesn't have retinal detachment, reassure him that his light flash-

es are temporary and don't indicate eye damage. For the patient with migraine headache, maintain a quiet, darkened environment, encourage sleep, and administer analgesics as ordered.

Pediatric pointers
Children usually experience light flashes after minor head trauma.

LOW BIRTH WEIGHT

Two groups of infants are born weighing less than the normal minimum birth weight of 5½ lb (2,500 g)—those who are born prematurely (before the 37th week of gestation) and those who are small for gestational age (SGA). The premature infant weighs an appropriate amount for his gestational age and probably would have matured normally if carried to term. However, the SGA infant weighs less than the normal amount for his age, even if carried to term, and his organs are mature.

In the premature infant, low birth weight usually results from a disorder that prevents the uterus from retaining the fetus, interferes with the normal course of pregnancy, causes premature separation of the placenta, or stimulates uterine contractions before term. In the SGA infant, intrauterine growth may be retarded by a disorder that interferes with placental circulation, fetal development, or maternal health. (See *Maternal causes of low birth weight and prematurity.*)

Low birth weight is linked with higher infant morbidity and mortality and can signal a life-threatening emergency.

Emergency interventions
 Because low birth weight is associated with poorly developed body systems, particularly the respiratory, your first priority is to monitor respiratory status. Be alert for signs

of distress, such as apnea, grunting respirations, intercostal or xiphoid retractions, or a respiratory rate exceeding 60 breaths/minute after the first hour of life. If you detect any of these signs, prepare to resuscitate the infant. Endotracheal intubation or supplemental oxygen with an oxygen hood may be necessary.

Monitor the infant's axillary temperature. Decreased fat reserves may keep him from maintaining a normal body temperature, and a drop below 97.8° F (36.5° C) will exacerbate respiratory distress by increasing oxygen consumption. To maintain a normal body temperature, use an overbed warmer or an isolette. (If these are unavailable, use a wrapped rubber bottle filled with warm water, but be careful to avoid hyperthermia.) Cover the infant's head to prevent heat loss.

History and physical examination

As soon as possible, evaluate the infant's neuromuscular and physical maturity to determine his gestational age. (See *Ballard Scale: Calculating gestational age,* pages 352 and 353.) Follow with a routine neonatal examination.

Common medical causes

This section lists the fetal and placental causes of low birth weight as well as the associated signs and symptoms present in the infant at birth.

● *Chromosomal aberrations.* Abnormalities in chromosomal number, size, or configuration cause low birth weight and possibly multiple congenital anomalies in a premature or SGA infant. For example, the infant with Down syndrome may be SGA and have prominent epicanthal folds, a flat-bridged nose, a protruding tongue, palmar simian creases, muscular hypotonia, and an umbilical hernia.

● *Placental dysfunction.* Low birth weight and a wasted appearance occur in an infant who's SGA. The infant may be symmetrically short or may appear relatively long for his low weight. Addi-

---

MATERNAL CAUSES OF LOW BIRTH WEIGHT AND PREMATURITY

If the infant is small for his gestational age, consider these possible maternal causes:
● acquired immunodeficiency syndrome
● alcohol or narcotics abuse
● chronic maternal illness
● cigarette smoking
● hypertension
● hypoxemia
● malnutrition
● toxemia.

If the infant is born prematurely, consider these common maternal causes:
● abruptio placentae
● amnionitis
● cocaine or crack use
● incompetent cervix
● placenta previa
● polyhydramnios
● preeclampsia
● premature rupture of membranes
● severe maternal illness
● urinary tract infection.

---

tional findings reflect the underlying cause. For example, if maternal hyperparathyroidism caused placental dysfunction, the infant may have muscle jerking and twitching, carpopedal spasm, ankle clonus, vomiting, tachycardia, and tachypnea.

● *Rubella (congenital).* Usually, the low-birth-weight infant with this disease is born at term but is SGA. A characteristic "blueberry muffin" rash accompanies cataracts, purpuric lesions, hepatosplenomegaly, and a large anterior fontanel. Abnormal heart sounds, if present, vary with the type of associated congenital heart defect.

(Text continues on page 354.)

BALLARD SCALE: CALCULATING GESTATIONAL AGE

To use this tool, the examiner evaluates and scores the neuromuscular and physical maturity criteria, totals the scores, then plots the sum in the maturity rating box to determine gestational age. Unlike portions of the Dubowitz neurologic examination, the Ballard neuromuscular examination can be done even if the neonate is not alert.

Neuromuscular maturity

Neuromuscular maturity sign	Score							Record score here
	−1	0	1	2	3	4	5	
Posture	—						—	
Square window (wrist)	>90°	90°	60°	45°	30°	0°	—	
Arm recoil	—	180°	140° to 180°	110° to 140°	90° to 110°	<90°	—	
Popliteal angle	180°	160°	140°	120°	100°	90°	<90°	
Scarf sign							—	
Heel to ear							—	
Total neuromuscular maturity score								

Physical maturity

Physical maturity sign	Score							Record score here
	−1	0	1	2	3	4	5	
Skin	Sticky, friable, transparent	Gelatinous, red, translucent	Smooth, pink, visible vessels	Superficial peeling or rash; few visible vessels	Cracking; pale areas; rare visible vessels	Parchment-like; deep cracking; no visible vessels	Leathery, cracked, wrinkled	
Lanugo	None	Sparse	Abundant	Thinning	Bald area	Mostly bald	—	

Physical maturity sign	Score							Record score here
	−1	0	1	2	3	4	5	
Plantar surface	Heel-toe 40 to 50 mm: −1; <40 mm: −2	> 50 mm; no crease	Faint red marks	Anterior transverse crease only	Creases over anterior two-thirds	Creases over entire sole	—	
Breast	Imperceptible	Barely perceptible	Flat areola; no bud	Stippled areola: 1- to 2-mm bud	Raised areola; 3- to 4-mm bud	Full areola; 5- to 10-mm bud	—	
Eye and ear	Lids fused: loosely: −1; tightly: −2	Lids open; pinna; flat, stays folded	Slightly curved pinna; soft, slow recoil	Well-curved pinna; soft but ready recoil	Formed and firm; instant recoil	Thick cartilage; ear stiff	—	
Genitalia (male)	Scrotum flat, smooth	Scrotum empty; faint rugae	Testes in upper canal; rare rugae	Testes descending; few rugae	Testes down; good rugae	Testes pendulous; deep rugae	—	
Genitalia (female)	Prominent clitoris; flat labia	Prominent clitoris; small labia minora	Prominent clitoris; enlarging labia minora	Equally prominent labia majora and minora	Large labia majora; small labia minora	Large labia majora covers clitoris and labia minora	—	

Total physical maturity score

Maturity rating

Total maturity score	−10	−5	0	5	10	15	20	25	30	35	40	45	50
Gestational age (weeks)	20	22	24	26	28	30	32	34	36	38	40	42	44

SCORE
Neuromuscular _____
Physical _____
Total _____

GESTATIONAL AGE (weeks)
By dates _____
By ultrasound _____
By score _____

- *Varicella (congenital).* Low birth weight is accompanied by cataracts and skin vesicles.

Special considerations
To make up for low fat and glycogen stores in the low-birth-weight infant, initiate feedings as soon as examination reveals that peristalsis and the suck, swallow, and gag reflexes are present, and continue to feed the infant every 2 to 3 hours. Provide gavage or I.V. feeding for the sick or premature infant. Check abdominal girth with each feeding, and check stools for blood because increasing girth and bloody stools may indicate necrotizing enterocolitis. A sepsis workup may be necessary if there are signs of infection associated with low birth weight.

Check the infant's vital signs every 15 minutes for the first hour and at least once every hour thereafter until his condition stabilizes. Be alert for changes in temperature or behavior, feeding problems, or periods of apnea—possible indications of infection. Also monitor blood glucose levels and watch for signs of hypoglycemia, such as irritability, jitteriness, tremors, seizures, irregular respirations, lethargy, and a high-pitched or weak cry. And if the infant is receiving supplemental oxygen, carefully monitor arterial blood gas values and the oxygen concentration of inspired air to prevent retinopathy.

Monitor the infant's urine output by weighing diapers before and after voiding. Check urine color, measure specific gravity, and test for the presence of glucose, blood, or protein. Also watch for changes in the infant's skin color because increasing jaundice may indicate hyperbilirubinemia.

Encourage the parents to participate in their infant's care to strengthen bonding, and allow ample time for their questions.

LYMPHADENOPATHY

Lymphadenopathy—enlargement of one or more lymph nodes—may result from increased production of lymphocytes or reticuloendothelial cells, or from infiltration of cells not normally present. This sign may be generalized (involving three or more node groups) or localized. Generalized lymphadenopathy may be caused by an inflammatory process, such as bacterial or viral infection; connective tissue disease; endocrine disorder; or neoplasm. Localized lymphadenopathy most commonly results from infection or trauma affecting the drained area. (See *Reviewing common areas and causes of localized lymphadenopathy,* pages 356 and 357.)

Normally, lymph nodes range from $1/4''$ to $1''$ (0.5 to 2.5 cm) and are discrete, mobile, nontender and, except in children, nonpalpable. Nodes larger than $1\,1/4''$ (3 cm) are cause for concern. They may be tender and erythematous, suggesting a draining lesion. Or they may be hard and fixed, tender or nontender, suggesting malignancy.

History and physical examination
Ask the patient when he first noticed the swelling and if the swelling is on one side of his body or both. Are the swollen areas sore, hard, or red? Ask the patient if he has recently had a cold or virus, or any other health problems. Also ask if a biopsy has ever been done on any nodes because this may indicate a previously diagnosed malignant tumor. Find out if the patient has a family history of cancer.

Palpate the entire lymph node system to determine the extent of lymphadenopathy and detect any other areas of local enlargement. Use the pads of your index and middle fingers to move the skin over underlying tissues at the nodal area. If you detect enlarged nodes, note their size in centimeters and whether they're fixed or mobile, tender or nontender. Also note texture: Is the node discrete or does the area feel matted? If you detect tender, erythematous lymphadenopathy, check the area drained by that part of the lymph system for signs of infection, such as swelling.

Common medical causes
● *Brucellosis.* Generalized lymphadenopathy usually affects cervical and axillary lymph nodes, making them tender. The disease usually begins insidiously with easy fatigability, headache, backache, anorexia, and arthralgias; it may also begin abruptly with chills, fever, and diaphoresis.
● *Cytomegalovirus infection.* Generalized lymphadenopathy occurs in the immunocompromised patient. It's accompanied by fever, malaise, rash, and hepatosplenomegaly.
● *Hodgkin's disease.* The extent of lymphadenopathy determines the stage of malignancy—from stage I involvement of a single lymph node region to stage IV generalized lymphadenopathy. Usually, nodes in the neck enlarge first and become hard, swollen, movable, nontender, and discrete. Other common early signs and symptoms include pruritus and, in older patients, fatigue, weakness, night sweats, malaise, weight loss, and unexplained fever (usually as high as 101° F [38.3° C]). Also, if mediastinal lymph nodes enlarge, tracheal and esophageal pressure produces dyspnea and dysphagia.
● *Infectious mononucleosis.* Characteristic painful lymphadenopathy involves cervical, axillary, and inguinal nodes. Typically, prodromal symptoms, such as headache, malaise, and fatigue, occur 3 to 5 days before the appearance of the classic triad of sore throat, lymphadenopathy, and temperature fluctuations with an evening peak of about 102° F (38.9° C). Hepatosplenomegaly

may develop, along with stomatitis, exudative tonsillitis, or pharyngitis.
● *Leukemia (acute lymphocytic).* Generalized lymphadenopathy is accompanied by fatigue, malaise, pallor, and low fever. The patient also experiences prolonged bleeding time, swollen gums, weight loss, bone or joint pain, and hepatosplenomegaly.
● *Leukemia (chronic lymphocytic).* Generalized lymphadenopathy appears early, along with fatigue, malaise, and fever. As the disease progresses, hepatosplenomegaly, severe fatigue, and weight loss occur. Other late findings include bone tenderness, edema, pallor, dyspnea, tachycardia, palpitations, bleeding, and macular or nodular lesions.
● *Malignant lymphoma.* Painless enlargement of one or more peripheral lymph nodes is the most common sign of this disease, with generalized lymphadenopathy characterizing stage IV. Dyspnea, cough, and hepatosplenomegaly occur, along with such systemic complaints as night sweats, fever up to 101° F (38.3° C), fatigue, malaise, and weight loss.
● *Sarcoidosis.* Generalized, bilateral hilar, and right paratracheal lymphadenopathy with splenomegaly are common. Initial findings are arthralgia, fatigue, malaise, and weight loss. Other findings vary with the site and extent of fibrosis. Typical cardiopulmonary findings include breathlessness, cough, substernal chest pain, and arrhythmias. Musculoskeletal and cutaneous features may include muscle weakness and pain, phalangeal and nasal mucosal lesions, and subcutaneous skin nodules. Common ophthalmic findings include eye pain, photophobia, and nonreactive pupils. Central nervous system involvement may produce cranial or peripheral nerve palsies and seizures.
● *Systemic lupus erythematosus.* Generalized lymphadenopathy commonly accompanies the hallmark butterfly rash, photosensitivity, Raynaud's phenome-

REVIEWING COMMON AREAS AND CAUSES OF LOCALIZED LYMPHADENOPATHY

When you detect an enlarged lymph node, palpate the entire lymph node system to determine the extent of lymphadenopathy. Include the lymph nodes indicated below in your examination.

Localized lymphadenopathy may be caused by a variety of disorders, but it usually results from infection or trauma affecting the drained area. The list at right matches some common causes with the areas they affect.

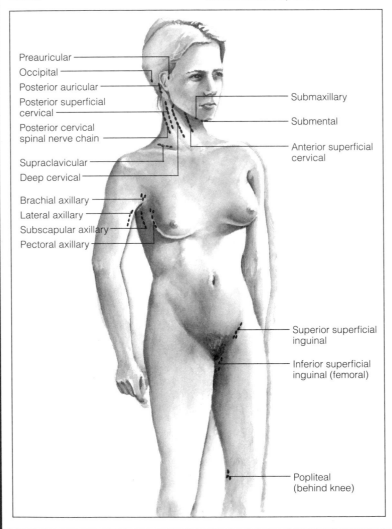

Preauricular

Occipital

Posterior auricular

Posterior superficial cervical

Posterior cervical spinal nerve chain

Supraclavicular

Deep cervical

Brachial axillary

Lateral axillary

Subscapular axillary

Pectoral axillary

Submaxillary

Submental

Anterior superficial cervical

Superior superficial inguinal

Inferior superficial inguinal (femoral)

Popliteal (behind knee)

Occipital
Roseola
Scalp infection
Seborrheic dermatitis
Tick bite
Tinea capitis

Auricular
Erysipelas
Herpes zoster ophthalmicus
Infection
Mastoiditis
Otitis media
Rubella
Squamous cell carcinoma
Styes or chalazion
Tularemia

Cervical
Cat-scratch fever
Facial or oral cancer
Infection
Mucocutaneous lymph node
    syndrome
Rubella
Rubeola
Thyrotoxicosis
Tonsillitis
Tuberculosis
Varicella

Submaxillary and submental
Cystic fibrosis
Dental infection
Gingivitis
Glossitis

Supraclavicular
Neoplastic disease

Axillary
Breast cancer
Lymphoma

Inguinal and femoral
Carcinoma
Chancroid
Lymphogranuloma venereum
Syphilis

Popliteal
Infection

non, and joint pain and stiffness. Pleuritic chest pain and cough may appear with systemic findings, such as fever, anorexia, and weight loss.

● *Tuberculous lymphadenitis.* Lymphadenopathy may be restricted to superficial lymph nodes, or it may be generalized. Affected lymph nodes may become fluctuant and drain to surrounding tissue, and may occur with fever, chills, weakness, and fatigue.

● *Waldenström's macroglobulinemia.* Lymphadenopathy may appear with hepatosplenomegaly. Associated findings include retinal hemorrhage, pallor, and signs of heart failure, such as neck vein distention and crackles. The patient shows decreased level of consciousness, abnormal reflexes, and signs of peripheral neuritis. Weakness, fatigue, weight loss, epistaxis, and GI bleeding may also occur.

Other causes
● *Drugs.* Phenytoin may cause generalized lymphadenopathy.
● *Immunizations.* Typhoid vaccination may also cause generalized lymphadenopathy.

Special considerations
If the patient has a fever exceeding 101° F (38.3° C), provide antipyretics, tepid sponge baths, or a hypothermia blanket.

Expect to obtain blood for routine blood work, a platelet count, and liver and renal function studies. Prepare the patient for other scheduled diagnostic tests, such as chest X-ray, liver and spleen scan, lymph node biopsy, or lymphography to visualize the lymphatic system. If tests reveal infection, check institutional policy regarding infection control.

Pediatric pointers
Infection is the most common cause of lymphadenopathy in children. The condition is commonly associated with otitis media and pharyngitis.

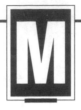

McBURNEY'S SIGN

A telltale indicator of localized peritoneal inflammation in appendicitis, McBurney's sign is tenderness elicited by palpating the right lower quadrant over McBurney's point. Before McBurney's sign is elicited, the abdomen is inspected for distention and auscultated for hypoactive or absent bowel sounds. (See *Eliciting McBurney's sign.*)

History and physical examination

Ask the patient about abdominal pain. When did it begin? Does coughing, movement, eating, or elimination worsen or help relieve it? Also ask about the development of any other signs and symptoms.

Continue light palpation of the patient's abdomen to detect additional tenderness, rigidity, guarding, or pain. Observe the patient's facial expression for signs of pain, such as grimacing or wincing.

EXAMINATION TIP

 ELICITING McBURNEY'S SIGN

To elicit McBurney's sign, place the patient in the supine position with his knees slightly flexed and his abdominal muscles relaxed. Then palpate deeply and slowly in the right lower quadrant over McBurney's point—located one-third of the distance from the anterior superior iliac spine to the umbilicus. Point tenderness, a positive McBurney's sign, indicates appendicitis.

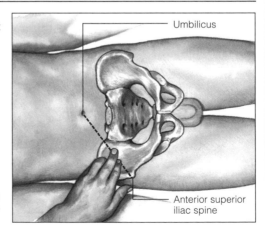

Umbilicus

Anterior superior iliac spine

Common medical causes

● *Appendicitis.* McBurney's sign appears within the first 2 to 12 hours, after initial pain in the epigastric and periumbilical area shifts to the right lower quadrant (McBurney's point). This persistent point pain increases with walking or coughing. Nausea and vomiting may be present from the start. Boardlike abdominal rigidity and rebound tenderness accompany cutaneous hyperalgia, fever, constipation or diarrhea, tachycardia, retractive respirations, anorexia, and moderate malaise.

Rupture of the appendix causes a sudden cessation of pain. Then signs and symptoms of peritonitis develop, such as severe abdominal pain, pallor, hypoactive or absent bowel sounds, diaphoresis, and high fever.

Special considerations

Draw blood for laboratory tests and prepare the patient for abdominal X-rays to confirm appendicitis. Expect to prepare the patient for appendectomy.

Pediatric pointers

McBurney's sign is also elicited in children with appendicitis.

McMURRAY'S SIGN

Commonly an indicator of medial meniscal injury, McMurray's sign is a palpable, audible click or pop elicited by manipulating the leg. It results when gentle manipulation of the leg traps torn cartilage and then lets it snap free. Because eliciting this sign forces the surface of the tibial plateau against the femoral condyles, it's contraindicated in patients with suspected fractures of the tibial plateau or femoral condyles. (See *Eliciting McMurray's sign,* page 360.)

A positive McMurray's sign augments other findings commonly associated with meniscal injury, such as severe knee pain and decreased range of motion (ROM).

History and physical examination

After McMurray's sign has been elicited, find out if the patient is experiencing acute knee pain. Then ask him to describe any recent knee injury. For example, did his injury place twisting external or internal force on the knee, or did he experience blunt knee trauma from a fall? Also ask about previous knee injuries, surgery, or prosthetic replacement as well as other joint problems that could have weakened the knee, such as arthritis. Ask if anything aggravates or relieves the pain and if he needs assistance to walk.

Have the patient point to the exact area of pain. Assess the leg's ROM, both passive and with resistance. Next check for cruciate ligament stability by noting anterior or posterior movement of the tibia on the femur (drawer sign). Finally, measure the quadriceps muscles in both legs for symmetry.

Common medical causes

● *Meniscal tear.* McMurray's sign can usually be elicited in this injury. Associated signs and symptoms include acute knee pain at the medial or lateral joint line (depending on injury site) and decreased ROM or locking of the knee joint. Quadriceps weakening and atrophy commonly occur.

Special considerations

Prepare the patient for knee X-rays, arthroscopy, and arthrography and obtain any previous X-rays for comparison. If trauma precipitated the knee pain and McMurray's sign, an effusion or hemarthrosis may occur. Prepare the patient for aspiration of the joint. Immobilize and apply ice to the knee, and apply a cast or a knee immobilizer.

EXAMINATION TIP

ELICITING McMURRAY'S SIGN

Eliciting this sign requires special training and gentle manipulation of the patient's leg to avoid extending a meniscal tear or locking the knee. If you've been trained to elicit McMurray's sign, place the patient in a supine position and flex the affected knee until the heel nearly touches the buttock. Place your thumb and index finger on either side of the knee joint space and grasp the heel with your other hand. Then rotate the foot and lower leg laterally to test the posterior meniscus. Keeping the patient's foot in a lateral position, extend the knee to a 90-degree angle to test the anterior meniscus. A palpable or audible click—a positive McMurray's sign—indicates a meniscal tear.

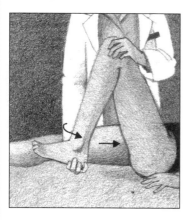
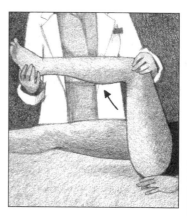

Instruct the patient to elevate the affected leg and to perform straight leg–raising exercises up to 200 times a day. As appropriate, teach him how to use crutches. Also tell him the prescribed dosage and schedule of analgesics and anti-inflammatory drugs. Help him adjust to lifestyle changes by providing support and including significant others in teaching.

Pediatric pointers
McMurray's sign in adolescents is most commonly elicited in meniscal tear from sports injury. It may also be elicited in children with congenital discoid meniscus.

MELENA

A common sign of upper GI bleeding, melena is the passage of black, tarry stools. The characteristic color results from bacterial degradation and hydrochloric acid acting on the blood as it travels through the GI tract. At least 2 oz (60 ml) of blood is needed to produce this sign.

Severe melena can signal acute bleeding and life-threatening hypovolemic shock. In most cases, melena indicates bleeding from the esophagus, stomach, or duodenum, although it can also indicate bleeding from the jejunum, ileum, or ascending colon. In addition, this sign can result from swallowing blood (as in epistaxis) or from the use of certain drugs or alcohol. Because false melena may occur from ingestion of lead, iron, bismuth, or licorice (which produces black stools without blood), all black stools should be tested for occult blood.

Emergency interventions

 If the patient is experiencing severe melena, quickly take his orthostatic vital signs to detect hypovolemic shock. A drop of 10 mm Hg or more in systolic pressure or an increase of 10 beats or more in pulse rate indicates volume depletion. Quickly look for other signs of shock, such as tachycardia, tachypnea, and cool, clammy skin. Insert a large-bore I.V. catheter to administer replacement fluids and allow blood transfusion. Place the patient flat with his head turned to the side and his feet elevated. Administer supplemental oxygen as needed.

History and physical examination

If the patient's condition permits, ask when he discovered his stools were black and tarry. Ask about the frequency and amount of bowel movements. Has he had melena before? Ask about other signs and symptoms, notably hematemesis or hematochezia, and about use of anti-inflammatory drugs, alcohol, and other GI irritants. Also find out if he has a history of GI lesions. (See *Comparing melena and hematochezia*, page 362.)

Next, inspect the patient's mouth and nasopharynx for evidence of bleeding. Perform an abdominal examination that includes auscultation, palpation, and percussion.

Common medical causes

● *Colon cancer.* On the right side of the colon, early tumor growth may cause melena accompanied by abdominal aching, pressure, or cramps. As the disease progresses, the patient develops weakness, fatigue, and anemia. Eventually, he also develops diarrhea or obstipation, anorexia, weight loss, vomiting, and other signs of intestinal obstruction.

On the left side, melena is a rare sign. Early tumor growth commonly causes rectal bleeding with intermittent abdominal fullness or cramping and rectal pressure. As the disease progresses, the patient may develop obstipation, diarrhea, or pencil-shaped stools. At this stage, bleeding from the colon is signaled by melena or bloody stools.

● *Ebola virus.* Melena, hematemesis, and bleeding from the nose, gums, and vagina may occur later with this disorder. Patients usually present with a history of abrupt onset of headache, malaise, myalgia, high fever, diarrhea, abdominal pain, dehydration, and lethargy on the 5th day of illness. Pleuritic chest pain, dry hacking cough, and pharyngitis have also been noted. A maculopapular rash develops within 5 to 7 days of illness onset.

● *Esophageal varices (ruptured).* This life-threatening disorder can produce melena, hematochezia, and hematemesis. Melena is preceded by signs of shock, such as tachycardia, tachypnea, hypotension, and cool, clammy skin. Agitation or confusion signals developing hepatic encephalopathy.

● *Gastritis.* Melena and hematemesis are common. The patient may also experience mild epigastric or abdominal discomfort, belching, nausea, vomiting, and malaise.

● *Mallory-Weiss syndrome.* Melena and hematemesis follow vomiting. Severe upper abdominal bleeding leads to signs and symptoms of shock, such as tachycardia, tachypnea, hypotension, and cool, clammy skin. The patient may also have epigastric or back pain.

● *Mesenteric vascular occlusion.* This life-threatening disorder produces slight melena with 2 to 3 days of persistent, mild abdominal pain. Later, abdominal pain becomes severe and may be ac-

COMPARING MELENA AND HEMATOCHEZIA

With GI bleeding, the site, amount, and rate of blood flow through the GI tract determine if a patient will develop melena (black, tarry stools) or hematochezia (bright red, bloody stools). Usually, melena indicates *upper* GI bleeding, and hematochezia indicates *lower* GI bleeding. However, in some disorders, melena may alternate with hematochezia. This chart helps differentiate these two commonly related signs.

	SIGN	SITES	CHARACTERISTICS
	Melena	Esophagus, stomach, duodenum; rarely, jejunum, ileum, ascending colon	Black, loose tarry stools; delayed or minimal passage of blood through GI tract
	Hematochezia	Usually distal to or affecting the colon; rapid hemorrhage of 1 qt (1 L) or more is associated with esophageal, stomach, or duodenal bleeding	Bright red or dark mahogany–colored stools; pure blood; blood mixed with formed stool; or bloody diarrhea; reflects lower GI bleeding or rapid blood loss and passage of undigested blood through GI tract

companied by tenderness, distention, guarding, and rigidity. The patient may also experience anorexia, vomiting, fever, and profound shock.

• *Peptic ulcer.* Melena may signal life-threatening hemorrhage from vascular penetration. The patient may also have nausea, vomiting, hematemesis, hematochezia, and diffuse epigastric pain that's gnawing, burning, or sharp. With hypovolemic shock comes tachycardia, tachypnea, hypotension, and cool, clammy skin.

• *Small-bowel tumors.* These tumors may bleed and produce melena. Other signs and symptoms include abdominal pain, distention, and increasing frequency and pitch of bowel sounds.

• *Thrombocytopenia.* Melena or hematochezia may accompany other manifes-tations of bleeding tendency, such as hematemesis, epistaxis, petechiae, ecchymoses, hematuria, vaginal bleeding, and characteristic blood-filled oral bullae. Typically, the patient has malaise, fatigue, weakness, and lethargy.

• *Typhoid fever.* Melena or hematochezia occurs late in this disorder and may occur with hypotension and hypothermia. Other late findings include mental dullness or delirium, marked abdominal distention and diarrhea, marked weight loss, and profound fatigue.

• *Yellow fever.* Melena, hematochezia, and hematemesis are ominous signs of hemorrhage, a classic feature, along with jaundice. Other findings include nausea, fever, headache, epistaxis, and dizziness.

Other causes
- **Drugs and alcohol.** Aspirin, other non-steroidal anti-inflammatories, and alcohol can all cause melena as a result of gastric irritation.

Special considerations
Monitor vital signs and look closely for signs of hypovolemic shock. For general comfort, encourage bed rest, and keep the patient's perianal area clean and dry to prevent skin irritation and breakdown. Prepare him for diagnostic tests, including blood studies, gastroscopy or other endoscopic studies, barium swallow, and upper GI series.

Pediatric pointers
Newborns may experience melena neonatorum due to extravasation of blood into the alimentary canal. In older children, melena most commonly results from peptic ulcer, gastritis, or Meckel's diverticulum.

MENORRHAGIA

Profuse or extended menstrual bleeding, menorrhagia may occur as a single episode or a chronic condition. Normal menstrual flow lasts about 5 days and produces a total blood loss of $2^{3}/_{4}$ to $8^{1}/_{2}$ oz (80 to 250 ml). In menorrhagia, the menstrual period may be extended and total blood loss can range from 80 ml to overt hemorrhage. A form of dysfunctional uterine bleeding, menorrhagia can also result from endocrine and hematologic disorders, stress, and certain drugs and procedures.

Emergency interventions

Evaluate hemodynamic status by taking orthostatic vital signs. Insert a large-gauge I.V. catheter to begin fluid replacement if the patient shows an increase of 10 beats/minute in pulse rate, a decrease of 10 mm Hg in systolic blood pressure, or any other signs of hypovolemic shock, such as pallor, tachycardia, tachypnea, and cool, clammy skin. Place the patient in a supine position with her feet elevated, and administer supplemental oxygen as needed.

Then prepare the patient for a pelvic examination to help determine the cause of bleeding.

History
When the patient's condition permits, obtain a history. Determine her age at menarche, the duration of menstrual periods, and the interval between them. Establish the date of the patient's last menses and ask about any recent changes in her normal menstrual pattern. Have the patient describe the character and amount of bleeding. For example, how many pads or tampons does the patient use? Has she noted clots or tissue in the blood? Also ask about the development of other signs and symptoms prior to and during the menstrual period.

Next, ask if the patient is sexually active. Does she use birth control? If so, what kind? Could the patient be pregnant? Be sure to note the number of pregnancies, the outcome of each, and any pregnancy-related complications. Find out the dates of her most recent pelvic examination and Papanicolaou smear and the details of any previous gynecologic infections or neoplasms. In addition, be sure to ask about any previous episodes of abnormal bleeding and the outcome of any treatment. If possible, obtain a pregnancy history of the patient's mother, and determine if the patient was exposed to diethylstilbestrol in utero.

Be sure to ask the patient about her general health and past medical history. Note particularly if she or any member of her family has a history of thyroid, adrenal, or hepatic disease, blood dyscrasias, or tuberculosis because these may predispose to menorrhagia. Also ask about the patient's past surgical procedures and any recent emotional stress. In addition, find out about any past radiation therapy because this may indicate prior treatment for menorrhagia.

Common medical causes

• *Blood dyscrasias.* Menorrhagia is one of several possible signs of a bleeding disorder. Other possible associated findings include epistaxis, bleeding gums, purpura, hematemesis, hematuria, or melena.

• *Hypothyroidism.* Menorrhagia is a common early sign and is accompanied by such nonspecific findings as fatigue, cold intolerance, constipation, and weight gain despite anorexia. As hypothyroidism progresses, intellectual and motor activity decrease, the hair becomes dry and sparse, the nails become thick and brittle, and the skin becomes dry, pale, cool, and doughy. Myalgia, hoarseness, decreased libido, and infertility commonly occur. Eventually, the patient will develop a characteristic dull, expressionless face; edema of the face, hands, and feet; and delayed deep tendon reflexes. Bradycardia and abdominal distention also may occur.

• *Uterine fibroids.* Menorrhagia is the most common sign, but other forms of abnormal uterine bleeding as well as dysmenorrhea or leukorrhea can also occur. Possible related findings include abdominal pain, a feeling of abdominal heaviness, backache, constipation, urinary urgency or frequency, and an enlarged uterus.

Other causes

• *Drugs.* Use of oral contraceptives may cause sudden onset of profuse, prolonged menorrhagia. Anticoagulants have also been associated with excessive menstrual flow.

• *Intrauterine devices.* Menorrhagia can result from the use of intrauterine contraceptive devices.

Special considerations

Continue to monitor the patient closely for signs of hypovolemia. Monitor intake and output, and estimate uterine blood loss by recording the number of sanitary napkins or tampons used during an abnormal period and comparing this to usage during a normal period. To help decrease blood flow, encourage the patient to rest and to avoid strenuous activities.

Prepare the patient for a pelvic examination if one hasn't already been performed, and obtain blood and urine samples for pregnancy testing.

Pediatric pointers

Irregular menstrual function in young girls may be accompanied by hemorrhage and resulting anemia.

METRORRHAGIA

Metrorrhagia—uterine bleeding that occurs irregularly between menstrual periods—is usually light, although it can range from staining to hemorrhage. In most cases, this common sign reflects slight physiologic bleeding from the endometrium during ovulation. However, metrorrhagia may be the only indication of an underlying gynecologic disorder and can also result from stress, treatments, and use of certain drugs or intrauterine devices.

History

Begin your evaluation by obtaining a thorough menstrual history. Ask the patient when she began menstruating and about the duration of menstrual periods, the interval between them, and the average number of tampons or pads she uses. When does metrorrhagia usually occur in relation to her period? Does she experience any other signs and symptoms? Find out the date of her last menses, and ask about any other recent changes in her normal menstrual pattern. Get details of any previous gynecologic problems. If applicable, obtain a contraceptive and obstetric history. Record the dates of her last Pap smear and pelvic examination.

Next, ask about her general health and any recent changes. Is she under emotional stress? If possible, obtain a pregnancy history of the patient's mother. Was the patient exposed to diethylstilbestrol in utero? (This drug has been linked to vaginal adenosis.)

Common medical causes

● *Cervicitis.* This nonspecific infection may cause spontaneous bleeding, spotting, or posttraumatic bleeding. Assessment reveals red, granular, irregular lesions on the external cervix. Purulent vaginal discharge, lower abdominal pain, and fever may occur.

● *Dysfunctional uterine bleeding.* Abnormal uterine bleeding not caused by pregnancy or major gynecologic disorders usually occurs as metrorrhagia, although menorrhagia is possible. Bleeding may be profuse or scant, intermittent or constant.

● *Endometrial polyps.* This disorder may produce metrorrhagia, but most patients are asymptomatic.

● *Endometriosis.* Metrorrhagia (usually premenstrual) may be the only indication of this disorder, or it may accompany pelvic discomfort and dyspareunia.

● *Endometritis.* This causes metrorrhagia and purulent vaginal discharge. It also produces fever, lower abdominal pain, and abdominal muscle spasm.

● *Gynecologic carcinoma.* Metrorrhagia is a common early sign of cervical or uterine carcinomas. Later, the patient may experience weight loss, pelvic pain, fatigue, and possibly an abdominal mass.

● *Uterine leiomyomas.* Besides metrorrhagia, these tumors may cause backache, constipation, signs of ureteral obstruction, and lower abdominal pain that worsens with menses.

● *Vaginal adenosis.* This disorder commonly produces metrorrhagia. Palpation reveals roughening or nodules in affected vaginal areas.

Other causes

● *Drugs.* Anticoagulants and oral contraceptives may cause metrorrhagia.

● *Surgery and procedures.* Cervical conization and cauterization may cause metrorrhagia.

Special considerations

Obtain blood and urine samples for pregnancy testing. A pelvic examination may be indicated. Encourage bed rest to reduce bleeding. Give analgesics for discomfort. Monitor bleeding by recording the number of pads or tampons used.

Pediatric pointers

Girls who have recently begun menstruating may mistake irregular periods for metrorrhagia.

MIOSIS

Miosis pupillary constriction caused by contraction of the sphincter muscle in the iris—occurs normally as a response to fatigue, increased light, and administration of miotic drugs; as part of the eye's accommodation reflex; and as part of the aging process (pupil size steadily decreases from adolescence to about age 60). However, it can also stem from ocular and neurologic disorders, trauma, systemic drugs, and contact lens overuse. A rare form of miosis—Argyll Robertson pupils—can stem from tabes dorsalis and diverse neurologic disorders. Occurring bilaterally, these miotic (commonly pinpoint), unequal, and irregularly shaped pupils don't dilate properly with mydriatic drug use and fail to react to light, although they do constrict on accommodation.

History and physical examination

Begin by asking the patient if he's experiencing other ocular symptoms, and have him describe their onset, duration, and intensity. Does he wear contact lenses? During your history, be sure to ask about trauma, serious systemic disease, and use of topical and systemic medications.

Now perform a thorough eye examination. Examine and compare both pupils for size (many persons have a normal discrepancy), color, shape, reaction to light, accommodation, and consensual light response. Examine both eyes for additional signs, and then evaluate extraocular muscle function by evaluating the six cardinal fields of gaze. Finally, test visual acuity in each eye, with and without correction, paying particular attention to blurred or decreased vision in the miotic eye.

Common medical causes

• *Cerebrovascular arteriosclerosis.* Miosis is usually unilateral, depending on the site and extent of vascular damage. Other findings may include visual blurring, slurred speech or possibly aphasia, loss of muscle tone, memory loss, vertigo, and headache.

• *Cluster headache.* Ipsilateral miosis, tearing, conjunctival injection, and ptosis commonly accompany a severe cluster headache, along with facial flushing and sweating, bradycardia, restlessness, and nasal stuffiness or rhinorrhea.

• *Corneal foreign body.* Miosis in the affected eye occurs with pain, a foreign body sensation, slight vision loss, conjunctival injection, photophobia, and profuse tearing.

• *Corneal ulcer.* Miosis in the affected eye appears with moderate pain, visual blurring and possibly some vision loss, and diffuse conjunctival injection.

• *Horner's syndrome.* Moderate miosis is common in this syndrome and occurs ipsilaterally to the lesion. Related ipsilateral findings include a sluggish pupillary reflex, slight enophthalmos, moderate ptosis, facial anhidrosis, transient conjunctival injection, and vascular headache. When the syndrome is congenital, the iris on the affected side may appear lighter.

• *Hyphema.* Usually the result of blunt trauma, hyphema can cause miosis with moderate pain, visual blurring, diffuse conjunctival injection, and slight eyelid swelling. The eyeball may feel harder than normal.

• *Iritis (acute).* Miosis typically occurs in the affected eye along with decreased pupillary reflex, severe eye pain, photophobia, visual blurring, conjunctival injection, and possibly pus accumulation in the anterior chamber.

• *Neuropathy.* Two forms of neuropathy occasionally produce Argyll Robertson pupils. In *diabetic neuropathy*, related effects may include paresthesia and other sensory disturbances, extremity pain, postural hypotension, impotence, incontinence, and leg muscle weakness and atrophy. In *alcoholic neuropathy*, related effects are progressive, variable muscle weakness and wasting, various sensory disturbances, and hypoactive deep tendon reflexes.

• *Parry-Romberg syndrome.* This facial hemiatrophy typically produces miosis, sluggish pupillary reflexes, enophthalmos, nystagmus, ptosis, and different-colored irises.

• *Pontine hemorrhage.* Bilateral miosis is characteristic, along with rapid onset of coma, total paralysis, decerebrate posture, absent doll's eye sign, and a positive Babinski's sign.

• *Uveitis.* Anterior uveitis commonly produces miosis in the affected eye, moderate to severe eye pain, severe conjunctival injection, and photophobia. In *posterior uveitis*, miosis is accompanied by gradual onset of eye pain, photophobia, visual floaters, visual blurring, conjunctival injection and, commonly, distorted pupil shape.

Other causes

• *Drugs.* Such topical drugs as acetylcholine, carbachol, demecarium bromide, echothiophate iodide, and pilocarpine are used to treat eye disorders specifically for their miotic effect. Such systemic drugs as barbiturates, cholinergics, cholinesterase inhibitors, clonidine (overdose), guanethidine, opiates, and reserpine also cause miosis, as does deep anesthesia.

Special considerations

Because any ocular abnormality can be a source of fear and anxiety, be sure to reassure and support the patient. Clearly explain any diagnostic tests ordered, which may include a complete ophthalmologic examination or a neurologic workup.

Pediatric pointers

Miosis is a common finding in neonates simply because they're asleep or sleepy most of the time. Bilateral miosis occurs in congenital microcoria.

MOUTH LESIONS

Mouth lesions include ulcers (the most common type), cysts, firm nodules, hemorrhagic lesions, papules, vesicles, bullae, and erythematous lesions. They may occur anywhere on the lips, cheeks, hard and soft palate, salivary glands, tongue, gingivae, or mucous membranes. Many are painful and readily detected. Some, however, produce no symptoms; when they occur deep in the mouth, they may be discovered only through a complete oral examination. (See *Common mouth lesions,* page 368.)

Mouth lesions can result from trauma, infection, systemic diseases, drugs, and radiation therapy.

History and physical examination

Begin your evaluation with a thorough history. Ask the patient when the lesions appeared and whether he's noticed any pain, odor, or drainage. Also ask about associated complaints, particularly skin lesions. Obtain a complete medication history, including drug allergies, and a complete medical history. Note especially any history of cancer, sexually transmitted disease, I.V. drug use, recent infection, or trauma. Ask about his dental history, including oral hygiene habits, frequency of dental examinations, and the date of his most recent dental visit.

Next, perform a complete oral examination, noting lesion sites and character. Examine the patient's lips for color and texture. Inspect and palpate the buccal mucosa and tongue for color, texture, and contour; note especially any painless ulcers on the sides or base of the tongue. Hold the tongue with a piece of gauze, lift it, and examine its underside and the floor of the mouth. Depress the tongue with a tongue blade and examine the oropharynx. Inspect teeth and gums, noting missing, broken, or discolored teeth; dental caries; excessive debris; and bleeding, inflamed, swollen, or discolored gums.

Common medical causes

• *Acquired immunodeficiency syndrome (AIDS).* Oral lesions may be an early indication of immunosuppression characteristic of this disease. Fungal infections—most commonly oral candidiasis—can occur. Bacterial infections (of oral mucosa, tongue, gingivae, and periodontal tissue) and viral infections may be seen. The primary oral neoplasm associated with AIDS is Kaposi's sarcoma. In the mouth, this tumor is most commonly found on the hard palate and may appear initially as an asymptomatic, flat or raised lesion, ranging in color from red to blue to purple. As it grows, it may ulcerate and become painful.

• *Actinomycosis (cervicofacial).* This chronic fungal infection typically produces small, firm, flat, painful or painless swellings on the oral mucosa and under the skin of the jaw and neck. Swellings may indurate and abscess, producing fistulas with a characteristic purulent yellow discharge.

COMMON MOUTH LESIONS

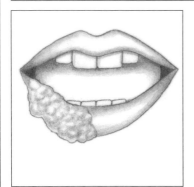

Squamous cell carcinoma

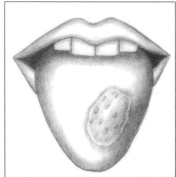

Lichen planus

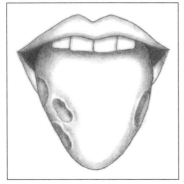

Ulceration from tongue biting

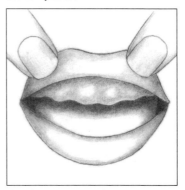

Gingival hyperplasia

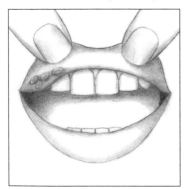

Recurrent aphthous stomatitis

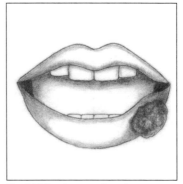

Syphilitic chancre (rare)

• *Behçet's syndrome.* This chronic, progressive syndrome produces small, painful ulcers on the lips, gums, buccal mucosa, and tongue. In severe cases, the ulcers also develop on the palate, pharynx, and esophagus. Typically, the ulcers have a reddened border and are covered with a gray or yellow exudate. Similar lesions appear on the scrotum and penis or labia majora; small pustules or papules on the trunk and limbs; and painful erythematous nodules on the shins. Ocular lesions may also be present.

• *Candidiasis.* This common fungal infection characteristically produces soft, elevated plaques on the buccal mucosa, tongue, and sometimes the palate, gingivae, and floor of the mouth; the plaques may be wiped away. The lesions of *acute atrophic candidiasis* are red and painful. The lesions of *chronic hyperplastic candidiasis* are white and firm. Localized areas of redness, pruritus, and foul odor may be present.

• *Discoid lupus erythematosus.* Oral lesions are common, typically appearing on the tongue, buccal mucosa, and palate as erythematous areas with white spots and radiating white striae. Associated findings include skin lesions on the face, possibly extending to the neck, ears, and scalp; if the scalp is involved, alopecia may result. Hair follicles are enlarged and filled with scale.

• *Erythema multiforme.* This acute inflammatory skin disease produces sudden onset of vesicles and bullae on the lips and buccal mucosa. Also, erythematous macules and papules form symmetrically on the hands, arms, feet, legs, face, and neck and possibly in the eyes and on the genitalia. Lymphadenopathy may also occur. With visceral involvement, other findings include fever, malaise, cough, throat and chest pain, vomiting, diarrhea, myalgias, arthralgias, fingernail loss, blindness, hematuria, and signs of renal failure.

• *Gingivitis (acute necrotizing ulcerative).* This condition causes a sudden onset of gingival ulcers covered with a grayish white pseudomembrane. Other findings may include tender or painful gingivae, intermittent gingival bleeding, and halitosis.

• *Herpes simplex.* In primary infection, a brief period of prodromal tingling and itching, accompanied by fever and pharyngitis, is followed by eruption of vesicles on any part of the oral mucosa, especially the tongue, gums, and cheeks. Vesicles form on an erythematous base, then rupture and leave a painful ulcer, followed by a yellowish crust. Other findings include submaxillary lymphadenopathy, increased salivation, halitosis, anorexia, and keratoconjunctivitis.

• *Herpes zoster.* This common viral infection may produce painful vesicles on the buccal mucosa, tongue, uvula, pharynx, and larynx. Small red nodules commonly erupt unilaterally around the thorax or vertically on the arms and legs, and rapidly become vesicles filled with clear fluid or pus; vesicles dry and form scabs about 10 days after eruption. Fever and general malaise accompany pruritus, paresthesia or hyperesthesia, and tenderness along the course of the involved sensory nerve.

• *Inflammatory fibrous hyperplasia.* This painless nodular swelling of the buccal mucosa typically results from cheek trauma or irritation. It's characterized by pink, smooth, pedunculated areas of soft tissue.

• *Mucous duct obstruction.* Obstruction produces a ranula—a painless, slow-growing mucocele on the floor of the mouth near the ducts of the submandibular and sublingual glands.

• *Pemphigoid (benign mucosal).* This autoimmune disease is characterized by vesicles on the oral mucous membranes, conjunctiva and, less commonly, the skin. Mouth lesions typically develop months or even years before other manifestations and may occur as desquamative patchy gingivitis or as a vesicobullous eruption. Secondary fibrous bands may lead to dysphagia, hoarseness, and blindness. Recurrent skin lesions include vesicobullous eruptions, usually on the inguinal area and extremities, and an erythematous, vesicobullous plaque on the scalp and face near the affected mucous membranes.

● *Pemphigus.* This chronic skin disease is characterized by vesicles and bullae that appear in cycles. On the oral mucosa, bullae rupture, leaving painful lesions that bleed easily. Associated findings include bullae anywhere on the body, denudation of the skin, and pruritus.

● *Pyogenic granuloma.* Commonly the result of trauma or irritation, this soft, painless nodule, papule, or polypoid mass usually appears on the gingivae but can also erupt on the lips, tongue, or buccal mucosa. The affected area may be smooth or have a warty surface; erythema develops in the surrounding mucosa. The lesions may ulcerate, producing a purulent exudate.

● *Squamous cell carcinoma.* This is typically a painless ulcer with an elevated, indurated border. It may erupt in areas of leukoplakia. It's most common on the lower lip but may also occur on the edge of the tongue or floor of the mouth. High risk factors include chronic smoking or alcohol intake.

● *Stomatitis (aphthous).* This common disease is characterized by recurrent, painful ulcerations of the oral mucosa, usually on the dorsum of the tongue, gingivae, and hard palate. In *recurrent aphthous stomatitis minor*, the ulcer begins as one or more erosions covered by a gray membrane and surrounded by a red halo. It is commonly found on the buccal and lip mucosa and junction, tongue, soft palate, pharynx, gingivae, and all places not bound to the periosteum. In *recurrent aphthous stomatitis major*, large, painful ulcers commonly occur on the lips, cheek, tongue, and soft palate; they may last up to 6 weeks and leave a scar.

● *Systemic lupus erythematosus.* Oral lesions are common and appear as erythematous areas associated with edema, petechiae, a tendency to bleed, and a superficial ulcer with a red halo. Primary effects include nondeforming arthritis, butterfly rash across the nose and cheeks, and photosensitivity.

Other causes

● *Drugs.* Various chemotherapeutic agents can directly produce stomatitis. Also, allergic reactions to penicillin, sulfonamides, gold, quinine, streptomycin, phenytoin, aspirin, and barbiturates commonly cause lesions to erupt.

● *Radiation therapy.* This treatment may produce oral lesions.

Special considerations

If the patient's mouth ulcers are painful, provide a topical anesthetic such as lidocaine. Instruct him to avoid irritants, such as highly seasoned foods, citrus fruits, alcohol, and tobacco. For mouth care, avoid using lemon-glycerin swabs because they can dry and irritate the lesions.

As appropriate, teach the patient proper oral hygiene. If toothbrushing is contraindicated, instruct him to use a mouth rinse, such as normal saline solution or half-strength hydrogen peroxide, and to avoid commercial mouthwashes that contain alcohol. Tell him to report any mouth lesions that don't heal within 2 weeks.

Elder tip

 Elderly people with a long-standing history of pipe smoking are at risk for lip lesions. Be sure to include an examination of the oral mucosa, including lips, in your assessment of an elderly person. Remember, some women have also been pipe and cigar smokers or tobacco chewers, so don't neglect women in this assessment.

Pediatric pointers

Causes of mouth ulcers in children include chickenpox, measles, scarlet fever, diphtheria, and hand-foot-and-mouth disease. In neonates, mouth ulcers can result from candidiasis or congenital syphilis.

MURMURS

Murmurs are auscultatory sounds heard within the heart chambers or major arteries. They're classified by their timing and duration in the cardiac cycle, auscultatory location, loudness, configuration, pitch, and quality. *Timing* can be characterized as systolic, holosystolic (continuous throughout systole), diastolic, or continuous throughout systole and diastole; systolic and diastolic murmurs can be further characterized as early, middle, or late. *Location* refers to the area of maximum loudness, such as the apex, the lower left sternal border, or an intercostal space. *Loudness* is graded on a scale of I to VI, with I signifying the faintest audible murmur. *Configuration,* or shape, refers to the nature of loudness—crescendo, decrescendo, crescendo-decrescendo, decrescendo-crescendo, plateau (even), or variable (uneven). The murmur's *pitch* may be high or low. Its *quality* may be described as harsh, rumbling, blowing, scratching, buzzing, musical, or squeaking.

Murmurs can reflect accelerated blood flow through normal or abnormal valves; forward blood flow through a narrowed or irregular valve or into a dilated vessel; blood backflow through an incompetent valve, septal defect, or patent ductus arteriosus; or decreased blood viscosity. Commonly the result of organic heart disease, murmurs occasionally may signal an emergency situation—for example, a loud holosystolic murmur after acute myocardial infarction (MI) may signal papillary muscle rupture or ventricular septal defect. (See *When murmurs signal an emergency*.) Murmurs

EMERGENCY INTERVENTIONS

WHEN MURMURS SIGNAL AN EMERGENCY

Although not normally a sign of an emergency, murmurs—especially newly developed ones—may signal a serious complication in patients with bacterial endocarditis or recent acute myocardial infarction (MI).

When caring for a patient with known or suspected bacterial endocarditis, carefully auscultate for any new murmurs. Their development along with crackles, distended neck veins, orthopnea, and dyspnea may herald heart failure.

Regular auscultation is also important in a patient who has experienced an acute MI. A loud decrescendo holosystolic murmur at the apex that radiates to the axilla and left sternal border or throughout the chest is significant, particularly in association with a widely split S_2 and an atrial gallop (S_4). This murmur, when accompanied by signs of acute pulmonary edema, usually indicates the development of acute mitral regurgitation due to rupture of the chordae tendineae—a medical emergency.

may also result from surgical implantation of a prosthetic valve.

Some murmurs are innocent or functional. An *innocent systolic murmur* is generally soft, medium-pitched, and loudest along the left sternal border at the second or third intercostal space. It's exacerbated by physical activity, excitement, fever, pregnancy, anemia, or thyrotoxicosis. Examples include *Still's murmur* in children and *mammary souffle,* com-

IDENTIFYING COMMON MURMURS

The timing and configuration of a murmur can help you identify its underlying cause. Learn to recognize the characteristics of these common murmurs.

Aortic insufficiency (chronic)
Thickened valve leaflets fail to close correctly, permitting backflow of blood into the left ventricle.

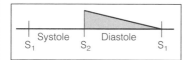

Mitral insufficiency (chronic)
Incomplete mitral valve closure permits backflow of blood into the left atrium.

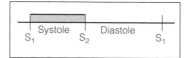

Aortic stenosis
Thickened, scarred, or a calcified valve leaflets impede ventricular systolic ejection.

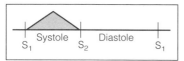

Mitral stenosis
Thickened or scarred valve leaflets cause valve stenosis and restrict blood flow.

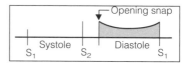

Mitral valve prolapse
Incompetent mitral valve bulges into the left atrium because of an enlarged posterior leaflet and elongated chordae tendineae.

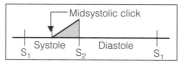

monly heard over either breast during late pregnancy and early postpartum.

History and physical examination
If you discover a murmur, try to determine its type through careful auscultation. (See *Identifying common murmurs.*) Use the bell of your stethoscope for low-pitched murmurs; the diaphragm for high-pitched murmurs.

Next, obtain a patient history. Ask if the murmur is a new discovery or has been known since birth or childhood. (See *Detecting congenital murmurs,* pages 374 and 375.) Find out if the patient has experienced any associated symptoms, particularly palpitations, dizziness, syncope, chest pain, dyspnea, and fatigue. Explore his medical history, noting especially any incidence of rheumatic fever, heart disease, or heart surgery, particularly prosthetic valve replacement.

Now perform a systematic physical examination. Note especially the presence of cardiac arrhythmias, jugular vein distention, and such pulmonary signs as dyspnea, orthopnea, and crackles. Is the patient's liver tender or palpable? Does he have peripheral edema?

Common medical causes

● *Aortic insufficiency (regurgitation).* *Acute aortic insufficiency* typically produces a soft, short diastolic murmur over the left sternal border that's best heard when the patient sits and leans forward and at the end of a forced held expiration. S_2 may be soft or absent. Sometimes, a soft, short midsystolic murmur may also be heard over the second right intercostal space. Associated findings may include tachycardia, dyspnea, distended neck veins, crackles, increased fatigue, and pale, cool extremities.

Chronic aortic insufficiency causes a high-pitched, blowing, decrescendo diastolic murmur that's best heard over the second or third right intercostal space or the left sternal border with the patient sitting, leaning forward, and holding his breath after deep expiration. An Austin Flint murmur—a rumbling, mid- to late diastolic murmur best heard at the apex—may also occur. Complications may not occur until age 40 to 50; then, typical findings include palpitations, tachycardia, anginal pain, increased fatigue, dyspnea, orthopnea, and crackles.

● *Cardiomyopathy (hypertrophic).* This disorder generates a harsh late systolic murmur, ending at S_2. Best heard over the left sternal border and at the apex, the murmur is commonly accompanied by an audible S_3 or S_4. Major associated symptoms are dyspnea and chest pain; palpitations, dizziness, and syncope may also occur.

● *Complete heart block.* This disorder commonly produces a short, crescendo-decrescendo diastolic murmur following atrial contraction, best heard at the apex. S_1 may be paradoxical. Associated signs and symptoms may include fatigue, dizziness, or syncope.

● *Mitral insufficiency (regurgitation).* *Acute mitral insufficiency* is characterized by an early systolic or holosystolic decrescendo murmur at the apex, along with a widely split S_2 and commonly an S_4. Accompanying findings typically include tachycardia and signs of acute pulmonary edema. *Chronic mitral insufficiency* produces a high-pitched, blowing, holosystolic plateau murmur that is loudest at the apex and usually radiates to the axilla or back. Fatigue, dyspnea, and palpitations may also occur.

● *Mitral valve prolapse.* This disorder generates a midsystolic to late systolic click with a high-pitched late systolic crescendo murmur, best heard at the apex. Occasionally, multiple clicks may be heard, with or without a systolic murmur. Accompanying findings may include cardiac awareness, migraine headaches, dizziness, weakness, syncope, palpitations, chest pain, dyspnea, severe episodic fatigue, mood swings, and anxiety.

● *Mitral stenosis.* In this valvular disorder, the murmur is soft, low-pitched, rumbling, decrescendo-crescendo, and diastolic, and is accompanied by a loud S_1 and an opening snap—a cardinal sign. It's best heard at the apex with the patient in the left lateral position. In severe stenosis, the murmur of mitral insufficiency may also be heard. Other findings may include hemoptysis, exertional dyspnea and fatigue, and signs of acute pulmonary edema.

● *Myxomas.* A *left atrial myxoma* (most common) usually produces a middiastolic murmur and a holosystolic murmur that's loudest at the apex, with an S_4, an early diastolic thudding sound (tu-

(Text continues on page 376.)

DETECTING CONGENITAL MURMURS

HEART DEFECT	TYPE OF MURMUR
Aorticopulmonary septal defect	*Small defect:* a continuous rough or crackling murmur best heard at the upper left sternal border and below the left clavicle, possibly accompanied by a systolic ejection click *Large defect:* a harsh systolic murmur heard at the left sternal border
Atrial septal defect	A midsystolic, spindle-shaped murmur of grade II to III intensity heard at the upper left sternal border, with a fixed splitting of S_2; large shunts may also produce a low- to medium-pitched early diastolic murmur over the lower left sternal border
Bicuspid aortic valve	An early systolic, loud, high-pitched ejection sound or click that's best heard at the apex; commonly accompanied by a soft, early or midsystolic murmur at the upper right sternal border; the aortic component of S_2 is usually accentuated at the apex
Coarctation of the aorta	Usually a systolic ejection click at the base of the heart, at the apex, and occasionally over the carotid arteries, commonly accompanied by a systolic ejection murmur at the base; this disorder may also produce a blowing diastolic murmur of aortic insufficiency or an apical pansystolic murmur of unknown origin
Common atrio-ventricular canal defects (endocardial cushion defect)	*With a competent mitral valve:* a midsystolic, spindle-shaped murmur of grade II to III intensity heard at the upper left sternal border, with a fixed splitting of S_2; may be accompanied by a low- to medium-pitched early diastolic murmur over the lower left sternal border *With an incompetent mitral valve:* an early systolic or holosystolic decrescendo murmur at the apex, along with a widely split S_2 and commonly an S_4
Ebstein's anomaly	A soft, high-pitched holosystolic blowing murmur that increases with inspiration (Carvallo's sign), best heard over the lower left sternal border and the xiphoid area; possibly accompanied by a low-pitched diastolic rumbling murmur at the apex; fixed splitting of S_2 and a loud split S_4 also occur
Left ventricular–right atrial communication	A holosystolic, grade II to IV, decrescendo murmur heard along the lower left sternal border, accompanied by a normal S_2; large shunts also produce a diastolic rumbling murmur over the apex

DETECTING CONGENITAL MURMURS *(continued)*

HEART DEFECT	TYPE OF MURMUR
Mitral atresia	A nonspecific systolic murmur and a diastolic flow rumble at the lower left sternal border, with a loud and single S_2
Partial anomalous pulmonary venous connection	A midsystolic, spindle-shaped, grade II to III murmur at the upper left sternal border, possibly accompanied by a low- to medium-pitched early diastolic murmur over the lower left sternal border
Patent ductus arteriosus	A continuous rough or crackling murmur best heard at the upper left sternal border and below the left clavicle
Pulmonic insufficiency	An early to middiastolic, soft, medium-pitched crescendo-decrescendo murmur best heard at the second or third right intercostal space
Pulmonic stenosis	An early systolic, harsh, grade IV to VI crescendo-decrescendo murmur at the second left intercostal space, possibly radiating along the left sternal border
Single atrium	A holosystolic regurgitant murmur at the apex, accompanied by a fixed splitting of S_2
Supravalvular aortic stenosis	A systolic ejection murmur best heard over the second right intercostal space or higher in the episternal notch or over the right lower neck; the aortic closure sound is usually preserved, and no ejection clicks are heard
Tetralogy of Fallot	A midsystolic murmur with a systolic thrill palpable at the left midsternal border; softer murmurs occurring earlier in systole generally indicate a more severe obstruction
Tricuspid atresia	Variable, depending on associated defects
Trilogy of Fallot	A systolic, harsh crescendo-decrescendo murmur, best heard at the upper left sternal border with radiation toward the left clavicle; the pulmonic component of S_2 becomes progressively softer with increasing degrees of obstruction
Ventricular septal defect	*Small defect:* usually a holosystolic (but may be limited to early or midsystole), grade II to IV decrescendo murmur heard along the lower left sternal border, accompanied by a normal S_2 *Large defect:* a holosystolic murmur at the lower left sternal border and a midsystolic rumbling murmur at the apex, accompanied by an increased S_1 at the lower left sternal border and an increased pulmonic component of S_2

mor plop), and a loud, widely split S_1. Related features may include dyspnea, orthopnea, chest pain, fatigue, weight loss, and syncope.

A *right atrial myxoma* causes a late diastolic rumbling murmur, a holosystolic crescendo murmur, and tumor plop, best heard at the lower left sternal border. Other findings include fatigue, peripheral edema, ascites, and hepatomegaly.

A *right ventricular myxoma* commonly generates a systolic ejection murmur with a delayed S_2 and a tumor plop, best heard at the left sternal border. It's accompanied by peripheral edema, hepatomegaly, ascites, dyspnea, and syncope.

● *Papillary muscle rupture.* In this life-threatening complication of acute MI, a loud holosystolic murmur can be auscultated at the apex. Related findings include severe dyspnea, chest pain, syncope, hemoptysis, tachycardia, and hypotension.

● *Tricuspid insufficiency (regurgitation).* This valvular abnormality is characterized by a soft, high-pitched, holosystolic blowing murmur that increases with inspiration (Carvallo's sign); it's best heard over the lower left sternal border and xiphoid area. After a lengthy asymptomatic period, exertional dyspnea and orthopnea may develop, along with neck vein distention, ascites, peripheral cyanosis and edema, and muscle wasting.

● *Tricuspid stenosis.* This valvular disorder produces a diastolic murmur similar to that of mitral stenosis, but louder with inspiration. S_1 may also be louder. Associated signs and symptoms may include fatigue, distended neck veins, ascites, hepatomegaly, and dyspnea.

Other causes
● *Surgery.* Prosthetic valve replacement may cause variable murmurs, depending on the location, valve composition, and method of operation.

Special considerations
Prepare the patient for diagnostic tests, such as electrocardiography and echocardiography. Because any cardiac abnormality will be frightening to the patient, provide emotional support.

Pediatric pointers
Innocent murmurs such as Still's murmur are commonly heard in young children and often disappear at puberty. Pathognomonic heart murmurs in infants and young children usually result from congenital heart disease, such as atrial and ventricular septal defects. Other murmurs can be acquired, as with rheumatic heart disease.

MUSCLE ATROPHY
[Muscle wasting]

Muscle atrophy results from denervation or prolonged muscle disuse. When deprived of regular exercise, muscle fibers lose both bulk and length, producing a visible loss of muscle size and contour and apparent emaciation or deformity in the affected area. Even slight atrophy usually causes some loss of motion or power.

Atrophy most commonly stems from neuromuscular disease or injury. However, it may also stem from certain metabolic and endocrine disorders and prolonged immobility. Some muscle atrophy also occurs with aging.

History and physical examination
Ask the patient when and where he first noticed the muscle wasting and how it has progressed. Also ask about any associated symptoms, such as weakness, pain, loss of sensation, and recent weight loss. Review the patient's medical history for chronic illnesses; musculoskeletal or neurologic disorders, including trauma; and endocrine and metabolic disor-

ders. Ask about his use of alcohol and drugs, particularly steroids.

Begin the physical examination by determining the location and extent of atrophy. Visually evaluate small and large muscles. Check all major muscle groups for size, tonicity, and strength. Measure the circumference of all limbs, comparing sides. (See *Measuring limb circumference*.) Check for muscle contractures in all limbs by fully extending joints and noting any pain or resistance. Complete the examination by palpating peripheral pulses for quality and rate, assessing sensory function in and around the atrophied area, and testing deep tendon reflexes.

Common medical causes

• *Amyotrophic lateral sclerosis.* Initial symptoms of this progressive disease include muscle weakness and atrophy that typically begin in one hand, spread to the arm, and then develop in the other hand and arm. Eventually, weakness and atrophy spread to the trunk, neck, tongue, larynx, pharynx, and legs; progressive respiratory muscle weakness leads to respiratory insufficiency. Other findings include muscle flaccidity, fasciculations, hyperactive deep tendon reflexes, slight leg muscle spasticity, dysphagia, impaired speech, excessive drooling, and depression.

• *Burns.* Fibrous scar tissue formation, pain, and loss of serum proteins from severe burns can limit muscle movement, resulting in atrophy.

• *Hypothyroidism.* Reversible weakness and atrophy of proximal limb muscles may occur in hypothyroidism. Accompanying findings commonly include muscle cramps and stiffness; cold intolerance; weight gain despite anorexia; mental dullness; dry, pale, cool, doughy skin; puffy face, hands, and feet; and bradycardia.

• *Meniscal tear.* Quadriceps muscle atrophy, resulting from prolonged knee immobility and muscle weakness, is a classic sign of this traumatic disorder.

EXAMINATION TIP

MEASURING LIMB CIRCUMFERENCE

To ensure accurate and consistent limb circumference measurements, use a consistent reference point each time and measure with the limb in full extension. The diagram below shows the correct reference points for arm and leg measurements.

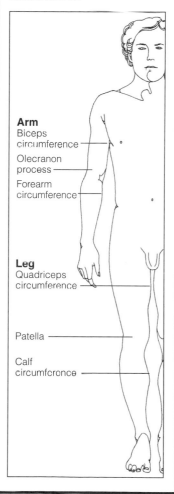

Arm
Biceps circumference
Olecranon process
Forearm circumference

Leg
Quadriceps circumference

Patella

Calf circumference

● *Multiple sclerosis.* This degenerative disease may produce arm and leg atrophy as a result of chronic progressive weakness; spasticity and contractures may also develop. Associated signs and symptoms typically wax and wane and may include diplopia and blurred vision, nystagmus, hyperactive deep tendon reflexes, sensory loss or paresthesia, dysarthria, dysphagia, incoordination, ataxic gait, intention tremors, emotional lability, impotence, and urinary dysfunction.

● *Osteoarthritis.* This chronic disorder eventually causes atrophy proximal to involved joints as a result of progressive weakness and disuse. Other late signs and symptoms include bony joint deformities, such as Heberden's nodes on the distal interphalangeal joints, crepitus and fluid accumulation, and contractures.

● *Parkinson's disease.* In this disorder, muscle rigidity, weakness, and disuse may produce muscle atrophy. The patient may have insidious tremors that usually begin in the fingers (pill-rolling tremor), worsen with stress, and ease with purposeful movement and sleep. He may also have bradykinesia, a characteristic propulsive gait, masklike facies, drooling, dysphagia, dysarthria, oculogyric crisis or blepharospasm (occasionally), and a high-pitched, monotone voice.

● *Peripheral neuropathy.* In this disorder, muscle weakness progresses slowly to flaccid paralysis and eventually atrophy. Distal extremity muscles are generally affected first. Associated findings may include loss of vibration sense; paresthesia, hyperesthesia, or anesthesia in the hands and feet; mild to sharp, burning pain; anhidrosis; glossy red skin; and diminished or absent deep tendon reflexes.

● *Protein deficiency.* If chronic, this may lead to muscle weakness and atrophy. Other findings include chronic fatigue, apathy, anorexia, dry skin, peripheral edema, and dull, sparse, dry hair.

● *Rheumatoid arthritis.* Muscle atrophy occurs in the late stages of this disorder, as joint pain and stiffness decrease range of motion (ROM) and discourage muscle use.

● *Spinal cord injury.* Trauma to the spinal cord can produce severe muscle weakness and flaccid, then spastic, paralysis, eventually leading to atrophy. Other signs and symptoms depend on the level of the injury but may include respiratory insufficiency or paralysis, sensory losses, bowel and bladder dysfunction, hyperactive deep tendon reflexes, positive Babinski's reflex, sexual dysfunction, priapism, hypotension, and anhidrosis (usually unilateral).

Other causes

● *Drugs.* Prolonged steroid therapy interferes with muscle metabolism and leads to atrophy, most prominently in the limbs.

● *Immobility.* Prolonged immobilization from bed rest, casts, splints, or traction may cause muscle weakness and atrophy.

Special considerations

Because contractures can occur as atrophied muscle fibers shorten, help the patient maintain muscle length by encouraging him to perform frequent active ROM exercises. If he's unable to actively move a joint, provide active-assistive or passive exercises, and apply splints or braces to maintain muscle length. If you find resistance to full extension during exercises, use heat, pain medication, or relaxation techniques to relax the muscle. Then slowly stretch it to full extension. (*Caution:* Do not pull or strain the muscle—you may tear muscle fibers and cause further contracture.)

If these techniques fail to correct the contracture, use moist heat, a whirlpool bath, resistive exercises, or ultrasound therapy. If these techniques aren't effective, surgical release of contractures may be necessary.

Prepare the patient for electromyography, nerve conduction studies, muscle biopsy, and X-rays or computed tomography scans.

Pediatric pointers

In young children, profound muscle weakness and atrophy can result from muscular dystrophy. Muscle atrophy may also result from cerebral palsy and poliomyelitis, and from paralysis associated with meningocele and myelomeningocele.

MUSCLE FLACCIDITY
[Muscle hypotonicity]

Flaccid muscles are profoundly weak and soft, with decreased resistance to movement, increased mobility, and greater-than-normal range of motion (ROM). The result of disrupted muscle innervation, flaccidity can be localized to a limb or muscle group or generalized over the entire body. Its onset may be acute, as in trauma, or chronic, as in neurologic disease.

Emergency interventions

 If the patient's flaccidity results from trauma, make sure that his cervical spine has been stabilized. Quickly determine his respiratory status. If you note signs of respiratory insufficiency—dyspnea, shallow respirations, nasal flaring, and cyanosis—administer oxygen by nasal cannula or mask. Intubation and mechanical ventilation may be necessary.

History and physical examination

If the patient isn't in distress, ask about the onset and duration of muscle flaccidity and any precipitating factors. Ask about associated symptoms, notably weakness, other muscle changes, and sensory losses or paresthesia.

Examine the affected muscles for atrophy, which indicates a chronic problem. Test muscle strength and check deep tendon reflexes in all limbs.

Common medical causes

● *Amyotrophic lateral sclerosis.* Progressive muscle weakness and paralysis are accompanied by generalized flaccidity. Typically, these effects begin in one hand, spread to the arm, and then develop in the other hand and arm. Eventually, they spread to the trunk, neck, tongue, larynx, pharynx, and legs; progressive respiratory muscle weakness leads to respiratory insufficiency. Other findings may include muscle cramps and coarse fasciculations, hyperactive deep tendon reflexes, slight leg muscle spasticity, dysphagia, dysarthria, excessive drooling, and depression.

● *Brain lesions.* Frontal and parietal lobe lesions may cause contralateral flaccidity, weakness or paralysis, and eventually spasticity. Other findings may include hyperactive deep tendon reflexes, positive Babinski's sign, loss of proprioception, analgesia, anesthesia, and thermoanesthesia.

● *Guillain-Barré syndrome.* This disorder causes muscle flaccidity. Progression is typically symmetrical and ascending, moving from the feet to the arms and facial nerves within 24 to 72 hours of onset. Associated findings include sensory loss or paresthesia, absent deep tendon reflexes, tachycardia (or, less commonly, bradycardia), fluctuating hypertension and postural hypotension, diaphoresis, incontinence, dysphagia, dysarthria, hypernasality, and facial diplegia. Weakness may progress to total motor paralysis and respiratory failure.

● *Huntington's disease.* Besides flaccidity, progressive mental status changes and choreiform movements are major symptoms. Others include poor balance, hesitant or explosive speech, dysphagia, impaired respirations, and incontinence.

● *Peripheral neuropathy.* Flaccidity usually occurs in the legs as a result of chronic progressive muscle weakness and paralysis. It may also cause mild to sharp burning pain, glossy red skin, anhidrosis, and loss of vibration sensation. Paresthesia, hyperesthesia, or anesthesia may affect the hands and feet. Deep tendon reflexes may be hypoactive or absent.

• *Seizure disorder.* Brief periods of syncope and generalized flaccidity commonly follow a generalized tonic-clonic seizure.

• *Spinal cord injury.* Spinal shock can result in acute muscle flaccidity or spasticity below the level of injury. Associated signs and symptoms also occur below the level of injury and may include paralysis, absent deep tendon reflexes, analgesia, thermoanesthesia, anhidrosis (usually unilateral), and loss of proprioception and vibration, touch, and pressure sensation. Hypotension, bowel and bladder dysfunction, and impotence or priapism may also occur. Injury in the C1 to C5 region can produce respiratory paralysis and bradycardia.

Special considerations

Provide regular, systematic, passive ROM exercises to preserve joint mobility and to increase circulation. Reposition a patient with generalized flaccidity every 2 hours to protect him from skin breakdown. Pad bony prominences and other pressure points, and prevent thermal injury by testing bathwater yourself before the patient bathes. Treat isolated flaccidity by supporting the affected limb in a sling or with a splint.

Prepare the patient for diagnostic tests, such as cranial and spinal X-rays or computed tomography scans and electromyography.

Pediatric pointers

Pediatric causes of muscle flaccidity include myelomeningocele, Lowe's disease, Werdnig-Hoffmann disease, and muscular dystrophy. An infant or young child with generalized flaccidity may lie in a froglike position, with his hips and knees abducted.

MUSCLE SPASMS
[Muscle cramps]

Muscle spasms are strong, painful contractions. They can occur in virtually any muscle but are most common in the calf and foot. Muscle spasms typically result from simple muscle fatigue, from exercise, and during pregnancy. However, they may also occur in electrolyte imbalances and neuromuscular disorders, or as the result of certain drugs. They're commonly precipitated by movement and can usually be relieved by slow stretching.

Emergency interventions

 If the patient complains of frequent or unrelieved spasms in many muscles, accompanied by paresthesia in his hands and feet, quickly attempt to elicit Chvostek's and Trousseau's signs. If these signs are present, suspect hypocalcemia. Evaluate respiratory function, watching for the development of laryngospasm; provide supplemental oxygen as necessary, and prepare to intubate the patient and provide mechanical ventilation. Draw blood for calcium levels and arterial blood gas analysis, and insert an I.V. for administration of a calcium supplement. Monitor cardiac status, and prepare to begin resuscitation if necessary.

History and physical examination

If the patient isn't in distress, ask when the spasms began. How long did they last? How painful were they? Did anything worsen or lessen the pain? Ask about other symptoms, such as weakness, sensory loss, or paresthesia.

Evaluate muscle strength and tone. Then, check all major muscle groups, and note whether any movements precipitate spasms. Test the presence and quality of all peripheral pulses, and examine the limbs for color and temperature changes. Test capillary refill time and inspect for edema, especially in the involved area. Finally, test reflexes and sensory function in all extremities.

Common medical causes

• *Amyotrophic lateral sclerosis.* In this disorder, muscle spasms may accompany progressive muscle weakness and atrophy that typically begin in one hand, spread to the arm, and then spread to the other hand and arm. Eventually, muscle weakness and atrophy affect the trunk, neck, tongue, larynx, pharynx, and legs; progressive respiratory muscle weakness leads to respiratory insufficiency. Other findings may include muscle flaccidity progressing to spasticity, coarse fasciculations, hyperactive deep tendon reflexes, dysphagia, impaired speech, excessive drooling, and depression.

• *Arterial occlusive disease.* Arterial occlusion typically produces spasms and intermittent claudication in the leg, with residual pain. Associated findings are usually localized to the legs and feet and include loss of peripheral pulses, pallor or cyanosis, decreased sensation, hair loss, dry or scaling skin, edema, and ulcerations.

• *Dehydration.* Sodium loss may produce limb and abdominal cramps. Other findings may include a slight fever, decreased skin turgor, dry mucous membranes, tachycardia, postural hypotension, muscle twitching, seizures, nausea, vomiting, and oliguria.

• *Hypocalcemia.* The classic feature is tetany—a syndrome of muscle cramps and twitching, carpopedal and facial muscle spasms, and seizures, possibly with stridor. Both Chvostek's and Trousseau's signs may be elicited. Related findings include choreiform movements, hyperactive deep tendon reflexes, fatigue, palpitations, cardiac arrhythmias, and paresthesia of the lips, fingers, and toes.

• *Muscle trauma.* Excessive muscle strain may cause mild to severe spasms.

The injured area may be painful, swollen, reddened, and warm.

• *Respiratory alkalosis.* Acute onset of muscle spasms may be accompanied by twitching and weakness, carpopedal spasms, circumoral and peripheral paresthesia, vertigo, syncope, pallor, and extreme anxiety. In severe alkalosis, cardiac arrhythmias may occur.

• *Spinal injury or disease.* Muscle spasms can result from spinal injury, such as cervical extension injury or spinous process fracture, or from spinal disease such as infection.

Other causes

• *Drugs.* Common spasm-producing drugs include diuretics, corticosteroids, and estrogens.

Special considerations

Depending on the cause, help alleviate your patient's spasms by slowly stretching the affected muscle in the direction opposite the contraction. Or have the patient stand, preferably on a cold surface, such as tile or marble. If necessary, administer a mild analgesic.

Diagnostic studies may include serum calcium and sodium levels, thyroid function tests, and blood flow studies or arteriography.

Pediatric pointers

Muscle spasms rarely occur in children. However, their presence may indicate hypoparathyroidism, osteomalacia, rickets or, rarely, congenital torticollis.

MUSCLE SPASTICITY
[Muscle hypertonicity]

Spasticity is a state of excessive muscle tone manifested by increased resistance to stretching and heightened reflexes. It's commonly detected by evaluating a muscle's response to passive movement; a

HOW SPASTICITY DEVELOPS

Motor activity is controlled by pyramidal and extrapyramidal tracts that originate in the motor cortex, basal ganglia, brain stem, and spinal cord. Nerve fibers from the various tracts converge and synapse at the anterior horn in the spinal cord. Together, they maintain segmental muscle tone by modulating the *stretch reflex arc*. This arc, shown in simplified form below, is basically a negative feedback loop in which muscle stretch (stimulation) causes reflexive contraction (inhibition), thus maintaining muscle length and tone.

Damage to certain tracts results in loss of inhibition and disruption of the stretch reflex arc. Uninhibited muscle stretch produces exaggerated, uncontrolled muscle activity, accentuating the reflex arc and eventually resulting in spasticity.

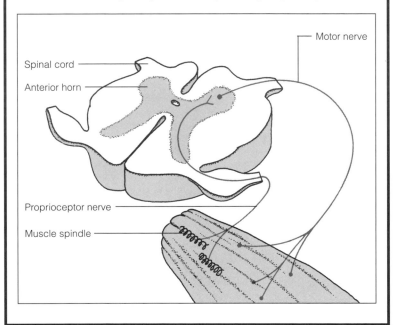

- Motor nerve
- Spinal cord
- Anterior horn
- Proprioceptor nerve
- Muscle spindle

spastic muscle offers more resistance when the passive movement is performed quickly. Caused by an upper motor neuron lesion, spasticity most commonly occurs in the arm and leg muscles. (See *How spasticity develops.*) Long-term spasticity results in muscle fibrosis and contractures.

History and physical examination

Once you detect spasticity, ask the patient about its onset, duration, and progression. What, if any, events precipitated onset? Has he experienced other muscular changes or related symptoms? Does his medical history reveal any incidence of trauma or degenerative or vascular disease?

Take the patient's vital signs and perform a complete neurologic examination.

Test reflexes and evaluate motor and sensory function in all limbs. Evaluate muscles for wasting and contractures.

During your examination, keep in mind that generalized spasticity and trismus in a patient with a recent skin puncture or laceration indicates tetanus. If you suspect this rare disorder, look for signs of respiratory distress. If necessary, provide ventilatory support and monitor the patient closely.

Common medical causes

• *Amyotrophic lateral sclerosis.* This disorder commonly produces spasticity, spasms, coarse fasciculations, hyperactive deep tendon reflexes, and a positive Babinski's sign. Earlier effects include progressive muscle weakness and flaccidity that typically begin in the hands and arms and eventually spread to the trunk, neck, larynx, pharynx, and legs; progressive respiratory muscle weakness leads to respiratory insufficiency. Other findings may include dysphagia, dysarthria, excessive drooling, and depression.

• *Cerebrovascular accident (CVA).* Spastic paralysis may develop on the affected side following the acute stage of CVA. Associated findings vary with the site and extent of vascular damage and may include dysarthria, aphasia, ataxia, apraxia, agnosia, ipsilateral paresthesia or sensory losses, visual disturbances, altered level of consciousness, amnesia and poor judgment, personality changes, emotional lability, bowel and bladder dysfunction, headache, vomiting, and seizures.

• *Epidural hemorrhage.* In this disorder, bilateral limb spasticity is a late and ominous sign. Other findings may include a momentary loss of consciousness after head trauma, followed by a lucid interval and then a rapid deterioration in consciousness. The patient may also have unilateral hemiparesis or hemiplegia, seizures, high fever, decreased and bounding pulse, widened pulse pressure, elevated blood pressure, irregular respiratory pattern, decerebrate posture, and

fixed, dilated pupils. A positive Babinski's sign can be elicited.

• *Spinal cord injury.* Spasticity commonly results from cervical and high thoracic spinal cord injury, especially from incomplete lesions. Spastic paralysis in the affected limbs follows initial flaccid paralysis; typically, spasticity and muscle atrophy increase for up to $1\frac{1}{2}$ to 2 years after the injury, then gradually regress to flaccidity. Associated signs and symptoms vary with the level of the injury but may include respiratory insufficiency or paralysis, sensory losses, bowel and bladder dysfunction, hyperactive deep tendon reflexes, positive Babinski's sign, sexual dysfunction, priapism, hypotension, anhidrosis, and bradycardia.

• *Tetanus.* This rare, life-threatening disease produces varying degrees of spasticity. In generalized tetanus, the most common form, early signs and symptoms include jaw and neck stiffness, trismus, headache, irritability, restlessness, low-grade fever with chills, tachycardia, diaphoresis, and hyperactive deep tendon reflexes. As the disease progresses, painful involuntary spasms may spread and cause boardlike abdominal rigidity, opisthotonos, and a characteristic grotesque grin known as risus sardonicus. Reflex spasms may occur in any muscle group with the slightest stimulus. Glottal, pharyngeal, or respiratory muscle involvement can cause death by asphyxia or cardiac failure.

Special considerations

Prepare the patient for diagnostic tests, which may include electromyography, muscle biopsy, or intracranial or spinal magnetic resonance imaging or computed tomography. Administer prescribed pain medications and antispasmodics. Passive range-of-motion exercises, splinting, traction, and application of heat may help relieve spasms and prevent contractures. Maintain a calm, quiet environment to help relieve spasms and prevent recurrence, and encourage bed rest. In cases of prolonged, uncontrollable spasticity, as in spastic paralysis, nerve blocks or surgical transection may be necessary for permanent relief.

Pediatric pointers
In children, muscle spasticity may be a sign of cerebral palsy.

MUSCLE WEAKNESS

Muscle weakness is detected by observing and measuring the strength of an individual muscle or muscle group. It can result from a malfunction in the cerebral hemispheres, brain stem, spinal cord, nerve roots, peripheral nerves, or myoneural junctions and within the muscle itself. Muscle weakness occurs as a response to certain drugs, after prolonged immobilization, and in certain neurologic, musculoskeletal, metabolic, endocrine, and cardiovascular disorders.

History and physical examination
Begin by determining the location of the patient's muscle weakness. Ask if he has difficulty with any specific movements such as rising from a chair. Find out when he first noticed the weakness; ask him whether it worsens with exercise or as the day progresses. Also ask about related symptoms, especially muscle or joint pain, altered sensory function, and fatigue.

Obtain a medical history, noting especially chronic diseases such as hyperthyroidism; musculoskeletal or neurologic problems, including recent trauma; family history of chronic muscle weakness, especially in males; and alcohol and drug use.

Focus your physical examination on evaluating muscle strength. Test all major muscles bilaterally. (See *Testing muscle strength.*) If the patient complains of pain, ease or discontinue testing and have

him try the movements again. Remember that the patient's dominant arm, hand, and leg are somewhat stronger than their nondominant counterparts. Besides testing individual muscle strength, test for range of motion (ROM) at all major joints (shoulder, elbow, wrist, hip, knee, ankle). Also test sensory function in the involved areas and test deep tendon reflexes bilaterally.

Common medical causes
• *Amyotrophic lateral sclerosis.* This disorder typically begins with muscle weakness and atrophy in one hand that rapidly spreads to the arm and then to the other hand and arm. Eventually, these effects spread to the trunk, neck, tongue, larynx, pharynx, and legs; progressive respiratory muscle weakness leads to respiratory insufficiency.
• *Anemia.* Varying degrees of muscle weakness and fatigue are exacerbated by exertion and temporarily relieved by rest. Other signs and symptoms may include pallor, tachycardia, paresthesia, and bleeding tendencies.
• *Brain tumor.* Signs and symptoms of muscle weakness vary with the location of the tumor. Other associated findings include headache, vomiting, diplopia, decreased visual acuity, decreased level of consciousness (LOC), pupillary changes, decreased motor strength, hemiparesis, hemiplegia, diminished sensations, ataxia, seizures, and behavioral changes.
• *Cerebrovascular accident (CVA).* Depending on the site and extent of damage, a CVA may produce contralateral or bilateral weakness of the arms, legs, face, and tongue, possibly progressing to hemiplegia and atrophy. Associated effects may include dysarthria, aphasia, ataxia, apraxia, agnosia, ipsilateral paresthesia or sensory losses, visual disturbances, altered LOC, amnesia and poor judgment, personality changes, bowel and bladder dysfunction, headache, vomiting, and seizures.

TESTING MUSCLE STRENGTH

Obtain an overall picture of your patient's motor function by testing strength in 10 selected muscle groups. Ask the patient to attempt normal range-of-motion movements against your resistance. If the muscle group is weak, vary the amount of resistance as necessary to permit accurate assessment. If necessary, position the patient so his limbs don't have to resist gravity, and repeat the test.

Arm muscles

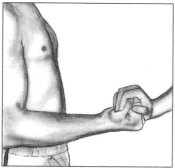

Biceps. With your hand on the patient's hand, have him flex his forearm against your resistance; observe for biceps contraction.

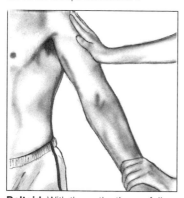

Deltoid. With the patient's arm fully extended, place one hand over his deltoid muscle and the other on his wrist. Ask him to abduct his arm to a horizontal position against your resistance; as he does so, palpate for deltoid contraction.

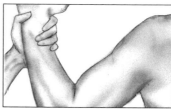

Triceps. Have the patient abduct and hold his arm midway between flexion and extension. Hold and support his arm at the wrist, and ask him to extend it against your resistance. Observe for triceps contraction.

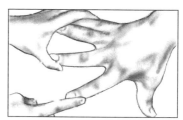

Dorsal interossei. Have the patient extend and spread his fingers, and tell him to try to resist your attempt to squeeze them together.

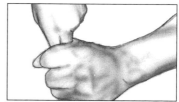

Forearm and hand (grip). Have the patient grasp your middle and index fingers and squeeze as hard as he can.

(continued)

TESTING MUSCLE STRENGTH *(continued)*

Rate muscle strength on a scale from 0 to 5:
0 = Total paralysis
1 = Visible or palpable contraction, but no movement
2 = Full muscle movement with force of gravity eliminated
3 = Full muscle movement against gravity, but no movement against resistance
4 = Full muscle movement against gravity; partial movement against resistance
5 = Full muscle movement against both gravity and resistance—normal strength.

Leg muscles

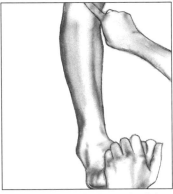

Anterior tibial. With the patient's leg extended, place your hand on his foot and ask him to dorsiflex his ankle against your resistance.

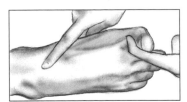

Extensor hallucis longus. With your finger on the patient's great toe, have him dorsiflex the toe against your resistance. Palpate for extensor hallucis contraction.

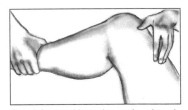

Quadriceps. Have the patient bend his knee slightly while you support his lower leg. Then ask him to extend the knee against your resistance; as he's doing so, palpate for quadriceps contraction.

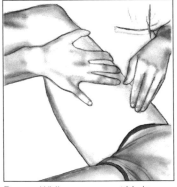

Psoas. While you support his leg, have the patient raise his knee and flex his hip against your resistance. Observe for psoas muscle contraction.

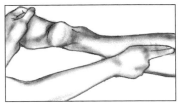

Gastrocnemius. With the patient on his side, support his foot and ask him to plantar-flex his ankle against your resistance. Palpate for gastrocnemius contraction.

- **Guillain-Barré syndrome.** Rapidly progressive, symmetrical weakness ascends from the feet to the arms and facial nerves and may progress to total motor paralysis and respiratory failure. Associated findings include sensory loss or paresthesia, muscle flaccidity, loss of deep tendon reflexes, tachycardia or bradycardia, fluctuating hypertension and postural hypotension, diaphoresis, bowel and bladder incontinence, facial diplegia, dysphagia, dysarthria, and hypernasality.

- **Herniated disk.** Pressure on nerve roots leads to muscle weakness, disuse, and ultimately atrophy. The primary symptom is severe low back pain, possibly radiating to the buttocks, legs, and feet—usually on one side. Diminished reflexes and sensory changes may also occur.

- **Hypercortisolism.** This disorder may cause limb weakness and eventually atrophy. Related cushingoid features include buffalo hump, moon face, truncal obesity, purple striae, thin skin, acne, elevated blood pressure, fatigue, hyperpigmentation, easy bruising, poor wound healing, and diaphoresis. The male patient may be impotent; the female patient may have hirsutism and menstrual irregularities.

- **Multiple sclerosis.** Muscle weakness in one or more limbs may progress to atrophy, spasticity, and contractures. Other findings typically wax and wane and may include diplopia and blurred vision, vision loss, nystagmus, hyperactive deep tendon reflexes, sensory loss or paresthesia, dysarthria, dysphagia, incoordination, ataxic gait, intention tremors, emotional lability, impotence, and urinary dysfunction.

- **Myasthenia gravis.** Gradually progressive skeletal muscle weakness and fatigue are the cardinal symptoms of this disorder. Typically, weakness is mild upon awakening but worsens during the day. Early signs may include weak eye closure, ptosis, and diplopia; a blank, masklike facies; difficulty chewing and swallowing; nasal regurgitation of fluid with hypernasality; and a hanging jaw and bobbing head. Respiratory muscle involvement may eventually lead to respiratory failure.

- **Osteoarthritis.** This chronic disorder causes progressive muscle disuse and weakness that leads to atrophy.

- **Parkinson's disease.** Muscle weakness accompanies rigidity in this degenerative disorder. Related findings include a pill-rolling tremor, propulsive gait, dysarthria, bradykinesia, drooling, dysphagia, masklike facies, and a high-pitched, monotonic voice.

- **Peripheral nerve trauma.** Prolonged pressure on or injury to a peripheral nerve causes muscle weakness and atrophy. Other findings include paresthesia or sensory loss, pain, and loss of reflexes supplied by the damaged nerve.

- **Peripheral neuropathy.** In this disorder, muscle weakness progresses slowly to flaccid paralysis, generally affecting distal extremities first. It may be accompanied by loss of vibration sense, hypoactive or absent deep tendon reflexes, mild to sharp and burning pain, anhidrosis, glossy red skin, and paresthesia, hyperesthesia, or anesthesia in the hands and feet.

- **Potassium imbalance.** In *hypokalemia,* temporary generalized muscle weakness may be accompanied by nausea, vomiting, diarrhea, decreased mentation, leg cramps, diminished reflexes, malaise, polyuria, dizziness, hypotension, and arrhythmias. In *hyperkalemia,* weakness may progress to flaccid paralysis accompanied by irritability and confusion, hyperreflexia, paresthesia or anesthesia, oliguria, anorexia, nausea, diarrhea, abdominal cramps, tachycardia or bradycardia, and arrhythmias.

- **Rheumatoid arthritis.** In this disorder, muscle weakness may accompany pain, stiffness that restricts motion, and increased warmth, swelling, and tenderness in involved joints.

• *Seizure disorder.* Temporary generalized muscle weakness may occur after a generalized tonic-clonic seizure; other postictal findings include headache, muscle soreness, and profound fatigue.

• *Spinal trauma and disease.* Trauma can cause severe muscle weakness, leading to flaccidity or spasticity and, eventually, paralysis. Infection, tumor, and cervical stenosis or spondylosis can also cause muscle weakness.

Other causes

• *Drugs.* Generalized muscle weakness can result from prolonged corticosteroid use, digitalis toxicity, and excessive doses of dantrolene. Aminoglycoside antibiotics may worsen weakness in patients with myasthenia gravis.

• *Immobility.* Immobilization in a cast, a splint, or traction can lead to muscle weakness in the involved extremity; prolonged bed rest or inactivity results in generalized muscle weakness.

Special considerations

Provide assistive devices as necessary, and protect the patient from injury. If he has concomitant sensory loss, guard against decubitus ulcer formation and thermal injury. With chronic weakness, provide ROM exercises or splint limbs as necessary. Arrange therapy sessions to allow for adequate rest periods, and administer pain medications, as needed.

Prepare the patient for blood tests, muscle biopsy, electromyography, nerve conduction studies, and X-rays or computed tomography scans.

Pediatric pointers

Muscular dystrophy, usually the Duchenne type, is a major cause of muscle weakness in children.

MYDRIASIS

Mydriasis—pupillary dilation caused by contraction of the dilator of the iris—is a normal response to decreased light, strong emotional stimuli, and topical administration of mydriatic and cycloplegic drugs. It can also result from ocular and neurologic disorders, eye trauma, and disorders that decrease level of consciousness (LOC). Mydriasis may be an adverse effect of antihistamines or other drugs.

History and physical examination

Begin by asking the patient about any other eye problems, such as pain, blurring, diplopia, or visual field defects. Obtain a health history, focusing on eye or head trauma, glaucoma and other ocular problems, and neurologic and vascular disorders. In addition, obtain a complete medication history.

Next, perform a thorough eye and pupil examination. Inspect and compare the pupils' size, color, and shape (many people normally have unequal pupils). (See *Grading pupil size.*) Also test each pupil for light reflex, consensual response, and accommodation. Be sure to check the eyes for ptosis, swelling, and ecchymosis. Test visual acuity in both eyes with and without correction. Evaluate extraocular muscle function by checking the six cardinal fields of gaze.

Keep in mind that mydriasis appears in two ocular emergencies: acute angle-closure glaucoma and traumatic iridoplegia.

Common medical causes

• *Adie's syndrome.* This disorder is characterized by abrupt unilateral mydriasis, poor or absent pupillary reflexes, visual blurring, and cramplike eye pain. Deep tendon reflexes may be hyperactive or absent.

• *Aortic arch syndrome.* Bilateral pupillary mydriasis commonly occurs late in this syndrome. Other ocular findings include visual blurring, transient vision loss, and diplopia. Related findings may include dizziness and syncope, bruits, loss of radial and carotid pulses, paresthesia, intermittent claudication, and neck, shoulder, and chest pain. Blood pressure may be decreased in the arms.

• *Botulism.* Botulinum toxin causes bilateral mydriasis, usually 12 to 36 hours after ingestion. Other early findings are loss of pupillary reflexes, visual blurring, diplopia, ptosis, strabismus and extraocular muscle palsies, anorexia, nausea, vomiting, diarrhea, and dry mouth. Vertigo, hearing loss, hoarseness, hypernasality, dysarthria, dysphagia, progressive muscle weakness, and loss of deep tendon reflexes soon follow.

• *Carotid artery aneurysm.* Here, unilateral mydriasis may be accompanied by bitemporal hemianopia, decreased visual acuity, hemiplegia, decreased LOC, headache, aphasia, behavioral changes, and hypoesthesia.

• *Glaucoma (acute angle-closure).* This ocular emergency is characterized by moderate mydriasis and loss of pupillary reflex in the affected eye, accompanied by abrupt onset of excruciating pain, decreased visual acuity, visual blurring, halo vision, conjunctival injection, and a cloudy cornea.

• *Oculomotor nerve palsy.* Unilateral mydriasis is commonly the first sign of this disorder. It's soon followed by ptosis, diplopia, decreased pupillary reflexes, exotropia, and complete loss of accommodation. Focal neurologic signs may accompany signs of increased intracranial pressure (ICP).

• *Traumatic iridoplegia.* Eye trauma commonly paralyzes the sphincter of the iris, causing mydriasis and loss of pupillary reflex; usually, this is transient. Associated findings may include a quivering iris (iridodonesis), ecchymosis, pain, and swelling.

GRADING PUPIL SIZE

To ensure accurate evaluation of pupillary size, compare your patient's pupils to the scale below. Keep in mind that maximum constriction may be less than 1 mm and maximum dilation greater than 9 mm.

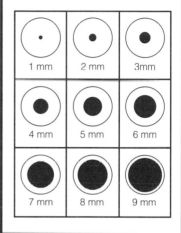

Other causes

• *Drugs.* Mydriasis can be caused by anticholinergics, antihistamines, sympathomimetics, barbiturates (in overdose), estrogens, and tricyclic antidepressants; it also occurs commonly early in anesthesia induction. Topical mydriatics and cycloplegics—such as phenylephrine, atropine, homatropine, scopolamine, cyclopentolate, and tropicamide—are administered specifically for their mydriatic effects.

• *Surgery.* Traumatic mydriasis commonly results from ocular surgery.

Special considerations

If the patient's mydriasis is the result of mydriatic drugs received during an eye examination, explain that he'll likely experience some photophobia and loss of accommodation. Instruct him to wear dark glasses and to avoid bright light, and reassure him that the condition is only temporary.

Diagnostic tests may vary, depending on your findings, but may include a complete ophthalmologic examination and a thorough neurologic workup. Explain any diagnostic tests to the patient.

Pediatric pointers
Mydriasis occurs in children as a result of ocular trauma, drugs, Adie's syndrome and, in most cases, increased ICP.

MYOCLONUS

Myoclonus—sudden, shocklike contractions of a single muscle or muscle group—occurs in various neurologic disorders and commonly heralds onset of a seizure. These contractions may be isolated or repetitive, rhythmic or arrhythmic, symmetrical or asymmetrical, synchronous or asynchronous, generalized or focal. They may be precipitated by bright flickering lights, a loud sound, or unexpected physical contact. One type, *intention myoclonus,* is evoked by intentional muscle movement.

Myoclonus occurs normally just before falling asleep and as a part of the natural startle reaction. It also occurs with some poisonings and, rarely, as a complication of hemodialysis.

Emergency interventions
 If you observe myoclonus, check for seizure activity. Take vital signs to rule out arrhythmias or a blocked airway. Have resuscitation equipment on hand.

If the patient has a seizure, gently help him lie down. (Place a pillow or a rolled-up towel under his head to prevent concussion.) Loosen any constrictive cloth-ing, especially around the neck, and turn his head (gently, if possible) to one side to prevent airway occlusion or aspiration of secretions. Insert an oral airway if the teeth aren't already clenched.

History and physical examination
If the patient is stable, evaluate level of consciousness (LOC) and mental status. Ask about the frequency, severity, location, and circumstances of the myoclonus. Has he ever had a seizure? If so, did myoclonus precede it? Is the myoclonus ever precipitated by a sensory stimulus? During the physical examination, check for muscle rigidity and wasting, and test deep tendon reflexes.

Common medical causes
• *Alzheimer's disease.* Generalized myoclonus may occur in advanced stages of this slowly progressive dementia. Other late findings may include mild choreoathetoid movements, muscle rigidity, bowel and bladder incontinence, delusions, and hallucinations.

• *Creutzfeldt-Jakob disease.* Diffuse myoclonic jerks appear early in this rapidly progressive dementia. Initially random, they gradually become more rhythmic and symmetrical, commonly occurring in response to sensory stimuli. Associated effects may include ataxia, aphasia, hearing loss, muscle rigidity and wasting, fasciculations, hemiplegia, and visual disturbances or, possibly, blindness.

• *Encephalitis (viral).* In this disease, myoclonus is usually intermittent and either localized or generalized. Associated findings vary but may include rapidly decreasing LOC, fever, headache, irritability, nuchal rigidity, vomiting, seizures, aphasia, ataxia, hemiparesis, facial muscle weakness, nystagmus, ocular palsies, and dysphagia.

• *Encephalopathy.* *Hepatic encephalopathy* occasionally produces myoclonic jerks in association with asterixis and focal or generalized seizures.

Hypoxic encephalopathy may produce generalized myoclonus or seizures almost immediately after restoration of cardiopulmonary function. The patient may also have a residual intention myoclonus.

Uremic encephalopathy commonly produces myoclonic jerks and seizures. Other signs and symptoms include apathy, fatigue, irritability, headache, confusion, gradually decreasing LOC, nausea, vomiting, oliguria, edema, and papilledema. The patient may also have elevated blood pressure, dyspnea, arrhythmias, and abnormal respirations.

● *Epilepsy.* In *idiopathic epilepsy,* localized myoclonus is usually confined to an arm or leg and occurs singly or in short bursts, typically upon awakening. It's generally more common and severe during the prodromal stage of a major generalized seizure, after which it diminishes in frequency and intensity.

Myoclonic jerks are usually the first signs of *myoclonic epilepsy,* the most common cause of progressive myoclonus. At first, myoclonus is infrequent and localized, but over a period of months it becomes more common and involves the entire body, disrupting voluntary movement (intention myoclonus). As the disease progresses, myoclonus is accompanied by generalized seizures and dementia.

● *Poisoning.* Acute intoxication with methyl bromide, bismuth, or strychnine may produce an acute onset of myoclonus and confusion.

Other causes

● *Drug withdrawal.* Myoclonus may be seen in patients with alcohol, narcotic, or sedative withdrawal, and in delirium tremens.

Special considerations

If your patient's myoclonus is progressive, take seizure precautions. Keep an oral airway, suction equipment, and padded tongue blade at his bedside, and pad the side rails. Because myoclonus may cause falls, remove potentially harmful objects from the patient's environment, and remain with him while he walks. Be sure to instruct the patient and his family about the need for safety precautions.

As needed, administer drugs that suppress myoclonus: ethosuximide, phenobarbital, clonazepam, or carbidopa. An EEG may be needed to evaluate myoclonus and related brain activity.

Pediatric pointers

Although myoclonus is relatively uncommon in infants and children, it can result from subacute sclerosing panencephalitis, severe meningitis, progressive poliodystrophy, childhood myoclonic epilepsy, and encephalopathies such as Reye's syndrome.

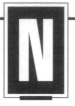

NASAL FLARING

Nasal flaring is the abnormal dilation of the nostrils. It usually occurs during inspiration but may occasionally occur during expiration or throughout the respiratory cycle. Nasal flaring indicates respiratory dysfunction, ranging from mild difficulty to potentially life-threatening respiratory distress.

Emergency interventions

 If you note nasal flaring in the patient, quickly evaluate his respiratory status. Inspiratory chest movement, absent breath sounds, cyanosis, diaphoresis, and tachycardia point to complete airway obstruction. As necessary, you'll need to deliver back blows or abdominal thrusts (Heimlich maneuver) to relieve the obstruction. If these don't clear the airway, emergency intubation or tracheostomy and mechanical ventilation may be necessary.

If the patient's airway is not obstructed but he displays breathing difficulty, administer oxygen by nasal cannula or face mask. Intubation and mechanical ventilation may be necessary. Insert an I.V. line for fluid and medication access, and begin cardiac monitoring. Obtain a chest X-ray and blood samples for arterial blood gas (ABG) and electrolyte studies.

History

Once the patient is stabilized, obtain a pertinent history. Ask about cardiac and pulmonary disorders such as asthma. Does the patient have allergies? Has he recently experienced a traumatic injury or an illness such as a respiratory infection?

Common medical causes

• **Adult respiratory distress syndrome (ARDS).** ARDS causes increased respiratory difficulty, with nasal flaring, dyspnea, tachypnea, diaphoresis, cyanosis, scattered crackles, and rhonchi. It also causes tachycardia, anxiety, and decreased level of consciousness (LOC).

• **Airway obstruction.** *Complete obstruction* above the tracheal bifurcation causes sudden nasal flaring, absent breath sounds despite intercostal retractions and marked accessory muscle use, tachycardia, diaphoresis, cyanosis, decreasing LOC, and eventually respiratory arrest.

Partial obstruction causes nasal flaring with inspiratory stridor, gagging, wheezing, violent cough, marked accessory muscle use, agitation, cyanosis, and hoarseness.

• **Anaphylaxis.** Severe reactions can produce respiratory distress with nasal flaring, stridor, wheezing, accessory muscle use, intercostal retractions, and dyspnea. Associated signs and symptoms may include nasal congestion, sneezing, pruritus, urticaria, erythema, diaphoresis, angioedema, weakness, hoarseness, dysphagia, and, rarely, vomiting, nausea, diarrhea, urinary urgency, and incontinence. Cardiac arrhythmias and signs of shock may occur late.

• **Asthma (acute).** An asthma attack can cause nasal flaring, dyspnea, tachypnea, prolonged expiratory wheezing, accessory muscle use, cyanosis, and a dry or productive cough. Auscultation may reveal rhonchi, crackles, and decreased or absent breath sounds. Other findings include anxiety, tachycardia, and increased blood pressure.

• *Chronic obstructive pulmonary disease.* This disorder can lead to acute respiratory failure secondary to pulmonary infection or edema. Nasal flaring is accompanied by prolonged pursed-lip expiration, accessory muscle use, cyanosis, crackles, rhonchi, reduced chest expansion, wheezing, dyspnea, and a loose, rattling, productive cough.

• *Pneumothorax.* This acute disorder can result in respiratory distress with nasal flaring, dyspnea, tachypnea, shallow respirations, hyperresonance or tympany on percussion, agitation, distended neck veins, tracheal deviation, and cyanosis. Other findings typically include sharp chest pain, tachycardia, hypotension, cold and clammy skin, diaphoresis, and subcutaneous crepitation. Breath sounds may be decreased or absent on the affected side; similarly, chest wall motion may be decreased on the affected side.

Similar findings can occur with hydrothorax, chylothorax, or hemothorax, depending on the amount of fluid accumulation.

• *Pulmonary edema.* This disorder typically produces nasal flaring, severe dyspnea, wheezing, and a cough that produces frothy, pink sputum. Increased accessory muscle use may occur with tachycardia, cyanosis, hypotension, crackles, distended neck veins, peripheral edema, and decreased LOC.

• *Pulmonary embolus.* Signs of this potentially life-threatening disorder may include nasal flaring, dyspnea, tachypnea, wheezing, cyanosis, pleural friction rub, and productive cough (possibly hemoptysis). Other possible effects include sudden chest tightness or pleuritic pain, tachycardia, hypotension, low-grade fever, syncope, marked anxiety, and restlessness.

Other causes

• *Diagnostic tests.* Pulmonary function tests, such as vital capacity testing, can produce nasal flaring with forced inspiration or expiration.

• *Treatments.* Certain respiratory treatments, such as deep breathing, can cause nasal flaring.

Special considerations

To help ease breathing, place the patient in a high Fowler position. If he's at risk for aspirating secretions, place him in a modified Trendelenburg or side-lying position. If necessary, suction frequently to remove oropharyngeal secretions. Administer humidified oxygen to thin secretions and decrease airway drying and irritation. Provide adequate hydration to liquefy secretions. Reposition the patient every hour and encourage coughing and deep breathing. Avoid administering sedatives or opiates, which can depress both the cough reflex and respirations. Continually assess the patient's respiratory status, and check his vital signs every 30 minutes or as necessary.

Prepare the patient for diagnostic tests, such as chest X-rays, lung scan, pulmonary arteriography, sputum culture, complete blood count, ABG analysis, and 12-lead electrocardiogram.

Pediatric pointers

Nasal flaring is an important sign of respiratory distress in infants and very young children, who can't verbalize their discomfort. Common causes include airway obstruction, hyaline membrane disease, croup, and acute epiglottitis.

NAUSEA

Nausea is a sensation of profound revulsion to food or of impending vomiting. Commonly accompanied by autonomic signs, such as hypersalivation, diaphoresis, tachycardia, pallor, and tachypnea, it's closely associated with both anorexia and vomiting.

Nausea is a common symptom of GI disorders, but it also occurs in fluid and electrolyte imbalances, infections, and metabolic, endocrine, labyrinthine, and cardiac disorders. It may also result from drug therapy, surgery, or radiation. Commonly present during the first trimester of pregnancy, nausea may also arise from severe pain, anxiety, alcohol intoxication, overeating, or ingestion of distasteful food or liquids.

History and physical examination

Begin by obtaining a complete medical history. Focus on recent infections, treatment for cancer, and GI, endocrine, and metabolic disorders. Ask about medication use and alcohol consumption. If the patient is a female of childbearing age, ask if she is or could be pregnant. Have her describe the onset, duration, and intensity of the nausea as well as what causes or relieves it. Ask about related complaints, particularly vomiting (color, amount), abdominal pain, anorexia and weight loss, changes in bowel habits or stool character, excessive belching or flatus, and a sensation of bloating.

Inspect the skin for jaundice, bruises, and spider angiomas, and assess skin turgor. Next, inspect the abdomen for distention, auscultate for bowel sounds and bruits, palpate for rigidity and tenderness, and test for rebound tenderness. Palpate and percuss the liver for enlargement. Assess other body systems as appropriate.

Common medical causes

• *Adrenal insufficiency.* Common GI findings in this endocrine disorder include nausea, vomiting, anorexia, and diarrhea. Other findings may include weakness, fatigue, weight loss, bronze skin, hypotension, and a weak, irregular pulse.

• *Appendicitis.* With acute appendicitis, a brief period of nausea may accompany onset of abdominal pain. Pain typically begins as vague epigastric or periumbilical discomfort and rapidly progresses to severe stabbing pain localized in the right lower quadrant (McBurney's sign). Associated findings usually include abdominal rigidity and tenderness, cutaneous hyperalgesia, fever, constipation or diarrhea, tachycardia, anorexia, and moderate malaise.

• *Cholecystitis (acute).* In this disorder, nausea commonly follows severe right upper quadrant pain that may radiate to the back or shoulders. Associated findings include mild vomiting, abdominal tenderness and, possibly, rigidity and distention, fever with chills, and diaphoresis.

• *Cholelithiasis.* In this disorder, nausea accompanies attacks of severe right upper quadrant or epigastric pain after ingestion of fatty foods. Other associated findings include vomiting, abdominal tenderness and guarding, flatulence, belching, epigastric burning, tachycardia, and restlessness. Occlusion of the common bile duct may cause jaundice, clay-colored stools, fever, and chills.

• *Cirrhosis.* Insidious early symptoms of cirrhosis typically include nausea and vomiting, anorexia, abdominal pain, and constipation or diarrhea. As the disease progresses, jaundice and hepatomegaly may occur with abdominal distention, spider angiomas, palmar erythema, severe pruritus, dry skin, fetor hepaticus, enlarged superficial abdominal veins, mental changes, and bilateral gynecomastia and testicular atrophy or menstrual irregularities.

• *Diverticulitis.* In addition to nausea, diverticulitis causes intermittent abdominal pain, constipation or diarrhea, low-grade fever and, commonly, a palpable mass.

• *Gastritis.* Nausea is common in gastritis, especially after ingestion of alcohol, aspirin, spicy foods, or caffeine. Vomiting of mucus or blood, epigastric pain, belching, fever, and malaise may also occur.

• *Gastroenteritis.* Usually viral, this disorder causes nausea, vomiting, diarrhea, and abdominal cramping. Fever, malaise, hyperactive bowel sounds, abdominal pain and tenderness, and dehydration may also develop.

• **Heart failure.** This disorder may produce nausea and vomiting, particularly with right-sided heart failure. Associated findings include tachycardia, ventricular gallop, profound fatigue, dyspnea, crackles, peripheral edema, and jugular vein distention.

• **Hepatitis.** Nausea is an insidious early symptom of viral hepatitis. Vomiting, fatigue, myalgia and arthralgia, headache, anorexia, photophobia, pharyngitis, cough, and fever also occur early in the preicteric phase.

• **Hyperemesis gravidarum.** Unremitting nausea and vomiting that persist beyond the first trimester are characteristic of this disorder of pregnancy. Vomitus ranges from undigested food, mucus, and bile early in the disorder to a coffee-ground appearance in later stages. Associated findings include weight loss, signs of dehydration, headache, and delirium.

• **Intestinal obstruction.** Nausea is common, especially in a high obstruction of the small intestine. Vomiting may be bilious or fecal; abdominal pain is usually episodic and colicky but can become severe and steady with strangulation. Constipation occurs early in large-intestinal and later in small-intestinal obstruction; obstipation may signal complete obstruction. Bowel sounds are typically hyperactive in partial obstruction, and hypoactive or absent in complete obstruction. Abdominal distention and tenderness occur, possibly with visible peristaltic waves and a palpable abdominal mass.

• **Labyrinthitis.** Nausea and vomiting commonly occur with this acute inner ear inflammation. More significant findings include severe vertigo, progressive hearing loss, nystagmus, and possibly otorrhea.

• **Ménière's disease.** This inner ear disorder causes sudden, brief, recurrent attacks of nausea, vomiting, vertigo, tinnitus, diaphoresis, and nystagmus. Hearing loss may also occur.

• **Mesenteric venous thrombosis.** Insidious or acute onset of nausea, vomiting, and abdominal pain occur here, with diarrhea or constipation, abdominal distention, hematemesis, and melena.

• **Metabolic acidosis.** This acid-base imbalance may produce nausea and vomiting, anorexia, diarrhea, Kussmaul's respirations, and decreased level of consciousness.

• **Migraine headache.** Nausea and vomiting may occur in the prodromal stage, along with photophobia, light flashes, increased sensitivity to noise, and possibly partial vision loss and paresthesia of the lips, face, and hands.

• **Motion sickness.** In this disorder, nausea and vomiting are brought on by motion or rhythmic movement. Headache, dizziness, fatigue, diaphoresis, and dyspnea may also occur.

• **Pancreatitis (acute).** Nausea, usually followed by vomiting, is an early symptom of pancreatitis. Common associated findings include abdominal tenderness and rigidity, diminished bowel sounds, fever, and steady, severe pain in the epigastrium or left upper quadrant that may radiate to the back. Tachycardia, restlessness, hypotension, skin mottling, and cold, sweaty extremities may occur in severe cases.

• **Peptic ulcer.** In this disorder, nausea and vomiting may follow attacks of sharp or burning epigastric pain. Attacks typically occur when the stomach is empty or after ingestion of alcohol, caffeine, or aspirin; they're relieved by eating or antacids. Hematemesis or melena may also occur.

• **Peritonitis.** Nausea and vomiting usually accompany acute abdominal pain localized to the area of inflammation. Other findings may include high fever with chills, tachycardia, hypoactive or absent bowel sounds, abdominal distention and tenderness (including rebound tenderness), weakness, diaphoresis, hypotension, shallow respirations, hiccups, and pale, cold skin.

• **Preeclampsia.** Nausea and vomiting commonly occur in this disorder of pregnancy, along with rapid weight gain, epigastric pain, generalized edema, elevated blood pressure, oliguria, severe frontal headache, and blurred or double vision.

Other causes

• **Drugs.** Common nausea-producing drugs include antineoplastic agents, opiates, ferrous sulfate, levodopa, oral potassium chloride replacements, estrogens, sulfasalazine, antibiotics, quinidine, and anesthetic agents. An overdose of digitalis glycosides or theophylline may also cause nausea.

• **Radiation and surgery.** Radiation therapy may cause nausea and vomiting. Postoperative nausea and vomiting are common, especially after abdominal surgery.

Special considerations

If your patient is experiencing severe nausea, prepare him for blood tests to determine fluid, electrolyte, and acid-base balance. Have him breathe deeply to ease his nausea; keep his room air fresh and clean-smelling by removing bedpans and emesis basins promptly after use and by providing adequate ventilation. Because he could easily aspirate vomitus when supine, elevate his head or position him on his side.

Because pain can precipitate or intensify nausea, administer pain medications promptly, as needed. If possible, give medications by injection or suppository to prevent exacerbating nausea. Be alert for abdominal distention and hypoactive bowel sounds when you administer antiemetics: These signs may indicate gastric retention. If you detect these, immediately insert a nasogastric tube, as required.

Pediatric pointers

Nausea, generally described as stomachache, is one of the most common childhood complaints. Commonly the result of overeating, it can also occur with diverse disorders, ranging from acute infections to a conversion reaction caused by fear.

NECK PAIN

Neck pain may originate from any neck structure, ranging from the meninges and cervical vertebrae to its blood vessels, muscles, and lymphatic tissue. This symptom can also be referred from other areas of the body. Its location, onset, and pattern help determine its origin and underlying causes. Neck pain usually results from traumatic injury and from degenerative, congenital, inflammatory, metabolic, and neoplastic disorders.

Emergency interventions

 If the patient's neck pain is due to trauma, first ensure proper cervical spine immobilization, preferably with a long backboard and a Philadelphia collar. (See *Applying a Philadelphia collar.*) Then take vital signs, and perform a quick neurologic evaluation. If he shows signs of respiratory distress, give oxygen. Intubation and mechanical ventilation may be necessary. Ask the patient (or his companion, if the patient can't answer) how the injury occurred. Then examine the neck for abrasions, swelling, lacerations, erythema, and ecchymoses.

History and physical examination

If the patient hasn't sustained trauma, find out the severity and onset of his neck pain. Where in the neck does he feel pain? Does anything relieve or worsen the pain? Also ask about the development of other symptoms. Next, focus on the patient's current and past illnesses and injuries, diet, medication use, and family health history.

Thoroughly inspect the patient's neck, shoulders, and cervical spine for swelling, masses, erythema, and ecchymoses. Assess range of motion (ROM) in his neck by having him turn his head from side to side; note the degree of pain produced by these movements. Check the sensation in his arms and assess his hand grasp and arm reflexes. Attempt to elicit Brudzinski's and Kernig's signs, and palpate the cervical lymph nodes for enlargement.

Common medical causes

● *Ankylosing spondylitis.* Intermittent, moderate to severe neck pain and stiffness with severely restricted ROM is characteristic of this disorder. Related findings also occur intermittently and may include low back pain and stiffness, arm pain, low-grade fever, limited chest expansion, malaise, anorexia, fatigue, and occasionally iritis.

● *Cervical extension injury.* Anterior or posterior neck pain may develop within hours or days following a whiplash injury. Anterior pain usually diminishes within several days, but posterior pain persists and may even intensify. Associated findings include tenderness, swelling and nuchal rigidity, arm or back pain, occipital headache, muscle spasms, visual blurring, and unilateral miosis on the affected side.

● *Cervical spine fracture.* A fracture at C1 to C4 commonly causes sudden death; survivors may have severe neck pain that restricts all movement, intense occipital headache, quadriplegia, deformity, and respiratory paralysis.

● *Cervical spine tumor. Metastatic tumors* typically produce persistent neck pain that increases with movement and isn't relieved by rest; *primary tumors* cause mild to severe pain along a specific nerve root. Other findings depend on the lesions and may include paresthesia, arm and leg weakness that progresses to atrophy and paralysis, and bladder and bowel incontinence.

● *Cervical spondylosis.* This degenerative process produces posterior neck pain that restricts movement and is aggravat-

APPLYING A PHILADELPHIA COLLAR

A lightweight molded polyethylene collar designed to hold the neck straight with the chin slightly elevated and tucked in, the Philadelphia cervical collar immobilizes the cervical spine, decreases muscle spasms, and relieves some pain. It also prevents further injury and promotes healing.

When applying the collar, fit it snugly around the patient's neck and attach the Velcro fasteners or buckles at the back. Be sure to check the patient's airway and his neurovascular status to ensure that the collar isn't too tight. Also make sure that the collar isn't placed too high in front, which could hyperextend the neck. In a patient with a neck sprain, hyperextension may cause the ligaments to heal in a shortened position; in a patient with a cervical spine fracture, it could cause serious neurologic damage.

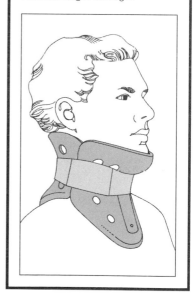

NECK PAIN: COMMON CAUSES AND ASSOCIATED FINDINGS

CAUSES	Arm pain	Back pain	Brudzinski's sign	Decreased level of consciousness	Decreased range of motion	Deformity	Dysphagia	Dyspnea	Ecchymoses	Fatigue	Fever	Headache	Hemoptysis	Hoarseness
MAJOR ASSOCIATED SIGNS AND SYMPTOMS														
Ankylosing spondylitis	●	●			●					●	●			
Cervical extension injury	●	●										●		
Cervical fibrositis														
Cervical spine fracture					●	●						●		
Cervical spine tumor					●									
Cervical spondylosis	●				●									
Esophageal trauma							●						●	
Hemorrhage (subarachnoid)			●	●								●		
Herniated cervical disk	●	●			●									
Laryngeal cancer							●	●					●	●
Lymphadenitis											●			
Meningitis			●	●							●	●		
Neck sprain					●				●					
Rheumatoid arthritis					●	●				●	●			
Spinous process fracture					●	●								
Thyroid trauma							●	●						
Torticollis														
Tracheal trauma							●	●					●	●

Kernig's sgn	Lymphadenopathy	Malaise	Muscle spasms	Nuchal rigidity	Paralysis	Paresthesia	Swelling	Tenderness	Weakness
			•	•					
			•	•			•		
									•
				•					
					•	•			•
				•					•
							•		
•				•					
							•		•
		•							
			•	•				•	
•				•					
				•	•		•		
		•				•	•	•	•
				•			•	•	
							•		
				•	•	•			

ed by it. Pain may radiate down either arm and may accompany paresthesia and weakness.

• *Esophageal trauma.* An esophageal mucosal tear or a pulsion diverticulum may produce mild neck pain, chest pain, edema, hemoptysis, and dysphagia.

• *Hemorrhage (subarachnoid).* This life-threatening condition may cause moderate to severe neck pain and rigidity, headache, and a decreased level of consciousness (LOC). Kernig's and Brudzinski's signs are present.

• *Herniated cervical disk.* This disorder characteristically causes variable neck pain that restricts movement and is aggravated by it. It also causes referred pain, paresthesia and other sensory disturbances, and arm weakness.

• *Laryngeal cancer.* Neck pain that radiates to the ear develops late in this disorder. The patient may also have dysphagia, dyspnea, hemoptysis, stridor, hoarseness, and cervical lymphadenopathy.

• *Lymphadenitis.* In this disorder, enlarged and inflamed cervical lymph nodes cause acute pain and tenderness. Fever, chills, and malaise may also occur.

• *Meningitis.* Neck pain may accompany characteristic nuchal rigidity. Related findings include fever, headache, photophobia, positive Brudzinski's and Kernig's signs, and decreased LOC.

• *Neck sprain.* *Minor sprains* typically produce pain, slight swelling, stiffness, and restricted ROM. *Ligament rupture* causes pain, marked swelling, ecchymosis, muscle spasms, and nuchal rigidity with head tilt.

• *Rheumatoid arthritis.* This disorder usually affects peripheral joints, but it can also involve the cervical vertebrae. Acute inflammation may cause moderate to severe pain that radiates along a specific nerve root; increased warmth, swelling, and tenderness in involved joints; stiffness restricting ROM; paresthesia and muscle weakness; low-grade fever; anorexia; malaise; fatigue; and pos-

ALTERNATIVE THERAPY

THERAPEUTIC TOUCH FOR NECK PAIN

Therapeutic touch can be used to treat pain and reduce inflammation. This alternative therapy is a combination of body work and visualization in which the practitioner assesses the patient's energy field by slowly moving his hands a few inches over the patient's body. (Therapeutic touch is a misnomer because body contact is rare.) Blocked energy fields, as evidenced by a feeling of radiant heat or unusual pressure, indicate an underlying disorder.

Energy fields are believed to be linked to hemoglobin levels in circulating blood. By dissipating the blocked energy to other parts of the body, therapeutic touch is believed to restore the patient's vitality and well-being.

sibly neck deformity. Some pain and stiffness remain after the acute phase.

• *Spinous process fracture.* Fracture near the cervicothoracic junction produces acute pain radiating to the shoulders. Associated findings include swelling, exquisite tenderness, restricted ROM, muscle spasms, and deformity.

• *Thyroid trauma.* Besides mild to moderate neck pain, thyroid trauma may cause local swelling and ecchymosis. If a hematoma forms, it can cause dyspnea.

• *Torticollis.* In this neck deformity, severe neck pain accompanies recurrent unilateral stiffness and muscle spasms that produce a characteristic head tilt.

• *Tracheal trauma.* Fracture of the tracheal cartilage, a life-threatening condition, produces moderate to severe neck pain and respiratory difficulty. Torn tra-*cheal mucosa* produces mild to moderate pain and may result in airway occlusion, hemoptysis, hoarseness, and dysphagia.

Special considerations
Promote patient comfort by providing anti-inflammatory drugs and analgesics, as needed. Prepare him for diagnostic tests, such as X-rays, computed tomography scan, blood tests, and cerebrospinal fluid analysis. Alternative therapies may also prove helpful. (See *Therapeutic touch for neck pain.*)

Pediatric pointers
The most common causes of neck pain in children are meningitis and trauma. A rare cause of neck pain is congenital torticollis.

NIPPLE DISCHARGE

Nipple discharge can occur spontaneously or can be elicited by nipple stimulation. It's characterized as intermittent or constant, unilateral or bilateral, and by color, consistency, and composition. Its incidence increases with age and parity. This sign rarely occurs (but is more likely to be pathologic) in men or in nulligravid, regularly menstruating women, but it's relatively common and generally normal in parous women. A thick, grayish discharge—benign epithelial debris from inactive ducts—is common in middle-aged parous women. Colostrum, a thin, yellowish or milky discharge, commonly occurs in the last weeks of pregnancy.

Nipple discharge can signal serious underlying disease, particularly when accompanied by other breast changes. Significant causes include endocrine disorders, cancer, blocked lactiferous ducts, and use of certain drugs.

History and physical examination

Ask the patient when she first noticed the discharge, and determine its duration, extent, quantity, color, and consistency. Has she had other nipple and breast changes, such as pain, tenderness, itching, warmth, changes in contour, and lumps? If she reports a lump, question her about its onset, location, size, and consistency.

Obtain a complete gynecologic and obstetric history, and determine her normal menstrual cycle and the date of her last menses. Ask the patient if she experiences breast swelling and tenderness, bloating, irritability, headaches, abdominal cramping, nausea, or diarrhea before or during menses. Note the number, date, and outcome of her pregnancies and, if she breast-fed, the approximate time of her last lactation. Also check for any risk factors of breast cancer—family history, previous or current malignancies, nulliparity or first pregnancy after age 30, early menarche, or late menopause.

Start your physical examination by characterizing the discharge. If the discharge isn't frank, try to elicit it. (See *Eliciting nipple discharge.*) Then examine the nipples and breasts with the patient in four different positions: sitting with her arms at her sides, with her arms overhead, and with her hands pressing on her hips; and leaning forward so her breasts hang. Check for nipple deviation, flattening, retraction, redness, asymmetry, thickening, excoriation, erosion, or cracking. Inspect her breasts for asymmetry, irregular contours, peau d'orange, dimpling, and erythema. With the patient supine, palpate the breasts and axilla for lumps, giving special attention to the areolae. Note the size, location, delineation, consistency, and mobility of any lump you find.

Common medical causes

• **Breast abscess.** This disorder, most common in lactating women, may produce a thick, purulent discharge from a

 ELICITING NIPPLE DISCHARGE

If your patient has a history or evidence of nipple discharge, you can attempt to elicit it during your examination. Position the patient supine, and gently squeeze her nipple between your thumb and index finger; note any discharge through the nipple. Then place your fingers on the areola, as shown, and palpate the entire areolar surface, watching for any discharge through areolar ducts.

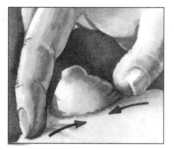

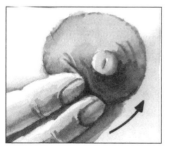

cracked nipple or an infected duct. Associated findings include abrupt onset of high fever with chills, a palpable soft nodule or generalized induration, possibly nipple retraction, and breast pain, tenderness, and erythema.

• *Breast cancer.* This may cause bloody, watery, or purulent discharge from a normal appearing nipple. More characteristic findings include a hard, irregular, fixed lump; erythema; dimpling; peau d'orange; changes in contour; nipple deviation, flattening, or retraction; axillary lymphadenopathy; and possibly breast pain.

• *Choriocarcinoma.* Galactorrhea (a white or grayish milky discharge) may result from this highly malignant neoplasm, which can follow pregnancy. Other characteristics include persistent uterine bleeding and bogginess after delivery or curettage.

• *Intraductal papilloma.* Unilateral serous, serosanguineous, or bloody nipple discharge is the predominant sign of this disorder. The discharge may be intermittent or profuse and constant; it can usually be stimulated by gentle pressure around the areola. Subareolar nodules, breast pain, and tenderness may occur.

• *Mammary duct ectasia.* A thick, sticky, grayish discharge may be the first sign of this disorder; it may be bilateral and is usually spontaneous. Other findings include a rubbery, poorly delineated lump beneath the areola, with a blue-green discoloration of the overlying skin; nipple retraction and redness, swelling, tenderness, and burning pain in the areola and nipple.

• *Paget's disease.* Serous or bloody discharge emits from denuded skin on the nipple, which is red, intensely itchy, and possibly eroded or excoriated.

• *Prolactin-secreting pituitary tumor.* Bilateral galactorrhea may occur with this tumor. Other findings include amenorrhea, infertility, and decreased libido and vaginal secretions.

Other causes
• *Drugs.* Galactorrhea can be caused by some antihypertensives (reserpine and methyldopa), oral contraceptives, cimetidine, metoclopramide, verapamil, and psychotropic agents, particularly phenothiazines and tricyclic antidepressants.

• *Surgery.* Chest wall surgery may stimulate the thoracic nerves, causing intermittent bilateral galactorrhea.

Special considerations
Although nipple discharge is usually insignificant, it can be frightening to the patient. Help relieve the patient's anxieties by clearly explaining the nature and origin of her discharge. Apply a breast binder, which may reduce discharge by eliminating nipple stimulation.

Diagnostic tests may include tissue biopsy (if a breast lump is found), cytologic study of discharge, mammography, ultrasonography, transillumination, and serum prolactin.

Pediatric pointers
Nipple discharge in children and adolescents is rare. When it does occur, it's almost always nonpathologic, as in the bloody discharge that sometimes accompanies onset of menarche. Infants of both sexes may experience a milky breast discharge beginning 3 days after birth and lasting up to 2 weeks.

NIPPLE RETRACTION

Nipple retraction, the inward displacement of the nipple below the level of surrounding breast tissue, may indicate an inflammatory breast lesion or cancer. It results from scar tissue formation within a lesion or large mammary duct. As the scar tissue shortens, it pulls adjacent tissue in, causing nipple deviation, flattening, and finally retraction.

History and physical examination
Ask the patient when she first noticed retraction of the nipple. Has she experienced other nipple changes, such as itching, discoloration, discharge, or excori-

ation? Has she had breast pain, lumps, redness, swelling, or warmth? Obtain a history, noting risk factors of breast cancer, such as a family history or a previous malignant tumor.

Carefully examine both nipples and breasts with the patient sitting upright with her arms at her sides, with her hands pressing on her hips, and with her arms overhead; then examine the breasts with the patient leaning forward so that they hang. Look for redness, excoriation, discharge, nipple flattening and deviation, breast asymmetry, dimpling, and contour differences. (See *Comparing nipple anomalies*.)

Try to evert the nipple by gently squeezing the areola. With the patient supine, palpate both breasts for lumps, especially beneath the areola. Mold breast skin over the lump or gently pull it up toward the clavicle, looking for accentuated nipple retraction. Also palpate axillary lymph nodes.

Common medical causes

● ***Breast abscess.*** This disorder, which is most common in lactating women, occasionally produces unilateral nipple retraction. More common findings include high fever with chills; breast pain, erythema, and tenderness; breast induration or soft mass; and cracked, sore nipples, possibly accompanied by purulent discharge.

● ***Breast cancer.*** Unilateral nipple retraction is commonly accompanied by a hard, fixed nodule beneath the areola as well as other breast nodules. Other nipple changes include itching, burning, erosion, and watery or bloody discharge. Breast changes commonly include dimpling, altered contour, peau d'orange, ulceration, tenderness (possibly pain), redness, and warmth. Axillary lymph nodes may be enlarged.

● ***Mammary duct ectasia.*** Nipple retraction commonly occurs along with a poorly defined, rubbery nodule beneath the areola, with a blue-green skin dis-

 COMPARING NIPPLE ANOMALIES

Nipple retraction is often confused with nipple inversion, a common abnormality that's generally congenital and doesn't usually signal underlying disease. A *retracted* nipple appears flat and broad, whereas an *inverted* nipple can be pulled out from the sulcus where it hides.

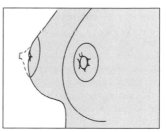

Nipple retraction

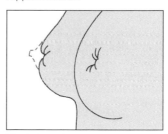

Nipple inversion

coloration; areolar burning, itching, swelling, tenderness, and erythema; and nipple pain with a thick, sticky, grayish discharge.

● ***Mastitis.*** Nipple retraction, deviation, cracking, or flattening may occur in this disorder with a breast nodule, warmth, erythema, tenderness, and edema. Fatigue, high fevers, and chills may also be present.

Other causes
● *Surgery.* Previous breast surgery may cause underlying scarring and retraction.

Special considerations
Prepare the patient for diagnostic tests, including mammography, cytology of nipple discharge, and biopsy.

Pediatric pointers
Nipple retraction doesn't occur in prepubescent females.

NOCTURIA

Nocturia—excessive urination at night—may result from disruption of the normal diurnal pattern of urine concentration or from overstimulation of the nerves and muscles that control urination. Normally, more urine is concentrated during the night than during the day. As a result, most persons excrete three to four times more urine during the day, and can sleep for 6 to 8 hours during the night without being awakened. In nocturia, the patient may awaken one or more times during the night to empty his bladder and excrete 700 ml or more of urine.

Although nocturia usually results from renal and lower urinary tract disorders, it may result from certain cardiovascular, endocrine, and metabolic disorders. This common sign may also result from drugs that induce diuresis, particularly when they're taken at night, and from the ingestion of large quantities of fluids, especially caffeinated beverages or alcohol, at bedtime.

History and physical examination
Begin by exploring the history of the patient's nocturia. When did it begin? How often does it occur? Can the patient identify a specific pattern? Precipitating factors? Also note the volume of urine voided. Ask the patient about any change in the color, odor, or consistency of his urine. Has the patient changed his usual pattern or volume of fluid intake? Next, explore associated symptoms. Ask about pain or burning on urination, difficulty initiating a urine stream, costovertebral angle tenderness, and flank, upper abdominal, or suprapubic pain.

Determine if the patient or his family has a history of renal or urinary tract disorders or endocrine and metabolic diseases, particularly diabetes. Is the patient taking drugs that increase urine output, such as diuretics, digitalis glycosides, and antihypertensives?

Focus your physical examination on palpating and percussing the kidneys, the costovertebral angle (CVA), and the bladder. Carefully inspect the urinary meatus. Inspect a urine specimen for color, odor, and the presence of sediment.

Common medical causes
● *Benign prostatic hyperplasia.* Common in men older than age 50, this disorder produces nocturia when significant urethral obstruction develops. Typically, it causes frequency, hesitancy, incontinence, reduced force and caliber of the urine stream, and possibly hematuria. Oliguria may also occur. Palpation reveals a distended bladder and an enlarged prostate. The patient may also complain of lower abdominal fullness, perineal pain, and constipation.
● *Cystitis.* All three forms of cystitis may cause nocturia marked by frequent, small voidings and accompanied by dysuria and tenesmus. *Bacterial cystitis* may also cause urinary urgency, hematuria, fatigue, occasionally low-grade fever, and suprapubic, perineal, flank, and low back pain. Most common in women between ages 25 and 60, *chronic interstitial cystitis* is characterized by Hunner's ulcers—small, punctate, bleeding lesions in the bladder; it also causes gross hematuria. *Viral cystitis* also causes urinary urgency, hematuria, and fever.

• **Diabetes insipidus.** The result of antidiuretic hormone deficiency, this disorder usually produces nocturia early in its course. It's characterized by periodic voiding of moderate to large amounts of urine. Diabetes insipidus can also produce polydipsia.

• **Diabetes mellitus.** An early sign of diabetes mellitus, nocturia involves frequent, large voidings. Associated features include daytime polyuria, polydipsia, polyphagia, weakness, fatigue, weight loss and, possibly, signs of dehydration, such as dry mucous membranes and poor skin turgor.

• **Hypercalcemic nephropathy.** In this disorder, nocturia involves the periodic voiding of moderate to large amounts of urine. Related findings include daytime polyuria, polydipsia, and occasionally hematuria and pyuria.

• **Prostatic cancer.** The second leading cause of cancer deaths in men, this disorder is usually asymptomatic in early stages. Later, it produces nocturia characterized by infrequent voiding of moderate amounts of urine. Other characteristic signs and symptoms include dysuria (most common symptom), difficulty initiating a urine stream, bladder distention, urinary frequency, weight loss, pallor, weakness, perineal pain, and constipation. Palpation reveals a hard, irregularly shaped prostate.

• **Pyelonephritis (acute).** Nocturia is a common finding in this inflammatory disorder; it's usually characterized by infrequent voiding of moderate amounts of urine. The urine may appear cloudy. Associated signs and symptoms include a high, sustained fever with chills, fatigue, flank pain, CVA tenderness, weakness, dysuria, hematuria, urinary frequency and urgency, and tenesmus. Occasionally, anorexia, nausea, vomiting, and hypoactive bowel sounds may also occur.

• **Renal failure (chronic).** Nocturia occurs relatively early in this disorder and is usually characterized by infrequent voiding of moderate amounts of urine. As the disorder progresses, oliguria or even anuria develops. Other widespread signs and symptoms of chronic renal failure include fatigue, ammonia breath odor, Kussmaul's respirations, peripheral edema, elevated blood pressure, decreased level of consciousness, muscle twitching, anorexia, constipation or diarrhea, petechiae, ecchymoses, pruritus, yellow- or bronze-tinged skin, nausea, and vomiting.

Other causes

• **Drugs.** Any drug that mobilizes edematous fluid or produces diuresis (for example, diuretics and digitalis glycosides) may cause nocturia; obviously, this effect depends on when the drug is administered.

Special considerations

Patient care includes maintaining fluid balance, ensuring adequate rest, and providing patient education. Monitor vital signs, intake and output, and daily weight; continue to document the frequency of nocturia, amount, and specific gravity. Plan administration of diuretics for daytime hours, if possible. Also plan rest periods to compensate for sleep lost because of nocturia.

Prepare the patient for diagnostic tests, which may include routine urinalysis, urine concentration and dilution studies, and serum blood urea nitrogen, creatinine, and electrolyte levels.

Pediatric pointers

In children, nocturia may be voluntary or involuntary. The latter is commonly known as enuresis, or bedwetting. With the exception of prostate disorders, causes of nocturia are generally the same for children and adults.

NUCHAL RIGIDITY

A common early sign of meningeal irritation, nuchal rigidity is stiffness of the neck that prevents flexion. To elicit this sign, attempt to passively flex the patient's neck and touch his chin to his chest. If nuchal rigidity is present, this maneuver triggers pain and muscle spasms. (Be sure that there is no cervical spinal misalignment, such as a fracture or dislocation, before testing for nuchal rigidity. Severe spinal cord damage could result.) The patient may also notice nuchal rigidity when he attempts to flex his neck during daily activities.

Nuchal rigidity may herald life-threatening subarachnoid hemorrhage or meningitis. It may also be a late sign of cervical arthritis, in which joint mobility is gradually lost.

Emergency interventions

 After eliciting nuchal rigidity, attempt to elicit Kernig's and Brudzinski's signs. Quickly evaluate level of consciousness (LOC). Take vital signs. If you note signs of increased intracranial pressure (ICP), such as increased systolic pressure, bradycardia, and widened pulse pressure, start an I.V. line for drug administration and deliver oxygen, as necessary. Draw a specimen for routine blood studies.

History and physical examination

Obtain a patient history, relying on family members if altered LOC prevents the patient from responding. Ask about the onset and duration of neck stiffness. Were there any precipitating factors? Also ask about associated symptoms, such as headache, fever, nausea and vomiting, and motor and sensory changes. Check for a history of hypertension, head trauma, cerebral aneurysm or arteriovenous malformation, endocarditis, recent infection (such as sinusitis or pneumonia), or recent dental work. Then obtain a complete drug history.

If the patient has no other signs of meningeal irritation, ask about a history of arthritis or neck trauma. Can the patient recall pulling a muscle in his neck? Inspect the patient's hands for swollen, tender joints, and palpate the neck for pain or tenderness.

Common medical causes

● *Cervical arthritis.* In this disorder, nuchal rigidity develops gradually. Initially, the patient may complain of neck stiffness in the early morning or after a period of inactivity. Stiffness then becomes increasingly severe and frequent. Pain on movement, especially with lateral motion or head turning, is common. Typically, arthritis also affects other joints, especially in the hands.

● *Encephalitis.* This viral infection may cause nuchal rigidity accompanied by other signs of meningeal irritation, such as positive Kernig's and Brudzinski's signs. Usually, nuchal rigidity appears abruptly and is preceded by headache, vomiting, and fever. The patient may display a rapidly decreasing LOC, progressing from lethargy to coma within 24 to 48 hours of onset. Associated features include seizures, ataxia, hemiparesis, nystagmus, and cranial nerve palsies, such as dysphagia and ptosis.

● *Meningitis.* Nuchal rigidity is an early sign in this disorder. It's accompanied by other signs of meningeal irritation—positive Kernig's and Brudzinski's signs, hyperreflexia, and possibly opisthotonos. Other early features include fever with chills, headache, photophobia, and vomiting. Initially, the patient is confused and irritable; later, he may stuporous and seizure-prone or may slip into coma. Cranial nerve involvement may cause ocular palsies, facial weakness, and hearing loss. An erythematous papular rash may occur in viral meningitis; a purpuric rash may occur in meningococcal meningitis.

• **Subarachnoid hemorrhage.** Nuchal rigidity develops immediately after bleeding into the subarachnoid space. Examination may detect positive Kernig's and Brudzinski's signs. The patient may experience abrupt onset of severe headache, photophobia, fever, nausea and vomiting, dizziness, cranial nerve palsies, and focal neurologic signs, such as hemiparesis or hemiplegia. His LOC deteriorates rapidly, possibly progressing to coma. Signs of increased ICP, such as bradycardia and altered respirations, may also occur.

Special considerations

Prepare the patient for diagnostic tests, such as computed tomography scans, magnetic resonance imaging, and cervical spinal X-rays.

Monitor vital signs, intake and output, and neurologic status closely. Avoid routine administration of narcotic analgesics because they may mask signs of increasing ICP. Enforce strict bed rest; keep the head of the bed elevated at least 30 degrees to help reduce ICP.

Pediatric pointers

Nuchal rigidity reliably indicates meningeal irritation in children, unless they are paralyzed or comatose.

NYSTAGMUS

Nystagmus refers to the involuntary oscillations of one or—more commonly—both eyeballs. These oscillations are usually rhythmical and may be horizontal, vertical, or rotary. They may be transient or sustained and may occur spontaneously or on deviation or fixation of the eyes. Although nystagmus is fairly easy to identify, the patient may be unaware of it unless it affects his vision.

Nystagmus may be classified as pendular or jerk. *Pendular nystagmus* consists of horizontal (pendular) or vertical (seesaw) oscillations that are equal in both directions and resemble the movements of a clock's pendulum. *Jerk nystagmus* (convergence-retraction, downbeat, and vestibular) has a fast component and then a slow—perhaps unequal—corrective component in the opposite direction. (See *Classifying nystagmus,* page 408.)

Nystagmus is considered a *supranuclear* ocular palsy—that is, it results from pathology in the visual perceptual area, vestibular system, cerebellum, or brain stem rather than in the extraocular muscles or cranial nerves III, IV, and VI. Its causes are varied and include brain stem or cerebellar lesions, multiple sclerosis, encephalitis, labyrinthine disease, and drug toxicity. Occasionally, nystagmus is entirely normal; it's also considered a normal response in the unconscious patient during the doll's eye test (oculocephalic stimulation) or the cold caloric water test (oculovestibular stimulation).

History and physical examination

Begin by asking the patient how long he's had nystagmus. Does it occur intermittently? Does it affect his vision? Ask about recent infection, especially of the ear or respiratory tract, and about head trauma and cancer. Does the patient or anyone in his family have a history of cerebrovascular accident (CVA)? Then explore associated signs and symptoms. Ask about vertigo, dizziness, tinnitus, nausea or vomiting, numbness, weakness, bladder dysfunction, and fever.

Begin the physical examination by assessing the patient's level of consciousness (LOC) and vital signs. Be alert for signs of increased intracranial pressure (ICP), such as pupillary changes, drowsiness, elevated systolic pressure, and altered respiratory pattern. Next, assess nystagmus fully by testing extraocular muscle function: Ask the patient to focus straight ahead and then to follow your finger up, down, and in an *X* across his

CLASSIFYING NYSTAGMUS

PENDULAR NYSTAGMUS
Oscillating nystagmus refers to slow, steady oscillations of equal velocity around a center point. It can indicate congenital loss of visual acuity or multiple sclerosis.

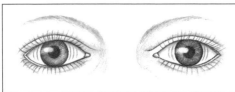

Vertical, or seesaw, nystagmus is the rapid, seesaw movement of the eyes: one eye appears to rise while the other appears to fall. It suggests an optic chiasm lesion.

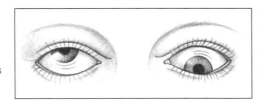

JERK NYSTAGMUS
Convergence-retraction nystagmus refers to the irregular jerking of the eyes back into the orbit during upward gaze. It can indicate midbrain tegmental damage.

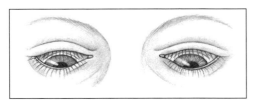

Downbeat nystagmus refers to the irregular downward jerking of the eyes during downward gaze. It can signal lower medullary damage.

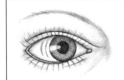
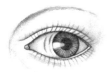

Vestibular nystagmus, the horizontal or rotary movements of the eyes, suggests vestibular disease or cochlear dysfunction.

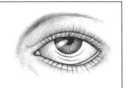

face. Note when nystagmus occurs as well as its velocity and direction. Finally, test reflexes, motor and sensory function, and the cranial nerves.

Common medical causes
• *Brain tumor.* Insidious onset of jerk nystagmus may occur with tumors of the brain stem and cerebellum. Associated characteristics include deafness, dysphagia, nausea and vomiting, vertigo, and ataxia. Brain stem compression by the tumor may cause signs of increased ICP, such as altered LOC, bradycardia, widening pulse pressure, and elevated systolic blood pressure.

• *Cerebrovascular accident.* A CVA involving the posterior inferior cerebellar artery may cause sudden horizontal or vertical jerk nystagmus that may be gaze-dependent. Other findings include dysphagia, dysarthria, loss of pain and temperature sensation on the ipsilateral face and contralateral trunk and limbs, ipsilateral Horner's syndrome (unilateral ptosis, pupillary constriction, and facial anhidrosis), and cerebellar signs, such as ataxia and vertigo. Signs of increased ICP, such as altered LOC, bradycardia, widening pulse pressure, and elevated systolic pressure, may also occur.

• *Encephalitis.* In this disorder, jerk nystagmus is typically accompanied by altered LOC, ranging from lethargy to coma. Usually, it's preceded by sudden onset of fever, headache, and vomiting. Among other features are nuchal rigidity, seizures, aphasia, ataxia, photophobia, and cranial nerve palsies, such as dysphagia and ptosis.

• *Head trauma.* Brain stem injury may cause jerk nystagmus, which is usually horizontal. The patient may also display pupillary changes, altered respiratory pattern, coma, and decerebrate posture.

• *Labyrinthitis (acute).* This inner ear inflammation causes sudden onset of jerk nystagmus, accompanied by dizziness, vertigo, tinnitus, nausea, and vomiting. The fast component of the nystagmus is toward the unaffected ear. Gradual sensorineural hearing loss may also occur.

• *Ménière's disease.* This inner ear disorder is characterized by acute attacks of jerk nystagmus, severe nausea and vomiting, dizziness, vertigo, progressive hearing loss, tinnitus, and diaphoresis. Typically, the direction of jerk nystagmus varies from one attack to the next. Attacks may last from 10 minutes to several hours.

Other causes
• *Drugs and alcohol.* Jerk nystagmus may result from barbiturate, phenytoin, or carbamazepine toxicity or from alcohol intoxication.

Special considerations
Prepare the patient for diagnostic tests, such as electronystagmography and a cerebral computed tomography scan.

Pediatric pointers
In children, pendular nystagmus may be idiopathic, or it may sometimes result from early impaired vision associated with such disorders as optic atrophy, albinism, congenital cataracts, and severe astigmatism.

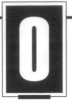

OCULAR DEVIATION

Ocular deviation refers to abnormal eye movement that may be *conjugate* (both eyes move together) or *dysconjugate* (one eye moves differently from the other). This common sign may result from ocular, neurologic, endocrine, and systemic disorders that interfere with the muscles, nerves, or brain centers that govern eye movement. Occasionally, it signals a life-threatening disorder such as ruptured cerebral aneurysm.

Normally, eye movement is directly controlled by the extraocular muscles innervated by the oculomotor, trochlear, and abducens nerves (cranial nerves III, IV, and VI). Together, these muscles and nerves direct a visual stimulus to fall on corresponding parts of the retina. Dysconjugate ocular deviation may result from unequal muscle tone (nonparalytic strabismus) or from muscle paralysis associated with cranial nerve damage (paralytic strabismus). Conjugate ocular deviation may result from disorders that affect the centers in the cerebral cortex and brain stem responsible for conjugate eye movement. Typically, such disorders cause *gaze palsy*—difficulty moving the eyes in one or more directions. (See *Ocular deviation: Characteristics and causes.*)

Emergency interventions

If the patient displays ocular deviation, quickly take his vital signs and look for altered level of consciousness (LOC), pupil changes, motor or sensory dysfunction, and severe headache. If possible, ask the patient's family about behavioral changes. Is there a history of recent head trauma? Respiratory support may be necessary. Also prepare the patient for emergency neurologic tests such as a computed tomography (CT) scan.

History and physical examination
If the patient isn't in distress, find out how long he's had the ocular deviation. Is it accompanied by double vision, eye pain, or headache? Also ask if he's noticed any associated motor or sensory changes, or fever.

Check for a history of hypertension, diabetes, allergies, and thyroid, neurologic, or muscular disorders. Then obtain a thorough ocular history. Has the patient ever had extraocular muscle imbalance, eye or head trauma, or eye surgery?

During the physical examination, observe the patient for partial or complete ptosis. Does he spontaneously tilt his head or turn his face to compensate for ocular deviation? Check for eye redness or periorbital edema. Assess visual acuity, then evaluate extraocular muscle function by testing the six cardinal fields of gaze.

OCULAR DEVIATION: CHARACTERISTICS AND CAUSES

CRANIAL NERVE AND EXTRAOCULAR MUSCLES INVOLVED	CHARACTERISTICS	PROBABLE CAUSES
Oculomotor nerve (III); medial rectus, superior rectus, inferior rectus, and inferior oblique muscles	Inability to focus the eye upward, downward, inward, and outward; drooping eyelid; and, except in diabetes, a dilated pupil in the affected eye	Cerebral aneurysm, diabetes, brain tumor, temporal lobe herniation from increased intracranial pressure
Trochlear nerve (IV), superior oblique muscle	Loss of downward and outward movement in the affected eye	Head trauma
Abducens nerve (VI), lateral rectus muscle	Loss of outward movement in the affected eye	Brain tumor

Common medical causes

• *Brain tumor.* Ocular deviation varies, depending upon the site and extent of the tumor. Associated signs and symptoms may include headache that's most severe in the morning, behavioral changes, memory loss, dizziness, confusion, vision loss, motor and sensory dysfunction, aphasia, and possibly signs of hormonal imbalance. The patient's LOC may slowly deteriorate from lethargy to coma. Late signs include papilledema, vomiting, increased systolic blood pressure, widening pulse pressure, and decorticate posture.

• *Cavernous sinus thrombosis.* In this disorder, ocular deviation may be accompanied by diplopia, photophobia, exophthalmos, orbital and eyelid edema, corneal haziness, diminished or absent pupillary reflexes, and impaired visual acuity. Other features may include high fever, headache, malaise, nausea and vomiting, seizures, and tachycardia. Retinal hemorrhages and papilledema are late signs.

• *Cerebrovascular accident.* This life-threatening disorder may cause ocular deviation, depending on the site and extent of the stroke. Accompanying features may include altered LOC, contralateral hemiplegia and sensory loss, dysarthria, dysphagia, homonymous hemianopia, blurred vision, diplopia, urine retention, incontinence, constipation, behavioral changes, headache, vomiting, and seizures.

• *Diabetes mellitus.* A leading cause of isolated third cranial nerve palsy, especially in the middle-aged patient with long-standing mild diabetes, this disorder may cause ocular deviation and ptosis. Typically, the patient also complains of sudden onset of diplopia and pain.

• *Encephalitis.* This infection causes ocular deviation and diplopia in some patients. Typically, it begins abruptly with fever, headache, and vomiting, followed by signs of meningeal irritation (such as nuchal rigidity) and of neuronal damage (such as seizures, aphasia, ataxia, hemiparesis, cranial nerve palsies, and photophobia). The patient's LOC may rapidly deteriorate from lethargy to coma within 24 to 48 hours after onset.

● *Head trauma.* Ocular deviation varies with the site and extent of head trauma. The patient may have visible soft-tissue injury, bony deformity, facial edema, and clear or bloody otorrhea or rhinorrhea. Besides these obvious signs of trauma, he may also have blurred vision, diplopia, nystagmus, behavioral changes, headache, motor and sensory dysfunction, and a decreased LOC that may progress to coma. Signs of increased intracranial pressure—bradycardia, increased systolic pressure, and widening pulse pressure—may also occur.

● *Orbital blow-out fracture.* In this fracture, the inferior rectus muscle may become entrapped, resulting in limited extraocular movements and ocular deviation. Typically, the patient's upward gaze is absent; other directions of gaze may be affected if edema is dramatic. The globe may also be displaced downward and inward. Associated signs and symptoms include pain, diplopia, nausea, periorbital edema, and ecchymosis.

● *Orbital tumor.* Ocular deviation occurs as the tumor gradually enlarges. Associated findings include proptosis, diplopia, and possibly blurred vision.

● *Thyrotoxicosis.* This disorder may produce exophthalmos—protruding eyes—which, in turn, causes limited extraocular movements and ocular deviation. Usually, the patient's upward gaze weakens first, followed by diplopia. Other features are lid retraction, a wide-eyed staring gaze, excessive tearing, edematous eyelids and, sometimes, inability to close the eyes. Cardinal features of thyrotoxicosis include tachycardia, palpitations, weight loss despite increased appetite, diarrhea, tremors, an enlarged thyroid, dyspnea, nervousness, diaphoresis, heat intolerance, and an atrial or ventricular gallop.

Special considerations

Continue to monitor the patient's vital signs and neurologic status if you suspect an acute neurologic disorder. Take seizure precautions, if necessary. Also prepare the patient for diagnostic tests, such as blood studies, orbital and skull X-rays, and a CT scan.

Pediatric pointers

In children, the most common cause of ocular deviation is nonparalytic strabismus. Normally, children achieve binocular vision by age 3 to 4 months. Although severe strabismus is readily apparent, mild strabismus must be confirmed by tests for misalignment, such as the corneal light reflex test and the cover test. Testing is crucial—early corrective measures help preserve binocular vision and cosmetic appearance. Also, mild strabismus may indicate retinoblastoma, a tumor that may be asymptomatic before age 2, except for a characteristic whitish reflex in the pupil.

OLIGOMENORRHEA

In most women, menstrual bleeding occurs every 28 days plus or minus 4 days. Although some variation is normal, menstrual bleeding at intervals of greater than 36 days may indicate oligomenorrhea—abnormally infrequent menstrual bleeding characterized by three to six menstrual cycles per year. When menstrual bleeding does occur, it's usually profuse, prolonged (up to 10 days), and laden with clots and tissue. Occasionally, scant bleeding or spotting occurs between these heavy menses.

Oligomenorrhea may develop suddenly, or it may follow a period of gradually lengthening cycles. Although oligomenorrhea may alternate with normal menstrual bleeding, it can progress to secondary amenorrhea.

Because oligomenorrhea is commonly associated with anovulation, it's common in infertile, early postmenarchal, and perimenopausal women. Usually, this sign reflects abnormalities of the hormones that govern normal endometrial function. It may result from ovarian, hypothalamic, pituitary, or other metabolic disorders and from the effects of certain drugs. It may also result from emotional or physical stress—such as sudden weight change, debilitating illness, or rigorous physical training.

History and physical examination

Find out the patient's age and when menarche occurred. Has she ever had normal menstrual cycles? When did she begin having abnormal cycles? Ask her to describe the bleeding pattern. How many days does the bleeding last, and how often does it occur? Does her menstrual flow contain clots and tissue fragments? When was her last period?

Next, determine if she's having symptoms of ovulatory bleeding. Does she have mild abdominal cramps 14 days before she bleeds? Is the bleeding accompanied by premenstrual symptoms, such as breast tenderness, irritability, bloating, and weight gain? Does she have cramping or pain with bleeding? Also check for a history of infertility. Does the patient have any children? Is she trying to conceive? Ask if she's currently using oral contraceptives or if she's ever used them in the past. If she has, find out when she stopped taking them.

Then ask about previous gynecologic disorders such as ovarian cysts. If the patient is breast-feeding, has she had any problems with milk production? If she hasn't been breast-feeding recently, has she noticed milk leaking from her breasts? Ask about recent weight gain or loss. Does the patient weigh less than 80% of her ideal weight? If so, does she

claim that she's overweight? Ask if she's exercising more vigorously than usual.

Screen for metabolic disorders by asking about excessive thirst, frequent urination, or fatigue. Has the patient been jittery or had palpitations? Ask about headache, dizziness, and impaired peripheral vision. Complete the history by asking what drugs the patient is taking.

Begin the physical examination by taking the patient's vital signs and weighing her. Inspect for increased facial hair growth, sparse body hair, male distribution of fat and muscle, acne, and clitoral enlargement. Note if the skin is abnormally dry or moist, and check hair texture. Also be alert for signs of psychological or physical stress.

Common medical causes

• *Adrenal hyperplasia.* In this disorder, oligomenorrhea may occur with signs of androgen excess, such as clitoral enlargement and male distribution of hair, fat, and muscle mass.

• *Anorexia nervosa.* Anorexia nervosa may cause sporadic oligomenorrhea or amenorrhea. Its cardinal symptom, however, is a morbid fear of being fat associated with weight loss of more than 20% of ideal body weight. Typically, the patient displays dramatic skeletal muscle atrophy and loss of fatty tissue, dry or sparse scalp hair, lanugo on the face and body, and blotchy or sallow, dry skin.

• *Diabetes mellitus.* Oligomenorrhea may be an early sign in this disorder. In juvenile-onset diabetes, the patient may have never had normal menses. Associated findings include excessive hunger, polydipsia, polyuria, weakness, fatigue, dry mucous membranes, poor skin turgor, and weight loss.

• *Hypothyroidism.* Besides oligomenorrhea, this disorder may result in fatigue; forgetfulness; cold intolerance; unexplained weight gain; constipation; bradycardia; decreased mental acuity; dry, flaky, inelastic skin; puffy face, hands, and feet; hoarseness; periorbital edema; ptosis; dry, sparse hair; and thick, brittle nails.

• *Prolactin-secreting pituitary tumor.* Oligomenorrhea or amenorrhea may be the first sign of a prolactin-secreting pituitary tumor. Accompanying findings include unilateral or bilateral galactorrhea, infertility, loss of libido, and sparse pubic hair. Headache and visual field disturbances—such as diminished peripheral vision, blurred vision, diplopia, and hemianopia—signal tumor expansion.

• *Thyrotoxicosis.* This disorder may produce oligomenorrhea along with reduced fertility. Cardinal findings include irritability, weight loss despite increased appetite, dyspnea, tachycardia, palpitations, diarrhea, tremors, diaphoresis, heat intolerance, an enlarged thyroid, and possibly exophthalmos.

Other causes

• *Drugs.* Drugs that increase androgen levels—such as corticosteroids, corticotropin, anabolic steroids, and danocrine—may cause oligomenorrhea. Discontinuation of oral contraceptives may result in delayed resumption of normal menses; however, 95% of women resume normal menses within 3 months. Other drugs that may cause oligomenorrhea include phenothiazine derivatives, amphetamines, and antihypertensive drugs.

Special considerations

Prepare the patient for diagnostic tests, such as blood hormone levels, thyroid studies, or pelvic imaging studies. The patient also may be asked to record her basal body temperature to determine if she's having ovulatory cycles. Provide her with blank charts, and teach her how to keep them accurately.

Remind the patient that she may become pregnant even though she isn't menstruating normally. Discuss contraceptive measures, as appropriate.

Pediatric pointers

Teenage girls may experience oligomenorrhea associated with immature hormonal function. However, prolonged oligomenorrhea or the development of amenorrhea may signal congenital adrenal hyperplasia or Turner's syndrome.

OLIGURIA

A cardinal sign of renal and urinary tract disorders, oliguria is clinically defined as urine output of less than 400 ml per 24 hours. Typically, this sign occurs abruptly and may herald serious—and possibly life-threatening—hemodynamic instability. Its causes can be classified as prerenal (decreased renal blood flow), intrarenal (intrinsic renal damage), or postrenal (urinary tract obstruction); the pathophysiology differs for each classification. (See *How oliguria develops,* pages 416 and 417.)

Oliguria associated with a prerenal or postrenal cause is usually promptly reversible with treatment, although it may lead to intrarenal damage if untreated. However, oliguria associated with an intrarenal cause is usually more persistent and may be irreversible.

History and physical examination

Begin by asking the patient about his usual daily voiding pattern, including frequency and amount. When did he first notice changes in this pattern or in the color, odor, or consistency of his urine? Ask about pain or burning on urination. Note his normal daily fluid intake. Has he recently been drinking more or less? Has he recently had diarrhea or vomiting that might cause fluid loss? Next, explore associated complaints, especially fatigue, loss of appetite, thirst, dyspnea, chest pain, or recent weight gain.

Check for a history of renal, urinary tract, or cardiovascular disorders. Note recent traumatic injuries or surgery associated with significant blood loss as well as recent blood transfusions. Was the patient exposed to nephrotoxic agents, such as heavy metals, organic solvents, anesthetics, or radiographic contrast media? Next, obtain a drug history.

Begin the physical examination by taking the patient's vital signs and weighing him. Assess his overall appearance for edema. Palpate both kidneys for tenderness and enlargement, and percuss for costovertebral angle (CVA) tenderness. Also inspect the flank area for edema or erythema. Auscultate the heart and lungs for abnormal sounds, and the flank area for renal artery bruits.

Obtain a urine specimen and inspect it for abnormal color, odor, or sediment. Use reagent strips to test for glucose, protein, and blood. Also, use a urinometer to measure specific gravity.

Common medical causes

● *Acute tubular necrosis.* An early sign of this renal disorder, oliguria may occur abruptly (in shock) or gradually (in nephrotoxicity). It usually persists for about 2 weeks and is followed by polyuria. Related features may include signs of hyperkalemia (muscle weakness and cardiac arrhythmias), uremia (anorexia, confusion, lethargy, twitching, seizures, pruritus, and Kussmaul's respirations), and heart failure (edema, jugular vein distention, crackles, and dyspnea).

● *Calculi.* Oliguria or anuria may result from stones lodging in the kidneys, ureters, bladder outlet, or urethra. Associated signs and symptoms include urinary urgency and frequency, dysuria, and hematuria or pyuria. Usually, the patient experiences renal colic—excruciating pain that radiates from the CVA to the flank, the suprapubic region, and the external genitalia. This pain may be accompanied by nausea, vomiting, hypoactive bowel sounds, abdominal distention and, occasionally, fever and chills.

● *Glomerulonephritis (acute).* This disorder produces oliguria or anuria. Other features are mild fever, fatigue, hematuria, generalized edema, elevated blood pressure, headache, nausea and vomiting, flank and abdominal pain, and signs of pulmonary congestion (dyspnea and a productive cough).

● *Heart failure.* Oliguria may occur in left-sided failure as a result of low cardiac output and decreased renal perfusion. Accompanying signs and symptoms include dyspnea, fatigue, weakness, peripheral edema, distended jugular veins, tachycardia, tachypnea, crackles, and a dry or productive cough. In advanced heart failure, the patient may also have orthopnea, cyanosis, clubbing, ventricular gallop, and hemoptysis.

● *Hypovolemia.* Any disorder that decreases circulating fluid volume can produce oliguria. Associated findings may include orthostatic hypotension, apathy, fatigue, muscle weakness, anorexia, nausea, profound thirst, dizziness, sunken eyeballs, poor skin turgor, and dry mucous membranes.

● *Pyelonephritis (acute).* Accompanying the sudden onset of oliguria in this disorder are high fever with chills, fatigue, flank pain, CVA tenderness, weakness, nocturia, dysuria, hematuria, urinary frequency and urgency, and tenesmus. The urine may appear cloudy. Some patients also experience anorexia, nausea, and vomiting.

● *Renal failure (chronic).* Oliguria is a major sign of end-stage chronic renal failure. Associated findings reflect progressive uremia and may include fatigue, weakness, irritability, uremic fetor, ecchymoses and petechiae, peripheral edema, elevated blood pressure, confusion, drowsiness, coarse muscle twitching, muscle cramps, peripheral neuropathies, anorexia, nausea and vomiting, constipation or diarrhea, stomatitis, pruritus,

(Text continues on page 418.)

HOW OLIGURIA DEVELOPS

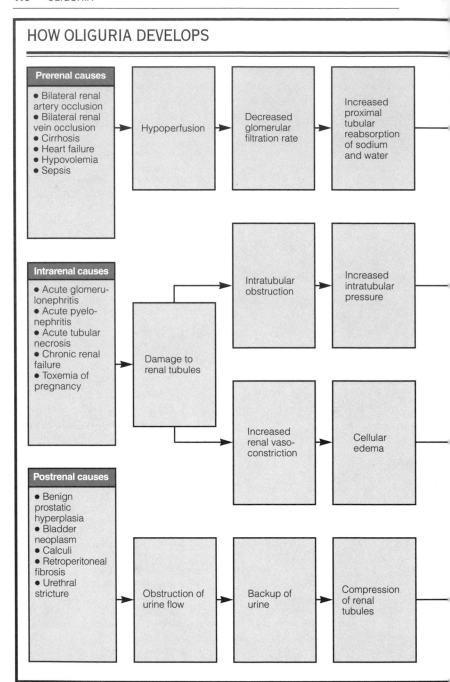

Prerenal causes

- Bilateral renal artery occlusion
- Bilateral renal vein occlusion
- Cirrhosis
- Heart failure
- Hypovolemia
- Sepsis

Hypoperfusion → Decreased glomerular filtration rate → Increased proximal tubular reabsorption of sodium and water →

Intrarenal causes

- Acute glomerulonephritis
- Acute pyelonephritis
- Acute tubular necrosis
- Chronic renal failure
- Toxemia of pregnancy

Damage to renal tubules →

Intratubular obstruction → Increased intratubular pressure →

Increased renal vasoconstriction → Cellular edema →

Postrenal causes

- Benign prostatic hyperplasia
- Bladder neoplasm
- Calculi
- Retroperitoneal fibrosis
- Urethral stricture

Obstruction of urine flow → Backup of urine → Compression of renal tubules →

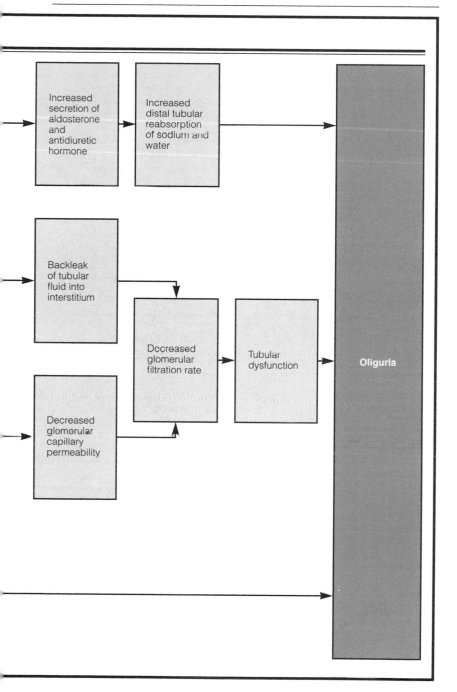

pallor, and yellow- or bronze-tinged skin. Eventually, seizures, coma, and uremic frost may develop.

● *Renal vein occlusion (bilateral).* This disorder occasionally causes oliguria accompanied by acute low back and flank pain, CVA tenderness, fever, pallor, hematuria, enlarged, palpable kidneys, and possibly signs of uremia.

● *Toxemia of pregnancy.* In severe preeclampsia, oliguria may be accompanied by elevated blood pressure, dizziness, diplopia, blurred vision, epigastric pain, nausea and vomiting, irritability, and severe frontal headache. In most cases, oliguria is preceded by generalized edema and a sudden weight gain of more than 3 lb (1.5 kg)/week during the second trimester or more than 1 lb (0.5 kg)/week during the third trimester. If preeclampsia progresses to eclampsia, the patient has seizures and may slip into a coma.

● *Urethral stricture.* This disorder rarely produces oliguria. Frequency and urgency, dysuria, and diminished urine stream are more common.

Other causes

● *Diagnostic studies.* Radiographic studies that use contrast media may cause nephrotoxicity and oliguria.

● *Drugs.* Oliguria may result from the use of drugs that cause decreased renal perfusion (diuretics), nephrotoxicity (most notably, aminoglycosides and chemotherapeutic agents), urine retention (adrenergic and anticholinergic agents) or urinary obstruction associated with precipitation of urine crystals (sulfonamides and acyclovir).

Special considerations

Monitor vital signs, intake and output, and daily weight. Depending on the oliguria's cause, fluid intake is normally restricted to 600 ml to 1 L more than the patient's urine output for the previous day. But you may encourage fluids if he's hypokalemic. Provide a diet low in sodium, potassium, and protein.

Laboratory tests may be needed to determine if oliguria is reversible. Such tests may include serum blood urea nitrogen and creatinine levels, urea and creatinine clearance, urine sodium levels, and urine osmolality. Abdominal X-rays, ultrasound, computed tomography scan, and a renal scan may be required.

Pediatric pointers

In neonates, oliguria may result from edema or dehydration. Major causes include congenital heart disease, respiratory distress syndrome, sepsis, congenital hydronephrosis, acute tubular necrosis, and renal vein thrombosis. Common causes of oliguria in children ages 1 to 5 are acute poststreptococcal glomerulonephritis and hemolytic uremic syndrome. After age 5, causes of oliguria are similar to those in adults.

OPISTHOTONOS

A sign of severe meningeal irritation, opisthotonos is marked by a strongly arched, rigid back; a hyperextended neck; the heels bent back; and the arms and hands flexed at the joints. This posture usually occurs spontaneously and continuously; however, it may be aggravated by movement. (See *Recognizing opisthotonos.*) Opisthotonos is believed to represent a protective reflex because it immobilizes the spine, alleviating the pain associated with meningeal irritation.

Usually caused by meningitis, opisthotonos may also result from subarachnoid hemorrhage, Arnold-Chiari syndrome, and tetanus. Occasionally, it occurs in achondroplastic dwarfism, but not necessarily as an indicator of meningeal irritation.

Opisthotonos is far more common in children—especially infants—than in adults. It's also more exaggerated in chil-

RECOGNIZING OPISTHOTONOS

In this characteristic sign of severe meningeal irritation, the back is severely arched and the neck is hyperextended. The heels bend back on the legs, and the arms and hands flex rigidly at the joints, as shown.

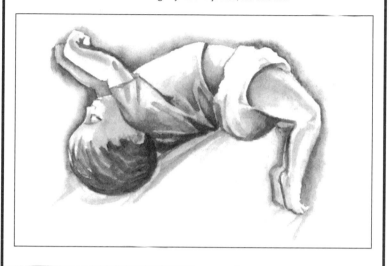

dren—the result of nervous system immaturity.

Emergency interventions

 If the patient is stuporous or comatose, quickly evaluate his vital signs and perform resuscitative measures as appropriate. Place the patient in a bed, with side rails raised and padded, or in a crib.

History and physical examination

If the patient's condition permits, obtain a history. Consult with the parents of a young child or an infant. Ask about a history of cerebral aneurysm or arteriovenous malformation and about hypertension. Note any recent infection that may have spread to the nervous system. Explore associated findings, such as headache, chills, and vomiting.

Focus the physical examination on the patient's neurologic status. Evaluate level of consciousness (LOC), and test sensorimotor and cranial nerve function. Then check for Brudzinski's and Kernig's signs and for nuchal rigidity.

Common medical causes

● *Arnold-Chiari syndrome.* In this disorder, opisthotonos is typically accompanied by hydrocephalus, with its characteristic, enlarged head; thin, shiny scalp with distended veins; and underdeveloped neck muscles. The infant usually also has a high-pitched cry, abnormal leg muscle tone, anorexia, vomiting, nuchal rigidity, irritability, noisy respirations, and a weak sucking reflex.

• *Meningitis.* In this infection, opisthotonos accompanies other signs of meningeal irritation, including nuchal rigidity, positive Brudzinski's and Kernig's signs, and hyperreflexia. Meningitis also causes cardinal signs of infection—moderate to high fever with chills and malaise—and of increased intracranial pressure (ICP)—headache, vomiting and, eventually, papilledema. Other features include irritability, photophobia, decreased LOC that may progress to seizures and coma, and diplopia, deafness, and other cranial nerve palsies.

• *Subarachnoid hemorrhage.* This disorder may also produce opisthotonos along with other signs of meningeal irritation, such as nuchal rigidity and positive Kernig's and Brudzinski's signs. Focal signs of hemorrhage—severe headache, hemiplegia or hemiparesis, aphasia, and photophobia—and other vision problems may also occur. With increasing ICP, the patient may develop bradycardia, elevated blood pressure, altered respiratory pattern, seizures, and vomiting. His LOC may rapidly deteriorate, resulting in coma; then, decerebrate posture may alternate with opisthotonos.

• *Tetanus.* This life-threatening infection can cause opisthotonos. Initially, trismus occurs. Eventually, muscle spasms may affect the abdomen, producing boardlike rigidity; the back, resulting in opisthotonos; or the face, producing risus sardonicus. Spasms may affect the respiratory muscles, causing distress. Tachycardia, diaphoresis, hyperactive deep tendon reflexes, and seizures may develop.

Other causes
• *Drugs.* Phenothiazines and other antipsychotic drugs may cause opisthotonos, usually as part of an acute dystonic reaction.

Special considerations
Assess neurologic status and vital signs frequently. Make the patient as comfortable as possible; place him in a side-lying position with pillows for support. If meningitis is suspected, institute respiratory isolation. Lumbar puncture may be ordered to identify pathogens and analyze cerebrospinal fluid. If subarachnoid hemorrhage is suspected, prepare the patient for a computed tomography scan or magnetic resonance imaging.

ORTHOPNEA

Orthopnea—difficulty breathing in the supine position—is a common symptom of cardiopulmonary disorders that produce dyspnea. It's typically a subtle symptom; the patient may complain that he can't catch his breath when lying down or mention that he sleeps most comfortably in a reclining chair or propped up by pillows.

Orthopnea presumably results from increased hydrostatic pressure in the pulmonary vasculature related to gravitational effects in the supine position. It may be aggravated by obesity, which restricts diaphragmatic excursion. Assuming the upright position relieves orthopnea by placing much of the pulmonary vasculature above the left atrium, which reduces mean hydrostatic pressure, and by enhancing diaphragmatic excursion, which increases inspiratory volume.

History and physical examination
Begin by asking about a history of cardiopulmonary disorders, such as myocardial infarction, rheumatic heart disease, valvular disease, emphysema, or chronic bronchitis. Does the patient smoke? If so, how much? Explore associated symptoms, especially complaints of cough, nocturnal or exertional dyspnea, fatigue, weakness, loss of appetite, or chest pain.

When examining the patient, check for other signs of increased respiratory effort, such as accessory muscle use, shallow respirations, and tachypnea. Also note barrel chest. Inspect the patient's skin for pallor or cyanosis, and the fingers for clubbing. Observe and palpate for edema, and check for jugular vein distention. Auscultate the lungs and heart.

Common medical causes

• *Chronic obstructive pulmonary disease (COPD).* This disorder typically produces orthopnea and other dyspneic complaints, accompanied by accessory muscle use, tachypnea, tachycardia, and paradoxical pulse. Auscultation may reveal diminished breath sounds, rhonchi, crackles, and wheezing. The patient may also have a dry or productive cough with copious sputum. Other features include anorexia, weight loss, and edema. Barrel chest, cyanosis, and clubbing are usually late signs.

• *Left-sided heart failure.* Orthopnea occurs late in this disorder. If heart failure is acute, orthopnea may begin suddenly; if chronic, it may be constant. The earliest symptom of this disorder is progressively severe dyspnea. Other common early symptoms include Cheyne-Stokes respirations, paroxysmal nocturnal dyspnea, fatigue, weakness, and a cough that may produce clear or blood-tinged sputum. Tachycardia, tachypnea, and crackles may also occur.

Late findings may include cyanosis, clubbing, ventricular gallop, and hemoptysis. Signs of shock—hypotension, thready pulse, and cold, clammy skin—may also occur.

• *Mediastinal tumor.* Orthopnea is an early sign of this disorder, resulting from pressure of the tumor against the trachea, bronchus, or lung when the patient lies down. However, many patients are asymptomatic until the tumor enlarges, when it produces retrosternal chest pain, dry cough, hoarseness, dysphagia, stertorous

respirations, palpitations, and cyanosis. Examination reveals suprasternal retractions on inspiration, bulging of the chest wall, tracheal deviation, dilated jugular and superficial chest veins, and edema of the face, neck, and arms.

Special considerations

To relieve orthopnea, place the patient in semi-Fowler's or high Fowler's position; if this does not help, have him lean over a bedside table with his chest forward. You may need to administer oxygen via nasal cannula. (Patients with COPD require a low flow rate of 1 to 3 L/minute.)

An electrocardiogram, chest X-ray, and pulmonary function tests may be necessary for further evaluation.

Pediatric pointers

Common causes of orthopnea in children include heart failure, croup, cystic fibrosis, and asthma.

ORTHOSTATIC HYPOTENSION
[Postural hypotension]

In orthostatic hypotension, the patient's blood pressure drops 15 to 20 mm Hg or more when he rises from a supine to a sitting or standing position. This common sign indicates failure of compensatory vasomotor responses to adjust to position changes. It's typically associated with light-headedness, syncope, or blurred vision and may occur in a hypotensive, normotensive, or hypertensive patient. Although a nonpathologic sign in many elderly people, orthostatic hypotension may result from prolonged bed rest, fluid and electrolyte imbalance, endocrine or systemic disorders, and the effects of drugs.

To detect orthostatic hypotension, take and compare blood pressure readings with the patient supine, sitting, and then standing.

Emergency interventions

 If you detect orthostatic hypotension, quickly check for tachycardia, altered level of consciousness (LOC), and pale, clammy skin. If these signs are present, suspect hypovolemic shock. Insert a large-bore I.V. catheter for fluid or blood replacement. Take the patient's vital signs every 15 minutes, and monitor intake and output.

History and physical examination

If the patient is in no danger, obtain a history. Ask him if he frequently experiences dizziness, weakness, or fainting when he stands. Also ask about related symptoms, particularly fatigue, orthopnea, impotence, nausea, headache, abdominal or chest discomfort, and GI bleeding. Then obtain a complete drug history.

Begin the physical examination by checking the patient's skin turgor. Palpate peripheral pulses and auscultate the heart and lungs. Finally, test muscle strength and observe his gait for unsteadiness.

Common medical causes

• **Adrenal insufficiency.** This disorder typically begins insidiously, with progressively severe signs and symptoms. Orthostatic hypotension may be accompanied by fatigue, muscle weakness, anorexia, nausea and vomiting, weight loss, abdominal pain, irritability, and a weak, irregular pulse. Another common feature is hyperpigmentation—bronze coloring of the skin—which is especially prominent on the face, lips, gums, tongue, buccal mucosa, elbows, palms, knuckles, waist, and knees. Diarrhea, constipation, decreased libido, amenorrhea, and syncope may also occur along with enhanced taste, smell, and hearing.

• **Amyloidosis.** Orthostatic hypotension is commonly associated with amyloid infiltration of the autonomic nerves. As-sociated signs and symptoms vary widely and may include anginal chest pain, tachycardia, dyspnea, orthopnea, fatigue, and cough.

• **Hyperaldosteronism.** This disorder typically produces orthostatic hypotension with sustained elevated blood pressure. Most other clinical effects of hyperaldosteronism result from hypokalemia, which increases neuromuscular irritability and produces muscle weakness, intermittent flaccid paralysis, fatigue, headache, paresthesia, and possibly tetany with positive Trousseau's and Chvostek's signs. The patient may also have visual disturbances, nocturia, polydipsia, and personality changes.

• **Hyponatremia.** In this disorder, orthostatic hypotension is typically accompanied by headache, profound thirst, tachycardia, nausea and vomiting, abdominal cramps, muscle twitching and weakness, fatigue, oliguria or anuria, cold clammy skin, poor skin turgor, irritability, seizures, and decreased LOC. Cyanosis, thready pulse, and eventually vasomotor collapse may occur in severe sodium deficit.

• **Hypovolemia.** Mild to moderate hypovolemia may cause orthostatic hypotension associated with apathy, fatigue, muscle weakness, anorexia, nausea, and profound thirst. The patient may also develop dizziness, oliguria, sunken eyeballs, poor skin turgor, and dry mucous membranes.

Other causes

• **Drugs.** Certain drugs may cause orthostatic hypotension by reducing circulating blood volume, causing blood vessel dilation, or depressing the sympathetic nervous system. These drugs include antihypertensives (especially guanethidine and the initial dosage of prazosin), tricyclic antidepressants, phenothiazines, levodopa, nitrates, monoamine oxidase inhibitors, morphine, bretylium, and spinal anesthesia. Large

doses of diuretics can also cause orthostatic hypotension.
- ***Treatments.*** Orthostatic hypotension often occurs with prolonged bed rest (24 hours or longer). It may also result from sympathectomy, which disrupts normal vasoconstrictive mechanisms.

Special considerations
Monitor the patient's fluid balance by carefully recording his intake and output and weighing him daily. To help minimize orthostatic hypotension, advise the patient to change his position *gradually.* Elevate the head of the patient's bed, and help him to a sitting position with his feet dangling over the side of the bed. If he can tolerate this position, have him sit in a chair for brief periods. Return him to bed at once if he becomes dizzy or pale or shows other signs of hypotension.

Always keep the patient's safety in mind. Never leave him unattended while he's sitting or walking; evaluate his need for assistive devices such as a cane.

Prepare the patient for diagnostic tests, such as hematocrit, serum electrolyte and drug levels, urinalysis, 12-lead electrocardiogram, and chest X-ray.

Pediatric pointers
Because normal blood pressure is lower in children than in adults, you must be familiar with normal age-specific values to detect orthostatic hypotension. From birth to age 3 months, normal systolic pressure is 40 to 80 mm Hg; from ages 3 months to 1 year, 80 to 100 mm Hg; and from ages 1 to 12, 100 mm Hg plus 2 mm Hg for every year over age 1. Diastolic blood pressure is first heard at about age 4; it's normally 60 mm Hg at this age and slowly rises to 70 mm Hg by age 12.

Orthostatic hypotension has the same causes in children as in adults.

ORTOLANI'S SIGN

Ortolani's sign—a click or popping sensation that's felt and commonly heard on abduction of a neonate's thighs—is an indication of developmental dysplasia of the hip. Screening for this sign is an important part of newborn care because early detection and treatment of developmental dysplasia of the hip improves the infant's chances of growing with a correctly formed, functional joint. (See *Detecting developmental dysplasia of the hip,* pages 424 and 425.)

History and physical examination
After eliciting Ortolani's sign, evaluate the infant for asymmetrical gluteal folds, limited hip abduction, and unequal leg length.

Common medical causes
- ***Developmental dysplasia of the hip.*** Most common in females and in Native Americans, this disorder produces Ortolani's sign, which may be accompanied by limited hip abduction and unequal gluteal folds. Usually, the infant with developmental hip dysplasia has no gross deformity or pain.

In complete dysplasia, the affected leg may appear shorter, or the affected hip more prominent.

Special considerations
Ortolani's sign can be elicited only during the first 4 to 6 weeks of life—the optimum time for effective corrective treatment. If treatment is delayed, developmental dysplasia of the hip may cause degenerative hip changes, lordosis, joint malformation, and soft-tissue damage. Various methods of abduction can be used to produce a stable joint. These methods include double-diapering, soft splinting devices, and a plaster hip spica cast.

DETECTING DEVELOPMENTAL DYSPLASIA OF THE HIP

When assessing a neonate, attempt to elicit *Ortolani's sign* to detect developmental dysplasia of the hip. Begin by placing the infant supine with his knees and hips flexed. Observe for symmetry.

Place your hands on the infant's knees, with your index fingers along his lateral thighs. Then raise his knees to a 90-degree angle with his back.

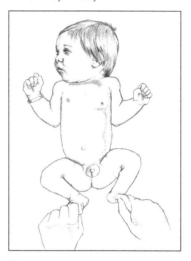

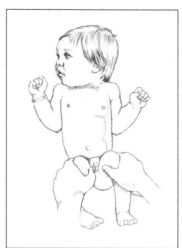

Abduct the infant's thighs so that the lateral aspect of his knees lies almost flat on the table. If the infant has a dislocated hip, you'll feel and commonly hear a click or popping sensation (Ortolani's sign) as the head of the femur moves out of the acetabulum. The infant may also give a sudden cry of pain.

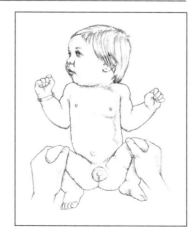

DETECTING DEVELOPMENTAL DYSPLASIA OF THE HIP *(continued)*

If you elicit a positive Ortolani's sign, look for these other signs of developmental dysplasia of the hip:

Observe for asymmetry of the infant's gluteal or thigh folds.

Flex the infant's hips to detect limited abduction.

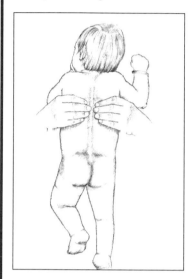

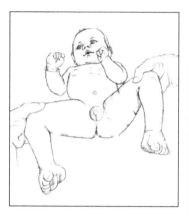

Flex the infant's knees, and observe for apparent shortening of the femur.

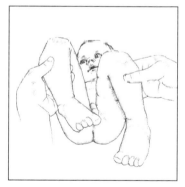

OTORRHEA

Otorrhea—drainage from the ear—may be bloody (otorrhagia), purulent, clear, or serosanguineous. Its onset, duration, and severity provide clues to the underlying cause. This sign may result from disorders that affect the external ear canal or the middle ear, including allergy, infection, neoplasms, trauma, and collagen diseases. Otorrhea may occur alone or with other symptoms such as ear pain.

History and physical examination

Begin your evaluation by asking the patient when the otorrhea began and how he recognized it. Did he clean the drainage from deep within the ear canal or wipe it from the auricle? Have him describe the color, consistency, and odor of the drainage. Is it clear, purulent, or bloody? Does it occur in one or both ears? Is it continuous or intermittent? If the patient puts cotton in his ear to absorb the drainage, ask how often he changes it.

Then explore associated otologic symptoms, especially pain. Does the patient feel tenderness on movement of the pinna or tragus? Ask about vertigo, which is absent in disorders of the external ear canal, and about tinnitus.

Next, check the patient's medical history for recent upper respiratory infection or head trauma. Also ask how he cleans his ears and if he's an avid swimmer. Note a history of cancer, dermatitis, or immunosuppressive therapy.

Focus the physical examination on the patient's external ear, middle ear, and tympanic membrane. (If his symptoms are unilateral, examine the uninvolved ear first.) Inspect the external ear, and apply pressure on the tragus and mastoid area to elicit tenderness. Then insert an otoscope, using the largest speculum that will comfortably fit into the ear canal. If necessary, clean cerumen, pus, or other debris from the canal. Observe for edema, erythema, crusts, or polyps. Inspect the tympanic membrane, which should look like a shiny, pearl gray cone. Note color changes, perforation, absence of the normal light reflex (a cone of light appearing toward the bottom of the drum), or a bulging membrane.

Next, test hearing acuity. Have the patient occlude one ear while you whisper some common two-syllable words toward the unoccluded ear. Stand behind him so he doesn't read your lips, and ask him to repeat what he hears. Perform the test on the other ear using different words. Then use a tuning fork to perform the Weber and Rinne tests.

Finally, palpate the patient's neck and his preauricular, parotid, and postauricular (mastoid) areas for lymphadenopathy. Also test the function of cranial nerves VII, IX, X, and XI.

Common medical causes

● *Aural polyps.* These polyps may produce foul, purulent, and perhaps blood-streaked discharge. If they occlude the external ear, the polyps may cause partial hearing loss.

● *Basilar skull fracture.* In this disorder, otorrhea may be clear and watery, representing cerebrospinal fluid (CSF) leakage, or bloody, representing hemorrhage. Occasionally, inspection reveals blood behind the eardrum. Otorrhea may be accompanied by hearing loss, CSF or bloody rhinorrhea, periorbital ecchymosis (raccoon eyes), and mastoid ecchymosis (Battle's sign). Cranial nerve palsies, decreased level of consciousness, and headache are other common findings.

● *Epidural abscess.* In this disorder, profuse, creamy otorrhea is accompanied by steady, throbbing ear pain; fever; and a temporal or temporoparietal headache on the ipsilateral side.

● *Myringitis (infectious).* In myringitis, small, reddened, blood-filled blebs erupt in the external ear canal, the tympanic membrane and, occasionally, the middle ear. Spontaneous rupture of these blebs causes serosanguineous otorrhea. Other features are severe ear pain, tenderness over the mastoid process and, rarely, fever and hearing loss.

● *Otitis externa.* Acute otitis externa, commonly known as swimmer's ear, usually causes purulent, yellow, sticky, foul-smelling otorrhea. Inspection may reveal white-green debris in the external ear canal. Associated findings include edema, erythema, pain, and itching of the auricle and external ear canal; severe tenderness with movement of the mastoid, tragus, mouth, or jaw; tenderness and swelling of surrounding nodes; and partial conductive hearing loss. The patient may also have a low-grade fever and a headache ipsilateral to the affected ear.

• *Otitis media.* In acute otitis media, rupture of the tympanic membrane produces bloody, purulent otorrhea and relieves ear pain. Conductive hearing loss typically worsens over several hours.

In acute suppurative otitis media, the patient may also have signs and symptoms of upper respiratory infection—sore throat, cough, nasal discharge, headache. Other features may include dizziness, fever, nausea, and vomiting.

Chronic otitis media causes intermittent, purulent, foul-smelling otorrhea associated with frequent perforation of the tympanic membrane. Conductive hearing loss occurs gradually and may be accompanied by pain, nausea, and vertigo.

• *Trauma.* Bloody otorrhea may result from trauma, such as a blow to the external ear, a foreign body in the ear, or barotrauma. Usually, the bleeding is minimal or moderate; it may be accompanied by partial hearing loss.

• *Tumor (malignant).* Squamous cell carcinoma of the external ear causes purulent otorrhea with itching; deep, boring ear pain; hearing loss; and, in late stages, facial paralysis. In squamous cell carcinoma of the middle ear, blood-tinged otorrhea occurs early, typically with hearing loss on the affected side. Pain and facial paralysis are late features.

Special considerations

Apply warm, moist compresses, heating pads, or hot-water bottles to the patient's ears to relieve inflammation and pain. Use cotton wicks to gently clean the draining ear or to apply topical drugs. Keep ear drops at room temperature; cold ear drops may cause vertigo.

Advise the patient with chronic ear problems to avoid forceful nose blowing when he has an upper respiratory infection, to avoid channeling infectious secretions to the middle ear. Instruct him to blow his nose with his mouth open. Also remind him to clean his ear with a washcloth only and not to stick anything in his ear that could cause injury, such as a hairpin or a cotton-tipped applicator. If the patient is a swimmer, instruct him to wear earplugs and to dry his ears thoroughly after swimming. Have him report recurring ear pain and drainage, especially in the absence of upper respiratory infection, because this may be a sign of cancer.

A ruptured tympanic membrane usually heals spontaneously. However, tell the patient to avoid water while it heals; instruct him to insert lubricated cotton balls into his ear canal before he showers or shampoos.

Pediatric pointers

When you examine or clean a child's ear, remember that the auditory canal lies horizontally and that the pinna must be pulled *downward* and *backward*. Restrain a child during an ear procedure by having him sit on a parent's lap with the ear to be examined facing you. Have him put one arm around the parent's waist and the other down at his own side, and then ask the parent to hold the child in place. Or, if you're alone with the child, you can have him lie on his abdomen with his arms at his sides and his head turned so the affected ear faces the ceiling. Bend over him, restraining his upper body with your elbows and upper arms.

Otitis media is the most common cause of otorrhea in infants and young children. Children are also likely to insert foreign bodies into their ears, resulting in infection, pain, and purulent discharge.

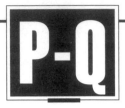

PALLOR

Pallor is an abnormal paleness or loss of skin color, which may develop suddenly or gradually. Although generalized pallor affects the entire body, it's most apparent on the face, conjunctivae, oral mucosa, and nail beds. Localized pallor commonly affects a single limb.

How easily pallor is detected varies with the patient's skin color and the thickness and vascularity of underlying subcutaneous tissue. At times, it's merely a subtle lightening of skin color. It may be difficult to detect in dark-skinned persons; sometimes it's only evident on their conjunctiva and oral mucosa.

Pallor may result from decreased peripheral oxyhemoglobin or decreased total oxyhemoglobin. The former reflects diminished peripheral blood flow associated with peripheral vasoconstriction or arterial occlusion or with low cardiac output. (Transient peripheral vasoconstriction may occur with exposure to cold, causing nonpathologic pallor.) The latter usually results from anemia, the chief cause of pallor. (See *How pallor develops*.)

Emergency interventions

If generalized pallor develops suddenly, quickly look for signs of shock, such as tachycardia, hypotension, oliguria, and decreased level of consciousness (LOC). Prepare to infuse fluids or blood rapidly, and keep emergency resuscitation equipment nearby.

History and physical examination

If the patient's condition permits, take a complete history. Does the patient or anyone in his family have a history of anemia? What about chronic disorders that might lead to pallor, such as renal failure, heart failure, or diabetes? Ask about the patient's diet, particularly his intake of green vegetables.

Then explore the pallor more fully. Find out when the patient first noticed it. Is pallor constant or intermittent? Does it occur when he's exposed to the cold? Does it occur when he's under emotional stress? Explore associated signs and symptoms, such as dizziness, fainting, orthostasis, weakness and fatigue on exertion, chest pain, palpitations, menstrual irregularities, or loss of libido. If the pallor is confined to one or both legs, ask the patient if walking is painful. Do his legs feel cold or numb? If the pallor is confined to his fingers, ask about tingling and numbness.

Start the physical examination by taking the patient's vital signs. Be sure to check for orthostatic hypotension. Auscultate the heart for gallops and murmurs and the lungs for crackles. Check the patient's skin temperature—cold extremities commonly occur with vasoconstriction or arterial occlusion. Also note skin ulceration. Finally, palpate peripheral pulses. An absent pulse in a pale extremity may indicate arterial occlusion, whereas a weak pulse may indicate low cardiac output.

HOW PALLOR DEVELOPS

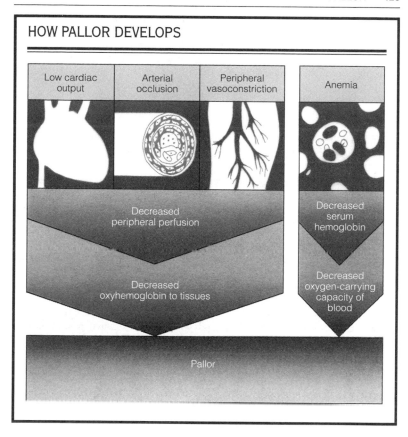

Low cardiac output	Arterial occlusion	Peripheral vasoconstriction	Anemia

Decreased peripheral perfusion

Decreased serum hemoglobin

Decreased oxyhemoglobin to tissues

Decreased oxygen-carrying capacity of blood

Pallor

Common medical causes

• *Anemia.* Typically, pallor develops gradually in this disorder. The patient's skin color may also appear sallow or grayish. Other effects may include fatigue, dyspnea, tachycardia, bounding pulse, atrial gallop, systolic bruit over the carotid arteries, and possibly crackles and bleeding tendencies.

• *Arterial occlusion (acute).* Pallor develops abruptly in the extremity with the occlusion, which usually results from an embolus. A line of demarcation develops, separating the cool, pale, cyanotic, and mottled skin below the occlusion from the normal skin above it. Accompanying the pallor may be severe pain, intense intermittent claudication, pares-

thesia, and paresis in the affected extremity. Absent pulses and diminished capillary refill below the occlusion are also characteristic.

• *Arterial occlusive disease (chronic).* In this disorder, pallor is also specific to an extremity—usually one leg, but occasionally both legs or an arm. It develops gradually from obstructive arteriosclerosis or thrombus formation and is aggravated by elevating the extremity. Associated findings include intermittent claudication, weakness, cool skin, diminished pulses in the extremity, and possibly ulceration and gangrene.

• *Frostbite.* Pallor is localized to the frostbitten area, such as the feet, hands, or ears. Typically, the area feels cold, waxy and, perhaps, hard in deep frostbite. The skin doesn't blanch and sensation may be absent. As the area thaws, the skin turns purplish blue. Blistering and gangrene may then follow if the frostbite was severe.

• **Orthostatic hypotension.** In this condition, pallor occurs abruptly on rising from a recumbent position to a sitting or standing position. A precipitous drop in blood pressure, an increase in heart rate, and dizziness are also characteristic. At times, the patient loses consciousness for several minutes.

• **Raynaud's disease.** Pallor of the fingers upon exposure to cold or stress is a hallmark of this disease. Typically, the fingers abruptly turn pale, then cyanotic; with rewarming, they become red and paresthetic. In chronic disease, ulceration may occur.

• **Shock.** Two forms of shock initially cause acute onset of pallor and cool, clammy skin. In *hypovolemic shock,* other early signs and symptoms include restlessness, thirst, slight tachycardia, and tachypnea. As shock progresses, the skin becomes increasingly clammy, pulse becomes more rapid and thready, and hypotension develops with narrowing pulse pressure. Other signs may include oliguria, subnormal body temperature, and decreased LOC. In *cardiogenic shock,* the signs and symptoms are similar, but usually more profound.

Special considerations

If the patient has chronic *generalized pallor,* prepare him for blood studies and, possibly, bone marrow biopsy. If he has *localized pallor,* he may require arteriography to accurately determine the cause.

When pallor results from low cardiac output, administer blood and fluid replacements, as needed, or such drugs as diuretics, cardiotonics, and antiarrhythmics, as prescribed. Frequently monitor the patient's vital signs, intake and out-

put, electrocardiogram, and hemodynamic status.

Pediatric pointers

In children, pallor stems from the same causes as it does in adults. It can also stem from congenital heart defects and chronic lung disease.

PALPITATIONS

Defined as a conscious awareness of one's heartbeat, palpitations are usually felt over the precordium or in the throat or neck. The patient may describe them as pounding, jumping, turning, fluttering, flopping, or as missing or skipping beats. They may be regular or irregular, fast or slow, paroxysmal or sustained.

Although usually insignificant, this common symptom may result from cardiac and metabolic disorders and from the effects of certain drugs. Nonpathologic palpitations may occur with a newly implanted prosthetic valve because its clicking sound heightens the patient's awareness of his heartbeat. Transient palpitations may accompany emotional stress, such as fright, anger, and anxiety, or physical stress, such as exercise and fever. They can also accompany use of stimulants, such as tobacco and caffeine.

To help characterize the palpitations, ask the patient to simulate their rhythm by tapping his finger on a hard surface. An irregular "skipped beat" rhythm points to premature ventricular contractions, whereas an episodic racing rhythm that ends abruptly suggests paroxysmal atrial tachycardia.

Emergency interventions

 If the patient complains of palpitations, ask him if he feels dizzy and short of breath. Then inspect for pale, cool, clammy skin. Also, take the patient's vital signs, noting hypotension and irregular or abnormal pulse. If these signs are present, suspect cardiac arrhythmias. Prepare to begin cardiac monitoring and, if necessary, to deliver cardioversion. Start an I.V. line to administer antiarrhythmic drugs, if needed.

History and physical examination

If the patient is not in distress, perform a more complete cardiac history and physical examination. Ask about cardiovascular or pulmonary disorders, which may produce arrhythmias. Does the patient have a history of hypertension or hypoglycemia? Be sure to obtain a drug history. Has the patient recently started digitalis therapy? In addition, ask about caffeine, tobacco, and alcohol consumption.

Then explore associated symptoms, such as weakness, fatigue, and anginal pain. Finally, auscultate for gallops, murmurs, and abnormal breath sounds.

Common medical causes

● *Acute anxiety attack.* In this disorder, palpitations may be accompanied by diaphoresis, facial flushing, trembling, and an impending sense of doom. Almost invariably, the patient hyperventilates, which may lead to dizziness, weakness, and syncope. Other typical findings include tachycardia, precordial pain, shortness of breath, restlessness, and insomnia.

● *Cardiac arrhythmias.* Paroxysmal or sustained palpitations may occur with cardiac arrhythmias, accompanied by dizziness, weakness, and fatigue. Patients also may experience diaphoresis, decreased blood pressure, confusion, pallor, oliguria, and irregular, rapid, or slow pulse.

● *Hypertension.* The patient with hypertension may be asymptomatic or may complain of sustained palpitations alone or with headache, dizziness, tinnitus, and fatigue. Typically, the patient's blood pressure exceeds 140/90 mm Hg. The patient

may also experience nausea and vomiting, seizures, and decreased level of consciousness.

● *Hypocalcemia.* Typically, this disorder produces palpitations, weakness, and fatigue. It progresses from paresthesia to muscle tension and carpopedal spasms. The patient may also have muscle twitching, hyperactive deep tendon reflexes, chorea, and positive Chvostek's and Trousseau's signs.

● *Mitral valve prolapse.* This valvular disorder may cause paroxysmal palpitations accompanied by sharp, stabbing, or aching precordial pain. The hallmark of this disorder, though, is a midsystolic click followed by an apical systolic murmur. Associated signs and symptoms may include dyspnea, dizziness, severe fatigue, migraine headache, anxiety, paroxysmal tachycardia, crackles, and peripheral edema.

● *Mitral stenosis.* Early features of this disorder typically include sustained palpitations accompanied by dyspnea and fatigue on exertion. Auscultation reveals a loud S_1 or opening snap and a rumbling diastolic murmur at the apex. Related effects may include atrial gallop and, in advanced mitral stenosis, orthopnea, dyspnea at rest, paroxysmal nocturnal dyspnea, and atrial fibrillations.

● *Thyrotoxicosis.* A characteristic symptom in this disorder, sustained palpitations may be accompanied by tachycardia, dyspnea, weight loss despite increased appetite, diarrhea, tremors, nervousness, diaphoresis, heat intolerance and, possibly, exophthalmos and an enlarged thyroid. In addition, the patient may experience an atrial or ventricular gallop.

Other causes

● *Drugs.* Palpitations may result from drugs that precipitate cardiac arrhythmias or increase cardiac output, such as digitalis glycosides, sympathomimetics (such as cocaine), ganglionic blockers, and atropine.

Special considerations

Prepare the patient for diagnostic tests, such as an electrocardiogram and Holter monitoring. Remember that even mild palpitations may cause the patient much concern. In addition, maintain a quiet, comfortable environment to minimize anxiety and perhaps decrease palpitations.

Pediatric pointers

Palpitations in children commonly result from fever and congenital heart defects, such as patent ductus arteriosus and septal defects. Because many children are unable to describe this complaint, you'll have to focus your attention on objective measurements. These include cardiac monitoring, physical examination findings, and laboratory tests.

PAPULAR RASH

A papular rash consists of small, raised, circumscribed—and perhaps discolored—lesions known as papules. It may erupt anywhere on the body in various configurations and may be acute or chronic. Papular rashes characterize many cutaneous disorders; they may also result from allergy and from infectious, neoplastic, and systemic disorders.

History and physical examination

First, evaluate the papular rash fully: Note its color, configuration, and location on the patient's body. (See *Recognizing common skin lesions,* pages 434 and 435.) Find out when it erupted. Has the patient noticed any changes in the rash since then? Is it itchy or burning? Painful or tender? Also have him describe associated signs and symptoms, such as fever, headache, and GI distress.

Next, obtain a medical history, including allergies, previous rashes or skin

disorders, infections, childhood diseases, sexually transmitted diseases, and neoplasms. Has the patient recently been bitten by an insect or a rodent or been exposed to anyone with an infectious disease? Finally, obtain a complete drug history.

Common medical causes

- *Acne vulgaris.* In this disorder, rupture of enlarged comedones produces inflamed—and, perhaps, painful and pruritic—papules, pustules, nodules, or cysts on the face and sometimes the shoulders, chest, and back.

- *Dermatomyositis.* Grotton's papules—flat, violet lesions on the dorsum of the finger joints—are pathognomonic of this disorder, as is the dusky lilac discoloration of periorbital tissue and lid margins. These signs may be accompanied by a transient, erythematous, macular rash in a malar distribution on the face and sometimes on the scalp, forehead, neck, upper torso, and arms. This rash may be preceded by symmetrical muscle soreness and weakness in the pelvis, upper extremities, shoulders, neck, and possibly the face.

- *Follicular mucinosis.* In this cutaneous disorder, perifollicular papules or plaques are accompanied by prominent alopecia.

- *Granuloma annulare.* This benign, chronic disorder produces papules that usually coalesce to form plaques. The papules spread peripherally to form a ring with a normal or slightly depressed center. They usually appear on the feet, legs, hands, or fingers and may be pruritic or asymptomatic.

- *Infectious mononucleosis.* A maculopapular rash that resembles rubella is an early sign of this infection in 10% of patients. Typically, the rash is preceded by a headache, malaise, and fatigue. It may be accompanied by sore throat, cervical lymphadenopathy, and fluctuating temperature with an evening peak of 101°

to 102° F (38.3° to 38.9° C). Splenomegaly and hepatomegaly may also develop.

• *Insect bites.* Venom from insect bites—especially ticks, lice, flies, and mosquitoes—may produce an allergic reaction associated with a papular, macular, or petechial rash. The rash is usually accompanied by nonspecific signs and symptoms, such as fever, myalgia, headache, lymphadenopathy, nausea, and vomiting.

• *Kaposi's sarcoma.* This neoplastic disorder is characterized by purple or blue papules or macules on the extremities, ears, and nose. These lesions decrease in size upon firm pressure and then return to their original size within 10 to 15 seconds. They may become scaly and ulcerate with bleeding. Two variants—classic and acute generalized—affect elderly people and patients with acquired immunodeficiency syndrome.

• *Lichen planus.* Discrete, flat, angular or polygonal, violet papules, many of which are marked with white lines or spots, characterize this disorder. They may be linear or coalesce into plaques and most commonly appear on the lumbar region, genitalia, ankles, anterior tibiae, and the wrists. Lesions usually develop first on the buccal mucosa as a lacy network of white or gray threadlike papules or plaques. Pruritus, distorted fingernails, and atrophic alopecia commonly occur.

• *Necrotizing vasculitis.* In this systemic disorder, crops of purpuric, but otherwise asymptomatic, papules are typical. Some patients also have low-grade fever, headache, myalgia, arthralgia, and abdominal pain.

• *Pityriasis rosea.* This disorder begins with an erythematous "herald patch"—a slightly raised, oval lesion about 2 to 6 cm in diameter that may appear anywhere on the body. A few days to weeks later, yellow-to-tan or erythematous patches with scaly edges appear on the trunk, arms, and legs, often erupting along body cleavage lines in a characteristic "pine tree" pattern. These pruritic patches are about 0.6 to 1 cm in diameter.

• *Polymorphic light eruption.* Abnormal reactions to light may produce papular, vesicular, or nodular rashes on sun-exposed areas. Other symptoms may include pruritus, headache, and malaise.

• *Psoriasis.* This common, chronic disorder begins with small, erythematous papules on the scalp, chest, elbows, knees, back, buttocks, and genitalia. These papules sometimes are pruritic and sometimes painful. Eventually they enlarge and coalesce, forming elevated, red, scaly plaques covered by characteristic silver scales, except in moist areas such as the genitalia. These scales may flake off easily or thicken, covering the plaque. Associated features include pitted fingernails and arthralgia.

• *Rosacea.* This hyperemic disorder is characterized by persistent erythema, telangiectasia, and recurrent eruption of papules and pustules on the forehead, malar areas, nose, and chin. Eventually, eruptions recur more frequently and erythema deepens. Rhinophyma may occur in severe cases.

• *Seborrheic keratosis.* In this cutaneous disorder, benign skin tumors begin as small, yellow-brown papules on the chest, back, or abdomen; they eventually enlarge and become deeply pigmented. In blacks, these papules may remain small and affect only the malar part of the face (dermatosis papulosa nigra).

• *Syringoma.* In this disorder, adenoma of the sweat glands produces a yellowish or erythematous papular rash on the face (especially the eyelids), neck, and upper chest.

• *Systemic lupus erythematosus.* This disorder is characterized by a "butterfly rash" of erythematous maculopapules or discoid plaques that appears in a malar distribution across the nose and cheeks. Similar rashes may appear elsewhere, especially on exposed body areas. Other cardinal features include photosensitivity and nondeforming arthritis, especially

RECOGNIZING COMMON SKIN LESIONS

Macule

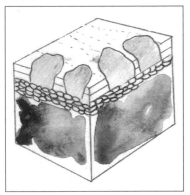

A flat blemish or discoloration, usually less than 1 cm in diameter, that can be brown, tan, red, or white; texture is the same as surrounding skin

Bulla

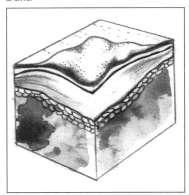

A raised, thin-walled blister greater than 0.6 cm in diameter, containing clear or serous fluid

Vesicle

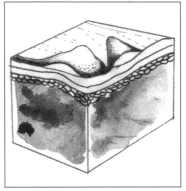

A thin-walled, raised blister less than 0.5 cm in diameter, containing clear, serous, purulent, or bloody fluid

Pustule

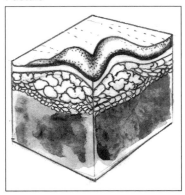

A circumscribed, pus- or lymph-filled elevation that varies in diameter and may be firm or soft and white or yellow

in the hands, feet, and large joints. Among widespread effects are patchy alopecia, mucous membrane ulceration, low-grade or spiking fever, chills, lymphadenopathy, anorexia, weight loss, abdominal pain, diarrhea or constipation, dyspnea, tachycardia, hematuria, headache, and irritability.

Wheal

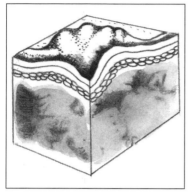

A slightly raised, firm lesion of variable size and shape, surrounded by edema; skin may be red or pale

Papule

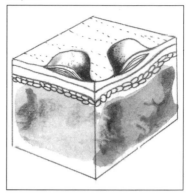

A small, solid, raised lesion less than 1 cm in diameter, with red-to-purple skin discoloration

Nodule

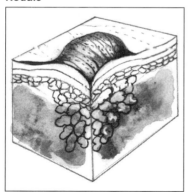

A small, firm, circumscribed elevation approximately 1 to 2 cm in diameter; skin discoloration may be present

Tumor

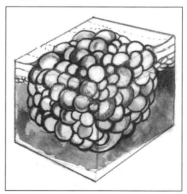

A solid, raised mass, usually larger than 2 cm in diameter; skin discoloration may be present

Other causes

● **Drugs.** A transient maculopapular rash, usually on the trunk, may accompany reactions to many drugs, including salicylates, benzodiazepines such as diazepam, lithium, phenylbutazone, gold salts, allopurinol, isoniazid, and antibiotics, such as tetracycline, ampicillin, cephalosporins, and sulfonamides.

Special considerations

Advise the patient to keep his skin clean and dry, to avoid scratching his rash, and to wear loose-fitting, nonirritating clothing. Instruct him to promptly report any change in its color, size, or configuration and the onset of itching or bleeding. Also have him avoid excessive exposure to direct sunlight and apply a protective sunscreen before going outdoors.

Apply cool compresses or an antipruritic lotion such as Aveeno lotion. Administer antihistamines for allergic reactions and antibiotics for infections.

Pediatric pointers

Common causes of papular rashes in children are infectious diseases, such as molluscum contagiosum and scarlet fever; scabies; insect bites; allergies or drug reactions; and miliaria, which occurs in three forms, depending on the depth of sweat gland involvement.

PARALYSIS

Paralysis, the total loss of voluntary motor function, results from severe cortical or pyramidal tract damage. It can occur in cerebrovascular disorders, degenerative neuromuscular disease, trauma, tumors, or central nervous system infection. Acute paralysis may be an early indicator of a life-threatening disorder such as Guillain-Barré syndrome. Paralysis can be local or widespread, symmetrical or asymmetrical, transient or permanent, and spastic or flaccid. It's commonly classified according to location and severity as paraplegia (sometimes transient paralysis of the legs), quadriplegia (permanent paralysis of the arms, legs, and body below the level of the spinal lesion), or hemiplegia (unilateral paralysis of vary-

ing severity and permanence). Incomplete paralysis with profound weakness (paresis) may precede total paralysis in some patients.

Emergency interventions

 If the patient's paralysis has developed suddenly, suspect trauma or an acute vascular insult. After ensuring that the patient's spine is properly immobilized, quickly determine his level of consciousness (LOC) and take his vital signs. Elevated systolic blood pressure, widening pulse pressure, and bradycardia may signal increasing intracranial pressure (ICP). If possible, elevate the patient's head 30 degrees to decrease ICP. Evaluate respiratory status, and be prepared to administer oxygen, insert an artificial airway, or provide intubation and mechanical ventilation, as needed. To help determine the nature of his injury, try to elicit an account of the precipitating events. If he's unable to respond, try to find an eyewitness.

History and physical examination

If the patient is in no immediate danger, perform a complete neurologic assessment. Start with the history, relying on family members for information, if necessary. Ask about the onset, duration, intensity, and progression of paralysis and about the events preceding its development. Focus medical history questions on the incidence of degenerative neurologic or neuromuscular disease, recent infectious illness, sexually transmitted disease, cancer, or recent injury. Explore related symptoms, noting fever, headache, visual disturbances, dysphagia, nausea and vomiting, bowel or bladder dysfunction, muscle pain or weakness, and fatigue.

Next, perform a complete neurologic examination, testing cranial nerve, motor, and sensory function and deep tendon reflexes. Assess strength in all major muscle groups, and note any muscle atrophy. Document all findings to serve as a baseline.

Common medical causes

● *Amyotrophic lateral sclerosis.* This fatal disorder produces spastic or flaccid paralysis in the body's major muscle groups, eventually progressing to total paralysis. Earlier findings include progressive muscle weakness, fasciculations, and muscle atrophy, commonly beginning in the arms and hands. Cramping and hyperreflexia are also common. Respiratory muscle and brain stem involvement produces dyspnea and possibly respiratory distress. Developing cranial nerve paralysis causes dysarthria, dysphagia, drooling, choking, and difficulty chewing.

● *Bell's palsy.* This disorder of cranial nerve VII causes transient, unilateral facial muscle paralysis. The affected muscles sag and eyelid closure is impossible. Other signs include increased tearing, drooling, and a diminished or absent corneal reflex.

● *Brain abscess.* Advanced abscess in the frontal or temporal lobe can cause hemiplegia accompanied by other late findings, such as ocular disturbances, unequal pupils, decreased LOC, ataxia, tremors, and signs of infection.

● *Brain tumor.* A tumor affecting the motor cortex of the frontal lobe may cause contralateral hemiparesis that progresses to hemiplegia. Onset is gradual, but paralysis is permanent without treatment. In early stages, a frontal headache and behavioral changes may be the only indicators. Eventually, seizures, aphasia, and signs of increased ICP (decreased LOC and vomiting) develop.

● *Cerebrovascular accident (CVA).* A CVA involving the motor cortex can produce contralateral paresis or paralysis. Onset may be sudden or gradual, and paralysis may be transient or permanent. Associated signs and symptoms vary widely and may include headache, vomiting, seizures, decreased LOC and mental acuity, dysarthria, dysphagia, ataxia, contralateral paresthesia or sensory loss, apraxia, agnosia, aphasia, visual disturbances, emotional lability, and bowel and bladder dysfunction.

● *Conversion disorder.* Hysterical paralysis, a classic conversion symptom, is characterized by the loss of voluntary movement with no obvious physical cause. It can affect any muscle group, appears and disappears unpredictably, and may occur with histrionic behavior (manipulative, dramatic, vain, irrational) or a strange indifference.

● *Encephalitis.* Variable paralysis develops in the late stages of this disorder. Earlier signs and symptoms include rapidly decreasing LOC (possibly coma), fever, headache, photophobia, vomiting, signs of meningeal irritation (nuchal rigidity, positive Kernig's and Brudzinski's signs), aphasia, ataxia, nystagmus, ocular palsies, myoclonus, and seizures.

● *Guillain-Barré syndrome.* This syndrome is characterized by a rapidly developing, but reversible, ascending paralysis. It commonly begins as leg muscle weakness and progresses symmetrically, sometimes affecting even the cranial nerves, producing dysphagia, nasal speech, and dysarthria. Respiratory muscle paralysis may be life-threatening. Other effects include transient paresthesia, orthostatic hypotension, tachycardia, diaphoresis, and bowel and bladder incontinence.

● *Head trauma.* Cerebral injury can cause paralysis due to cerebral edema and increased ICP. Onset is usually sudden. Location and extent vary, depending on the injury. Associated findings also vary but may include decreased LOC, focal neurologic disturbances, headache, blurred or double vision, nausea and vomiting, and sensory disturbances, such as paresthesia and loss of sensation.

● *Multiple sclerosis.* In this disorder, paralysis commonly waxes and wanes until the later stages, when it may become permanent. Its extent can range from monoplegia to quadriplegia. In most patients, visual and sensory disturbances (such as paresthesia) are the earliest symptoms. Later findings are widely variable and may include muscle weakness and spasticity, nystagmus, hyperreflexia, intention tremor, gait ataxia, dysphagia, dysarthria, impotence, and constipation. Urinary frequency, urgency, and incontinence may also occur.

• *Myasthenia gravis.* In this neuromuscular disease, profound muscle weakness and abnormal fatigability may produce paralysis of certain muscle groups. Paralysis is usually transient in early stages but becomes more persistent as the disease progresses. Associated findings depend on the areas of neuromuscular involvement; they may include weak eye closure, ptosis, diplopia, lack of facial mobility, dysphagia, nasal speech, and frequent nasal regurgitation of fluids. Neck muscle weakness may cause the patient's jaw to drop and his head to bob. Respiratory muscle involvement can lead to respiratory distress—dyspnea, shallow respirations, and cyanosis.

• *Parkinson's disease.* Tremor, bradykinesia, and lead-pipe or cogwheel rigidity are the classic signs of Parkinson's disease. Extreme rigidity can progress to paralysis, particularly in the extremities. In most cases, paralysis resolves with prompt treatment of the disease.

• *Peripheral neuropathy.* Typically, this syndrome produces muscle weakness that may lead to flaccid paralysis and atrophy. Related effects may include paresthesia, loss of vibration sensation, hypoactive or absent deep tendon reflexes, neuralgia, and skin changes such as anhidrosis.

• *Rabies.* This acute disorder produces progressive flaccid paralysis, vascular collapse, coma, and death within 2 weeks of contact with an infected animal. Prodromal signs and symptoms—fever; headache; hyperesthesia; paresthesia, coldness, and itching at the bite site; photophobia; tachycardia; shallow respirations; and excessive salivation, lacrimation, and perspiration—develop almost immediately. Within 2 to 10 days, a phase of excitement begins with agitation, cranial nerve dysfunction (pupil changes, hoarseness, facial weakness, ocular palsies), tachycardia or bradycardia, cyclic respirations, high fever, urine retention, drooling, and hydrophobia.

• *Seizure disorders.* Seizures, particularly focal seizures, can cause transient local paralysis (Todd's paralysis). Any part of the body may be affected, although paralysis tends to occur contralateral to the side of the irritable focus.

• *Spinal cord injury.* Complete spinal cord transection results in permanent spastic paralysis below the level of injury. Reflexes may return after resolution of spinal shock. Partial transection causes variable paralysis and paresthesia, depending on the location and extent of injury. (See *Understanding spinal cord syndromes.*)

• *Spinal cord tumors.* Paresis, pain, paresthesia, and variable sensory loss may occur along the nerve distribution pathway served by the affected cord segment. Eventually, these symptoms may progress to spastic paralysis with hyperactive deep tendon reflexes (unless the tumor is in the cauda equina, which produces hyporeflexia) and, perhaps, bladder and bowel incontinence. Paralysis is permanent without treatment.

• *Subarachnoid hemorrhage.* This potentially life-threatening disorder can produce sudden paralysis. Duration may be temporary, resolving with decreasing edema, or permanent, if tissue destruction has occurred. Other acute effects are severe headache, mydriasis, photophobia, aphasia, sharply decreased LOC, nuchal rigidity, vomiting, and seizures.

• *Transient ischemic attack (TIA).* Episodic TIAs may cause transient unilateral paresis or paralysis accompanied by paresthesia, blurred or double vision, dizziness, aphasia, dysarthria, decreased LOC, and other site-dependent effects.

UNDERSTANDING SPINAL CORD SYNDROMES

When the patient's spinal cord is incompletely severed, he will have partial motor and sensory loss. Most incomplete cord lesions fit into one of the syndromes described below.

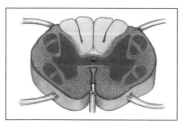

Anterior cord syndrome, most commonly resulting from a flexion injury, causes motor paralysis and loss of pain and temperature sensation below the level of injury. Touch, proprioception, and vibration sensation are usually preserved.

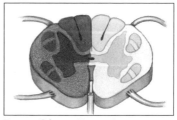

Brown-Séquard's syndrome can result from flexion, rotation, or penetration injuries. It's characterized by unilateral motor paralysis ipsilateral to the injury and loss of pain and temperature sensation contralateral to the injury.

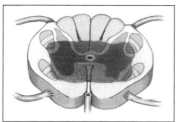

Central cord syndrome is caused by hyperextension or flexion injuries. Motor loss is variable and greater in the arms than in the legs; sensory loss is usually slight.

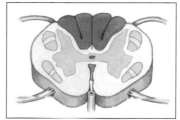

Posterior cord syndrome, produced by a cervical hyperextension injury, causes only a loss of proprioception and loss of light touch sensation. Motor function remains intact.

Other causes

- *Drugs.* Therapeutic use of neuromuscular blocking agents, such as pancuronium or curare, produces paralysis.
- *Electroconvulsive therapy.* This therapy can produce acute, transient paralysis.

Special considerations

Because a paralyzed patient is particularly susceptible to the complications of prolonged immobility, provide frequent position changes, meticulous skin care, and frequent chest physiotherapy. He may benefit from passive range-of-motion exercises to maintain muscle tone, application of splints to prevent contractures, and the use of footboards or other devices to prevent footdrop.

If his cranial nerves are affected, the patient will have difficulty chewing and swallowing. Provide a liquid or soft diet, and keep suction equipment on hand in case aspiration occurs. Feeding tubes or total parenteral nutrition may be necessary in severe paralysis. Paralysis and accompanying visual disturbances may make ambulation hazardous; provide a call light and show the patient how to call for help. As appropriate, arrange for physical, speech, or occupational therapy.

Pediatric pointers

Besides the obvious causes—trauma, infection, or tumors—children may contract paralysis from hereditary and congenital disorders, such as Tay-Sachs disease, Werdnig-Hoffmann disease, spina bifida, and cerebral palsy.

PARESTHESIA

Paresthesia is a combination of abnormal sensations—commonly described as numbness, prickling, or tingling—felt along peripheral nerve pathways. These sensations are generally not painful; unpleasant or painful sensations are termed *dysesthesia*. Paresthesia may develop suddenly or gradually and may be transient or permanent.

A common symptom of many neurologic disorders, paresthesia may also result from certain systemic disorders or drug effects. It may reflect damage or irritation of the parietal lobe, thalamus, spinothalamic tract, or spinal or peripheral nerves—the neural circuit that transmits and interprets sensory stimuli.

History and physical examination

First explore the paresthesia. When did the sensations begin? Have the patient describe their character and distribution. Also ask about associated signs and symptoms, such as sensory loss and paresis or paralysis. Next, take a medical history, including neurologic, cardiovascular, metabolic, renal, and chronic in-

flammatory disorders, such as arthritis or lupus. Has the patient sustained trauma or had recent surgery or invasive procedures that may have injured peripheral nerves?

Focus the physical examination on the patient's neurologic status. Assess his level of consciousness (LOC) and cranial nerve function. Test muscle strength and deep tendon reflexes in limbs affected by paresthesia. Systematically evaluate light touch, pain, temperature, vibration, and position sensation. Also note skin color and temperature, and palpate pulses.

Common medical causes

● *Arterial occlusion (acute).* In this disorder, sudden paresthesia and coldness may develop in one or both legs with a saddle embolus. Paresis, intermittent claudication, and aching pain at rest are also characteristic. The extremity becomes mottled with a line of temperature and color demarcation at the level of occlusion. Pulses are absent below the occlusion, and capillary refill is diminished.

● *Arteriosclerosis obliterans.* This disorder produces paresthesia, intermittent claudication (most common symptom), diminished or absent popliteal and pedal pulses, pallor, paresis, and coldness in the affected leg.

● *Arthritis.* Rheumatoid or osteoarthritic changes in the cervical spine may cause paresthesia in the neck, shoulders, and arms. Sometimes, the lumbar spine is affected, causing paresthesia in one or both legs and feet.

● *Brain tumor.* Tumors affecting the sensory cortex in the parietal lobe may cause progressive contralateral paresthesia accompanied by agnosia, apraxia, agraphia, homonymous hemianopia, and loss of proprioception.

● *Buerger's disease.* In this smoking-related inflammatory occlusive disorder, exposure to cold makes the feet cold, cyanotic, and numb; later, they redden, become hot, and tingle. Intermittent claudication, which is aggravated by exercise and relieved by rest, is also common. Other findings include weak peripheral pulses, migratory superficial thrombophlebitis and, later, ulceration, muscle atrophy, and gangrene.

● *Cerebrovascular accident (CVA).* Although contralateral paresthesia may occur in CVA, sensory loss is more common. Associated features vary with the artery affected and may include contralateral hemiplegia, decreased LOC, and homonymous hemianopia.

● *Diabetes mellitus.* Glove and stocking paresthesia of diabetic neuropathy commonly produces a burning sensation. Other findings include insidious, permanent anosmia, fatigue, polyuria, polydipsia, weight loss, and polyphagia.

● *Guillain-Barré syndrome.* In this syndrome, transient paresthesia may precede muscle weakness, which usually begins in the legs and ascends to the arms and facial nerves. Weakness may progress to total paralysis. Other clinical features may consist of dysarthria, dysphagia, nasal speech, orthostatic hypotension, bladder and bowel incontinence, diaphoresis, tachycardia, and possibly signs of life-threatening respiratory muscle paralysis.

● *Head trauma.* Unilateral or bilateral paresthesia may occur when head trauma causes concussion or contusion; however, sensory loss is more common. Other findings may include variable paresis or paralysis, decreased LOC, headache, blurred or double vision, nausea and vomiting, dizziness, and seizures.

● *Herniated disk.* Herniation of a lumbar or cervical disk may cause acute or gradual onset of paresthesia along the distribution pathways of affected spinal nerves. Other neuromuscular effects include severe pain, muscle spasms, and weakness that may progress to atrophy unless herniation is relieved.

● *Herpes zoster.* An early symptom of this disorder, paresthesia occurs in the dermatome supplied by the affected spinal nerve. Within several days, this dermatome is marked by a pruritic, erythematous, vesicular rash associated with sharp, shooting, or burning pain.

● *Hyperventilation syndrome.* Usually triggered by acute anxiety, this syndrome may produce transient paresthesia in the hands, feet, and perioral area, accompanied by agitation, vertigo, syncope, pallor, muscle twitching and weakness, carpopedal spasm, and cardiac arrhythmias.

● *Migraine headache.* Paresthesia in the hands, face, and perioral area may herald an impending migraine headache. Other prodromal symptoms may include scotomas, hemiparesis, confusion, dizziness, and photophobia. These effects may persist during the characteristic throbbing headache and continue after it subsides.

● *Multiple sclerosis (MS).* In this disorder, demyelination of the sensory cortex or spinothalamic tract may produce paresthesia—commonly one of the earliest symptoms of MS. Like other effects of MS, paresthesia commonly waxes and wanes until the later stages, when the sensations may become permanent. Associated findings include muscle weakness, spasticity, hyperreflexia, and others.

● *Peripheral nerve trauma.* Injury to any of the major peripheral nerves may cause paresthesia in the area supplied by that nerve. Paresthesia begins shortly after trauma and may be permanent. Other effects may include dysesthesia, flaccid paralysis or paresis, hyporeflexia, and variable sensory loss.

● *Peripheral neuropathy.* This syndrome may cause progressive paresthesia in all extremities. The patient also commonly displays muscle weakness, which may lead to flaccid paralysis and atrophy, loss of vibration sensation, diminished or absent deep tendon reflexes, neuralgia, and cutaneous changes, such as glossy, red skin and anhidrosis.

● *Rabies.* Paresthesia, coldness, and itching at the site of an animal bite herald the prodromal stage of rabies. Other prodromal effects are fever, headache, photophobia, hyperesthesia, tachycardia, shallow respirations, and excessive salivation, lacrimation, and perspiration.

- **Raynaud's disease.** Exposure to cold or stress makes the fingers turn pale, cold, and cyanotic; with rewarming, they become red and paresthetic. Ulceration may occur in chronic cases.
- **Seizure disorders.** Seizures originating in the parietal lobe usually cause paresthesia of the lips, fingers, and toes. These sensations may act as auras that lead to tonic-clonic seizures.
- **Spinal cord injury.** Paresthesia may occur in partial spinal cord transection, after spinal shock resolves. It may be unilateral or bilateral, occurring at or below the level of the lesion. Associated sensory and motor loss is variable. Spinal cord disorders may be associated with paresthesia on head flexion (Lhermitte's sign).
- **Spinal cord tumors.** Paresthesia, paresis, pain, and sensory loss along nerve pathways served by the affected cord segment result from such tumors. Eventually, paresis may cause spastic paralysis with hyperactive deep tendon reflexes (unless the tumor is in the cauda equina, which produces hyporeflexia) and, possibly, bladder and bowel incontinence.
- **Systemic lupus erythematosus.** This disorder may cause paresthesia. Primary clinical features include nondeforming arthritis (usually of hands, feet, and large joints), photosensitivity, and a butterfly rash that appears across the nose and cheeks.
- **Tabes dorsalis.** In this disorder, paresthesia—especially of the legs—is a common, but late, symptom. Other effects include ataxia, loss of proprioception and pain and temperature sensation, absent deep tendon reflexes, Charcot's joints, Argyll Robertson pupils, incontinence, and impotence.
- **Transient ischemic attack.** Typically, paresthesia occurs abruptly in an attack and is limited to one arm or another isolated part of the body. The sensations usually last about 10 minutes and are accompanied by paralysis or paresis. Associated findings may include decreased LOC, dizziness, unilateral vision loss, nystagmus, aphasia, dysarthria, tinnitus, facial weakness, dysphagia, and ataxic gait.

Other causes

- **Drugs.** Phenytoin, chemotherapeutic agents (such as vincristine, vinblastine, and procarbazine), D-penicillamine, isoniazid, nitrofurantoin, chloroquine, and parenteral gold therapy may produce transient paresthesia that disappears when the drug is discontinued.
- **Radiation therapy.** Long-term radiation therapy may eventually cause peripheral nerve damage, producing paresthesia.

Special considerations

Because paresthesia is commonly accompanied by patchy sensory loss, teach the patient safety measures. For example, have him test bathwater with a thermometer and and wear shoes at all times to protect his feet.

Pediatric pointers

Although children may experience paresthesia associated with the same causes as adults, they're frequently unable to describe this symptom. Nevertheless, hereditary polyneuropathies are usually first recognized in childhood.

PAROXYSMAL NOCTURNAL DYSPNEA

Typically dramatic and terrifying to the patient, this sign refers to an attack of dyspnea that abruptly awakens the patient and typically causes diaphoresis, coughing, wheezing, and chest discomfort. It abates after the patient sits up or stands for several minutes but may recur every 2 to 3 hours.

Paroxysmal nocturnal dyspnea is a sign of left-sided heart failure. It can reflect decreased respiratory drive, impaired left-sided heart function, enhanced reabsorption of interstitial fluid, and increased thoracic blood volume. All of these pathophysiologic mechanisms cause dyspnea to worsen when the patient lies down.

History and physical examination
Begin by exploring the patient's complaint of dyspnea. Does he have dyspneic attacks at other times, such as after exertion or while sitting down? If so, what type of activity triggers the attack? Does he have coughing, wheezing, fatigue, or weakness during an attack? Find out if he has a history of lower extremity edema. Ask if he sleeps with his head elevated and, if so, on how many pillows. Obtain a cardiopulmonary history. Does the patient or a family member have a history of myocardial infarction, coronary artery disease, or hypertension? Chronic bronchitis, emphysema, or asthma? Has the patient had cardiac surgery?

Now perform a physical examination. Begin by taking the patient's vital signs and forming an overall impression of his appearance. Is he noticeably cyanotic or edematous? Auscultate the lungs for crackles and wheezing and the heart for gallops and arrhythmias.

Common medical causes
● *Left-sided heart failure.* Dyspnea—on exertion, during sleep, and eventually even at rest—is an early sign of left-sided heart failure. It's characteristically accompanied by Cheyne-Stokes respirations, diaphoresis, weakness, wheezing, and a persistent, nonproductive cough or a cough that produces clear or blood-tinged sputum.

As the patient's condition worsens, he develops tachycardia, tachypnea, pulsus alternans (commonly initiated by a pre-mature beat), a ventricular gallop, crackles, and peripheral edema.

In advanced left-sided heart failure, the patient may also have severe orthopnea, cyanosis, clubbing, hemoptysis, and cardiac arrhythmias. He also may develop signs and symptoms of shock, such as hypotension, weak pulse, and cold, clammy skin.

Special considerations
Prepare the patient for diagnostic tests, such as chest X-ray, echocardiography, exercise electrocardiography, and cardiac blood pool imaging.

If the hospitalized patient experiences paroxysmal nocturnal dyspnea, assist him to a sitting position or help him walk around the room. If necessary, provide supplemental oxygen. Try to calm him because anxiety can exacerbate dyspnea.

Pediatric pointers
In a child, paroxysmal nocturnal dyspnea usually stems from congenital heart defects that precipitate heart failure. Help relieve the child's dyspnea by elevating his head and calming him.

PEAU D'ORANGE
[Orange-peel skin]

Usually a late sign of breast cancer, peau d'orange is the edematous thickening and pitting of breast skin. This slowly developing sign can also occur with breast or axillary lymph node infection. Its striking orange-peel appearance stems from lymphatic edema around deepened hair follicles. (See *Recognizing peau d'orange,* page 444.)

History and physical examination
Ask the patient when she first detected peau d'orange. Has she noticed any lumps, pain, or other breast changes? Does she have related symptoms, such

RECOGNIZING PEAU D'ORANGE

Usually a late sign of breast cancer, peau d'orange is characterized by a thickening and pitting of breast skin that produces an orange peel–like appearance— hence the name "peau d'orange" (French for skin of an orange).

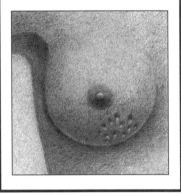

as malaise and achiness? Is she lactating or has she recently weaned her infant? Has she had previous axillary surgery that might have impaired lymphatic drainage of a breast?

In a well-lit examining room, observe the patient's breasts. Estimate the extent of the peau d'orange and check for erythema. Assess the nipples for discharge, deviation, retraction, dimpling, and cracking. Now gently palpate the area of peau d'orange, noting warmth or induration. Then palpate the entire breast, noting any fixed or mobile lumps, and the axillary lymph nodes, noting enlargement. Finally, take the patient's temperature.

Common medical causes

● *Breast abscess.* Usually affecting lactating women with milk stasis, this infectious disorder causes peau d'orange, malaise, breast tenderness and erythema, and a sudden fever possibly accompanied by shaking chills. A cracked nipple may produce a purulent discharge, and an indurated or palpable soft mass may be present.

● *Breast cancer.* Advanced breast cancer is the most common cause of peau d'orange, which usually begins in the dependent part of the breast or the areola. Palpation typically reveals a firm, immobile mass that adheres to the skin above the area of peau d'orange. Inspection of the breasts may reveal changes in contour, size, or symmetry. Inspection of the nipples may reveal deviation, erosion, retraction, and a thin and watery, bloody, or purulent discharge. The patient may report a burning and itching sensation in the nipples as well as a sensation of warmth or heat in the breast. Breast pain may occur, but it's not a reliable indicator of cancer.

Special considerations

Because peau d'orange usually signals advanced breast cancer, you'll need to provide emotional support for the patient. Encourage her to express her fears and concerns. Clearly explain expected diagnostic tests, such as mammography and breast biopsy.

PERICARDIAL FRICTION RUB

Commonly transient, a pericardial friction rub is a scratching, grating, or crunching sound that occurs when two inflamed layers of the pericardium slide over one another. Ranging from faint to loud, this abnormal sound is best heard along the lower left sternal border during deep inspiration. It indicates pericarditis, which can result from acute infection, cardiac and renal disorders, postpericardiotomy syndrome, and use of certain drugs, such as procainamide and antineoplastic agents.

Occasionally, a pericardial friction rub can resemble a murmur (see *Pericardial friction rub or murmur?*) or a pleural friction rub. However, the classic pericardial friction rub has three components. (See *Understanding pericardial friction rubs,* page 446.)

History and physical examination

Obtain a complete medical history, noting especially cardiac dysfunction. Has the patient recently had a myocardial infarction or cardiac surgery? Has he ever had pericarditis or rheumatic disorders, such as rheumatoid arthritis or systemic lupus erythematosus? Does he have chronic renal failure or an infection? If the patient complains of chest pain, ask him to describe its character and location. What relieves the pain? What worsens it?

Take the patient's vital signs, noting especially hypotension, tachycardia, irregular pulse, tachypnea, and fever. Inspect for jugular vein distention, edema, ascites, and hepatomegaly. Auscultate the lungs for crackles.

Common medical causes

• *Pericarditis.* A pericardial friction rub is the hallmark of *acute pericarditis.* This disorder also causes sharp precordial or retrosternal pain that usually radiates to the left shoulder and neck. The pain worsens when the patient breathes deeply, coughs, or lies flat and, possibly, when he swallows. It abates when he sits up and leans forward. He may also have fever, dyspnea, tachycardia, and arrhythmias.

In *chronic constrictive pericarditis,* a pericardial friction rub develops gradually. It's accompanied by signs of decreased cardiac filling and output, such as peripheral edema, ascites, jugular vein distention on inspiration (Kussmaul's

sign), and hepatomegaly. Dyspnea, orthopnea, pulsus paradoxus, and chest pain may also develop.

UNDERSTANDING PERICARDIAL FRICTION RUBS

The complete, or classic, pericardial friction rub is triphasic. Its three sound components are linked to phases of the cardiac cycle: The *presystolic* component (A) reflects atrial systole and precedes the first heart sound (S_1). The *systolic* component (B)—usually the loudest—reflects ventricular systole and occurs between the first and second heart sounds (S_2). The *early diastolic* component (C) reflects ventricular diastole and follows the second heart sound.

Sometimes, the early diastolic component merges with the presystolic component, producing a diphasic to-and-fro sound on auscultation. In other patients, auscultation may detect only one component—a monophasic rub, typically during ventricular systole.

Triphasic rub

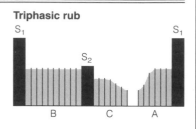

Diphasic rub

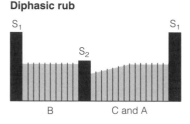

Monophasic rub

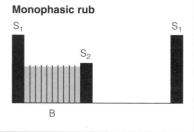

Special considerations

Continue to monitor the patient's cardiovascular status. If the pericardial friction rub disappears, be alert for signs of cardiac tamponade: pallor, increased jugular vein distention, hypotension, tachycardia, tachypnea, pulsus paradoxus, and cool, clammy skin. If these signs occur, prepare the patient for pericardiocentesis to prevent cardiovascular collapse.

Ensure that the patient gets adequate rest. Give anti-inflammatory drugs, antiarrhythmics, diuretics, or antimicrobials to treat the underlying cause. If necessary, prepare him for a pericardiectomy to promote adequate cardiac filling and contraction.

Pediatric pointers

Bacterial pericarditis may develop during the first two decades of life, most commonly before age 6. Although a pericardial friction rub may occur, other signs and symptoms—fever, tachycardia, dyspnea, chest pain, jugular vein distention, and hepatomegaly—more reliably indicate this life-threatening disorder.

A pericardial friction rub may occur after surgery to correct congenital cardiac anomalies, but it usually vanishes without development of pericarditis.

PERISTALTIC WAVES, VISIBLE

In intestinal obstruction, peristalsis temporarily increases in strength and frequency as the intestine tries to force its contents past the obstruction. As a result, visible peristaltic waves may roll across the abdomen. Typically, these waves appear suddenly and vanish quickly because increased peristalsis overcomes the obstruction or the GI tract becomes atonic. Peristaltic waves are best detected by stooping at the patient's side (he should be in a supine position) and inspecting the abdominal contour.

Visible peristaltic waves may also reflect normal stomach and intestinal contractions in thin patients or in malnourished patients with abdominal muscle atrophy.

History and physical examination

After observing peristaltic waves, collect pertinent history data. For example, ask about a history of pyloric ulcer, stomach cancer, or chronic gastritis, which can lead to pyloric obstruction. Ask about conditions leading to intestinal obstruction, such as intestinal tumors or polyps, gallstones, chronic constipation, and a hernia. Has the patient had abdominal surgery?

Determine if the patient has related symptoms. Spasmodic abdominal pain, for example, accompanies small-bowel obstruction, whereas colicky pain accompanies pyloric obstruction. Is the patient nauseated? Has he vomited? If he has vomited, ask about the consistency,

amount, and color of the vomitus. Lumpy vomitus may contain undigested food particles. Green or brown vomitus may contain bile or fecal matter.

Now, with the patient supine, inspect the abdomen for distention, surgical scars and adhesions, or visible loops of bowel. Auscultate for bowel sounds, noting high-pitched, tinkling sounds. Next, jar the patient's bed (or roll the patient from side to side) and auscultate for a succussion splash—a splashing sound in the stomach from retained secretions due to pyloric obstruction. Palpate the abdomen for rigidity and tenderness, and percuss for tympany. Check the skin and mucous membranes for dryness and poor skin turgor, indicating dehydration. Take the patient's vital signs, noting especially tachycardia and hypotension, which indicate hypovolemia.

Common medical causes

- *Large-bowel obstruction.* Visible peristaltic waves in the upper abdomen are an early sign of this obstruction. Obstipation, however, may be the earliest finding. Other characteristic signs and symptoms develop more slowly than in small-bowel obstruction. They may include nausea, colicky abdominal pain (milder than in small-bowel obstruction), gradual and eventually marked abdominal distention, and hyperactive bowel sounds.
- *Pyloric obstruction.* Peristaltic waves may be detected in a swollen epigastrium or in the left upper quadrant, usually beginning near the left rib margin and rolling from left to right. Related findings include vague epigastric discomfort or colicky pain after eating, nausea, vomiting, anorexia, and weight loss. Auscultation reveals a loud succussion splash.
- *Small-bowel obstruction.* Early signs of mechanical obstruction of the small bowel include peristaltic waves rolling across the upper abdomen and intermittent, cramping periumbilical pain. Associated signs and symptoms include nau-

sea, vomiting of bilious or, later, fecal material, and constipation; in partial obstruction, diarrhea may be present. Hyperactive bowel sounds and slight abdominal distention also occur early.

Special considerations

Because visible peristaltic waves are a common early sign of intestinal obstruction, you'll need to monitor the patient's status and prepare him for diagnostic evaluation and treatment. Withhold food and fluids, and explain the purpose and procedure of abdominal X-rays and barium studies, which can confirm obstruction.

If tests confirm obstruction, nasogastric suctioning may be used to decompress the stomach and small bowel. Provide frequent oral hygiene, and watch for a thick, swollen tongue and dry mucous membranes, indicating dehydration. Monitor vital signs and intake and output frequently.

Pediatric pointers

In infants, visible peristaltic waves may indicate pyloric stenosis. In small children, peristaltic waves may normally be visible because of their protuberant abdomens. Or visible waves may indicate bowel obstruction stemming from congenital anomalies, volvulus, or swallowing a foreign body.

PHOTOPHOBIA

A common symptom, photophobia is an abnormal sensitivity to light. In many patients, photophobia simply indicates increased eye sensitivity without an underlying pathology. In some patients, it can indicate excessive wearing of contact lenses or poorly fitted lenses. But in others, this symptom can indicate systemic disorders, ocular disorders or trauma, or an adverse reaction to certain drugs.

History and physical examination

If your patient reports photophobia, find out when it began and how severe it is. Did it follow eye trauma? A chemical splash or exposure to the rays of a sun lamp? If photophobia results from trauma, avoid eye manipulation. Ask the patient about eye pain and have him describe its location, duration, and intensity. Does he have a sensation of a foreign body in his eye? Does he have any other signs and symptoms, such as increased tearing and vision changes?

Next, take the patient's vital signs and assess his neurologic status. Follow this with a careful eye examination, inspecting the eyes' external structures for any abnormalities. Examine the conjunctiva and sclera, noting especially their color. Characterize the amount and consistency of any discharge. Then check pupillary reaction to light. Evaluate extraocular muscle function by testing the six cardinal fields of gaze, and test visual acuity in both eyes.

During your assessment, keep in mind that photophobia can accompany life-threatening meningitis, although it's not a cardinal sign of meningeal irritation.

Common medical causes

● *Burns.* In *chemical burns,* photophobia and eye pain may be accompanied by erythema and blistering on the face and lids, miosis, diffuse conjunctival injection, and corneal changes. The patient may be unable to keep the eye(s) open, and his vision is blurred.

In *ultraviolet radiation burns,* photophobia occurs with moderate to severe eye pain. These symptoms develop about 12 hours after exposure to the rays of a welding arc or sun lamp.

● *Conjunctivitis.* When conjunctivitis affects the cornea, it causes photophobia. Other common findings include con-

PHOTOPHOBIA: COMMON CAUSES AND ASSOCIATED FINDINGS

CAUSES	Conjunctival injection	Corneal changes	Eye discharge	Eyelid edema	Eye pain	Foreign body sensation	Nuchal rigidity	Pupillary changes	Tearing, increased	Vision changes	Visual floaters	Vomiting
Burns (chemical)	●	●			●	●		●	●	●		
Burns (ultraviolet)	●	●			●	●			●			
Conjunctivitis	●		●		●	●			●			
Corneal abrasion	●	●			●	●			●	●		
Corneal foreign body	●	●			●	●		●	●	●		
Corneal ulcer	●	●	●		●				●	●		
Interstitial keratitis	●	●			●					●		
Iritis (acute)	●				●			●		●		
Meningitis (acute bacterial)							●	●				●
Migraine headache										●		●
Sclerokeratitis		●			●							
Uveitis (anterior)	●				●			●				
Uveitis (posterior)	●				●			●		●	●	

junctival injection, increased tearing, a foreign body sensation, a feeling of fullness around the eyes, and eye pain, burning, and itching. *Allergic conjunctivitis* is distinguished by a stringy eye discharge and milky red injection. *Bacterial conjunctivitis* tends to cause a copious, mucopurulent, flaky eye discharge that may make the eyelids stick together as well as brilliant red conjunctiva. *Fungal conjunctivitis* produces a thick, purulent discharge, extreme redness, and crusting, sticky eyelids. *Viral conjunctivitis* causes copious tearing with little discharge as well as enlargement of the preauricular lymph nodes.

● *Corneal abrasion.* A common finding in corneal abrasion, photophobia is usually accompanied by excessive tearing, conjunctival injection, visible corneal damage, and a foreign body sensation in the eye. Blurred vision and eye pain may occur.

● *Corneal ulcer.* This vision-threatening disorder causes severe photophobia and eye pain that's aggravated by blinking. Impaired visual acuity may accompany blurring, eye discharge, and sticky eyelids. Conjunctival injection may occur even though the cornea appears white and opaque. A *bacterial ulcer* may also cause an irregularly shaped corneal ulcer and unilateral pupillary constriction. A *fungal ulcer* may be surrounded by progressively clearer rings.

• *Iritis (acute).* Severe photophobia may result from this disorder, along with marked conjunctival injection, moderate to severe eye pain, and blurred vision. The pupil may be constricted and may respond poorly to light.

• *Keratitis (interstitial).* This corneal inflammation causes photophobia, eye pain, blurred vision, dramatic conjunctival injection, and grayish pink corneas.

• *Meningitis (acute bacterial).* A common symptom of this disorder, photophobia may occur with other signs of meningeal irritation, such as nuchal rigidity, hyperreflexia, and opisthotonos. Brudzinski's and Kernig's signs can be elicited. Fever, an early finding, may be accompanied by chills. Related effects may include headache, vomiting, ocular palsies, facial weakness, pupillary abnormalities, and hearing loss. In severe meningitis, seizures may occur along with stupor progressing to coma.

• *Migraine headache.* Photophobia and noise sensitivity are prominent features of a common migraine. Typically severe, this aching or throbbing headache may also cause fatigue, blurred vision, nausea, and vomiting.

• *Sclerokeratitis.* Inflammation of the sclera and cornea causes photophobia, eye pain, burning, and irritation.

• *Uveitis.* Both anterior and posterior uveitis can cause photophobia. Typically, *anterior uveitis* also produces moderate to severe eye pain, severe conjunctival injection, and a small, nonreactive pupil. *Posterior uveitis* develops slowly, causing visual floaters, eye pain, pupil distortion, conjunctival injection, and blurred vision.

Other causes

• *Drugs.* Mydriatics—such as phenylephrine, atropine, scopolamine, cyclopentolate, and tropicamide—can cause photophobia due to ocular dilation. Amphetamines, cocaine, and ophthalmic antifungal drugs—such as trifluridine, vidarabine, and idoxuridine—can also cause photophobia.

Special considerations

Promote patient comfort by darkening the room and telling him to close both eyes. If photophobia persists at home, suggest that he wear dark glasses.

Prepare the patient for diagnostic tests, such as corneal scraping and slit-lamp examination.

Pediatric pointers

Suspect photophobia in any child who squints, rubs his eyes frequently, or wears sunglasses indoors and outdoors. Congenital disorders, such as syphilis and albinism, and childhood diseases, such as measles and rubella, can cause photophobia.

PLEURAL FRICTION RUB

Commonly resulting from pulmonary disorders or trauma, this loud, coarse, grating, creaking, or squeaking sound may be auscultated over one or both lungs during late inspiration or early expiration. It's heard best over the low axilla or the anterior, lateral, or posterior bases of the lung fields with the patient upright. Sometimes intermittent, it may resemble crackles or a pericardial friction rub. (See *Comparing auscultation findings,* pages 452 and 453.)

A pleural friction rub indicates inflammation of the visceral and parietal pleural lining, which causes congestion and edema. The resultant fibrinous exudate covers both pleural surfaces, displacing the fluid that's normally between them and causing the surfaces to rub together.

Emergency interventions

 When you detect a pleural friction rub, quickly look for signs of respiratory distress: shallow or decreased respirations; crowing, wheezing, or stridor; dyspnea; increased accessory muscle use; intercostal or suprasternal retractions; cyanosis; and nasal flaring. Check for hypotension, tachycardia, and a decreased level of consciousness. If you detect signs of distress, open and maintain an airway. Endotracheal intubation and supplemental oxygen may be necessary. Insert a large bore I.V. catheter to deliver drugs and fluids. Elevate the patient's head 30 degrees. Monitor cardiac status constantly and check vital signs frequently.

History and physical examination

If the patient isn't in severe distress, explore related symptoms. Find out if he has had chest pain. If so, ask him to describe its location and severity. How long does his chest pain last? Does it radiate to his shoulder, neck, or upper abdomen? Does the pain worsen with breathing, movement, coughing, or sneezing? Does it abate if he splints his chest, holds his breath, or exerts pressure or lies on the affected side?

Ask the patient about a history of rheumatoid arthritis, respiratory or cardiovascular disorders, recent trauma, asbestos exposure, or radiation therapy. If he smokes, obtain a history in pack years.

Characterize the pleural friction rub by auscultating the lungs with the patient sitting upright and breathing deeply and slowly through his mouth. Is the friction rub unilateral or bilateral? Also listen for absent or diminished breath sounds, noting their location and timing in the respiratory cycle. Do abnormal breath sounds clear with coughing? Observe for clubbing and pedal edema, which may indicate a chronic disorder. Then palpate for decreased chest motion and percuss for flatness or dullness.

Common medical causes

• *Asbestosis.* Besides a pleural friction rub, this disorder may cause dyspnea on exertion, a cough, chest pain, and crackles. Clubbing is a late sign.

• *Lung cancer.* A pleural friction rub may be heard in the affected area of the lung. Other effects may include a cough (with possible hemoptysis), dyspnea, chest pain, weight loss, anorexia, fatigue, clubbing, fever, and wheezing.

• *Pleurisy.* A pleural friction rub occurs early in this disorder. However, the cardinal symptom is sudden, intense chest pain that's usually unilateral and located in the lower and lateral parts of the chest. Deep breathing, coughing, or thoracic movement aggravates the pain. Decreased breath sounds and inspiratory crackles may be heard over the painful area. Other findings include dyspnea, tachypnea, tachycardia, cyanosis, fever, and fatigue.

• *Pneumonia (bacterial).* A pleural friction rub occurs in this disorder, which usually starts with a dry, painful, hacking cough that rapidly becomes productive. Related effects develop suddenly: shaking chills, high fever, headache, dyspnea, pleuritic chest pain, tachypnea, tachycardia, grunting respirations, nasal flaring, dullness to percussion, and cyanosis. Auscultation reveals decreased breath sounds and fine crackles.

• *Pulmonary embolism.* An embolism can cause a pleural friction rub over the affected area of the lung. Usually, the first symptom is sudden dyspnea that may be accompanied by anginal or pleuritic chest pain. Other clinical features include a nonproductive cough or a cough that produces blood-tinged sputum, tachycardia, tachypnea, low-grade fever, restlessness, and diaphoresis. Less common findings include massive hemoptysis, chest splinting, leg edema and, with a large embo-

(Text continues on page 454.)

COMPARING AUSCULTATION FINDINGS

During auscultation, you may detect a pleural friction rub, a pericardial friction rub, or crackles—three abnormal sounds that are commonly confused. Use this chart to help identify auscultation findings.

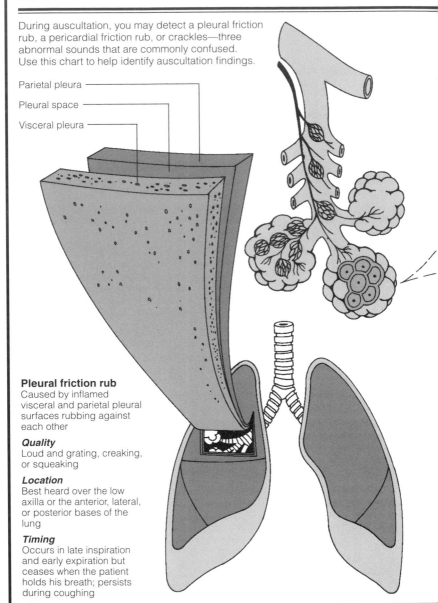

Parietal pleura

Pleural space

Visceral pleura

Pleural friction rub
Caused by inflamed visceral and parietal pleural surfaces rubbing against each other

Quality
Loud and grating, creaking, or squeaking

Location
Best heard over the low axilla or the anterior, lateral, or posterior bases of the lung

Timing
Occurs in late inspiration and early expiration but ceases when the patient holds his breath; persists during coughing

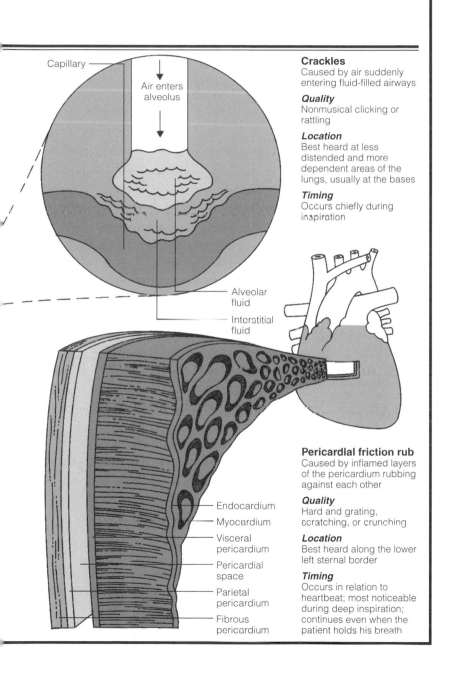

Capillary

Air enters alveolus

Alveolar fluid

Interstitial fluid

Crackles
Caused by air suddenly entering fluid-filled airways

Quality
Nonmusical clicking or rattling

Location
Best heard at less distended and more dependent areas of the lungs, usually at the bases

Timing
Occurs chiefly during inspiration

Endocardium
Myocardium
Visceral pericardium
Pericardial space
Parietal pericardium
Fibrous pericardium

Pericardial friction rub
Caused by inflamed layers of the pericardium rubbing against each other

Quality
Hard and grating, scratching, or crunching

Location
Best heard along the lower left sternal border

Timing
Occurs in relation to heartbeat; most noticeable during deep inspiration; continues even when the patient holds his breath

lus, cyanosis, syncope, and jugular vein distention. Crackles, diffuse wheezing, decreased breath sounds, and signs of circulatory collapse may also occur.

● *Systemic lupus erythematosus.* Pulmonary involvement can cause a pleural friction rub, hemoptysis, dyspnea, pleuritic chest pain, and crackles. More characteristic effects include a butterfly rash, nondeforming joint pain and stiffness, and photosensitivity. Fever, anorexia, weight loss, and lymphadenopathy may also occur.

● *Tuberculosis (pulmonary).* In this disorder, a pleural friction rub may occur over the affected part of the lung. Early signs and symptoms include weight loss, night sweats, low-grade fever in the afternoon, malaise, dyspnea, anorexia, and easy fatigability. Progression of the disorder usually produces pleuritic pain, fine crackles over the upper lobes, and a productive cough with blood-streaked sputum. Advanced tuberculosis can cause chest wall retraction, tracheal deviation, and dullness to percussion.

Other causes

● *Surgery and radiation therapy.* Thoracic surgery and radiation therapy can cause a pleural friction rub.

Special considerations

Continue to monitor the patient's respiratory status and vital signs.

Because pleuritic pain commonly accompanies a pleural friction rub, teach your patient splinting maneuvers to increase his comfort. Also apply a heating pad over the affected area and administer analgesics for pain relief.

Although coughing may be painful, instruct the patient not to suppress it because coughing and deep breathing help prevent respiratory complications. However, if the patient's persistent dry, hacking cough tires him, administer antitussives. (Avoid giving narcotics, which can further depress respirations.) Administer oxygen and antibiotics.

Prepare the patient for diagnostic tests such as chest X-rays.

Pediatric pointers

Auscultate for a pleural friction rub in any child who has grunting respirations, reports chest pain, or protects his chest by holding it or lying on one side. Usually, a pleural friction rub in a child is an early sign of pleurisy.

POLYDIPSIA

Polydipsia refers to excessive thirst—a common symptom associated with endocrine disorders and certain drugs. It may reflect decreased fluid intake, increased urine output, or excessive loss of water and salt.

History and physical examination

If the patient has polydipsia, you'll need to take his blood pressure and pulse when he's in the supine and standing positions. A decrease of 10 mm Hg in systolic pressure and a pulse rate increase of 10 beats/minute from the supine to the standing position may indicate hypovolemia. If you detect these changes, ask the patient about recent weight loss. Infuse I.V. replacement fluids as needed.

Next, obtain a history. Find out how much fluid the patient drinks each day. How often and how much does he typically urinate? Does the need to urinate awaken him at night? Ask about any recent weight loss or change in appetite. Determine if he or anyone in his family has diabetes or kidney disease. What medications does he use? Has his lifestyle changed recently? If so, have these changes upset him?

Finally, check for signs of dehydration, such as dry mucous membranes and decreased skin turgor.

Common medical causes

• *Diabetes insipidus.* This disorder characteristically produces polydipsia. It may also cause excessive voiding of dilute urine and mild to moderate nocturia. In severe cases, it causes fatigue and signs of dehydration.

• *Diabetes mellitus.* Polydipsia is a classic finding in this disorder. Other characteristic effects include polyuria, polyphagia, nocturia, weakness, fatigue, and weight loss. Signs of dehydration may occur.

• *Hypercalcemia.* As this disorder progresses, the patient develops polydipsia, polyuria, nocturia, constipation, paresthesia and, occasionally, hematuria and pyuria. Severe hypercalcemia can progress quickly to vomiting, decreased level of consciousness, and renal failure.

• *Hypokalemia.* This electrolyte imbalance can cause nephropathy, resulting in polydipsia, polyuria, and nocturia. Related hypokalemic effects include muscle weakness or paralysis, fatigue, decreased bowel sounds, hypoactive deep tendon reflexes, and arrhythmias.

• *Renal disorders (chronic).* Chronic renal disorders, such as glomerulonephritis and pyelonephritis, damage the kidneys, causing polydipsia and polyuria. Associated signs and symptoms may include nocturia, weakness, elevated blood pressure, pallor and, in later stages, oliguria.

• *Sheehan's syndrome.* Polydipsia, polyuria, and nocturia occur in this syndrome of postpartum pituitary necrosis. Other features include fatigue, failure to lactate, amenorrhea, decreased pubic and axillary hair growth, and reduced libido.

• *Sickle cell anemia.* As nephropathy develops, polydipsia and polyuria occur. They may be accompanied by abdominal pain and cramps, arthralgia and, occasionally, lower extremity skin ulcers and bone deformities, such as kyphosis and scoliosis.

Other causes

• *Drugs.* Diuretics and demeclocycline may produce polydipsia. Phenothiazines and anticholinergics can cause dry mouth, making the patient so thirsty that he drinks compulsively.

Special considerations

Carefully monitor the patient's fluid balance by recording his total intake and output. Weigh the patient at the same time each day, in the same clothing, and using the same scale. Regularly check blood pressure and pulse in the supine and standing positions to detect orthostatic hypotension, which may indicate hypovolemia. Because thirst is usually the body's way of compensating for water loss, give the patient ample liquids.

Pediatric pointers

In children, polydipsia usually stems from diabetes insipidus or diabetes mellitus. Rare causes include pheochromocytoma, neuroblastoma, and Prader-Willi syndrome. However, some children have habitual polydipsia that's unrelated to any disease.

POLYPHAGIA
[Hyperphagia]

Polyphagia refers to voracious or excessive eating before satiety. This common symptom can be persistent or intermittent, resulting primarily from endocrine and psychological disorders as well as from the use of certain drugs. Depending on the underlying cause, polyphagia may or may not cause weight gain.

History and physical examination

Begin your evaluation by asking the patient what he has eaten and drunk within the last 24 hours. (If the patient easily recalls this information, ask about the 2 previous days' intake for a broader view of his dietary habits.) Note the frequency of meals and the amount and types of food eaten. Find out if the patient's eating habits have changed recently. Has he always had a large appetite? Does his overeating alternate with periods of anorexia? Ask about conditions that may trigger overeating, such as stress, depression, or menstruation. Does the patient actually feel hungry, or does he eat simply because food is available? Does he ever vomit or have a headache after overeating?

Explore related signs and symptoms. Has the patient recently gained or lost weight? Does he feel tired, nervous, or excitable? Has he experienced heat intolerance, dizziness, or palpitations? Diarrhea or increased thirst or urination? Obtain a complete drug history, including use of laxatives or enemas.

During the physical examination, weigh the patient. Tell him his current weight, and watch for any expression of disbelief or anger. Inspect the skin to detect dryness or poor turgor. Palpate the thyroid for enlargement.

Common medical causes

● *Anxiety.* Polyphagia may result from mild to moderate anxiety or emotional stress. Typically, *mild anxiety* produces restlessness, sleeplessness, irritability, repetitive questioning, and constant seeking of attention and reassurance. In *moderate anxiety,* selective inattention and difficulty concentrating may also occur. Other effects of anxiety may include muscle tension, diaphoresis, GI distress, palpitations, tachycardia, and urinary and sexual dysfunction.

● *Bulimia.* Most common in women ages 18 to 29, bulimia causes polyphagia that alternates with self-induced vomiting, fasting, or diarrhea. The patient typically weighs less than normal but has a morbid fear of obesity. She appears depressed, has low self-esteem, and conceals her overeating.

● *Diabetes mellitus.* In this disorder, polyphagia occurs with weight loss, polydipsia, and polyuria. It's accompanied by nocturia, weakness, fatigue, and signs of dehydration, such as dry mucous membranes and poor skin turgor.

● *Premenstrual syndrome.* Appetite changes, typified by food cravings and binges, are common in this syndrome. Abdominal bloating, the most common associated finding, may occur with behavioral changes, such as depression and insomnia. Headache, paresthesia, and other neurologic symptoms may also occur. Related findings include diarrhea or constipation, edema and temporary weight gain, palpitations, back pain, breast swelling and tenderness, oliguria, and easy bruising.

Other causes

● *Drugs.* Corticosteroids and cyproheptadine may increase appetite, causing weight gain.

Special considerations

Offer the patient with polyphagia emotional support, and help him understand its underlying cause. As needed, refer the patient and his family for psychological counseling.

Pediatric pointers

In children, polyphagia commonly results from juvenile diabetes. In infants 6 to 18 months old, it can result from a malabsorptive disorder, such as celiac disease. However, polyphagia may occur normally in a child who's experiencing a sudden growth spurt.

POLYURIA

A relatively common sign, polyuria is the daily production and excretion of more than 3 qt (3 L) of urine. It's usually reported by the patient as increased voidings, especially when it occurs at night. Polyuria is aggravated by overhydration, consumption of caffeine or alcohol, and excessive ingestion of salt, glucose, or other hyperosmolar substances.

Polyuria usually results from the use of certain drugs, such as diuretics, or from psychological, neurologic, or renal disorders. It can reflect central nervous system dysfunction that diminishes or suppresses secretion of antidiuretic hormone (ADH), which regulates fluid balance. Or, when ADH levels are normal, it can reflect renal impairment. In both of these pathophysiologic mechanisms, the renal tubules fail to reabsorb sufficient water, causing polyuria.

History and physical examination

Because the patient with polyuria is at risk for developing hypovolemia, evaluate fluid status first. Take vital signs, noting especially increased body temperature, tachycardia, and orthostatic hypotension. Inspect for dry skin and mucous membranes, decreased skin turgor and elasticity, and reduced perspiration. Is the patient unusually tired or thirsty? Has he recently lost more than 5% of his body weight? If you detect these effects of hypovolemia, infuse replacement fluids.

If the patient doesn't display signs of hypovolemia, explore the frequency and pattern of the polyuria. When did it begin? How long has it lasted? Was it precipitated by a certain event? Ask the patient to describe the pattern and amount of his daily fluid intake. Find out about any current or past psychiatric disorders as well as chronic hypokalemia or hypercalcemia. Check for a history of visual deficits, headaches, or head trauma, which may precede diabetes insipidus. Also check for a history of urinary tract obstruction, diabetes mellitus, and renal disorders. Find out the schedule and dosage of any drugs the patient is currently taking.

Perform a neurologic examination, noting especially any change in the patient's level of consciousness (LOC). Then palpate the bladder and inspect the urethral meatus. Obtain a urine specimen and check its specific gravity.

Common medical causes

- *Acute tubular necrosis.* During the diuretic phase of this disorder, polyuria of less than 8 L/day gradually subsides after 8 to 10 days. Urine specific gravity (1.010 or less) increases as the polyuria subsides. Related findings include weight loss, decreasing edema, and nocturia.
- *Diabetes insipidus.* Extreme polyuria—up to 30 L/day—can occur in this disorder. However, polyuria of about 5 L/day with a specific gravity of 1.005 or less is a more common finding. Polyuria is commonly accompanied by polydipsia, nocturia, fatigue, and signs of dehydration, such as poor skin turgor and dry mucous membranes.
- *Diabetes mellitus.* In this disorder, polyuria seldom exceeds 5 L/day, while urine specific gravity typically exceeds 1.020. The patient usually has polydipsia, polyphagia, weight loss, weakness, fatigue, and nocturia. He may also display signs of dehydration.
- *Glomerulonephritis (chronic).* Polyuria gradually progresses to oliguria in this disorder. Urine output is usually less than 4 L/day; specific gravity is about 1.010. Related GI effects include anorexia, nausea, and vomiting. Other findings include drowsiness, fatigue, edema, headache, elevated blood pressure, and dyspnea. Nocturia, hematuria, and mild to severe proteinuria may occur.
- *Postobstructive uropathy.* After resolution of a urinary tract obstruction, polyuria—usually more than 5 L/day with a specific gravity of less than 1.010—occurs for several days before gradually subsiding. Resolving bladder distention and edema may occur with nocturia and weight loss. Occasionally, signs of dehydration appear.

POLYURIA: COMMON CAUSES AND ASSOCIATED FINDINGS

CAUSES	MAJOR ASSOCIATED SIGNS AND SYMPTOMS													
	Anorexia	Blood pressure increase	Constipation	Dyspnea	Dysuria	Edema	Fatigue	Fever	Flank pain	Headache	Hematuria	Level of consciousness, altered	Mucous membrane dryness	Nocturia
Acute tubular necrosis						•								•
Diabetes insipidus							•						•	•
Diabetes mellitus							•						•	•
Glomerulonephritis (chronic)	•	•		•		•	•			•	•			•
Postobstructive uropathy							•						•	•
Psychogenic polydipsia		•				•				•		•		
Pyelonephritis (acute)	•				•			•	•		•			•
Pyelonephritis (chronic)	•	•					•							
Sickle cell anemia							•							

• **Psychogenic polydipsia.** Most common in women over age 30, this disorder usually produces dilute polyuria of 3 to 15 L/day, depending on fluid intake. The patient may appear depressed and have a headache and blurred vision. She may have weight gain, edema, elevated blood pressure and, occasionally, stupor or coma. In severe overhydration, she may display signs of heart failure.

• **Pyelonephritis.** *Acute pyelonephritis* usually results in polyuria of less than 5 L/day with a low but variable specific gravity. Other findings may include persistent high fever, flank pain, hematuria, costovertebral angle tenderness, chills, weakness, dysuria, urinary frequency and urgency, tenesmus, and nocturia. Occasionally, nausea, anorexia, vomiting, and hypoactive bowel sounds may occur.

Chronic pyelonephritis produces polyuria of less than 5 L/day that declines as renal function worsens. Usually, urine specific gravity is about 1.010, but it may be higher if proteinuria is present. Other effects include irritability, paresthesia, fatigue, nausea, vomiting, drowsiness, anorexia, pyuria and, in late stages, elevated blood pressure.

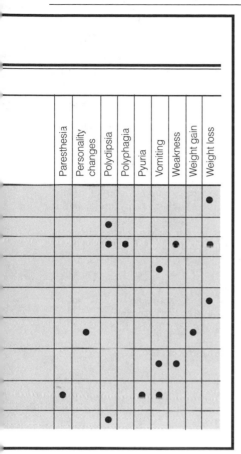

ly monitor the patient's vital signs to detect fluid imbalance, and encourage him to drink adequate fluids.

Prepare the patient for serum electrolyte, osmolality, blood urea nitrogen, and creatinine studies to monitor fluid and electrolyte status. Prepare him for a fluid deprivation test to determine the cause of polyuria.

Pediatric pointers
The major causes of polyuria in children are congenital nephrogenic diabetes insipidus, medullary cystic disease, polycystic renal disease, and distal renal tubular acidosis.

Because a child's fluid balance is more delicate than an adult's, check his urine specific gravity at each voiding, and be alert for signs of dehydration.

PRIAPISM

A urologic emergency, priapism is a persistent, painful erection that's unrelated to sexual excitation. This relatively rare sign may begin during sleep and appear to be a normal erection, but it may last for several hours or days. It's usually accompanied by a severe, constant, dull aching in the penis. Despite this, the patient may be too embarrassed to seek medical help and may try to achieve detumescence through continued sexual activity.

Priapism occurs when the veins of the corpora cavernosa fail to drain correctly, resulting in persistent engorgement of the tissues. Without prompt treatment, penile ischemia and thrombosis occur. In about half of all cases, priapism is idiopathic and develops without apparent predisposing factors. Secondary priapism results from blood disorders, neoplasms, trauma, and the use of certain drugs.

Other causes
• *Diagnostic tests.* Transient polyuria can result from radiographic tests that use contrast media.
• *Drugs.* Diuretics characteristically produce polyuria. Cardiotonics, vitamin D, demeclocycline, phenytoin, lithium, methoxyflurane, and propoxyphene can also produce polyuria.

Special considerations
Maintaining an adequate fluid balance is your primary concern when the patient has polyuria. Record intake and output accurately, and weigh him daily. Close-

Emergency interventions

 If the patient has priapism, apply an ice pack to the penis, administer analgesics, and insert an indwelling catheter to relieve urine retention. Procedures to remove blood from the corpora cavernosa, such as irrigation and surgery, may be required.

History and physical examination

When the patient's condition permits, ask him when the priapism began. Is it continuous or intermittent? Has he had a prolonged erection before? If so, what did he do to relieve it? How long did he remain detumescent? Does he have pain or tenderness when he urinates? Has he noticed any changes in sexual function?

Explore the patient's medical history. If he reports sickle cell anemia, find out about any factors that could precipitate a crisis, such as dehydration and infections. Ask if he has recently suffered genital trauma, and obtain a thorough drug history.

Examine the patient's penis, noting its color and temperature. Check for any loss of sensation, and look for signs of infection, such as redness or drainage. Finally, take his vital signs, particularly noting fever.

Common medical causes

● *Cerebrovascular accident (CVA).* A CVA may cause priapism, but sensory loss and aphasia may prevent the patient from noticing or describing it. Other findings depend on the CVA's location and extent but may include contralateral hemiplegia, seizures, headache, dysarthria, dysphagia, ataxia, apraxia, and agnosia. Visual deficits include homonymous hemianopia, blurring, decreased acuity, and diplopia. Urine retention or incontinence, constipation, and vomiting may also occur.

● *Penile carcinoma.* Carcinoma that exerts pressure on the corpora cavernosa can cause priapism. Usually, the first sign is a painless ulcerative lesion or an enlarging warty growth on the glans or foreskin, which may be accompanied by localized pain, a foul-smelling discharge from the prepuce, a firm lump near the glans, and lymphadenopathy. Later findings may include bleeding, dysuria, urine retention, and bladder distention.

● *Sickle cell anemia.* In this congenital disorder, painful priapism can occur without warning, usually on awakening. A history of priapism, impaired growth and development, and increased susceptibility to infection may be present. Related findings include tachycardia, pallor, weakness, hepatomegaly, dyspnea, joint swelling, joint or bone aching, chest pain, fatigue, murmurs, leg ulcers and, possibly, jaundice and gross hematuria.

In sickle cell crisis, signs and symptoms of sickle cell anemia may worsen and others, such as abdominal pain and low-grade fever, may appear.

● *Spinal cord injury.* In this condition, the patient may be unaware of the onset of priapism. Related effects depend on the extent and level of the injury and may include autonomic signs such as bradycardia.

Other causes

● *Drugs.* Priapism can result from phenothiazines, thioridazine, trazodone, androgenic steroids, and some antihypertensives. It may also occur after an intracorporeal injection of papaverine, which is a common treatment for impotence.

Special considerations

Prepare the patient for blood tests to help determine the cause of his priapism. If he requires surgery, keep his penis flaccid postoperatively by applying a pressure dressing. At least once every 30 minutes, inspect the glans for signs of vascular compromise, such as coolness or pallor.

Pediatric pointers

In neonates, priapism can result from hypoxia but is usually resolved with oxygen therapy. Priapism is more likely to develop in children who have sickle cell disease than in adults with the disease.

PRURITUS
[Itching]

Commonly provoking scratching in an attempt to gain relief, this unpleasant itching sensation affects the skin, the eyes, and certain mucous membranes. Pruritus tends to be most severe at night, but it may also worsen with increased skin temperature, poor skin turgor, local vasodilation, dermatoses, and stress.

The most common symptom of dermatologic disease, pruritus may also result from local and systemic disorders and from drug use. Physiologic pruritus, such as pruritic urticarial papules and plaques of pregnancy, may occur in primigravidas late in the third trimester. It can also stem from emotional upsets or contact with skin irritants.

History and physical examination

If the patient reports pruritus, have him describe its onset, frequency, and intensity. If pruritus occurs at night, ask him whether it prevents him from falling asleep or awakens him after he falls asleep. (Generally, pruritus related to dermatoses prevents—but doesn't disturb—sleep.) Does exercise, stress, fear, depression, or illness seem to aggravate the itching? Ask about contact with skin irritants, previous skin disorders, and related symptoms. Then obtain a complete drug history.

Examine the patient for signs of scratching, such as excoriation, purpura, scabs, scars, or lichenification. Look for primary lesions to help confirm dermatoses.

Common medical causes

- *Anemia (iron deficiency).* This disorder occasionally produces pruritus. Initially asymptomatic, anemia can later cause dyspnea on exertion, fatigue, listlessness, pallor, irritability, headache, tachycardia, poor muscle tone, and possibly murmurs. Chronic anemia causes spoon-shaped and brittle nails, cracked mouth corners, a smooth tongue, and dysphagia.

- *Cimex lectularius (bedbugs).* Typically, bedbug bites produce itching and burning over the ankles and lower legs, along with clusters of purpuric spots.

- *Conjunctivitis.* Regardless of the type, conjunctivitis causes eye itching, burning, and pain along with photophobia, conjunctival injection, a foreign body sensation, excessive tearing, and a feeling of fullness around the eye.

Allergic conjunctivitis may also cause milky redness and a stringy eye discharge. *Bacterial conjunctivitis* typically causes brilliant redness and a mucopurulent, flaky discharge that may make the eyelids stick together. *Fungal conjunctivitis* produces a thick, purulent discharge and crusting and sticking of the eyelid. *Viral conjunctivitis* may cause copious tearing—but little discharge—and preauricular lymph node enlargement.

- *Dermatitis.* Several types of dermatitis can cause pruritus accompanied by a skin lesion. *Atopic dermatitis* begins with intense, severe pruritus and an erythematous rash on dry skin at flexion points (antecubital fossa, popliteal area, and neck). During a flare-up, scratching may produce edema, scaling, and pustules. In chronic atopic dermatitis, lesions may progress to dry, scaly skin with white dermatographia, blanching, and lichenification.

Mild irritants and allergies can cause *contact dermatitis,* with itchy small vesicles that may ooze and scale and are surrounded by redness. Severe reaction can produce marked localized edema.

Dermatitis herpetiformis, most common in men between the ages of 20 and 50, initially causes intense pruritus and stinging. Symmetrically distributed lesions form on the buttocks, shoulders, elbows, and knees 8 to 12 hours later. Sometimes, they also form on the neck, face, and scalp. These lesions are erythematous and papular, bullous, or pustular.

● **Hepatobiliary disease.** An important diagnostic clue to liver and gallbladder disease, pruritus is commonly accompanied by jaundice and may be generalized or localized to the palms and soles. Other characteristics may include right upper quadrant pain, clay-colored stools, chills and fever, flatus, belching and a bloated feeling, epigastric burning, and bitter fluid regurgitation. Later, liver disease may produce mental changes, ascites, bleeding tendencies, spider angiomas, palmar erythema, dry skin, fetor hepaticus, enlarged superficial abdominal veins, bilateral gynecomastia, testicular atrophy or menstrual irregularities, and hepatomegaly.

● **Herpes zoster.** Within 2 to 4 days of fever and malaise, pruritus, paresthesia or hyperesthesia, and severe, deep pain from cutaneous nerve involvement develop on the trunk or the arms and legs in a dermatome distribution. Up to 2 weeks after the initial symptoms, red, nodular skin eruptions appear on the painful areas and become vesicular. About 10 days later, the vesicles rupture and form scabs.

● **Leukemia (chronic lymphocytic).** Pruritus is an uncommon symptom in this disorder. More characteristic effects include fatigue, malaise, generalized lymphadenopathy, fever, hepatomegaly, splenomegaly, weight loss, pallor, bleeding, and palpitations.

● **Lichen simplex chronicus.** Persistent rubbing and scratching cause localized pruritus and a circumscribed scaling patch with sharp margins. Later, the skin thickens and papules form.

● **Myringitis (chronic).** This disorder produces pruritus in the affected ear, along with a purulent discharge and gradual hearing loss.

● **Pediculosis (lice).** A prominent symptom of this disorder, pruritus occurs in the area of infestation. *Pediculosis capitis* (head lice) may also cause scalp excoriation from scratching, along with matted, foul-smelling, lusterless hair; occipital and cervical lymphadenopathy; and oval, gray-white nits on hair shafts.

Pediculosis corporis (body lice) initially causes small red papules (usually on the shoulders, trunk, or buttocks), which become urticarial from scratching. Later, rashes or wheals may develop. Untreated, *pediculosis corporis* produces dry, discolored, thickly encrusted, scaly skin with bacterial infection and scarring. In severe cases, it produces headache, fever, and malaise.

In *pediculosis pubis* (pubic lice), scratching commonly produces skin irritation. Nits or adult lice and erythematous, itching papules may appear in pubic hair or hair around the anus, abdomen, or thighs.

● **Pityriasis rosea.** Typically, this disorder produces mild to severe pruritus that's aggravated by a hot bath or shower. Usually, it begins with an erythematous herald patch—a slightly raised, oval lesion about $3/4''$ to $2 1/4''$ (2 to 6 cm) in diameter. After a few days or weeks, scaly yellow-tan or erythematous patches erupt on the trunk and extremities and persist for 2 to 6 weeks. Occasionally, these patches are macular, vesicular, or urticarial.

● **Psoriasis.** Pruritus and pain are common in this skin disorder. Typically, psoriasis begins with small erythematous papules that enlarge or coalesce to form red elevated plaques with silver scales on the scalp, chest, elbows, knees, back, buttocks, and genitalia. Nail pitting may occur.

● **Scabies.** Typically, scabies causes localized pruritus that awakens the patient. It may become generalized and persist for up to 2 weeks after treatment. Thread-like lesions several millimeters long appear with a swollen nodule or red papule. In males, crusty lesions may form on the glans penis, penile shaft, and scrotum. In females, lesions may form on the wrists, elbows, axilla, waistline, and nipples. Excoriation from scratching is common.

• *Tinea pedis.* This fungal infection causes severe foot pruritus, pain with walking, scales and blisters between the toes, and a dry, scaly squamous inflammation on the entire sole.

• *Urticaria.* Severe pruritus and stinging occur as transient erythematous or whitish wheals form on the skin or mucous membranes. Prickly sensations typically precede the wheals, which may affect any part of the body and range from pinpoint to palm-size or larger.

Pruritus may also occur with *mastocytosis.* In this disorder, reddish brown macules or papules or, less commonly, nodules or plaques occur. Other signs and symptoms may include flushing, tachycardia, hypotension, and nausea.

• *Vaginitis.* This disorder commonly causes localized pruritus and a foul-smelling vaginal discharge that may be purulent, white or gray, and curdlike. Perineal pain and urinary dysfunction may also occur.

Other causes
• *Drugs.* When mild and localized, an allergic reaction to such drugs as penicillin and sulfonamides can cause pruritus, erythema, an urticarial rash, and edema. However, in a severe drug reaction, anaphylaxis may occur.

Special considerations
Administer topical corticosteroids, antihistamines, or tranquilizers, as ordered. Suggest ways to control pruritus.

If the patient doesn't have a localized infection or skin lesions, suspect a systemic disease and prepare him for a complete blood count and differential, ery-throcyte sedimentation rate, protein electrophoresis, and radiologic studies.

Pediatric pointers
Many adult disorders also cause pruritus in children. However, they may affect different parts of the body. For instance, scabies may affect the head in infants, but not in adults. Pityriasis rosea may affect the face, hands, and feet of adolescents.

Some childhood diseases, such as measles and chickenpox, can cause pruritus. Hepatic diseases can also produce pruritus in children as bile salts accumulate on the skin.

PSOAS SIGN

A positive psoas sign—increased abdominal pain when the patient moves his leg against resistance—indicates direct or reflexive irritation of the psoas muscles. This sign, which can be elicited on the right or left side, usually indicates appendicitis but may also occur with localized abscesses. It's elicited in a patient with abdominal or lower back pain *after* completion of the abdominal examination to prevent spurious assessment findings. (See *Eliciting psoas sign,* page 464.)

Emergency interventions
 If you elicit a positive psoas sign in a patient with abdominal pain, suspect appendicitis. Quickly check the patient's vital signs, and prepare him for surgery. Explain the procedure, restrict food and fluids, and withhold analgesics, which can mask symptoms. Administer I.V. fluids to prevent dehydration, but do *not* give cathartics or enemas, which can cause a ruptured appendix and lead to peritonitis.

Check for Rovsing's sign by deeply palpating the patient's *left* lower quadrant. If he reports *right* lower quadrant

EXAMINATION TIP

 ELICITING PSOAS SIGN

You can use two techniques to elicit psoas sign in an adult with abdominal pain. With either technique, increased abdominal pain is a positive result, indicating psoas muscle irritation from an inflamed appendix or a localized abscess.

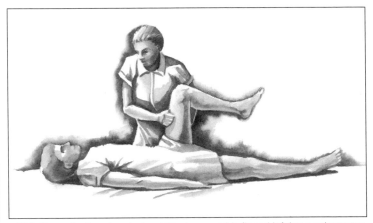

With the patient supine, instruct him to move his flexed left leg against your hand to test for a left psoas sign. Then perform this maneuver on the right leg to test for a right psoas sign.

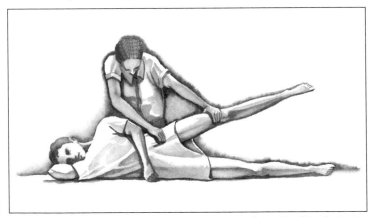

To test for a left psoas sign, turn the patient on his right side. Then instruct him to push his left leg upward from the hip against your hand. Next, turn the patient onto his left side and repeat this maneuver to test for a right psoas sign.

pain, the sign is positive, indicating peritoneal irritation.

Common medical causes
• *Appendicitis.* An inflamed retrocecal appendix can cause a positive right psoas sign. Early epigastric and periumbilical pain disappear only to worsen and localize in the right lower quadrant. This pain also worsens with walking or coughing. Related findings include nausea and vomiting, abdominal rigidity and rebound tenderness, and constipation or diarrhea. Fever, tachycardia, retractive respirations, anorexia, and malaise may also occur. If the appendix ruptures, additional findings may include sudden, severe pain, followed by signs of peritonitis, such as hypoactive or absent bowel sounds, high fever, and boardlike abdominal rigidity.
• *Retroperitoneal abscess.* After a lower retroperitoneal infection, an iliac or lumbar abscess can produce a positive right or left psoas sign and fever. An *iliac abscess* causes iliac or inguinal pain that may radiate to the hip, thigh, or knee; a tender mass in the lower abdomen or groin may be palpable. A *lumbar abscess* usually produces back tenderness and spasms on the affected side with a palpable lumbar mass; a tender abdominal mass without back pain may occur instead.

Special considerations
Monitor vital signs to detect complications such as peritonitis. Promote patient comfort through position changes. For example, have the patient lie down and flex his right leg. Then have him sit upright.

Prepare the patient for diagnostic tests, such as electrolyte studies and abdominal X-rays.

Pediatric pointers
Elicit psoas sign by asking the child to raise his head while you exert pressure on his forehead. Resulting right lower quadrant pain usually indicates appendicitis.

PSYCHOTIC BEHAVIOR

Psychotic behavior reflects an inability or unwillingness to recognize and acknowledge reality and to relate with others. It may begin suddenly or insidiously, progressing from vague complaints of fatigue, insomnia, or headache to withdrawal, social isolation, and preoccupation with certain issues.

Various behaviors together or separately can constitute psychotic behavior. These include delusions, illusions, hallucinations, bizarre language, and perseveration. *Delusions* are persistent beliefs that have no basis in reality or in the patient's knowledge or experience such as delusions of grandeur. *Illusions* are misinterpretations of external sensory stimuli, such as a mirage in the desert. In contrast, *hallucinations* are sensory perceptions that do not result from external stimuli. *Bizarre language* reflects a communication disruption. It can range from echolalia (purposeless repetition of a word or phrase) and clang association (repetition of words or phrases that sound similar) to neologisms (creation and use of words whose meaning only the patient knows). *Perseveration,* a persistent verbal or motor response, may indicate organic brain disease. Motor changes include inactivity, excessive activity, and repetitive movements.

History and physical examination
Because the patient's behavior can make it difficult—and even dangerous—to obtain pertinent information, conduct the interview in a calm, safe, and well-lit room. Provide enough personal space to avoid threatening or agitating him. Ask him to describe his problem and any circumstances that may have precipitated

DRUGS THAT CAN CAUSE PSYCHOTIC BEHAVIOR

Certain drugs can cause psychotic behavior and other psychiatric signs and symptoms, ranging from depression to violent behavior. These effects usually occur during therapy and resolve when the drug is discontinued. If your patient is receiving one of the following common drugs and exhibits the behavior described below, his drug dosage may have to be changed or another drug may have to be substituted.

DRUG	PSYCHIATRIC SIGNS AND SYMPTOMS
albuterol	Hallucinations, paranoia
alprazolam	Anger, hostility
amantadine	Visual hallucinations, nightmares
asparaginase	Confusion, depression, paranoia
atropine and anticholinergics	Auditory, visual, and tactile hallucinations; memory loss; delirium; fear; paranoia
bromocriptine	Mania, delusions, sudden relapse of schizophrenia, paranoia, aggressive behavior
cimetidine	Hallucinations, paranoia, confusion, depression, delirium
clonidine	Delirium, hallucinations, depression
corticosteroids (prednisone, corticotropin, cortisone)	Mania, catatonia, depression, confusion, paranoia, hallucinations
cycloserine	Anxiety, depression, confusion, paranoia, hallucinations
dapsone	Insomnia, agitation, hallucinations
diazepam	Suicidal thoughts, rage, hallucinations, depression
digitalis glycosides	Paranoia, euphoria, amnesia, visual hallucinations
disopyramide	Agitation, paranoia, auditory and visual hallucinations, panic
disulfiram	Delirium, auditory hallucinations, paranoia, depression
indomethacin	Hostility, depression, paranoia, hallucinations
lidocaine	Disorientation, hallucinations, paranoia
methyldopa	Severe depression, amnesia, paranoia, hallucinations

DRUGS THAT CAN CAUSE PSYCHOTIC BEHAVIOR (continued)

DRUG	PSYCHIATRIC SIGNS AND SYMPTOMS
methysergide	Depersonalization, hallucinations
propranolol	Severe depression, hallucinations, paranoia, confusion
thyroid hormones	Mania, hallucinations, paranoia
vincristine	Hallucinations

it. Obtain a medication history, focusing on antipsychotics, and explore his use of alcohol, noting duration of use and amount. Ask about any recent illnesses or accidents.

As the patient talks, watch for cognitive, linguistic, or perceptual abnormalities such as delusions. Do thoughts and actions seem to match? Look for unusual gestures, posture, gait, tone of voice, or mannerisms. Does the patient appear to be responding to external stimuli? For example, is he looking around the room? Interview the patient's family. Which family members does he seem closest to? How does the family describe the patient's relationships, communication patterns, and role? Ask about the patient's compliance with his medication regimen. Has any family member ever been hospitalized for psychiatric or emotional illness?

Finally, evaluate the patient's environment, educational and employment history, and socioeconomic status. Are community services available? How does the patient spend his leisure time? Does he have friends? Has he ever had a close emotional relationship?

Common medical causes

• *Organic disorders.* Various disorders may produce psychotic behavior. These include alcohol withdrawal syndrome, cerebral hypoxia, and nutritional disorders. Endocrine disorders (such as adrenal dysfunction) and severe infections (such as encephalitis) can also cause psychotic behavior. Neurologic causes include Alzheimer's disease and other dementias.

• *Psychiatric disorders.* Psychotic behavior usually occurs with bipolar disorders, personality disorders, schizophrenia, and traumatic stress disorders.

Other causes

• *Drugs.* Certain drugs can cause psychotic behavior. (See *Drugs that can cause psychotic behavior.*) However, almost any drug can provoke psychotic behavior as a rare, severe adverse or idiosyncratic reaction.

• *Surgery.* Postoperative delirium and depression may produce psychotic behavior.

Special considerations

Continuously evaluate the patient's orientation to reality. Help him build a conception of reality by calling him by his preferred name, telling him your name, describing where he is, and using clocks and calendars.

Encourage the patient's involvement in structured activities. However, if he's nonverbal or incoherent, be sure to spend time with him—simply sitting or walking with him, or talking about the day, the season, the weather, or other concrete topics. Avoid making time commitments that you can't keep: This will only upset the patient and may make him withdraw further.

Refer the patient for psychiatric evaluation. Administer antipsychotics or other drugs, as ordered, and prepare him for transfer to a mental health center, if necessary.

Don't overlook the patient's physiologic needs. Check his eating habits to avoid dehydration and malnutrition, and monitor his elimination patterns, especially if he's receiving psychotropic drugs, which can cause constipation.

Pediatric pointers

In children, psychotic behavior may result from early infantile autism, symbiotic infantile psychosis, and childhood schizophrenia—all of which can retard development of language, abstract thinking, and socialization.

The adolescent patient who exhibits psychotic behavior may have a history of several days' drug use or lack of sleep or food, which must be corrected before therapy can begin.

PTOSIS

Ptosis is the excessive drooping of the upper eyelid. In severe ptosis, the patient may be unable to raise his eyelids voluntarily.

This sign can be constant, progressive, or intermittent, and unilateral or bilateral. When it's unilateral, it's easy to detect by comparing the eyelids' relative positions. (See *Recognizing unilateral ptosis*.) When it's bilateral or mild, it's difficult to detect—the eyelids may be abnormally low, covering the upper part of the iris or even part of the pupil instead of overlapping the iris slightly. Other clues include a furrowed forehead or a tipped-back head—both of these help the patient see under his drooping lids. However, because ptosis can resemble enophthalmos, exophthalmometry may be required.

Ptosis can be classified as congenital or acquired. Congenital ptosis results from levator muscle underdevelopment or disorders of the third cranial (oculomotor) nerve. Acquired ptosis may result from trauma to or inflammation of these muscles and nerves, or from certain drugs, systemic diseases, intracranial lesions, and life-threatening aneurysms. But the most common cause is age, which reduces muscle elasticity and produces senile ptosis.

History and physical examination

Ask your patient when his ptosis began and if it has worsened or improved. Determine if he's had recent eye trauma. (If he has, avoid manipulating the eye to prevent further damage.) Ask about eye pain or headache and determine its location and severity. Has the patient experienced any vision changes? If so, have him describe them. Obtain a drug history, noting especially any chemotherapeutic agents.

Assess the degree of ptosis, and check for eyelid edema, exophthalmos, deviation, or conjunctival injection. Evaluate extraocular muscle function by testing the six cardinal fields of gaze. Test visual acuity and carefully examine the pupils' size, color, shape, and reaction to light.

Keep in mind that ptosis infrequently indicates a life-threatening condition. For example, sudden unilateral ptosis can herald a cerebral aneurysm.

Common medical causes

● *Botulism.* Acute cranial nerve dysfunction causes hallmark signs of ptosis, dysarthria, dysphagia, and diplopia. Other findings include dry mouth, sore throat, weakness, vomiting, diarrhea, hyporeflexia, and dyspnea.

EXAMINATION TIP

 RECOGNIZING UNILATERAL PTOSIS

Unilateral ptosis is easy to detect because you can compare the relative positions of both eyelids. In this illustration, the patient's left eyelid is clearly drooping.

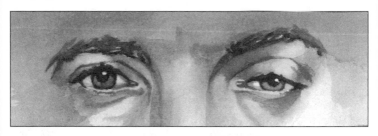

● *Cerebral aneurysm.* An aneurysm that compresses the oculomotor nerve can cause sudden ptosis, along with diplopia, a dilated pupil, and inability to rotate the eye. These may be the first signs of this life-threatening disorder.

With rupture, an aneurysm typically produces sudden severe headache, nausea, vomiting, and decreased level of consciousness (LOC). Other findings may include nuchal rigidity, back and leg pain, fever, restlessness, irritability, occasional seizures, blurred vision, hemiparesis, sensory deficits, dysphagia, and visual defects.

● *Lacrimal gland tumor.* This disorder commonly produces mild to severe ptosis, depending on the tumor's size and location. It may also cause brow elevation, exophthalmos, eye deviation, and possibly eye pain.

● *Lead poisoning.* Usually, ptosis develops over 3 to 6 months. Other effects include anorexia, nausea, vomiting, diarrhea, colicky abdominal pain, a lead line in the gums, decreased LOC, tachycardia, hypotension and, possibly, irritability and peripheral nerve weakness.

● *Myasthenia gravis.* Gradual bilateral ptosis is often the first sign of this disorder. It may be mild to severe and accompanied by weak eye closure and diplopia. Other characteristics include muscle weakness and fatigue that eventually may lead to paralysis. Depending on the muscles affected, other findings may include masklike facies, difficulty chewing or swallowing, dyspnea, cyanosis, and others.

● *Ocular muscle dystrophy.* In this disorder, bilateral ptosis progresses slowly to complete eyelid closure. Related signs and symptoms include progressive external ophthalmoplegia and muscle weakness and atrophy of the upper face, neck, trunk, and limbs.

● *Ocular trauma.* Trauma to the nerve or muscles that control the eyelids can cause mild to severe ptosis. Depending on the damage, eye pain, lid swelling, ecchymosis, and decreased visual acuity may also occur.

● *Parry-Romberg syndrome.* Unilateral ptosis and facial hemiatrophy occur with this disorder. Other signs may include miosis, sluggish pupil reaction to light, enophthalmos, irises that don't match in color, ocular muscle paralysis, nystagmus, and neck, shoulder, trunk, and extremity atrophy.

Other causes
• *Drugs.* Vinca alkaloids can produce ptosis.

Special considerations
Prepare the patient for diagnostic studies, such as the tensilon test and slit-lamp examination. If he needs surgery to correct levator muscle dysfunction, explain the procedure to him.

If the patient has decreased visual acuity, orient him to his surroundings. Provide special spectacle frames that suspend the eyelid by traction with a wire crutch. These frames are usually used to help patients with temporary paresis or those who aren't good candidates for surgery.

Pediatric pointers
Parents typically discover congenital ptosis when their child is an infant. Usually, the ptosis is unilateral, constant, and accompanied by lagophthalmos, which causes the infant to sleep with his eyes open. If this occurs, teach proper eye care to prevent drying.

PULSE, ABSENT OR WEAK

An absent or weak pulse may be generalized or may affect only one extremity. When generalized, this sign is an important indicator of such life-threatening conditions as shock and arrhythmia. Localized loss or weakness of a pulse that's normally present and strong may indicate acute arterial occlusion, which could require emergency surgery. However, the pressure of palpation may temporarily diminish or obliterate superficial pulses, such as the posterior tibial or the dorsal

pedal. Thus, bilateral weakness or absence of these pulses doesn't necessarily indicate underlying pathology.

History and physical examination
If you detect an absent or weak pulse, quickly palpate the remaining arterial pulses to distinguish between localized or generalized loss or weakness. Then quickly check other vital signs, evaluate cardiopulmonary status, and obtain a brief history. Based on your findings, proceed with emergency interventions. (See *Managing absent or weak pulse,* pages 472 and 473.)

Medical causes
• *Aortic aneurysm (dissecting).* When the dissecting aneurysm affects circulation to the innominate, left common carotid, subclavian, or femoral arteries, it causes weak or absent arterial pulses distal to the affected area. But 25% of patients with this life-threatening condition may have normal peripheral pulses. Tearing pain usually develops suddenly in the chest and neck and may radiate to the upper and lower back and abdomen. Blood pressure may be lower in the patient's legs than asymmetric brachial pulses in his arms. Other findings may include syncope, loss of consciousness, weakness or transient paralysis of the legs or arms, the diastolic murmur of aortic insufficiency, systemic hypotension, and mottled skin below the waist.
• *Aortic arch syndrome.* This syndrome produces weak or abruptly absent carotid pulses and unequal or absent radial pulses. These symptoms are usually preceded by night sweats, pallor, nausea, anorexia, weight loss, arthralgia, and Raynaud's phenomenon. Other findings may include hypotension in the arms, dizziness and syncope, paresthesia, intermittent claudication, bruits, visual disturbances, and neck, shoulder, and chest pain.
• *Aortic bifurcation occlusion (acute).* This rare disorder produces abrupt absence of all leg pulses. The patient re-

ports moderate to severe pain in the legs and, less commonly, in the abdomen, lumbosacral area, or perineum. In addition, his legs are cold, pale, numb, and flaccid.

● *Aortic stenosis.* In this disorder, the carotid pulse is sustained, but weak. Dyspnea, chest pain, and syncope dominate the clinical picture. The patient commonly has an atrial (S_4) gallop. He also may have a harsh systolic ejection murmur. Other findings may include crackles, palpitations, fatigue, and narrowed pulse pressure.

● *Arrhythmias.* Cardiac arrhythmias may produce generalized weak pulses accompanied by cool, clammy skin. Other findings reflect the arrhythmia's severity and may include hypotension, chest pain, dyspnea, dizziness, and decreased level of consciousness (LOC).

● *Arterial occlusion.* In *acute occlusion,* arterial pulses distal to the obstruction are unilaterally weak and then absent. The affected limb is cool, pale, and cyanotic, with prolonged capillary refill time, and the patient complains of moderate to severe pain and paresthesia. A line of color and temperature demarcation develops at the level of obstruction. Varying degrees of limb paralysis may also occur, along with intense intermittent claudication. In *chronic occlusion,* occurring in such disorders as arteriosclerosis and Buerger's disease, pulses in the affected limb weaken gradually.

● *Cardiac tamponade.* Life-threatening cardiac tamponade causes a weak, rapid pulse accompanied by these classic findings: pulsus paradoxus, jugular vein distention, hypotension, and muffled heart sounds. Narrowed pulse pressure, pericardial friction rub, and hepatomegaly may also occur. The patient may appear anxious, restless, and cyanotic. He may have chest pain, clammy skin, dyspnea, and tachypnea.

● *Coarctation of the aorta.* Findings in this disorder include bounding pulses in the arms and neck, with decreased pulsations and systolic pulse pressure in the lower extremities.

● *Peripheral vascular disease.* This disorder causes a weakening and loss of peripheral pulses. The patient complains of aching pain distal to the occlusion that worsens with exercise and abates with rest. The skin feels cool and shows decreased hair growth. If occlusion occurs in the descending aorta or femoral areas, the male patient may develop impotence.

● *Pulmonary embolism.* This disorder causes a generalized weak, rapid pulse. It also may cause abrupt onset of chest pain, tachycardia, dyspnea, apprehension, syncope, diaphoresis, and cyanosis. Acute respiratory effects may include tachypnea, dyspnea, decreased breath sounds, crackles, a pleural friction rub, and a cough—possibly with blood-tinged sputum.

● *Shock.* In *anaphylactic shock,* pulses become rapid and weak and then uniformly absent within seconds or minutes after exposure to an allergen. This is preceded by hypotension, anxiety, restlessness, feelings of doom, intense itching, a pounding headache, and possibly urticaria.

In *cardiogenic shock,* peripheral pulses are absent and central pulses are weak, depending on the degree of vascular collapse. A drop in systolic blood pressure to 30 mm Hg below baseline or a sustained reading below 80 mm Hg produces poor tissue perfusion. Resulting signs and symptoms include cold, pale, clammy skin; tachycardia; rapid, shallow respirations; oliguria; and restlessness, confusion, and obtundation.

In *hypovolemic shock,* all pulses in the extremities become weak and then uniformly absent, depending on the severity of hypovolemia. As shock progresses, remaining pulses become thready and more rapid. Early signs and symptoms of cardiogenic shock include tachypnea, restlessness, thirst, and cool, pale skin. Late signs include hypotension with nar-

(Text continues on page 474.)

MANAGING ABSENT OR WEAK PULSE

An absent or weak pulse can result from several life-threatening disorders. Your evaluation and interventions will vary, depending on whether the absent or weak pulse is generalized

ABSENT OR WEAK PULSE

Localized to one extremity.

Generalized

Patient is confused and restless; has hypotension and cool, pale, clammy skin.

Patient has a history of trauma, possibly with external bleeding, and reports thirst.	Patient has a history of myocardial infarction (MI) or heart failure.	Patient has a history of recent cardiac surgery or catheterization, chest trauma, pericardial effusion, or anticoagulant therapy.	Patient has a history of MI or chronic heart or lung disease.
Check for flat neck veins, low urine output, and narrowed pulse pressure.	Check for distended neck veins, ventricular (S_3) gallop, crackles, and narrowed pulse pressure.	Check for distended neck veins, pulsus paradoxus, and muffled heart sounds.	Check for irregular heart rate, severe tachycardia, and bradycardia.
If your examination reveals these findings, suspect *hypovolemic shock.*	If your examination reveals these findings, *suspect cardiogenic shock.*	If your examination reveals these findings, suspect *cardiac tamponade.*	If your examination reveals these findings, suspect *arrhythmias.*

Administer oxygen by nasal cannula and insert an I.V. line for fluid infusion. Begin cardiac monitoring and check vital signs every 5 to 15 minutes. A central venous pressure line, an arterial line, or a pulmonary artery catheter may have to be inserted. Be prepared for emergency resuscitation, if necessary.

Anticipate colloid or crystalloid replacement, or both.	Anticipate administering nitroprusside, dopamine, and dobutamine.	Anticipate pericardiocentesis.	Anticipate administering antiarrhythmics or delivering electroshock therapy, or both.

or affects one extremity. They'll also depend on associated signs and symptoms. Use the flowchart below to help you establish priorities for managing this emergency successfully.

Examine affected extremity for cool, mottled skin and pain.	If your examination reveals these findings, suspect *arterial occlusive disease*.	Prepare the patient for diagnostic tests, such as arteriography, aortography, or Doppler ultrasonography, to confirm or rule out arterial occlusion. Do not elevate the affected extremity. Start an I.V. line in an unaffected arm or leg, and administer heparin or streptokinase, as required. Anticipate preparing the patient for emergency embolectomy or peripheral angioplasty.

Patient has a history of trauma, congenital heart disease, or hypertension and reports severe, tearing chest pain.	Patient has a history of severe infection—commonly gram-negative, urinary, or respiratory infection.	Patient has a history of an insect sting, drug ingestion, or exposure to other possible allergen.	Patient has a history of venous stasis or deep vein thrombosis and reports sharp, substernal chest pain.
Check for pulse quality and blood pressure variation between extremities.	Check for fever, chills, and widened pulse pressure.	Check for urticaria, wheezing or stridor, and dyspnea.	Check for dyspnea, crackles, pleural friction rub, and hemoptysis.
If your examination reveals these findings, suspect *dissecting aortic aneurysm or aortic coarctation*.	If your examination reveals these findings, suspect *septic shock*.	If your examination reveals these findings, suspect *anaphylactic shock*.	If your examination reveals these findings, suspect *pulmonary embolism*.

Administer oxygen by nasal cannula and insert an I.V. line for fluid infusion. Begin cardiac monitoring and check vital signs every 5 to 15 minutes. A central venous pressure line, an arterial line, or a pulmonary artery catheter may have to be inserted. Be prepared for emergency resuscitation, if necessary.

Anticipate preparing the patient for surgery and administering an antihypertensive or nitroprusside.	Anticipate administering antibiotics and vasopressors.	Anticipate emergency intubation or cricothyrotomy and administration of epinephrine.	Anticipate possible intubation and anticoagulant or thrombolytic therapy.

rowing pulse pressure, clammy skin, a drop in urine output to less than 25 ml/hour, confusion, decreased LOC, and possibly hypothermia.

In *septic shock*, all pulses in the extremities first become weak. Depending on the degree of vascular collapse, pulses may then become uniformly absent. Shock is heralded by chills, sudden fever, and possibly nausea, vomiting, and diarrhea. Typically, the skin is flushed, warm, and dry, and tachycardia and tachypnea occur. As shock progresses, thirst, hypotension, anxiety, restlessness, and confusion develop. Pulse pressure narrows and the skin becomes cold, clammy, and cyanotic. The patient experiences severe hypotension, oliguria or anuria, respiratory failure, and coma.

● *Thoracic outlet syndrome.* A patient with this syndrome may have a gradual or abrupt weakness or loss of the pulses in the arms, depending on how quickly vessels in the neck compress. These pulse changes commonly occur after the patient works with his hands above his shoulders, lifts a weight, or abducts his arm. Paresthesia and pain occur along the ulnar distribution of the arm and disappear immediately when the patient returns his arm to a neutral position. In addition, the patient may have asymmetrical blood pressure and cool, pale skin.

Other causes
● *Treatments.* Localized pulse absence may occur distal to arteriovenous fistulas or shunts for dialysis.

Special considerations
Continue to monitor the patient's vital signs to detect untoward changes in his condition. Monitor hemodynamic status by measuring daily weight and hourly or daily intake and output and by assessing central venous pressure.

Pediatric pointers
Radial, dorsal pedal, and posterior tibial pulses aren't easily palpable in infants and small children, so be careful not to mistake these normally hard-to-find pulses for weak or absent pulses. Instead, palpate the brachial, popliteal, or femoral pulses to evaluate arterial circulation to the extremities. In children and young adults, weak or absent femoral and more distal pulses may indicate coarctation of the aorta.

PULSE, BOUNDING

Produced by large waves of pressure as blood ejects from the left ventricle with each contraction, a bounding pulse is strong and easily palpable and may be visible over superficial peripheral arteries. It's characterized by regular, recurrent expansion and contraction of the arterial walls and isn't obliterated by the pressure of palpation. (See *Evaluating peripheral pulses.*) A healthy person develops a bounding pulse during exercise, pregnancy, or periods of anxiety. However, this sign also results from fever and certain endocrine, hematologic, and cardiovascular disorders that increase the basal metabolic rate.

History and physical examination
After you detect a bounding pulse, check other vital signs, then auscultate the heart and lungs for any abnormal sounds, rates, or rhythms. Ask the patient if he's noticed any weakness, fatigue, shortness of breath, or other health changes. Review his medical history for hyperthyroidism, anemia, or cardiovascular disorders, and ask about his use of alcohol.

Common medical causes
● *Alcoholism (acute).* Vasodilation of acute alcoholism produces a rapid, bounding pulse and flushed face. An odor of alcohol on the breath and an ataxic gait are common. Other findings may include hypothermia, bradypnea, labored and

EXAMINATION TIP

EVALUATING PERIPHERAL PULSES

The rate, amplitude, and symmetry of peripheral pulses provide important clues to cardiac function and the quality of peripheral perfusion. To gather these clues, palpate peripheral pulses lightly with the pads of your index, middle, and ring fingers as space permits.

Rate. Count all pulses for at least 30 seconds (60 seconds when recording vital signs). The normal rate is between 60 and 100 beats/minute.

Amplitude. Palpate the blood vessel during ventricular systole. Describe pulse amplitude by using a scale like the one below:
4+ bounding

3+ normal

2+ difficult to palpate

1+ weak, thready

0 absent

Use a stick figure to easily document the location and amplitude of all pulses.

Symmetry. Simultaneously palpate pulses (except the carotid pulse) on both sides of the patient's body and note any inequality. Always assess peripheral pulses methodically, moving from the arms to the legs.

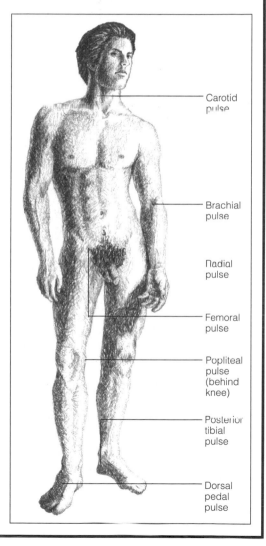

Carotid
pulse

Brachial
pulse

Radial
pulse

Femoral
pulse

Popliteal
pulse
(behind
knee)

Posterior
tibial
pulse

Dorsal
pedal
pulse

loud respirations, nausea, vomiting, diuresis, decreased level of consciousness, and seizures.

• *Aortic insufficiency.* Sometimes called a water-hammer pulse, the bounding pulse associated with this condition is characterized by a rapid, forceful expansion of the arterial pulse followed by rapid contraction. Widened pulse pressure also occurs. *Acute aortic insufficiency* may produce findings of left-sided heart failure and cardiovascular collapse, such as weakness, severe dyspnea, hypotension, a ventricular gallop (S_3), and tachycardia. Additional findings may include pallor, chest pain, palpitations, or strong, abrupt carotid pulsations. The patient may also have pulsus bisferiens, an early systolic murmur, a murmur heard over the femoral artery during systole and diastole, and a high-pitched diastolic murmur that starts with the second heart sound. An apical diastolic rumble (Austin Flint murmur) may also occur, especially with heart failure.

Most patients with *chronic aortic insufficiency* remain asymptomatic until age 40 or 50, when exertional dyspnea, increased fatigue, orthopnea and, eventually, paroxysmal nocturnal dyspnea may develop.

• *Febrile disorder.* Fever can cause a bounding pulse. Accompanying findings reflect the specific disorder.

• *Thyrotoxicosis.* This disorder produces a rapid, full, bounding pulse. Associated findings may include tachycardia, palpitations, an S3 or S4 gallop, weight loss despite increased appetite, and heat intolerance. The patient also may have diarrhea, an enlarged thyroid, dyspnea, tremors, nervousness, chest pain, exophthalmos, and signs of cardiovascular collapse. His skin will be warm, moist, and diaphoretic, and he may be hypersensitive to heat.

Special considerations
Prepare the patient for diagnostic laboratory and radiographic studies. If bounding pulse occurs with rapid or irregular heartbeat, you may need to connect him to a cardiac monitor for further evaluation.

Pediatric pointers
Bounding pulse can be normal in infants or children, because arteries lie close to the skin surface. It can also result from patent ductus arteriosus if the left-to-right shunt is large.

PULSE PRESSURE, NARROWED

Pulse pressure, the difference between systolic and diastolic blood pressures, is measured by sphygmomanometry or intra-arterial monitoring. Normally, systolic pressure exceeds diastolic by about 40 mm Hg. Narrowed pressure—a difference of less than 30 mm Hg—occurs when peripheral vascular resistance increases, cardiac output declines, or intravascular volume markedly decreases. (See *Understanding pulse pressure changes.*) In conditions that cause mechanical obstruction such as aortic stenosis, pulse pressure is directly related to the severity of the underlying condition. Usually a late sign, narrowed pulse pressure alone does not signal an emergency, even though it commonly occurs in shock and other life-threatening disorders.

History and physical examination
After you detect a narrowed pulse pressure, check for other signs of heart failure, such as hypotension, tachycardia, dyspnea, distended neck veins, pulmonary crackles, and decreased urine output. Also check for changes in skin temperature or color, strength of peripheral pulses, and level of consciousness (LOC). Auscultate the heart for murmurs. Ask about a history of chest pain, dizziness, or syncope.

UNDERSTANDING PULSE PRESSURE CHANGES

Two major factors affect pulse pressure: the amount of blood, or *stroke volume,* that the ventricles eject into the arteries with each beat and the arteries' *peripheral resistance* to blood flow. These two factors affect systolic and diastolic blood pressure and, as a result, pulse pressure.

For example, pulse pressure narrows when systolic pressure falls (lower right), diastolic pressure rises (upper left), or both. These changes reflect decreased stroke volume, increased peripheral resistance, or both.

Pulse pressure widens when systolic pressure rises (upper right), diastolic pressure falls (lower left), or both. These changes reflect increased stroke volume, decreased peripheral resistance, or both.

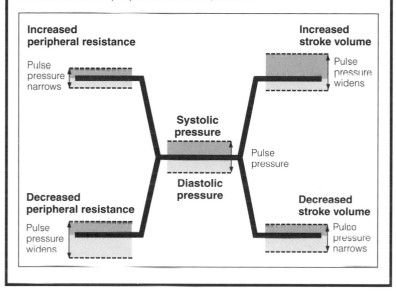

Common medical causes

• *Cardiac tamponade.* In this life-threatening disorder, pulse pressure narrows approximately 10 to 20 mm Hg. Pulsus paradoxus, neck vein distention, hypotension, and muffled heart sounds are classic. The patient may be anxious, restless, and cyanotic, with clammy skin and chest pain. He may exhibit dyspnea, tachypnea, decreased LOC, and a weak, rapid pulse. Pericardial friction rubs and hepatomegaly may also occur.

• *Heart failure.* Narrowed pulse pressure occurs relatively late in heart failure. It may accompany tachypnea, pal-

pitations, dependent edema, steady weight gain despite nausea and anorexia, chest tightness, slowed mental response, hypotension, diaphoresis, pallor, and oliguria. Assessment reveals a ventricular gallop, inspiratory crackles, and possibly a tender, palpable liver. Later, dullness develops over the lung bases, and hemoptysis, cyanosis, marked hepatomegaly, and marked pitting edema may occur.

• *Shock.* In *anaphylactic shock,* narrowed pulse pressure occurs late, preceded by a rapid, weak pulse that soon becomes uniformly absent. Within seconds or minutes after exposure to an allergen, the patient experiences hypotension, anxiety, restlessness, and feelings of doom, along with intense itching, a pounding headache, and possibly urticaria. Other possible findings include dyspnea, stridor, and hoarseness; chest or throat tightness; skin flushing; nausea, abdominal cramps, and urinary incontinence; and seizures.

In *cardiogenic shock*, narrowed pulse pressure occurs relatively late. Typically, peripheral pulses are absent and central pulses are weak. A drop in systolic pressure to 30 mm Hg below baseline, or a sustained reading below 80 mm Hg not attributable to medication produces poor tissue perfusion. Poor perfusion produces tachycardia, tachypnea, cyanosis, oliguria, restlessness, confusion, obtundation, and cold, pale, clammy skin.

In *hypovolemic shock*, narrowed pulse pressure occurs as a late sign. All peripheral pulses become first weak and then uniformly absent. Deepening shock leads to hypotension, urine output of less than 25 ml/hour, confusion, decreased LOC, and possibly hypothermia.

In *septic shock*, narrowed pulse pressure is a relatively late sign. All peripheral pulses become first weak and then uniformly absent. As shock progresses, the patient develops oliguria, thirst, anxiety, restlessness, confusion, and hypotension. Extremities become cool and cyanotic; the skin becomes cold and clammy. In time, he develops severe hypotension, persistent oliguria or anuria, respiratory failure, and coma.

Special considerations

Monitor closely for changes in pulse rate or quality and for hypotension or diminished consciousness. Prepare the patient for diagnostic studies, such as echocardiography, to detect valvular heart disease or cardiac tamponade secondary to a pericardial effusion.

Pediatric pointers

In children, narrowed pulse pressure can result from congenital aortic stenosis as well as from disorders that affect adults.

PULSE PRESSURE, WIDENED

Pulse pressure is the difference between systolic and diastolic blood pressures. In healthy adults, systolic pressure is about 40 mm Hg higher than diastolic. Widened pulse pressure—a difference greater than 50 mm Hg—commonly occurs as a physiologic response to fever, hot weather, exercise, anxiety, anemia, or pregnancy. However, it can also result from certain neurologic disorders—especially life-threatening increased intracranial pressure (ICP)—or from cardiovascular disorders that cause backflow of blood into the heart with each contraction, such as aortic insufficiency. Widened pulse pressure can easily be identified by monitoring arterial blood pressure and is commonly detected during routine sphygmomanometric recordings.

Emergency interventions

 If the patient's level of consciousness (LOC) is decreased and you suspect that his widened pulse pressure results from increased ICP, check his vital signs. Maintain a patent airway, and prepare to hyperventilate the patient with a handheld resuscitation bag to help reduce partial pressure of arterial carbon dioxide and, thus, ICP. Perform a thorough neurologic examination to serve as a baseline for assessing subsequent changes. Use the Glasgow Coma Scale to evaluate the patient's LOC. Also check cranial nerve function—especially in cranial nerves III, IV, and VI—and assess pupillary reactions, reflexes, and muscle tone. Insertion of an ICP monitor may be necessary.

If you don't suspect increased ICP, ask about associated symptoms, such as chest pain, shortness of breath, weakness, fatigue, or syncope. Check for edema and auscultate for murmurs.

Common medical causes

● *Aortic insufficiency.* In acute aortic insufficiency, pulse pressure widens progressively as the valve deteriorates, and a bounding pulse and an atrial gallop (S_4) or ventricular gallop (S_3) develop. These signs may occur with chest pain; palpitations; pallor; strong, abrupt carotid pulsations; pulsus bisferiens; and signs of heart failure, such as crackles, dyspnea, and distended neck veins. Auscultation may reveal an early diastolic murmur (common) and an apical diastolic rumble (Austin Flint murmur).

● *Arteriosclerosis.* In this disorder, reduced arterial compliance causes progressive widening of pulse pressure, which becomes permanent without treatment of the underlying disorder. It's preceded by moderate hypertension and accompanied by signs of vascular insufficiency, such as claudication, angina, and speech and visual disturbances.

● *Febrile disorders.* Fever can cause widened pulse pressure. Accompanying symptoms vary depending on the specific disorder.

● *Increased intracranial pressure.* Widening pulse pressure is an intermediate to late sign of increased ICP. Although decreased LOC is the earliest and most sensitive indicator of this life-threatening condition, the onset and progression of widening pulse pressure also parallel rising ICP. (Even a gap of only 50 mm Hg can signal a rapid deterioration in the patient's condition.) Assessment reveals Cushing's triad: bradycardia, hypertension, and respiratory pattern changes. Other findings may include headache, vomiting, impaired or unequal motor movement, pupillary changes, and visual disturbances, such as blurring or photophobia.

Special considerations

If the patient has increased ICP, continually reevaluate his neurologic status and compare your findings carefully with those of previous evaluations. Be alert for restlessness, confusion, unresponsiveness, or decreased LOC, but remember that *subtle changes* in the patient's condition, rather than the abrupt development of any one sign or symptom, commonly signal increasing ICP.

Pediatric pointers

Increased ICP causes widened pulse pressure in children. Patent ductus arteriosus (PDA) can also cause it, but this sign may not be evident at birth. The older child with PDA experiences exertional dyspnea, with pulse pressure that widens even further on exertion.

PULSE RHYTHM ABNORMALITY

An abnormal pulse rhythm is an irregular expansion and contraction of the peripheral arterial walls. It may be persistent or sporadic, and rhythmic or arrhythmic. Detected by palpating the radial or carotid pulse, an abnormal rhythm is typically reported first by the patient, who complains of feeling palpitations. This important finding reflects an underlying cardiac arrhythmia, which may range from benign to life-threatening. (See *Abnormal pulse rhythm: Clue to cardiac arrhythmias,* pages 480 to 483.) Arrhythmias are commonly associated with cardiovascular, renal, respiratory, metabolic, and neurologic disorders as well as with the effects of certain drugs, diagnostic tests, and treatments.

Emergency interventions

 Quickly look for signs of reduced cardiac output, such as decreased level of conscious-

(Text continues on page 482.)

ABNORMAL PULSE RHYTHM: CLUE TO CARDIAC ARRHYTHMIAS

An abnormal pulse rhythm may be your only clue that a patient has a cardiac arrhythmia. But this sign doesn't help you pinpoint the specific type of arrhythmia. For that, you need a cardiac monitor or an electrocardiogram (ECG) machine. These devices record the electrical current generated by the heart's con-

ARRHYTHMIA

Sinus arrhythmia

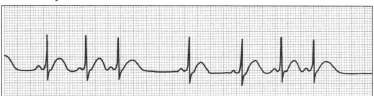

Premature atrial contractions (PACs)

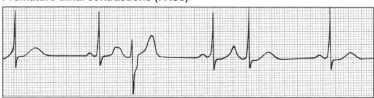

Paroxysmal atrial tachycardia

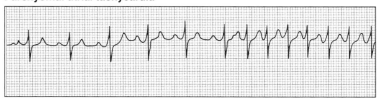

Atrial fibrillation

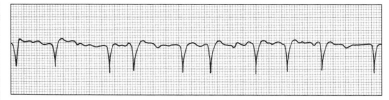

duction system and display this information on an oscilloscope screen or a strip-chart recorder. Besides rhythm disturbances, they can identify conduction defects and electrolyte imbalances. The ECG strips below show some common cardiac arrhythmias that can cause abnormal pulse rhythms.

PULSE RHYTHM AND RATE	CLINICAL IMPLICATIONS
Irregular rhythm; fast, slow, or normal rate	• Heart rate increases with inspiration and decreases with expiration. • May result from drugs, as in digitalis toxicity • Usually occurs in children and young adults
Irregular rhythm during PACs; fast, slow, or normal rate	• Occasional PAC may be normal. • Isolated PACs indicate atrial irritation—for example, from anxiety or excessive caffeine intake. Increasing PACs may herald other atrial arrhythmias • May result from heart failure, ischemic heart disease, acute respiratory failure, chronic obstructive pulmonary disease (COPD), or use of digitalis glycosides, aminophylline, or adrenergic drugs
Irregular rhythm at abrupt onset or end of arrhythmia; heart rate exceeds 140 beats/minute	• May occur in otherwise normal, healthy people with physical or psychological stress, hypoxia, or hypokalemia; may be associated with excessive use of caffeine or other stimulants, with use of marijuana, and with digitalis toxicity • May precipitate angina or heart failure
Irregular rhythm; atrial rate exceeds 400 beats/minute; ventricular rate usually 100 to 200 beats/minute	• May result from heart failure, COPD, hyperthyroidism, sepsis, pulmonary embolus, mitral valve disease, digitalis toxicity (rarely), atrial irritation, postcoronary bypass, or valve replacement surgery • Because atria don't contract, preload isn't consistent, so cardiac output changes with each beat. Emboli may also result.

(continued)

ABNORMAL PULSE RHYTHM: CLUE TO CARDIAC ARRHYTHMIAS *(continued)*

ARRHYTHMIA

Premature junctional contractions (PJCs)

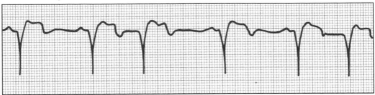

Second-degree atrioventricular (AV) heart block, Mobitz Type I (Wenckebach)

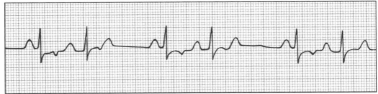

Second-degree AV heart block, Mobitz Type II

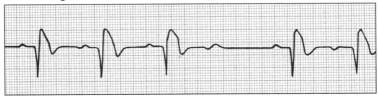

Premature ventricular contractions

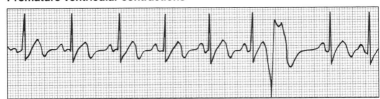

ness, hypotension, or dizziness. Promptly obtain an electrocardiogram and possibly a chest X-ray, and begin cardiac monitoring. Insert an I.V. line for emergency cardiac drugs, and give oxygen by nasal cannula or mask. Closely monitor vital signs, pulse quality, and cardiac rhythm because accompanying bradycardia or tachycardia may result in poor tolerance of the abnormal rhythm and cause further deterioration of cardiac output. Keep emergency intubation, cardioversion, and suction equipment handy.

PULSE RHYTHM AND RATE	CLINICAL IMPLICATIONS
Irregular rhythm during PJCs; fast, slow, or normal rate	● May result from myocardial infarction (MI) or ischemia, excessive caffeine intake, and most commonly digitalis toxicity (from enhanced automaticity)
Irregular rhythm; fast, slow, or normal rate	● Commonly transient; may progress to complete heart block ● May result from inferior wall MI, digitalis or quinidine toxicity, vagal stimulation, and arteriosclerotic heart disease
Irregular rhythm; slow or normal rate	● May progress to complete heart block ● May result from degenerative disease of conduction system, ischemia of AV node in anterior MI, anteroseptal infarction, or digitalis or quinidine toxicity
Usually irregular rhythm with a long pause after the premature beat; fast, slow, or normal rate	● Indicates ventricular irritability; may initiate ventricular tachycardia or ventricular fibrillation ● May result from heart failure, old or acute MI, contusion with trauma, myocardial irritation by a ventricular catheter, hypoxia, drug toxicity, electrolyte imbalance, or stress

History and physical examination

If the patient's condition permits, ask if he's experiencing any pain. If so, find out about onset and location. Does it radiate? Ask about a history of heart disease and treatments for arrhythmias. Obtain a medication history and check compliance. Also, ask about caffeine or alcohol use. Digitalis toxicity, cessation of antiarrhythmic drugs, and use of quinidine, sympathomimetics (such as epinephrine), caffeine, or alcohol may cause arrhythmias.

Now check the patient's apical and peripheral arterial pulses. An apical rate exceeding a peripheral arterial rate indicates a pulse deficit, which may also cause associated signs and symptoms of low cardiac output. Next, evaluate heart sounds: a long pause between S_1 (*lub*) and S_2 (*dub*) may indicate a conduction defect. A faint or absent S_1 and an easily audible S_2 may indicate atrial fibrillation or flutter. You may hear the two heart sounds close together on certain beats—possibly indicating premature atrial contractions—or other variations in heart rate or rhythm. Take the patient's apical and radial pulses while you listen for heart sounds. In some arrhythmias, such as premature ventricular contractions, you may hear the beat with your stethoscope but not feel it over the radial artery. This indicates an ineffective contraction that failed to produce a peripheral pulse. Now count the apical pulse for 60 seconds, noting the frequency of skipped peripheral beats. Report your findings to the doctor.

Common medical causes

• *Arrhythmias.* An abnormal pulse rhythm may be the only sign of a cardiac arrhythmia. The patient may complain of palpitations, a fluttering heartbeat, or weak and skipped beats. Pulses may be weak and rapid or slow. Depending on the specific arrhythmia, dull chest pain or discomfort and hypotension may occur. Associated findings, if any, reflect decreased cardiac output. Neurologic findings, for example, include confusion, dizziness, light-headedness, decreased LOC, and, sometimes, seizures. Other findings include decreased urine output, dyspnea, tachypnea, pallor, and diaphoresis.

Special considerations

The patient may require cardioversion therapy, before which he may need to be sedated. Prepare the patient for transfer to a cardiac or intensive care unit. If the patient remains in your care, he may require bed rest or help with ambulation,

depending on his condition. To prevent falls and injury, raise the side rails of the patient's bed and don't leave him unattended while he's sitting or walking. Check vital signs frequently to detect bradycardia, tachycardia, hypertension or hypotension, tachypnea, and dyspnea. Also monitor intake, output, and daily weight.

Collect blood samples for serum electrolyte, cardiac enzyme, and drug level studies. Prepare the patient for a chest X-ray and a 12-lead electrocardiogram (ECG). If possible, obtain a previous ECG to compare with current findings. Prepare the patient for 24-hour Holter monitoring. Stress to the patient the importance of keeping a diary of his activities and any symptoms that develop, to correlate with the incidence of arrhythmias.

Instruct the patient to avoid smoking and caffeine, which increase arrhythmias. If he has a history of failing to comply with prescribed antiarrhythmic therapy, help him develop strategies to overcome this.

Pediatric pointers

Arrhythmias also produce pulse rhythm abnormalities in children.

PULSUS ALTERNANS

A sign of severe left-sided heart failure, pulsus alternans is a beat-to-beat change in the size and intensity of a peripheral pulse. Although pulse rhythm remains regular, strong and weak contractions alternate. (See *Comparing arterial pressure waves.*) An alternation in the intensity of heart sounds and of existing heart murmurs may accompany this sign.

Pulsus alternans is thought to result from the change in stroke volume that occurs with beat-to-beat alteration in the left ventricle's contractility. Recumbency or exercise increases venous return

COMPARING ARTERIAL PRESSURE WAVES

The percussion wave in the *normal arterial pulse* reflects ejection of blood into the aorta (early systole). The tidal wave is the peak of the pulse wave (later systole). And the dicrotic notch marks the beginning of diastole.

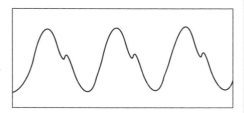

Pulsus alternans is a beat-to-beat alternation in pulse size and intensity. Although the rhythm of pulsus alternans is regular, the volume varies. If you take the blood pressure of a patient with this abnormality, you'll first hear a loud Korotkoff sound and then a soft sound, continually alternating. Pulsus alternans commonly accompanies states of poor contractility that occur with left-sided heart failure.

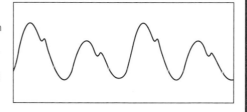

Pulsus paradoxus is an exaggerated drop in blood pressure during inspiration, resulting from an increase in negative intrathoracic pressure. A pulsus paradoxus that exceeds 10 mm Hg is considered abnormal and may result from cardiac tamponade, constrictive pericarditis, or severe lung disease.

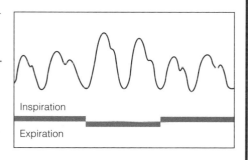

Inspiration

Expiration

and reduces the abnormal pulse, which commonly disappears with treatment for heart failure. Rarely, a patient with normal left ventricular function has pulsus alternans, but the abnormal pulse seldom persists for more than 10 to 12 beats.

Although most easily detected by sphygmomanometry, pulsus alternans can be detected by palpating the brachial, radial, or femoral artery when systolic pressure varies from beat to beat by more than 20 mm Hg. Because the small changes in arterial pressure that occur during normal respirations may obscure this abnormal pulse, you'll need to have the patient hold his breath during palpation. Apply *light* pressure to avoid obliterating the weaker pulse.

When using a sphygmomanometer to detect pulsus alternans, inflate the cuff 10 to 20 mm Hg above the systolic pressure as determined by palpation, then slowly deflate it. At first, you'll hear only the strong beats. With further deflation, all beats will become audible and palpable, and then equally intense. (The difference between this point and the peak systolic level is commonly used to determine the degree of pulsus alternans.) When the cuff is removed, pulsus alternans returns.

Occasionally, the weak beat is so small that no palpable pulse is detected at the periphery. This produces total pulsus alternans, an apparent halving of the pulse rate.

Emergency interventions

 Pulsus alternans indicates a critical change in the patient's status. After you detect it, be sure to quickly check other vital signs. Also closely evaluate the patient's heart rate, respiratory pattern, and blood pressure. In addition, auscultate for a ventricular gallop (S_3) and increased crackles.

Common medical causes

• *Left-sided heart failure.* In this disorder, pulsus alternans is commonly initiated by a premature beat. It's almost always associated with a ventricular gallop. Other findings may include hypotension and cyanosis. Possible respiratory findings include exertional and paroxysmal nocturnal dyspnea, orthopnea, tachypnea, Cheyne-Stokes respirations, hemoptysis, and crackles. Fatigue and weakness are common.

Special considerations

If left-sided heart failure develops suddenly, prepare the patient for transfer to an intensive or cardiac care unit. Meanwhile, elevate the head of his bed to promote respiratory excursion and increase oxygenation. Adjust the patient's current treatment plan to improve cardiac output, reduce the heart's workload, and promote diuresis.

Pediatric pointers

Pulsus alternans, which also occurs in a child with heart failure, may be difficult to assess if the child's crying or restless. Try to quiet the child by holding him, if his condition permits.

PULSUS PARADOXUS
[Paradoxical pulse]

Paradoxical pulse is an exaggerated decline in blood pressure during inspiration. Normally, systolic pressure decreases less than 10 mm Hg during inspiration. In pulsus paradoxus, however, it drops more than 10 mm Hg. When systolic pressure falls more than 20 mm Hg, the peripheral pulses may be barely palpable or may disappear during inspiration.

Pulsus paradoxus is thought to result from an exaggerated inspirational increase in negative intrathoracic pressure. Normally, systolic pressure drops during inspiration because of blood pooling in the pulmonary system. This, in turn, reduces left ventricular filling and stroke volume and transmits negative intrathoracic pressure to the aorta. Conditions associated with large intrapleural pressure swings, such as asthma, or those that reduce left heart filling, such as pericardial tamponade, produce paradoxical pulse.

To accurately detect and measure paradoxical pulse, use a sphygmomanometer or an intra-arterial monitoring device. Inflate the blood pressure cuff 10 to 20 mm Hg beyond the peak systolic pressure. Then deflate the cuff at a rate of 2 mm Hg/second until you hear the first Korotkoff sound during expiration. Note the systolic pressure. As you continue to slowly deflate the cuff, observe the patient's respiratory pattern. If a paradoxical pulse is present, the Korotkoff sounds will disappear with inspiration and return with expiration. Continue to deflate the cuff until you hear Korotkoff sounds during both inspiration and expiration, and again note the systolic pressure. Now subtract this reading from the first one to determine the degree of paradoxical pulse. A difference of more than 10 mm Hg is abnormal.

You can also detect paradoxical pulse by palpating the radial pulse over several cycles of slow inspiration and expiration. Marked pulse diminution during inspiration indicates paradoxical pulse. When you check for paradoxical pulse, remember that irregular heart rhythms and tachycardia cause variations in pulse amplitude and must be ruled out before a true paradoxical pulse can be identified.

Emergency interventions

 A paradoxical pulse may signal cardiac tamponade—a life-threatening complication of pericardial effusion that occurs when sufficient blood or fluid accumulates to compress the heart. After you detect paradoxical pulse, quickly take the patient's other vital signs. Check for additional signs and symptoms of cardiac tamponade, such as dyspnea, tachypnea, diaphoresis, distended neck veins, tachycardia, narrowed pulse pressure, and hypotension. Emergency pericardiocentesis to aspirate blood or fluid from the pericardial sac may be necessary. Then evaluate the effectiveness of pericardiocentesis by measuring the degree of pulsus paradoxus; it should decrease after aspiration.

History and physical examination

If the patient doesn't have cardiac tamponade, find out if he has a history of chronic cardiac or pulmonary disease. Ask about the development of associated signs and symptoms, such as a cough or chest pain. Then auscultate for abnormal breath sounds.

Common medical causes

● *Cardiac tamponade.* Pulsus paradoxus commonly occurs in this disorder. However, if intrapericardial pressure rises abruptly and profound hypotension occurs, paradoxical pulse may be difficult to detect. In severe tamponade, assessment also reveals these classic findings: hypotension, diminished or muffled heart sounds, and jugular vein distention. Related findings include chest pain, pericardial friction rub, narrowed pulse pressure, anxiety, restlessness, clammy skin, and hepatomegaly. Characteristic respiratory signs and symptoms include dyspnea, tachypnea, and cyanosis; the patient typically sits up and leans forward to facilitate breathing.

If cardiac tamponade develops gradually, paradoxical pulse may be accompanied by weakness, anorexia, and weight loss. The patient may also have chest pain, but he won't have muffled heart sounds or severe hypotension.

● *Chronic obstructive pulmonary disease (COPD).* The wide fluctuations in intrathoracic pressure that are characteristic of this disorder produce pulsus paradoxus and possibly tachycardia. Other findings vary but may include dyspnea, tachypnea, wheezing, productive or nonproductive cough, accessory muscle use, barrel chest, and clubbing. The patient may show labored, pursed-lip breathing after exertion or even at rest. Typically, he'll sit leaning forward to facilitate breathing. Auscultation reveals decreased breath sounds, rhonchi, and crackles. Weight loss, cyanosis, and edema may occur.

● *Pericarditis (chronic constrictive).* Paradoxical pulse can occur in up to 50% of patients with this disorder. Other findings include pericardial friction rub, chest pain, exertional dyspnea, orthopnea, hepatomegaly, and ascites. The patient also exhibits peripheral edema and Kussmaul's sign—distended neck veins that become more prominent on inspiration.

● *Pulmonary embolism (massive).* Decreased left ventricular filling and stroke volume in massive pulmonary embolism produces pulsus paradoxus. It also produces syncope and severe apprehension, dyspnea, tachypnea, and pleuritic chest pain. The patient appears cyanotic, with distended neck veins. He may succumb to circulatory collapse, with hypotension and a weak, rapid pulse. Infarction may produce hemoptysis, along with decreased breath sounds and a pleural friction rub over the affected area.

Special considerations

Prepare the patient for an echocardiogram to visualize cardiac motion and to help determine the causative disorder. Monitor his vital signs, and frequently check the degree of paradox. An increase in the degree of paradox may indicate recurring or worsening cardiac tamponade or impending respiratory arrest in severe COPD. Vigorous respiratory treatment—such as chest physiotherapy—may avert the need for endotracheal intubation.

Pediatric pointers

Paradoxical pulse commonly occurs in children with chronic pulmonary disease, especially during an acute asthma attack. Children with pericarditis may also develop pulsus paradoxus due to cardiac tamponade, although this disorder is more common in adults. A paradoxical pulse above 20 mm Hg is a reliable indicator of cardiac tamponade in these patients; a change of 10 to 20 mm Hg is equivocal.

PUPILS, NONREACTIVE

Nonreactive (fixed) pupils fail to constrict in response to light or dilate when the light is removed. The development of a unilateral or bilateral nonreactive response indicates an important change in the patient's condition and could signal a life-threatening emergency and possibly brain death. It also occurs with use of certain optic drugs.

To evaluate pupillary reaction to light, first test the patient's *direct light reflex.* Darken the room, and cover one of the patient's eyes while you hold open the opposite eyelid.

Using a bright penlight, bring the light toward the patient from the side and shine it directly into his opened eye. If normal, the pupil will promptly constrict. Now test the *consensual light reflex.* Hold the patient's eyelids open and shine the light into one eye while watching the pupil of the opposite eye. If normal, both pupils will promptly constrict. Repeat both procedures in the opposite eye. A unilateral or bilateral nonreactive response indicates dysfunction of cranial nerves II and III, which mediate the pupillary light reflex. (See *Innervation of direct and consensual light reflexes.*)

Emergency interventions

 If the patient is unconscious and develops unilateral or bilateral nonreactive pupil(s), quickly take his vital signs. Be alert for decerebrate or decorticate posture, bradycardia, elevated systolic blood pressure, widened pulse pressure, and the development of other untoward changes in the patient's condition. Remember, a unilateral dilated, nonreactive pupil may be an early sign of uncal brain herniation. Emergency surgery to try to decrease intracranial pressure (ICP) may be necessary. If the patient isn't already being treated for increased ICP, insert an I.V. line to administer diuretics, osmotics, and corticosteroids. You may also need to start the patient on controlled hyperventilation.

EXAMINATION TIP

INNERVATION OF DIRECT AND CONSENSUAL LIGHT REFLEXES

Two reactions—direct and consensual—constitute the pupillary light reflex. Normally, when a light is shined directly onto the retina of one eye, the parasympathetic nerves are stimulated to cause brisk constriction of that pupil—the *direct light reflex*. The pupil of the opposite eye also constricts— the *consensual light reflex*. The optic nerve (CN II) mediates the afferent arc of this reflex from each eye, while the oculomotor nerve (CN III) mediates the efferent arc to both eyes. A nonreactive or sluggish response in one or both pupils indicates dysfunction of these cranial nerves—usually due to degenerative disease of the central nervous system.

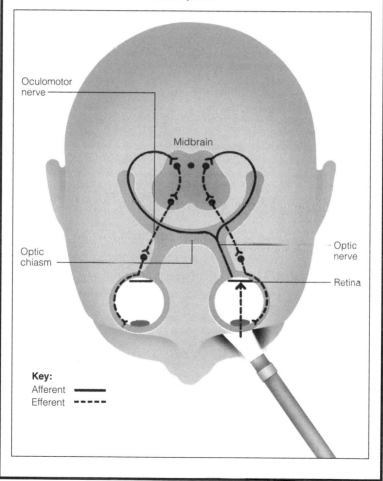

Oculomotor nerve

Midbrain

Optic chiasm

Optic nerve

Retina

Key:
Afferent ━━━━
Efferent ━ ━ ━ ━

History and physical examination

If the patient isn't unconscious, obtain a brief history. Ask him what type of eyedrops he's using, if any, and when they were last instilled. Also ask if he's experiencing any pain; if so, try to determine its location, intensity, and duration. Determine the patient's visual acuity in both eyes. Then test the pupillary reaction to accommodation: Normally, both pupils constrict equally as the patient shifts his glance from a distant to a near object.

Next, hold a penlight at the side of each eye and examine the cornea and iris for any abnormalities. Measure intraocular pressure with a tonometer. Or estimate intraocular pressure by placing your second and third fingers over the patient's closed eyelid. If the eyeball feels rock hard, suspect elevated intraocular pressure. Ophthalmoscopic and slit-lamp examinations of the eye will need to be performed. If the patient has experienced ocular trauma, don't manipulate the affected eye. After the examination, cover the affected eye with a protective metal shield, but don't let the shield rest on the globe.

Common medical causes

• *Botulism.* Bilateral mydriasis and nonreactive pupils usually appear 12 to 36 hours after ingestion of tainted food. Other early findings are blurred vision, diplopia, ptosis, strabismus, and extraocular muscle palsies, along with anorexia, nausea, vomiting, diarrhea, and dry mouth. Vertigo, deafness, hoarseness, nasal voice, dysarthria, and dysphagia follow. Progressive muscle weakness and absent deep tendon reflexes usually evolve over 2 to 4 days. This results in severe constipation and paralysis of respiratory muscles with respiratory distress.

• *Encephalitis.* As this disease progresses, initially sluggish pupils become dilated and nonreactive. Decreased accommodation and other symptoms of cranial nerve palsies, such as dysphagia, devel-

op. Within 48 hours after onset, encephalitis causes a decreased level of consciousness, a high fever, headache, vomiting, and nuchal rigidity. Aphasia, ataxia, nystagmus, hemiparesis, and photophobia may occur with seizures.

• *Glaucoma (acute angle-closure).* In this ophthalmic emergency, examination reveals a moderately dilated, nonreactive pupil in the affected eye. Conjunctival injection, corneal clouding, and decreased visual acuity also occur. The patient experiences sudden blurred vision, followed by excruciating pain in and around the affected eye. He typically reports seeing halos around white lights at night. Severely elevated intraocular pressure frequently induces nausea and vomiting.

• *Iridoplegia.* This disease causes pupillary nonreactivity in the affected eye(s). Visual acuity also may decrease.

• *Oculomotor nerve palsy.* In many cases, the first signs of this oculomotor ophthalmoplegia are a dilated, nonreactive pupil and loss of the accommodation reaction. These findings may occur in one eye or both, depending on whether the palsy is unilateral or bilateral. Among the causes of total third cranial nerve paralysis is life-threatening brain herniation. *Central herniation* causes bilateral midposition nonreactive pupils, whereas *uncal herniation* initially causes a unilateral dilated, nonreactive pupil. Other common findings include diplopia, ptosis, outward deviation of the eye, and inability to elevate or adduct the eye. Additional findings depend on the palsy's underlying cause.

• *Uveitis.* A small, nonreactive pupil typifies *anterior uveitis,* appearing suddenly with severe eye pain, conjunctival injection, and photophobia. In *posterior uveitis,* similar features develop insidiously, along with blurred vision and distorted pupil shape.

Other causes

• *Drugs.* Installation of topical mydriatics and cycloplegics may induce a temporarily nonreactive pupil in the affected eye. Use of glutethimide and deep ether anesthesia produces medium-sized or slightly enlarged pupils, which remain nonreactive for several hours. Opiates, such as heroin and morphine, cause pinpoint pupils with a minimal light response that can be seen only with a magnifying glass. And atropine poisoning produces widely dilated, nonreactive pupils.

Special considerations

If the patient is conscious, monitor his pupillary light reflex to detect changes. If he's unconscious, close his eyes to prevent corneal exposure. (Use tape to secure the eyelids, if needed.)

Pediatric pointers

Children have nonreactive pupils for the same reasons as adults. The most common cause is oculomotor nerve palsy from increased ICP.

PUPILS, SLUGGISH

A sluggish pupillary reaction is an abnormally slow pupil response to light. It can occur in one pupil or both, unlike the normal reaction, which is always bilateral. A sluggish reaction accompanies degenerative disease of the central nervous system and diabetic neuropathy. However, it can occur normally in elderly people, whose pupils become smaller and less responsive with age.

To assess pupillary reaction to light, first test the patient's *direct light reflex.* Darken the room, and cover one of the patient's eyes while you hold open the opposite eyelid. Using a bright penlight, bring the light toward the patient from the side and shine it directly into his opened eye. If normal, the pupil will promptly constrict. Now test the *consensual light reflex.* Hold both of the patient's eyelids open, and shine the light

into one eye while watching the pupil of the opposite eye. If normal, both pupils will promptly constrict. Repeat both procedures to test light reflexes in the opposite eye. A sluggish reaction in one or both pupils indicates dysfunction of cranial nerves II and III, which mediate the pupillary light reflex.

History and physical examination

After you detect a sluggish pupillary reaction, determine the patient's visual function. Start by testing visual acuity in both eyes. Then test the pupillary reaction to accommodation: The pupils should constrict equally as the patient shifts his glance from a distant to a near object.

Next, hold a penlight at the side of each eye and examine the cornea and iris for irregularities, scars, and foreign bodies. Measure intraocular pressure with a tonometer. Alternatively, you can estimate intraocular pressure without a tonometer by placing your fingers over the patient's closed eyelid. If the eyeball feels rock hard, suspect elevated intraocular pressure. An ophthalmoscopic and slit-lamp examination of the eye will also need to be performed.

Common medical causes

• *Adie's syndrome.* This syndrome produces abrupt onset of unilateral mydriasis and sluggish pupillary response, possibly progressing to a nonreactive response. The patient may complain of blurred vision and cramplike eye pain. Eventually, both eyes may be affected. Musculoskeletal assessment also reveals hypoactive or absent deep tendon reflexes in the arms and legs.

• *Encephalitis.* This disorder initially produces a bilateral sluggish pupillary response. Later, pupils become dilated and nonreactive, and decreased accommodation may occur, along with other cranial nerve palsies, such as dysphagia and facial weakness. Within 48 hours after onset, encephalitis causes a decreased level of consciousness, headache, high fever, vomiting, and nuchal rigidity. In addition, aphasia, ataxia, nystagmus, hemiparesis, and photophobia may occur. The patient may exhibit seizure activity and myoclonic jerks.

• *Herpes zoster.* The patient with herpes zoster affecting the nasociliary nerve may have a sluggish pupillary response. Examination of the conjunctiva will reveal follicles. Additional ocular findings include a serous discharge, absence of tears, ptosis, and extraocular muscle palsy.

• *Iritis (acute).* In this disorder, the affected eye exhibits a sluggish pupillary response and conjunctival injection. The pupil may remain constricted; if posterior synechiae have formed, the pupil will also be irregularly shaped. The patient will report sudden onset of eye pain and photophobia and may also have blurred vision.

• *Myotonic dystrophy.* In this disorder, sluggish pupillary reaction may be accompanied by lid lag, ptosis, miosis, and possibly diplopia. The patient may have decreased visual acuity from cataract formation. Muscular weakness and atrophy and testicular atrophy may occur.

• *Tertiary syphilis.* Sluggish pupillary reaction (especially in Argyll Robertson pupils) occurs in the late stage of neurosyphilis, along with marked weakness of the extraocular muscles, visual field defects, and possibly cataractous changes in the lens. The patient may complain of orbital rim pain, which worsens at night. Lid edema, decreased visual acuity, and exophthalmos may also occur. Tertiary lesions appear on the skin and mucous membranes. Liver, respiratory, cardiovascular, and additional neurologic dysfunction may also occur.

• *Wernicke's disease.* Initially, this disorder produces intention tremor accompanied by sluggish pupillary reaction. Later, pupils may become nonreactive. Additional ocular findings include diplopia, gaze paralysis, nystagmus, ptosis, decreased visual acuity, and conjunctival injection. The patient may also exhibit postural hypotension, tachycardia, ataxia, apathy, and confusion.

Special considerations
A sluggish pupillary reaction isn't diagnostically significant, although it occurs in a variety of disorders.

Pediatric pointers
Children experience sluggish pupillary reactions for the same reasons as adults.

PURPURA

Purpura is the extravasation of red blood cells from the blood vessels into the skin, subcutaneous tissue, or mucous membranes. It's characterized by discoloration—usually purplish or brownish red—that's easily visible through the epidermis. Purpuric lesions include petechiae, ecchymoses, and hematomas. (See *Identifying purpuric lesions*.) Purpura differs from erythema in that it doesn't blanch with pressure because it involves blood in the tissues, not just dilated vessels.

Purpura results from damage to the endothelium of small blood vessels, coagulation defects, ineffective perivascular support, capillary fragility and permeability, or a combination of these factors. In turn, these faulty hemostatic factors can result from thrombocytopenia or other hematologic disorders, invasive procedures, and the use of anticoagulant drugs.

Additional causes are nonpathologic. Purpura can be a consequence of aging, when loss of collagen decreases connective tissue support of upper skin blood vessels. In the elderly or cachectic person, skin atrophy and inelasticity and loss of subcutaneous fat increase susceptibility to minor trauma, causing purpura to appear along the veins of the forearms, hands, legs, and feet. Prolonged cough-

EXAMINATION TIP

IDENTIFYING PURPURIC LESIONS

Petechiae are painless, round, pinpoint lesions, 1 to 3 mm in diameter. Caused by extravasation of red blood cells into cutaneous tissue, these red or brown lesions usually arise on dependent portions of the body. They appear and fade in crops and can group to form ecchymoses.

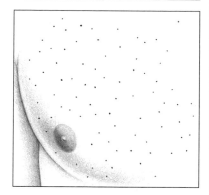

Ecchymoses, another form of blood extravasation, are larger than petechiae. These purple, blue, or yellow-green bruises vary in size and shape and can arise anywhere on the body as a result of trauma. Ecchymoses usually appear on the arms and legs of patients with bleeding disorders.

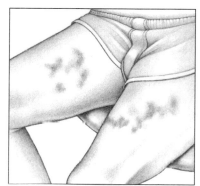

Hematomas are palpable ecchymoses that are painful and swollen. Usually the result of trauma, superficial hematomas are red, whereas deep hematomas are blue. Hematomas commonly exceed 1 cm in diameter, but their size varies widely.

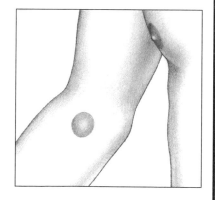

ing or vomiting can produce crops of petechiae in loose face and neck tissue. Violent muscle contraction, as occurs in seizures or weight lifting, sometimes results in localized ecchymoses from increased intraluminal pressure and rupture. High fever, which increases capillary fragility, can also produce purpura.

History and physical examination

After you detect purpura, ask the patient when he first noticed the lesion and if he has also noticed other lesions on his body. Does he or any member of his family have a history of bleeding disorders or easy bruising? Find out what medications the patient is taking, if any, and ask him to describe his diet. Ask about recent trauma or transfusions and the development of associated signs, such as epistaxis, bleeding gums, hematuria, and hematochezia. Also ask about systemic complaints such as fever, which may suggest infection. If the patient is female, ask about heavy menstrual flow.

Inspect the patient's entire skin surface to determine the type, size, location, distribution, and severity of purpuric lesions. Also inspect the mucous membranes. Remember that the same mechanisms that cause purpura can also cause internal hemorrhage, although purpura isn't a cardinal indicator of this condition.

Common medical causes

• *Autoerythrocyte sensitivity.* In this syndrome, painful ecchymoses appear either singly or in groups, usually preceded by local itching, burning, or pain. Common associated findings include epistaxis, hematuria, hematemesis, menometrorrhagia, abdominal pain, diarrhea, nausea, vomiting, syncope, headache, and chest pain. This syndrome can be linked to a psychiatric disorder, with associated anxiety, depression, hysteria, and masochism.

• *Disseminated intravascular coagulation.* This syndrome can cause varying degrees of purpura, depending on its severity and underlying cause. Rarely, the patient develops life-threatening purpura fulminans, with symmetrical cutaneous and subcutaneous lesions on the arms and legs. Or he may have cutaneous oozing, hematemesis, or bleeding from incision or needle insertion sites. Other findings may include acrocyanosis, nausea, dyspnea, seizures, signs of acute tubular necrosis (such as oliguria), and severe muscle, back, and abdominal pain.

• *Dysproteinemias.* In *multiple myeloma,* petechiae and ecchymoses accompany other bleeding tendencies: hematemesis, epistaxis, gum bleeding, and excessive bleeding after surgery. Similar findings occur in *cryoglobulinemia,* which may also produce malignant maculopapular purpura. *Hyperglobulinemia* typically begins insidiously with occasional attacks of purpura over the lower legs and feet. Attacks eventually become more frequent and extensive, involving the entire lower leg and possibly the trunk. Purpura usually occurs after prolonged standing or exercise and may be heralded by skin burning or stinging. Leg edema, knee or ankle pain, and low-grade fever may precede or accompany purpura, which gradually fades over 1 to 2 weeks. Persistent pigmentation develops after repeated attacks.

• *Easy bruising syndrome.* This syndrome is characterized by recurrent bruising on the legs, arms, and trunk, either spontaneously or following minor trauma. Bruising may be preceded by pain and is more common in women than in men, especially during menses.

• *Ehlers-Danlos syndrome.* Besides petechiae, this syndrome features easy bruising, epistaxis, gum bleeding, hematuria, melena, menorrhagia, and excessive bleeding after surgery. It characteristically produces hyperextensible joints, increased skin and blood vessel fragility, repeated dislocations of the temporomandibular joint, and soft, velvety, hyperelastic skin.

● *Idiopathic thrombocytopenic purpura (ITP).* Chronic ITP typically begins insidiously, with scattered petechiae that are most common on the distal arms and legs. Deep-lying ecchymoses may also occur. Other findings include epistaxis, easy bruising, hematuria, hematemesis, and menorrhagia.

● *Leukemia.* This neoplastic disorder produces widespread petechiae on the skin, mucous membranes, retina, and serosal surfaces that persist throughout the course of the disease. Confluent ecchymoses are uncommon but may occur. The patient may also have swollen and bleeding gums, epistaxis, and other bleeding tendencies. Lymphadenopathy and splenomegaly are common.

Acute leukemias also produce severe prostration and high fever and may cause dyspnea, tachycardia, palpitations, and abdominal or bone pain. Confusion, headache, seizures, vomiting, papilledema, and nuchal rigidity may occur late in the disease.

Chronic leukemias begin insidiously with minor bleeding tendencies, malaise, fatigue, pallor, low-grade fever, anorexia, and weight loss.

● *Myeloproliferative disorders.* These disorders, which include polycythemia vera, paradoxically can cause hemorrhage accompanied by ecchymoses and ruddy cyanosis. The oral mucosa takes on a deep purplish red hue, and slight trauma causes swollen gums to bleed. Other findings include pruritus, urticaria, and such nonspecific signs and symptoms as lethargy, weakness, fatigue, and weight loss. The patient typically complains of headache, a sensation of fullness in the head, and rushing in the ears; dizziness and vertigo; dyspnea; paresthesia of the fingers; double or blurred vision and scotoma; and epigastric distress. He may also experience intermittent claudication, hypertension, hepatosplenomegaly, and impaired mentation.

● *Nutritional deficiencies.* In *vitamin C deficiency,* the characteristic pattern of purpura is perifollicular petechiae, which coalesce to form ecchymoses, in the "saddle area" of the thighs and buttocks. Additional hemorrhage occurs in arm and leg muscles (with phlebothrombosis), viscera, joints (with limb and joint pain), and nail beds. Related findings include scaly dermatitis, pallor, dry mouth, poor wound healing, and tender, swollen, bleeding gums and loosened teeth. Nonspecific symptoms include weakness, lethargy, and anorexia. Irritability, depression, insomnia, and hysteria may also develop.

Vitamin K deficiency produces abnormal bleeding tendencies, such as ecchymosis, gum bleeding, epistaxis, and hematuria. It also causes GI and intracranial bleeding.

Vitamin B_{12} deficiency can cause varying degrees of purpura. Its GI effects include anorexia, nausea, vomiting, weight loss, abdominal discomfort, and jaundice. Dyspnea, peripheral neuropathies, ataxia, glossitis, and occasional depression also occur.

Folic acid deficiency also can cause varying degrees of purpura. The patient may complain of fatigue, weakness, dyspnea, palpitations, nausea, and anorexia. He may be irritable and forgetful and report headaches and fainting spells. Additional findings include pallor, slight jaundice, and glossitis.

● *Systemic lupus erythematosus.* This chronic inflammatory disorder may produce purpura accompanied by other cutaneous findings, such as ulceration, diffuse alopecia, telangiectasis, urticaria, and scaly patches on the scalp, face, neck, and arms. The characteristic butterfly rash appears in the disorder's acute phase. Commonly associated signs and symptoms include nondeforming joint pain and stiffness, Raynaud's phenomenon, seizures, psychotic behavior, photosensitivity, fever, anorexia, weight loss, and lymphadenopathy.

● *Thrombotic thrombocytopenic purpura.* Generalized purpura is usually a

ASSESSING FOR CHILD ABUSE

When caring for a child with non-pathologic purpuric lesions or other injuries, be sure to assess him for possible abuse. Abuse can be physical, psychological, emotional, or sexual. Be aware that an abuser can be anyone, not just a parent. Risk factors for abusers include high stress levels or poor coping skills, lack of social support, and a family history of abuse.

Try to examine the child in private. Suspect child abuse if you detect multiple bruises, lacerations, or abrasions in various stages of healing. Observe for unusual skin markings or scars that may indicate the object used, such as teeth, a hand, a belt, or a burning cigarette.

The child may have fractures, immersion (or "branding") burns, head trauma, retinal hemorrhages, oral irritation, internal injuries, or genital and rectal trauma. Check the child's records to see if he has been treated for similar injuries in the past. Observe his general appearance. He may seem unkempt, as if neglected, or be dressed inappropriately. Observe his behavior. The abused child may have a blank look, seem passive or anxious, display erratic or sexual behavior, cling to or move away from his parents, or avoid your touch. He may be developmentally delayed.

Note the parents' behavior. They may be uncooperative, evasive, or demanding, or they may not take the child's injuries seriously. The history they give may seem inconsistent with your findings. They may make excuses or blame others, including the child, for the injuries. Remain nonjudgmental even if you suspect abuse. Offer support through referrals to counselors and social workers.

Your priority is the safety of the child. After treating his injuries and collecting evidence when appropriate, make appropriate psychiatric and social support service referrals.

Document your assessment and actions thoroughly and objectively. Become familiar with your institution's protocol for notifying designated authorities because the law requires reporting of all incidents of suspected child abuse.

presenting sign in this disorder. Other presenting signs and symptoms vary but may include hematuria, vaginal bleeding, jaundice, and pallor. Most patients have fever, and some may also experience fatigue, weakness, headache, nausea, abdominal pain, and arthralgias. Hepatosplenomegaly may occur. Finally, neurologic changes—including seizures, paresthesia, cranial nerve palsies, vertigo, and altered level of consciousness—may develop along with renal failure.

● *Trauma.* Traumatic injury can cause local or widespread purpura.

Other causes

● *Diagnostic tests.* Invasive procedures, such as venipuncture and arterial catheterization, may produce local ecchymoses and hematomas due to extravasated blood.

● *Drugs.* The anticoagulants heparin and coumadin can produce purpura.

● *Surgery and other procedures.* Any procedures that disrupt circulation, coagulation, or platelet activity or production may cause purpura. These include pulmonary and cardiac surgery, radiation therapy, chemotherapy, hemodialysis, multiple blood transfusions with platelet-poor blood, and use of plasma expanders such as dextran.

Special considerations

Prepare the patient for diagnostic tests. These may include a peripheral blood smear, bone marrow examination, and blood tests to determine platelet count, bleeding and coagulation times, capillary fragility, clot retraction, one-stage prothrombin time, activated partial thromboplastin time, and fibrinogen levels.

Reassure the patient that purpuric lesions are not permanent and will fade if the underlying cause can be successfully treated. Warn the patient not to use cosmetic fade creams or other products in an attempt to reduce pigmentation. If the patient has a hematoma, apply pressure and cold compresses initially to help reduce bleeding and swelling. After the first 24 hours, apply hot compresses to help speed absorption of blood.

Pediatric pointers

Newborns commonly have petechiae, particularly on the head, neck, and shoulders, after vertex deliveries. Thought to result from the trauma of birth, these petechiae disappear within a few days. Other causes in infants include thrombocytopenia, vitamin K deficiency, and infantile scurvy.

The most common type of purpura in children is allergic purpura. Other causes in children include trauma, hemophilia, autoimmune hemolytic anemia, Gaucher's disease, thrombasthenia, congenital factor deficiencies, Wiskott-Aldrich syndrome, acute ITP, von Willebrand's disease, and the rare but life-threatening purpura fulminans, which usually follows bacterial or viral infection. As a child grows and tests his motor skills, the risk of accidents multiplies, and ecchymoses and hematomas commonly occur. However, when you assess a child with purpura, be alert for signs of possible child abuse: bruises in different stages of resolution, from repeated beatings; bruise patterns resembling a familiar object, such as a belt, hand, or thumb and finger; and bruises on the face, buttocks, or genitals, areas unlikely to be injured accidentally. (See *Assessing for child abuse.*)

PUSTULAR RASH

A pustular rash is made up of crops of pustules— vesicles and bullae that fill with purulent exudate. These lesions vary greatly in size and shape and can be generalized or localized to the hair follicles or sweat glands. Pustules appear in skin and systemic disorders, with use of certain drugs, and with exposure to skin irritants. For example, people who've been swimming in salt water commonly develop a papulopustular rash under the bathing suit or elsewhere on the body from irritation by sea organisms. Although many pustular lesions are sterile, a pustular rash usually indicates infection. Any vesicular eruption, or even acute contact dermatitis, can become pustular if a secondary infection occurs.

History and physical examination

Have the patient describe the appearance, location, and onset of the first pustular lesion. Did another type of skin lesion precede the pustule? Find out how the lesions spread. Ask what medications the patient takes and if he has applied any topical medication to his rash. If so, what type and when was it last applied? Find out if he has a family history of skin disorders.

Examine the entire skin surface, noting if it's dry, oily, moist, or greasy. Record the exact location and distribution of the skin lesions and their color, shape, and size.

Common medical causes

● *Acne vulgaris.* Pustules typify inflammatory lesions of this disorder, which occur with papules, nodules, cysts, and open comedones (blackheads). Lesions commonly appear on the face, shoulders, back, and chest. Other findings may include pain on pressure, pruritus, or burning. Chronic recurrent lesions produce scars.

● *Blastomycosis.* This fungal infection produces small, painless, nonpruritic macules or papules that can enlarge to well-circumscribed, verrucous, crusted, or ulcerated lesions edged by pustules. Localized infection may cause only one lesion; systemic infection, many lesions on the hands, feet, face, and wrists. Blastomycosis also produces signs and symptoms of pulmonary infection, such as pleuritic chest pain and a dry, hacking or productive cough with occasional hemoptysis.

● *Folliculitis.* This bacterial infection of hair follicles produces individual pustules, each pierced by a hair and possibly attended by pruritus. *Hot-tub folliculitis* produces pustules on areas covered by a bathing suit.

● *Furunculosis.* Crops of furuncles (purulent skin lesions involving hair follicles and sebaceous glands) typify this disorder. Furuncles usually begin as small, tender red pustules at the base of hair follicles. They typically occur on the face, neck, forearm, groin, axillae, buttocks, and legs and produce local pain, swelling, and redness. The pustules usually remain tense for 2 to 4 days and then become fluctuant. Rupture discharges pus and necrotic material. Then pain subsides, but erythema and edema may persist.

● *Impetigo contagiosa.* This vesiculopustular eruptive disorder, which occurs in nonbullous and bullous forms, usually is caused by streptococci or staphylococci. Vesicles form and break, and a crust forms from the exudate: a thick, yellow crust in streptococcal impetigo and a thin, clear crust in staphylococcal impetigo. Both forms usually produce pruritus.

● *Pompholyx.* This common recurrent disorder characteristically produces symmetrical vesicular lesions that can become pustular. The lesions appear on the palms and, less commonly, on the soles and may be accompanied by minimal erythema and recurrent pruritus.

● *Pustular miliaria.* This anhidrotic disorder causes pustular lesions that begin as tiny erythematous papulovesicles located at sweat pores. Diffuse erythema may radiate from the lesion. The rash and associated burning and pruritus worsen with perspiration.

● *Pustular psoriasis.* Small vesicles form and eventually become pustules in this disorder. The patient may report pruritus, burning, and pain. Localized pustular psoriasis usually affects the hands and feet. Generalized pustular psoriasis erupts suddenly in patients with psoriasis, psoriatic arthritis, or exfoliative psoriasis.

● *Rosacea.* This chronic hyperemic disorder commonly produces telangiectasia with acute episodes of pustules, papules, and edema. Characterized by persistent erythema, this disorder may begin as a flush covering the forehead, malar region, nose, and chin. Intermittent episodes gradually become more persistent, and the skin—instead of returning to its normal color—develops variations in the intensity of the erythema.

● *Scabies.* Threadlike channels or burrows under the skin characterize this disorder, which can also produce pustules, vesicles, and excoriations. The lesions are a few millimeters long, with a swollen nodule or red papule that contains the itch mite. In men, crusted lesions often develop on the glans, shaft, and scrotum. In women, lesions may form on the nipples. Lesions also develop on wrists, elbows, axillae, and waist. Related pruritus worsens with inactivity and warmth.

Other causes
• *Drugs.* Bromides and iodides commonly cause pustular rash. Other drug causes include adrenocorticotropic hormone, corticosteroids, dactinomycin, trimethadione, lithium, phenytoin, phenobarbital, isoniazid, oral contraceptives, androgens, and anabolic steroids.

Special considerations
Observe wound and skin isolation procedures until infection is ruled out by a Gram stain or culture and sensitivity test of the pustule's contents. If the organism is infectious, remember not to allow any drainage to touch unaffected skin. Instruct the patient to keep toilet articles and linen separate from those of other family members. Associated pain and itching, altered body image, or stress of isolation may result in loss of sleep, anxiety, and depression. Give medications as ordered to relieve pain and itching, and encourage the patient to express his feelings.

Pediatric pointers
Among the various disorders that produce pustular rash in children are varicella, erythema toxicum neonatorum, candidiasis, impetigo, and acrodermatitis enteropathica.

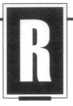

RACCOON EYES

Raccoon eyes refer to bilateral periorbital ecchymoses that don't result from facial trauma. Usually an indicator of basilar skull fracture, this sign develops when damage at the time of fracture tears the meninges and causes the venous sinuses to bleed into the arachnoid villi and the cranial sinuses. (See *Recognizing raccoon eyes*.)

Raccoon eyes may be the only indicator of basilar skull fracture, which isn't always visible on skull X-rays. Their appearance signals the need for careful assessment to detect any underlying trauma because a basilar skull fracture can injure cranial nerves, blood vessels, and the brain stem. Raccoon eyes can also occur after a craniotomy if the surgery causes a meningeal tear.

History and physical examination
After you detect raccoon eyes, check the patient's vital signs and try to find out when the head injury occurred. Then evaluate the extent of underlying trauma.

Start by evaluating the patient's level of consciousness (LOC) with the Glasgow Coma Scale. Next, evaluate function of the cranial nerves, especially the first (olfactory), third (oculomotor), fourth (trochlear), sixth (abducens), and seventh (facial). If the patient's condition permits, also test his visual acuity and gross hearing. Note any irregularities in the facial or skull bones as well as any swelling, localized pain, or lacerations of the face and scalp. Check for ecchymoses over the mastoid bone. Inspect for hemorrhage or cerebrospinal fluid (CSF) leakage from the nose or ears.

In addition, test any drainage with a sterile 4″ x 4″ gauze pad, and note if you find a halo sign—a circle of clear fluid that surrounds the drainage, indicating CSF. Also, use a Dextrostix to test any clear drainage for glucose. A positive test indicates CSF because mucus doesn't contain glucose.

Medical causes
• *Basilar skull fracture.* This injury produces raccoon eyes following head trauma that doesn't involve the orbital area. Associated signs and symptoms vary with the fracture site and may include pharyngeal hemorrhage, epistaxis, rhinorrhea, otorrhea, or a tympanic membrane bulging with blood or CSF. The patient may experience hearing difficulty, headache, nausea, vomiting, and altered LOC. He may also have a positive Battle's sign. In addition, most patients experience cranial nerve palsies.

Other causes
• *Surgery.* Raccoon eyes that occur after a craniotomy may indicate a meningeal tear and bleeding into the sinuses.

Special considerations
Keep the patient on complete bed rest. Perform a neurologic evaluation every hour to reevaluate his LOC. Also check vital signs hourly; be alert for such changes as bradypnea, bradycardia, hypertension, and fever. To avoid worsening a dural tear, instruct the patient not

RECOGNIZING RACCOON EYES

It's usually easy to differentiate raccoon eyes from the "black eye" associated with facial trauma. Raccoon eyes (below) are always bilateral. They develop 2 to 3 days after a closed head injury that results in basilar skull fracture. In contrast, the periorbital ecchymosis that occurs with facial trauma can affect one eye or both. It usually develops within hours of injury.

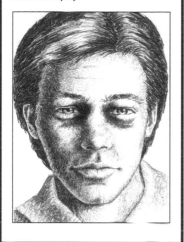

to blow his nose, cough vigorously, or strain. If otorrhea or rhinorrhea is present, don't attempt to stop the flow. Instead, place a sterile, loose gauze pad under the nose or ear to absorb the drainage. Monitor the amount and test it with a Dextrostix to confirm or rule out CSF leakage.

Never suction or pass a nasogastric tube through the patient's nose to prevent further tearing of the mucous membranes and infection. Observe the patient for signs and symptoms of meningitis, such as fever and nuchal rigidity, and expect to administer prophylactic antibiotics.

Prepare the patient for diagnostic tests, such as skull X-ray and possibly computed tomography. If the dural tear does not heal spontaneously, contrast cisternography may be performed to locate the tear, possibly followed by corrective surgery.

Pediatric pointers
Raccoon eyes in children are usually caused by basilar skull fracture following a fall.

REBOUND TENDERNESS
[Blumberg's sign]

A reliable indicator of peritonitis, rebound tenderness is intense, elicited abdominal pain caused by rebound of palpated tissue. (See *Eliciting rebound tenderness,* page 502.) The tenderness may be localized, as in an abscess, or generalized, as in perforation of an intra-abdominal organ. Rebound tenderness usually occurs with abdominal pain, tenderness, and rigidity. When a patient has sudden, severe abdominal pain, this symptom is usually elicited to detect peritoneal inflammation.

Emergency interventions
 If you elicit rebound tenderness in a patient who's experiencing constant, severe abdominal pain, quickly take his vital signs. Insert a large-bore I.V. catheter and begin administering I.V. fluids. Also insert an indwelling urinary catheter, and monitor intake and output. Give supplemental oxygen, as needed, and continue to monitor the patient for signs of shock, such as hypotension and tachycardia.

History and physical examination
When the patient's condition permits, ask him to describe the events that led up to the tenderness. Does movement, exer-

EXAMINATION TIP

ELICITING REBOUND TENDERNESS

To elicit rebound tenderness, place the patient in a supine position, and push your fingers deeply and steadily into the abdomen, as shown below. Then quickly release the pressure. Pain that results from the rebound of palpated tissue—rebound tenderness—indicates peritoneal inflammation or peritonitis.

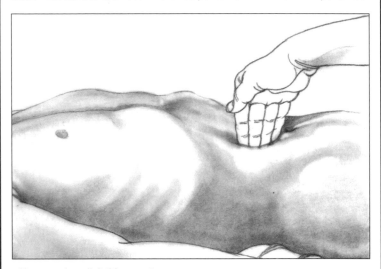

You can also elicit this symptom on a miniature scale by percussing the patient's abdomen lightly and indirectly (right). Better still, simply ask the patient to cough. This allows you to elicit rebound tenderness without having to touch the patient's abdomen and may also increase cooperation because he won't associate exacerbation of his pain with your actions.

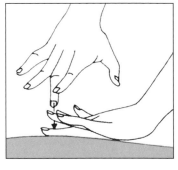

tion, or other activity relieve or aggravate the tenderness? Also ask about other signs and symptoms. Inspect the abdomen for distention, visible peristaltic waves, or scars. Then auscultate for bowel sounds and characterize their motili-

ty. Finally, palpate for associated rigidity or guarding.

Medical causes
• *Peritonitis.* In this life-threatening disorder, rebound tenderness is accompa-

nied by sudden and severe abdominal pain, which may be either diffuse or localized. Because movement worsens the patient's pain, he'll usually lie still. Typically, he'll display weakness, pallor, excessive sweating, and cold skin. He may also display hypoactive or absent bowel sounds; tachypnea; nausea; vomiting; abdominal distention, rigidity, and guarding; and a fever of 103° F (39.4° C) or higher. Inflammation of the diaphragmatic peritoneum may cause shoulder pain and hiccups.

Special considerations

Promote comfort by having the patient flex his knees or assume a semi-Fowler position. Be sure to administer analgesics carefully because these drugs could mask associated symptoms. In addition, you may administer antiemetics and antipyretics. However, because of decreased intestinal motility and the probability of surgery, do not give the patient *oral* drugs or fluids. Obtain samples of blood, urine, and feces for laboratory testing, and prepare the patient for chest and abdominal X-rays, sonograms, and computed tomography scans. Perform a rectal or pelvic examination.

Pediatric pointers

Eliciting rebound tenderness may be difficult in young children. Be alert for such clues as an anguished facial expression or intensified crying. When you elicit this symptom, use assessment techniques that produce minimal tenderness. For example, have the child hop or jump to allow tissue to rebound gently.

RETRACTIONS, COSTAL AND STERNAL

A cardinal sign of respiratory distress in infants and children, retractions are visible indentations of the soft tissue covering the chest wall. They may be suprasternal (directly above the sternum and clavicles), intercostal (between the ribs), subcostal (below the lower costal margin of the rib cage), or substernal (just below the xiphoid process). Retractions may be mild or severe, producing barely visible to deep indentations.

Emergency interventions

 If the child displays retractions, quickly check for other signs of respiratory distress, such as cyanosis, tachypnea, and tachycardia. In addition, prepare for suctioning, insertion of an artificial airway, and administration of oxygen.

Observe the depth and location of retractions. (See *Observing retractions,* page 504.) Also note the rate, depth, and quality of respirations. Look for accessory muscle use, nasal flaring during inspiration, or grunting during expiration. If the child has a cough, record the color, consistency, and odor of any sputum. Note if the child appears restless or lethargic. Finally, auscultate the child's lungs to detect abnormal breath sounds.

History and physical examination

When the child's condition permits, ask his parents about his medical history. Was he born prematurely? Was the delivery complicated? Ask about recent signs of an upper respiratory infection, such as a runny nose, cough, or low-grade fever. How often has the child had respiratory problems in the past year? Has he been in contact with anyone who has had a cold, the flu, or other respiratory ailments? Did he aspirate any food, liquid, or foreign body? Inquire about any personal or family history of allergies or asthma.

Common medical causes

• *Asthma attack.* Intercostal and suprasternal retractions may accompany an asthma attack. They are preceded by dyspnea, wheezing, a hacking cough, and pallor. Related features may include

OBSERVING RETRACTIONS

When observing retractions in infants and children, be sure to note their exact location—an important clue to the cause and severity of respiratory distress. For example, subcostal and substernal retractions usually result from lower respiratory tract disorders, whereas suprasternal retractions usually result from up- per respiratory tract disorders. Mild intercostal retractions alone may be normal. However, intercostal retractions accompanied by subcostal and substernal retractions may indicate moderate respiratory distress. Deep suprasternal retractions typically indicate severe distress.

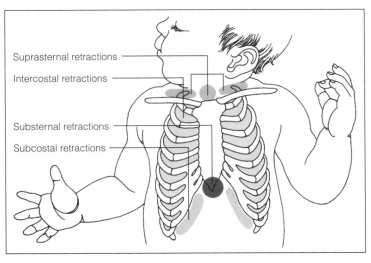

Suprasternal retractions

Intercostal retractions

Substernal retractions

Subcostal retractions

cyanosis or flushing, crackles, rhonchi, diaphoresis, tachycardia, tachypnea, a frightened, anxious expression and, in severe distress, nasal flaring.

● *Epiglottitis.* This life-threatening bacterial infection may precipitate severe respiratory distress with suprasternal, substernal, and intercostal retractions; stridor; nasal flaring; cyanosis; and tachycardia. Initially, it causes sudden onset of barking cough and high fever. Other early features include a sore throat, hoarseness, dysphagia, drooling, dyspnea, and restlessness. The child becomes panicky as edema makes breathing difficult. Total airway occlusion may occur in 2 to 5 hours.

● *Heart failure.* Usually linked to a congenital heart defect, this disorder may cause intercostal and substernal retractions along with nasal flaring, progressive tachypnea, and—in severe respiratory distress—grunting respirations, edema, and cyanosis. Other findings may include productive cough, crackles, jugular vein distention, tachycardia, right upper quadrant pain, anorexia, and fatigue.

● *Laryngotracheobronchitis (acute).* In this viral infection, substernal and intercostal retractions typically follow low to moderate fever, runny nose, poor appetite, barking cough, hoarseness, and inspiratory stridor. Associated signs and symptoms may include tachycardia; shallow, rapid respirations; restlessness; irritability; and pale, cyanotic skin.

• **Pneumonia (bacterial).** This disorder begins with signs of acute infection—such as high fever and lethargy—followed by subcostal and intercostal retractions, nasal flaring, dyspnea, tachypnea, grunting respirations, cyanosis, and productive cough. Auscultation may reveal diminished breath sounds, scattered crackles, and sibilant rhonchi over the affected lung. GI effects may include vomiting, diarrhea, and abdominal distention.

• **Respiratory distress syndrome.** Substernal and subcostal retractions are an early sign of this life-threatening syndrome, which affects premature infants shortly after birth. Associated early signs include tachypnea, tachycardia, and expiratory grunting. As respiratory distress worsens, intercostal and suprasternal retractions typically occur, and apnea or irregular respirations replace grunting. Other effects are nasal flaring, cyanosis, lethargy, and eventual unresponsiveness, bradycardia, and hypotension. Auscultation may detect crackles over the lung bases on deep inspiration and harsh, diminished breath sounds. Oliguria and peripheral edema may occur.

Special considerations

Continue to monitor the child's vital signs. Keep suction equipment and an appropriate-sized airway at bedside.

If the infant weighs less than 15 lb (6.8 kg), place him in an oxygen hood. If he weighs more, place him in a cool mist tent instead. Perform chest physical therapy with postural drainage to help mobilize and drain excess lung secretions.

Prepare the child for chest X-rays, cultures, and arterial blood gas analysis. Explain the procedures to his parents, too, and have them calm and comfort the child.

RHINORRHEA
[Nasal discharge]

Common but rarely serious, rhinorrhea is the free discharge of thin nasal mucus. It can be self-limiting or chronic, resulting from nasal, sinus, or systemic disorders or from basilar skull fracture. This sign can also result from sinus or cranial surgery, excessive use of vasoconstricting nose drops or sprays, or an irritant, such as tobacco smoke, dust, and fumes. Depending on the cause, the discharge may be clear, purulent, bloody, or serosanguineous.

History and physical examination

Begin the history by asking the patient if the discharge runs from both nostrils. Is the discharge intermittent or persistent? Did it begin suddenly or gradually? Does the position of his head affect the discharge?

Next, you should ask the patient to characterize the discharge. Is the discharge watery, bloody, purulent, or foul smelling? Is it copious or scanty? Does the discharge worsen or improve with the time of day?

In addition, find out if the patient is taking any medications, especially nose drops or sprays. Has the patient been exposed to nasal irritants at home or at work? Has he had a recent head injury?

Examine the patient's nose, checking airflow from each nostril. Evaluate the size, color, and condition of the turbinate mucosa (normally pale pink). Note if the mucosa is red, unusually pale, blue, or gray. Then examine the area beneath each turbinate. (See *Using a nasal speculum*, page 506.) Be sure to palpate over the frontal, ethmoid, and maxillary sinuses for tenderness.

To differentiate mucus from cerebrospinal fluid (CSF), collect a small amount of drainage on a glucose test strip.

USING A NASAL SPECULUM

To visualize the interior of the nares, you'll need a nasal speculum and a good light source such as a penlight. Hold the speculum in the palm of one hand and the penlight in the other hand. Have the patient tilt her head back slightly and rest it against a wall or other firm support, if possible. Insert the speculum blades about $1/2''$ (1.3 cm) into the nasal vestibule (as shown upper right).

Place your index finger on the tip of the patient's nose for stability. Carefully open the speculum blades. Shine the light source in the direction of the nares (as shown lower right).

Now, inspect the nares. The mucosa should be deep pink. Note any discharge, masses, lesions, or mucosal swellings. Check the nasal septum for perforation, bleeding, or crusting. Bluish turbinates suggest allergy. A rounded, elongated projection suggests a polyp.

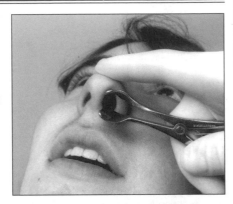

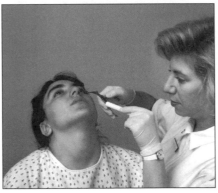

If CSF—which contains glucose—is present, the test will be positive. Finally, using a nonirritating substance, be sure to test for anosmia.

Common medical causes
- ***Basilar skull fracture.*** A tear in the dura can lead to cerebrospinal rhinorrhea, which increases when the patient lowers his head. Other findings may include epistaxis, otorrhea, and a bulging tympanum from blood or fluid.

In addition, a fracture may cause headache, facial paralysis, nausea, vomiting, impaired eye movement, ocular deviation, vision and hearing loss, depressed level of consciousness, Battle's sign, and raccoon eyes.
- ***Common cold.*** An initial watery nasal discharge may become thicker and mucopurulent. Related findings include sneezing, nasal congestion, a dry and hacking cough, sore throat, mouth breathing, and transient loss of smell and taste.

In addition, the patient may experience malaise, fatigue, myalgia, arthralgia, and a slight headache. The patient's lips will be dry, and his upper lip and nose red.

● ***Nasal or sinus tumors.*** Nasal tumors can produce intermittent, unilateral bloody or serosanguineous discharge, possibly purulent and foul smelling. Nasal congestion, postnasal drip, and headache may also occur. In advanced stages, paranasal sinus tumors may cause a cheek mass or eye displacement, facial paresthesia or pain, and nasal obstruction.

● ***Rhinitis.*** *Allergic rhinitis* produces an episodic, profuse watery discharge. (Mucopurulent discharge indicates infection.) Typical associated signs and symptoms include increased lacrimation; nasal congestion; itchy eyes, nose, and throat; postnasal drip; recurrent sneezing; mouth breathing; impaired sense of smell; and frontal or temporal headache. In addition, the turbinates are pale and engorged; the mucosa, pale and boggy.

In *atrophic rhinitis,* nasal discharge is scanty, purulent, and foul smelling. Nasal obstruction is common, and the crusts may bleed on removal. The mucosa is pale pink and shiny.

In *vasomotor rhinitis,* a profuse and watery nasal discharge accompanies chronic nasal obstruction, sneezing, recurrent postnasal drip, and pale, swollen turbinates. The nasal septum is pink; the mucosa, blue.

● ***Sinusitis.*** In *acute sinusitis,* nasal discharge is thick and purulent and leads to purulent postnasal drip resulting in throat pain and halitosis. Nasal congestion and severe pain and tenderness over the involved sinuses are also evident. The patient may also experience fever, headache, and malaise.

In *chronic sinusitis,* nasal discharge is usually a small amount, thick, and intermittently purulent. Nasal congestion and low-grade discomfort or pressure over the involved sinuses can be persistent or recurrent. The patient also may be suffering from a chronic sore throat. In addition, the patient may have nasal polyps.

In *chronic fungal sinusitis,* the clinical picture resembles that of chronic bacterial sinusitis. However, some cases—especially in the immunocompromised patient—may progress rapidly to exophthalmos, blindness, intracranial extension and, eventually, death.

Other causes

● ***Drugs.*** Nasal sprays or drops containing vasoconstrictors may cause rebound rhinorrhea (rhinitis medicamentosa) if used longer than 4 to 5 days.

● ***Surgery.*** Following sinus or cranial surgery, cerebrospinal rhinorrhea may occur.

Special considerations

You may have to prepare the patient for X-rays of the sinuses or the skull (in suspected skull fracture) and computed tomography scan.

In addition, you may need to administer antihistamines, decongestants, analgesics, or antipyretics. You should promote fluids to thin secretions. Be sure to warn the patient to avoid using over-the-counter nasal sprays for more than 5 days, unless required.

Pediatric pointers

Be aware that rhinorrhea may stem from choanal atresia, allergic or chronic rhinitis, acute ethmoiditis, or congenital syphilis. Unilateral rhinorrhea and nasal obstruction represents a foreign body in the nose until this is proven otherwise.

RHONCHI

Rhonchi are continuous adventitious breath sounds detected by auscultation. They're usually louder and lower pitched than crackles—more like a hoarse moan or a deep snore—though they may be described as rattling, sonorous, bubbling, rumbling, or musical. However, sibilant rhonchi, or wheezes, are high-pitched.

Rhonchi are heard over large airways such as the trachea. They occur in pulmonary disorders when air flows through passages that have been narrowed by secretions, a tumor or foreign body, bronchospasm, or mucosal thickening. The resulting vibration of airway walls produces the rhonchi.

History and physical examination

If you auscultate rhonchi, take the patient's vital signs and be alert for signs of respiratory distress. Characterize the patient's respirations as rapid or slow, shallow or deep, and regular or irregular. Inspect the chest, noting use of accessory muscles. Is the patient audibly wheezing or gurgling? Auscultate for other abnormal breath sounds, such as crackles and pleural friction rub. If you detect these, note the location. Are breath sounds diminished or absent? Next, percuss the chest.

If the patient has a cough, note its frequency and characterize its sound. If it's productive, examine the sputum for color, odor, consistency, and blood.

Ask related questions: Does the patient smoke? If so, obtain a smoking history. Has he recently lost weight or felt tired or weak? Does he have asthma or other pulmonary disorders? Is he currently taking any prescribed or over-the-counter drugs?

During the examination, keep in mind that thick or excessive secretions, bronchospasm, or inflammation of mucous membranes may lead to airway obstruction. If necessary, suction the patient and keep equipment available for inserting an airway. Also keep bronchodilators available to treat bronchospasm.

Common medical causes

• *Adult respiratory distress syndrome.* Fluid accumulation in this life-threatening disorder produces rhonchi and crackles. Initial features include rapid, shallow respirations and dyspnea, sometimes occurring after the patient appears to be stable. Developing hypoxemia leads to intercostal and suprasternal retractions, diaphoresis, and fluid accumulation. As hypoxemia worsens, the patient exhibits increased difficulty breathing, restlessness, apprehension, decreased level of consciousness, cyanosis, motor dysfunction, and possibly tachycardia.

• *Aspiration of a foreign body.* A foreign body retained in the bronchi can cause inspiratory and expiratory rhonchi and wheezing due to increased secretions. Diminished breath sounds may be auscultated over the obstructed area. Fever, pain, and a cough may also occur.

• *Asthma.* An asthma attack can cause rhonchi, crackles and, commonly, wheezing. Other features include apprehension, a dry cough that later becomes productive, prolonged expirations, and intercostal and supraclavicular retractions on inspiration. Increased accessory muscle use, nasal flaring, tachypnea, tachycardia, diaphoresis, and flushing or cyanosis may also occur.

• *Bronchiectasis.* This disorder causes lower-lobe rhonchi and crackles, which coughing may help relieve. Its classic sign is a cough that produces mucopurulent, foul-smelling, and possibly bloody sputum. Other findings include fever, weight loss, dyspnea on exertion, fatigue, malaise, halitosis, weakness, and late-stage clubbing.

• *Bronchitis.* Acute tracheobronchitis produces sonorous rhonchi and wheezing due to bronchospasm or increased mucus in the airways. Related findings include chills, sore throat, low-grade fever (rising up to 102° F [38.9° C] in severe illness), muscle and back pain, and substernal tightness. A cough becomes productive as secretions increase.

In *chronic bronchitis,* auscultation may reveal scattered rhonchi, coarse crackles, wheezing, high-pitched piping sounds, and prolonged expirations. An early hacking cough later becomes productive. The patient also displays exertional dyspnea, increased accessory muscle use, barrel chest, cyanosis, tachycardia, and late-stage clubbing.

• *Emphysema.* This disorder may cause sonorous rhonchi, but faint, high-pitched wheezing is more typical, along with weight loss; a mild, chronic, productive cough with scant sputum; exertional dyspnea; accessory muscle use on inspiration; tachypnea; and grunting expirations. Other features include anorexia, malaise, barrel chest, peripheral cyanosis, and late-stage clubbing.

• *Pneumonia.* Bacterial pneumonia can cause rhonchi and a dry cough that later becomes productive. Related signs and symptoms develop suddenly: shaking chills, high fever, myalgia, headache, pleuritic chest pain, tachypnea, tachycardia, dyspnea, cyanosis, diaphoresis, decreased breath sounds, and fine crackles.

Other causes

• *Diagnostic tests.* Pulmonary function tests and bronchoscopy can loosen secretions and mucus, causing rhonchi.

• *Respiratory therapy.* This treatment may produce rhonchi from loosened secretions and mucus.

Special considerations

Prepare the patient for diagnostic tests, such as arterial blood gas analysis, pulmonary function tests, sputum analysis, and chest X-rays.

To ease the patient's breathing, place him in semi-Fowler's position and reposition him every 2 hours. Or, if appropriate, encourage increased activity to promote drainage of secretions. Teach deep-breathing and coughing techniques and splinting, if necessary.

Administer antibiotics, bronchodilators, and expectorants, as ordered. Also, provide humidification to thin secretions, relieve inflammation, and prevent drying. Chest physiotherapy with postural drainage can also help loosen secretions. Encourage the patient to increase his intake of fluids to help liquefy secretions and prevent dehydration.

Pediatric pointers

Because a respiratory disorder may begin suddenly and progress rapidly in an infant or a child, observe carefully for signs of airway obstruction.

Rhonchi in children can result from bacterial pneumonia, cystic fibrosis, and croup.

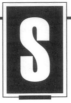

SCOTOMA

A scotoma is an area of partial or complete blindness within an otherwise normal or slightly impaired visual field. Usually located within the central 30-degree area, the defect ranges from absolute blindness to a barely detectable loss of visual acuity. Typically, the patient can pinpoint the scotoma's location in the visual field.

A scotoma can result from retinal, choroid, or optic nerve disorders. It can be classified as absolute, relative, or scintillating. An *absolute scotoma* refers to the total inability to see all sizes of test objects used in mapping the visual field. A *relative scotoma,* in contrast, refers to the ability to see only large test objects. A *scintillating scotoma* refers to the flashes or bursts of light commonly seen during a migraine headache.

History and physical examination
First, identify and characterize a scotoma, using such visual field tests as the tangent screen examination, the Goldmann perimeter test, and the automated perimetry test. (See *Locating scotomas.*) Two other visual field tests—confrontation testing and Amsler's charts—may also help identify a scotoma.

Next, test the patient's visual acuity and inspect his pupils for size, equality, and reaction to light. An ophthalmoscopic examination and measurement of intraocular pressure are necessary.

Explore the patient's history for eye disorders, vision problems, or chronic systemic disorders. Does he take medications or use eyedrops?

Common medical causes
• *Chorioretinitis.* Inflammation of the choroid produces a paracentral scotoma. Ophthalmoscopic examination reveals clouding and cells in the vitreous, subretinal hemorrhage, and neovascularization.
• *Macular degeneration.* Any degenerative process or disorder affecting the fovea centralis results in a central scotoma. Ophthalmoscopic examination reveals changes in the macular area. The patient may notice subtle changes in visual acuity, in color perception, and in the size and shape of objects.
• *Optic neuritis.* Inflammation, degeneration, or demyelination of the optic nerve produces central, circular, or centrocecal scotoma. The scotoma may be unilateral with involvement of one nerve or bilateral with involvement of both nerves. It can vary in size, density, and symmetry. The patient may have severe visual loss or blurring, lasting up to 3 weeks, and pain—especially with eye movement. Common ophthalmoscopic findings include hyperemia of the optic disk, retinal vein distention, blurred disk margins, and filling of the physiologic cup.
• *Retinal pigmentary degenerations.* These disorders cause premature retinal cell changes leading to cell death. One of these disorders, retinitis pigmentosa, initially involves loss of peripheral rods: The resulting annular scotoma progress-

LOCATING SCOTOMAS

Scotomas, or "blind spots," are classified according to the affected area of the visual field. The normal scotoma—shown in the temporal region of the right eye—appears in black in all the illustrations. In all illustrations but the normal eye, abnormal scotomas appear in gray.

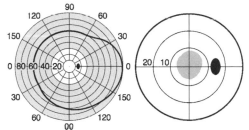

The *normally present scotoma* represents the position of the optic nerve head in the visual field. It appears between 10° and 20° on this chart of the normal visual field.

A *central scotoma* involves the point of central fixation. It's always associated with decreased visual acuity.

A *centrocecal scotoma* involves the point of central fixation and the area between the blind spot and the fixation point.

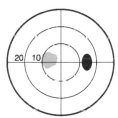

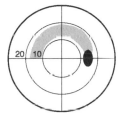

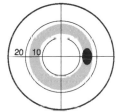

A *paracentral scotoma* affects an area of the visual field that is nasal or temporal to the point of central fixation.

An *arcuate scotoma* arches around the fixation point, usually ending on the nasal side of the visual field.

An *annular scotoma* forms a circular defect around the fixation point. It's common in retinal pigmentary degenerations.

es concentrically until only a central field of vision (tunnel vision) remains. The earliest symptom—impaired night vision—appears during adolescence. Associated signs include narrowing of the retinal blood vessels and pallor of the optic disk. Eventually, with invasion of the macula, blindness may occur.

Special considerations

For the patient with an arcuate scotoma associated with glaucoma, emphasize regular testing of intraocular pressure and visual fields. In addition, teach the patient with a disorder involving the fovea centralis (or the area surrounding it) to periodically use Amsler's charts to detect progression of macular degeneration.

Pediatric pointers

In young children, visual field testing is difficult and requires patience. Confrontation testing is the method of choice.

SCROTAL SWELLING

Scrotal swelling occurs when a condition affecting the testicles, epididymis, or scrotal skin produces edema or a mass; the penis may or may not be involved. Scrotal swelling can be unilateral or bilateral and painful or painless. It can affect males of any age.

The sudden onset of painful scrotal swelling suggests torsion of a testicle or testicular appendages, especially in the prepubescent male. This emergency requires immediate surgery to untwist and stabilize the spermatic cord or to remove the appendage.

Emergency interventions

 If severe pain accompanies scrotal swelling, ask when the swelling began. Using a Doppler stethoscope, evaluate blood flow to the testicle. If it's decreased or absent, suspect testicular torsion and prepare the patient for surgery. Withhold food and fluids, insert an I.V. line, and apply an ice pack to the scrotum to reduce pain and swelling. An attempt may be made to untwist the cord manually, but even if successful, the patient may still require surgery for stabilization.

History and physical examination

If the patient isn't in distress, proceed with the history. Ask about injury to the scrotum, about urethral discharge, and about cloudy urine, increased urinary frequency, and dysuria. Is the patient sexually active? When was his last sexual contact? Find out about recent illnesses, particularly mumps. Does he have a history of prostate surgery or prolonged catheterization? Does changing his body position or level of activity affect the swelling?

Take the patient's vital signs, noting especially fever, and palpate his abdomen for tenderness. Then examine the entire genital area. Assess the scrotum with the patient supine and standing. Note its size and color. Is the swelling unilateral or bilateral? Do you see signs of trauma or bruising? Gently palpate the scrotum for a cyst or a lump. Note especially tenderness or increased firmness. Check the testicles' position in the scrotum. Finally, transilluminate the scrotum to distinguish a fluid-filled cyst from a solid mass. (A solid mass can't be transilluminated.)

Common medical causes

• *Epididymal cysts.* Located in the head of the epididymis, these cysts produce painless scrotal swelling.

• *Epididymitis.* Key features of inflammation are pain, extreme tenderness, and swelling in the groin and scrotum. The patient waddles to avoid pressure on the groin and scrotum during walking. He may have high fever, malaise, urethral discharge and cloudy urine, and lower abdominal pain on the affected side. His scrotal skin may be hot, red, dry, flaky, and thin.

• *Hydrocele.* Fluid accumulation produces gradual scrotal swelling that's usually painless. The scrotum may be soft and cystic or firm and tense. Palpation reveals a round, nontender scrotal mass.

• *Idiopathic scrotal edema.* Swelling occurs quickly in this disorder and usually disappears within 24 hours. The affected testicle is pink.

• *Orchitis (acute).* Mumps may precipitate this disorder, which causes sudden painful swelling of one or, at times, both testicles. Related findings include a hot, reddened scrotum, fever of up to 104° F (40° C), chills, lower abdominal pain, nausea, vomiting, and extreme weakness. Urinary signs are usually absent.

● *Scrotal trauma.* Blunt trauma causes scrotal swelling with bruising and severe pain. The scrotum may appear dark or bluish.

● *Spermatocele.* This painless or painful cystic mass lies above and behind the testicle and contains opaque fluid and sperm. Its onset may be acute or gradual. Less than ⅜″ (1 cm) in diameter, it's movable and may be transilluminated.

● *Testicular torsion.* Most common before puberty, this urologic emergency causes scrotal swelling, sudden and severe pain, and possible elevation of the affected testicle within the scrotum. It may also cause nausea and vomiting.

● *Testicular tumor.* Typically painless, smooth, and firm, a testicular tumor produces swelling and a sensation of excessive weight in the scrotum.

● *Torsion of a hydatid of Morgagni.* Torsion of this small, pea-shaped cyst severs its blood supply, causing a hard, painful swelling on the testicle's upper pole.

Other causes

● *Surgery.* An effusion of blood from surgery can produce a hematocele, leading to scrotal swelling.

Special considerations

Keep the patient on bed rest and give antibiotics. Provide adequate fluids, fiber, and stool softeners. Place a rolled towel between the patient's legs and under the scrotum to help reduce severe swelling. Or, if the patient has mild or moderate swelling, advise him to wear a loose-fitting athletic supporter lined with soft cotton dressings. Administer analgesics for several days to relieve his pain. Encourage sitz baths, and apply heat or ice packs to decrease inflammation.

Prepare him for needle aspiration of fluid-filled cysts and other diagnostic tests, such as lung tomography and computed tomography of the abdomen, to rule out cancer.

Encourage the patient to perform testicular self-examination at home.

Pediatric pointers

Thorough physical assessment is especially important in children with scrotal swelling, who may be unable to give history data.

In children up to age 1, hernia or hydrocele of the cord may stem from abnormal fetal development. In infants, scrotal swelling may stem from ammonia-related dermatitis if diapers aren't changed often enough. In prepubescent males, it most commonly results from torsion of the spermatic cord.

Other disorders producing scrotal swelling in children include epididymitis (rare before age 10), traumatic orchitis from contact sports, and mumps, which usually occurs after puberty.

SEIZURE, ABSENCE
[Petit mal seizure]

Absence seizures are benign, generalized seizures thought to originate subcortically. These brief episodes of unconsciousness last 3 to 20 seconds and can occur 100 or more times a day, commonly causing periods of inattention. Absence seizures usually affect children between ages 4 and 12 and rarely persist beyond adolescence. Their first sign may be deteriorating schoolwork and behavior. Their cause isn't known.

Absence seizures occur without warning. The patient suddenly stops all purposeful activity and stares blankly ahead, as though daydreaming. Absence seizures may produce automatisms, such as repetitive lip smacking, or mild clonic or myoclonic movements, including mild jerking of the eyelids. The patient may drop objects he's holding, and muscle relaxation may cause him to drop his head or arms or to slump. After the attack, the patient resumes activity, typically unaware of the episode.

Absence status, a rare form of absence seizure, occurs as a prolonged absence seizure or as repeated episodes of these seizures. Usually not life-threatening, it occurs most commonly in patients with preexisting absence seizures.

History and physical examination
If you suspect a patient is having an absence seizure, evaluate its occurrence and duration by reciting a series of numbers and then asking him to repeat them after the attack ends. The patient will be unable to do this. Or, if the seizures are occurring within minutes of each other, ask the patient to count for about 5 minutes. He'll stop counting during a seizure, then resume when it's over. Look for accompanying automatisms. Find out if the family has noticed a change in behavior or deteriorating schoolwork.

Medical causes
● *Idiopathic epilepsy.* Some forms of absence seizures are accompanied by automatisms and learning disability.

Special considerations
Explain the purpose of any diagnostic tests, such as computed tomography scans, magnetic resonance imaging, and electroencephalography. Teach the patient and his family about these seizures and how to recognize their onset, pattern, and duration. Include the child's teacher and school nurse in the teaching process, if possible. If the seizures are being controlled with drug therapy, emphasize the importance of strict compliance.

SEIZURE, FOCAL
[Simple partial seizure]

Resulting from an irritable focus in the cerebral cortex, a focal seizure typically lasts about 30 seconds and doesn't alter the patient's level of consciousness (LOC). Its type and pattern reflect the location of the irritable focus. A focal seizure may be classified as motor or somatosensory. A focal motor seizure may be further classified as a jacksonian seizure or as epilepsia partialis continua. A somatosensory seizure may be further classified as a visual, olfactory, or auditory seizure.

A *focal motor seizure* is a series of unilateral clonic (muscle jerking) and tonic (muscle stiffening) movements of one part of the body. The patient's head and eyes characteristically turn away from the hemispheric focus—most commonly the frontal lobe near the motor strip. A tonic-clonic contraction of the trunk or extremities may follow.

A *jacksonian motor seizure* typically begins with a tonic contraction of a finger, the corner of the mouth, or one foot. Clonic movements follow, spreading to other muscles on the same side of the body, moving up the arm or leg, and eventually involving the whole side. Or clonic movements may spread to the opposite side, becoming generalized and leading to loss of consciousness. In the postictal phase, the patient may display paralysis (Todd's paralysis) in the affected limbs that usually resolves within 24 hours.

Epilepsia partialis continua causes clonic twitching of one muscle group, usually in the face, arm, or leg. Twitching occurs every few seconds and persists for hours, days, or months without spreading. Spasms affect the distal arm and leg muscles more frequently than the proximal ones; in the face, they affect

BODY FUNCTIONS AFFECTED BY FOCAL SEIZURES

The body function normally governed at the site of the irritable focus determines a focal seizure's signs and symptoms.

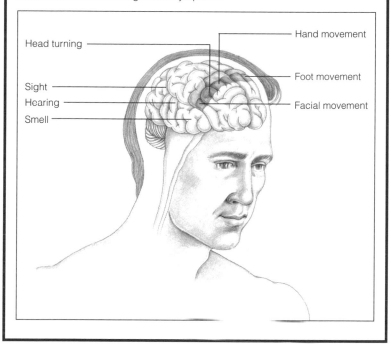

Head turning

Sight

Hearing

Smell

Hand movement

Foot movement

Facial movement

---

the corner of the mouth, one or both eyelids and, occasionally, the neck or trunk muscles unilaterally.

A *focal somatosensory seizure* affects a localized body area on one side. Usually, this seizure initially causes numbness, tingling, or crawling or "electric" sensations; rarely, it may cause pain or burning sensations in the lips, fingers, or toes. A *visual seizure* involves sensations of darkness or of stationary or moving lights or spots—usually red at first, then blue, green, and yellow. It can affect both visual fields or the visual field on the side opposite the lesion. The irritable focus is in the occipital lobe. In contrast, the irritable focus in an *auditory* or *olfacto-*

ry seizure is in the temporal lobe. (See *Body functions affected by focal seizures.*)

History and physical examination

Be sure to record the patient's behavior in detail; your data may be critical in locating the lesion in the brain. Does the patient turn his head and eyes? If so, to what side? Where does movement first start? Does it spread? Because a partial seizure may become generalized, you'll need to watch closely for loss of consciousness, bilateral tonicity and clonicity, cyanosis, tongue biting, and urinary incontinence. (See the entry "Seizure, generalized tonic-clonic.")

During the seizure, ask the patient to describe exactly what is happening. After the seizure, check the patient's LOC, and test for residual deficits (such as weakness in the involved extremity) and sensory disturbances.

Then obtain a history: What happened before the seizure? Did the patient recognize its onset? If so, how did the patient recognize it—a smell, a visual disturbance, or a sound or visceral phenomenon such as an unusual sensation in his stomach? How does this seizure compare with others the patient has had?

In addition, be sure to explore fully any history, recent or remote, of head trauma. Also check for a history of stroke or recent infection—especially with fever, headache, or a stiff neck.

Common medical causes

• *Brain abscess.* Seizures can occur in the acute stage of abscess formation or after resolution of the abscess. Decreased LOC varies from drowsiness to deep stupor. Early signs and symptoms reflect increased intracranial pressure and include constant, intractable headache, nausea, and vomiting. Later symptoms include ocular disturbances—such as nystagmus, decreased visual acuity, and unequal pupils. Other findings differ with the abscess site and may include aphasia, hemiparesis, and personality changes.

• *Brain tumor.* Focal seizures are commonly the earliest indicators of a brain tumor. The patient may report morning headache, dizziness, confusion, vision loss, and motor and sensory disturbances. He may also have aphasia, generalized seizures, ataxia, decreased LOC, papilledema, vomiting, increased systolic blood pressure, and widening pulse pressure. Eventually, he may assume a decorticate posture.

• *Cerebrovascular accident (CVA).* A major cause of seizures in patients over age 50, a CVA may induce focal seizures within 6 months after its onset. Related effects depend on the type and extent of the CVA but may include decreased LOC, contralateral hemiplegia, dysarthria, dysphagia, ataxia, unilateral sensory loss, apraxia, agnosia, and aphasia. A CVA may also cause visual deficits, memory loss, poor judgment, personality changes, emotional lability, headache, urine retention or incontinence, and vomiting. It may cause generalized seizures.

• *Head trauma.* Any head injury can cause seizures, but penetrating wounds are characteristically associated with focal seizures. These seizures most commonly arise 3 to 15 months after injury, decrease in frequency after several years, and eventually stop. The patient may have generalized seizures and a decreased LOC that may progress to coma.

Special considerations

No emergency care is necessary during a focal seizure, unless it progresses to a generalized seizure. However, you should remain with the patient during the seizure, and reassure him. After the seizure, instruct the patient to observe and record his seizures. Also emphasize the importance of complying with prescribed drug therapy.

Prepare the patient for such diagnostic tests as a computed tomography scan and EEG.

Pediatric pointers

In children more than in adults, focal seizures are likely to spread and become generalized. They typically cause the child's eyes, or his head and eyes, to turn to the side; in neonates, they cause mouth twitching, staring, or both.

Focal seizures in children can result from hemiplegic cerebral palsy, head trauma, child abuse, arteriovenous malformation, and Sturge-Weber syndrome. About 25% of febrile seizures may present as focal seizures.

SEIZURE, GENERALIZED TONIC-CLONIC
[Major seizure]

Like other types of seizure, a generalized tonic-clonic seizure is caused by the paroxysmal, uncontrolled discharge of central nervous system neurons, leading to neurologic dysfunction. Unlike most other types of seizure, this cerebral hyperactivity isn't confined to the original focus or to a localized area but extends to the entire brain.

A generalized tonic-clonic seizure may begin with or without an aura. As seizure activity spreads to the subcortical structures, the patient loses consciousness, falls to the ground, and may utter a loud cry that's precipitated by air rushing from the lungs through the vocal cords. His body stiffens (tonic phase); then he undergoes rapid, synchronous muscle jerking and hyperventilation (clonic phase). Tongue biting, incontinence, diaphoresis, profuse salivation, and signs of respiratory distress may also occur. The seizure usually stops after 2 to 5 minutes. The patient then regains consciousness but displays confusion. He may complain of headache, fatigue, muscle soreness, and arm and leg weakness. (See *What happens in a generalized seizure,* page 518.)

Generalized tonic-clonic seizures usually occur singly. The patient may be awake and active or sleeping. Possible complications include respiratory arrest due to airway obstruction from secretions, status epilepticus (occurring in 5% to 8% of patients), head or spinal injuries and bruises, Todd's paralysis and, rarely, cardiac arrest. Life-threatening status epilepticus is marked by prolonged seizure activity or by rapidly recurring seizures with no intervening periods of recovery. It's most commonly triggered by abrupt discontinuation of anticonvulsant drugs.

Generalized seizures may be caused by brain tumors, vascular disorders, head trauma, infections, metabolic defects, drug and alcohol withdrawal syndromes, toxins, and genetic defects. Generalized seizures may also result from a focal seizure. In recurring seizures, or epilepsy, the cause may be unknown.

Emergency interventions

 If you witness the beginning of the seizure, stay with the patient and ensure a patent airway. Focus your care on observing the seizure and protecting the patient. Place a towel under his head to prevent injury, loosen his clothing, and move any sharp or hard objects out of his way. Never try to restrain him or force a hard object into his mouth; you may chip his teeth or fracture his jaw. Only at the start of the ictal phase can you safely insert a soft object into his mouth.

If possible during the seizure, turn the patient to one side to allow secretions to drain. Otherwise, do this at the end of the clonic phase when respirations return. (If they fail to return, check for airway obstruction and suction the patient, if necessary. Intubation and mechanical ventilation may be needed.)

Protect the patient after the seizure by providing a safe area in which he can rest. As the patient awakens, you should reassure and reorient him. Check the patient's vital signs and neurologic status. Be sure to carefully record these and your observations made during the seizure.

If the seizure lasts longer than 4 minutes or if a second seizure occurs before full recovery from the first, suspect status epilepticus. Establish an airway, start an I.V. line, give supplemental oxygen, and begin cardiac monitoring. Draw blood for appropriate studies. Turn the patient on his side, with his head in a semidependent position, to drain secretions and prevent aspiration. Periodical-

WHAT HAPPENS IN A GENERALIZED SEIZURE

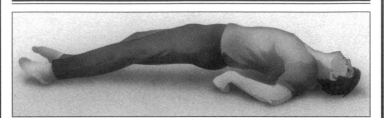

Before the seizure
Prodromal signs and symptoms, such as myoclonic jerks, throbbing headache, and mood changes, may occur over several hours or days. The patient may have premonitions of the seizure. For example, he may report an *aura,* such as seeing a flashing light or smelling a characteristic odor.

During the seizure
If a generalized seizure begins with an aura, this indicates that irritability in a specific area of the brain quickly became widespread. Common auras include palpitations, epigastric distress rapidly rising to the throat, head or eye turning, and sensory hallucinations.

Next, loss of consciousness occurs as a sudden discharge of intense electrical activity overwhelms the brain's subcortical center. The patient falls and experiences brief, bilateral myoclonic contractures. Air forced through spasmodic vocal cords may produce a birdlike, piercing cry.

During the *tonic phase* skeletal muscles contract for about 10 to 20 seconds. The patient's eyelids are drawn up, his arms are flexed, and his legs are extended. His mouth opens wide, then snaps shut; he may bite his tongue. His respirations cease because of respiratory muscle spasm, and initial pallor of the skin and mucous membranes (the result of impaired venous return)

changes to cyanosis secondary to apnea. The patient arches his back and slowly lowers his arms (as shown above). Other effects include dilated, nonreactive pupils; greatly increased heart rate and blood pressure; increased salivation and tracheobronchial secretions; and profuse diaphoresis.

During the *clonic phase,* lasting about 60 seconds, mild trembling progresses to violent contractures or jerks. Other motor activity includes facial grimaces (with possible tongue biting) and violent expiration of bloody, foamy saliva from clonic contractures of thoracic cage muscles. Clonic jerks slowly decrease in intensity and frequency. The patient is still apneic.

After the seizure
The patient's movements gradually cease and he becomes unresponsive to external stimuli. Other postseizure features include stertorous respirations from increased tracheobronchial secretions, equal or unequal pupils (but becoming reactive), and urinary incontinence due to brief muscle relaxation. After about 5 minutes, the patient's level of consciousness increases, and he appears confused and disoriented. His muscle tone, heart rate, and blood pressure return to normal.

After several hours' sleep, the patient awakens exhausted and may have a headache, sore muscles, and amnesia regarding the seizure.

ly turn the patient to the opposite side, check his arterial blood gas levels for hypoxemia, and give oxygen by mask, increasing the flow rate if necessary. Administer diazepam by slow I.V. push, repeated two or three times at 10- to 20-minute intervals, to stop the seizures. If the patient is not a known epileptic, an I.V. bolus of dextrose 50% (50 ml) with thiamine (100 mg) may be ordered. Dextrose may stop the seizures if the patient is hypoglycemic; thiamine, if he is alcoholic or malnourished.

If the patient is intubated, expect to insert a nasogastric (NG) tube to prevent vomiting and aspiration. However, if the patient has not been intubated, the NG tube itself can trigger the gag reflex and cause vomiting. Be sure to record your observations and the intervals between seizures.

History and physical examination
If you didn't witness the seizure, obtain a description from the patient's companion. Ask when the seizure started and how long it lasted. Did the patient report any unusual sensations before the seizure began? Did the seizure start in one area of the body and spread, or did it affect the entire body right away? Did the patient fall on a hard surface? Did his eyes or head turn? Did he turn blue? Did he lose bladder control? Did he have any other seizures before recovering?

If the patient possibly has a head injury, observe him closely for loss of consciousness, unequal or nonreactive pupils, and focal neurologic signs. Does he complain of headache and muscle soreness? Is he increasingly difficult to arouse when you check on him at 20-minute intervals? Examine his arms, legs, and face (including tongue) for injury, residual paralysis, or limb weakness.

Now obtain a history. Has the patient ever had generalized or focal seizures before? Are they frequent? Do other family members also have them? Is the patient receiving drug therapy? Is he compliant? Also ask about any sleep deprivation, or emotional or physical stress at the time the seizure occurred.

Common medical causes
● *Barbiturate withdrawal.* In chronically intoxicated patients, barbiturate withdrawal may produce generalized seizures 2 to 4 days after the last dose. Status epilepticus is possible.
● *Brain abscess.* Generalized seizures may occur in the acute stage of abscess formation or after the abscess disappears. Depending on the size and location of the abscess, decreased level of consciousness (LOC) varies from drowsiness to deep stupor. Early signs and symptoms reflect increased intracranial pressure (ICP) and include constant headache, nausea, vomiting, and focal seizures. Typical later features include ocular disturbances—such as nystagmus, impaired vision, and unequal pupils. Other findings differ with the abscess site but may include aphasia, hemiparesis, abnormal behavior, and personality changes.
● *Brain tumor.* Generalized seizures may occur, depending on the tumor's location and type. Other findings include a slowly decreasing LOC, morning headache, dizziness, confusion, focal seizures, vision loss, motor and sensory disturbances, aphasia, and ataxia. Papilledema, vomiting, increased systolic blood pressure, widening pulse pressure, and (eventually) decorticate posture may occur later.
● *Cerebrovascular accident (CVA).* Seizures (focal more often than generalized) occur within 6 months of an ischemic CVA. Associated signs and symptoms vary with the location and extent of brain damage. They include decreased LOC, contralateral hemiplegia, dysarthria, dysphagia, ataxia, unilateral sensory loss, apraxia, agnosia, and aphasia. There may also be visual deficits, memory loss, poor judgment, personality changes, emotional lability, urine retention or incontinence, constipation, headache, and vomiting.

• *Chronic renal failure.* End-stage renal failure produces rapid onset of twitching, trembling, myoclonic jerks, and generalized seizures. Related signs and symptoms include anuria or oliguria, fatigue, malaise, irritability, decreased mental acuity, muscle cramps, peripheral neuropathies, anorexia, and constipation or diarrhea. Integumentary effects include skin color changes (yellow, brown, or bronze), pruritus, and uremic frost. Other effects include ammonia breath odor, nausea and vomiting, ecchymoses, petechiae, GI bleeding, mouth and gum ulcers, hypertension, and Kussmaul's respirations.

• *Eclampsia.* Generalized seizures are a hallmark of this disorder. Related findings include severe frontal headache, nausea and vomiting, vision disturbances, increased blood pressure, peripheral edema, and sudden weight gain. The patient may also have oliguria, irritability, hyperactive deep tendon reflexes, and a decreased LOC.

• *Encephalitis.* Seizures are an early sign of this disorder, indicating a poor prognosis; they may also occur after recovery as a result of residual damage. Other findings include fever, headache, photophobia, nuchal rigidity, vomiting, aphasia, ataxia, hemiparesis, nystagmus, irritability, cranial nerve palsies (causing facial weakness, ptosis, dysphagia), and myoclonic jerks.

• *Head trauma.* In severe cases, generalized seizures may occur at the time of injury. (Months later, focal seizures may occur.) Severe head trauma may also cause a decreased LOC leading to coma; soft-tissue injury of the face, head, or neck; clear or bloody drainage from the mouth, nose, or ears; facial edema; bony deformity of the face, head, or neck; Battle's sign; and lack of response to oculocephalic and oculovestibular stimulation. Motor and sensory deficits may occur along with altered respirations. Examination may reveal signs of increasing ICP, such as decreased response to painful stimuli, nonreactive pupils, bradycardia, increased systolic pressure, and widening pulse pressure. If the patient is conscious, he may have visual deficits, behavioral changes, and headache.

• *Hypertensive encephalopathy.* This life-threatening disorder may cause seizures, along with severely increased blood pressure, decreased LOC, intense headache, vomiting, transient blindness, paralysis, and (eventually) Cheyne-Stokes respirations.

• *Hypoglycemia.* Generalized seizures usually occur in severe hypoglycemia, accompanied by blurred or double vision, motor weakness, hemiplegia, trembling, excessive diaphoresis, tachycardia, myoclonic twitching, and decreased LOC.

• *Hyponatremia.* Seizures develop when serum sodium levels fall below 125 mEq/L, especially if the decrease is rapid. Hyponatremia also causes postural hypotension, headache, muscle twitching and weakness, fatigue, oliguria or anuria, cold and clammy skin, decreased skin turgor, irritability, lethargy, confusion, and stupor or coma. Excessive thirst, tachycardia, nausea, vomiting, and abdominal cramps may also occur. Severe hyponatremia may cause cyanosis and vasomotor collapse, with a thready pulse.

• *Hypoparathyroidism.* Worsening tetany causes generalized seizures. Chronic hypoparathyroidism produces neuromuscular irritability and hyperactive deep tendon reflexes.

• *Hypoxic encephalopathy.* Besides generalized seizures, this disorder may produce myoclonic jerks and coma. After the patient has recovered, dementia, visual agnosia, choreoathetosis, and ataxia may occur.

• *Idiopathic epilepsy.* In most cases, the cause of recurrent seizures is unknown.

• *Neurofibromatosis.* Multiple brain lesions in this disorder cause focal and generalized seizures. Inspection reveals café-au-lait spots, multiple skin tumors, scoliosis, and kyphoscoliosis. Related findings include dizziness, ataxia, monocular blindness, and nystagmus.

Other causes

- *Diagnostic tests.* Contrast agents used in radiologic tests may cause generalized seizures.
- *Drugs.* Toxic blood levels of some drugs—such as theophylline, lidocaine, meperidine, penicillin, and cimetidine—may cause generalized seizures. Phenothiazines, tricyclic antidepressants, amphetamines, isoniazid, and vincristine may cause seizures in patients with pre-existing epilepsy.

Special considerations

Closely monitor the patient after the seizure for recurring seizure activity. Prepare him for a computed tomography scan or magnetic resonance imaging, and electroencephalography.

Emphasize the importance of strict compliance with drug therapy, and warn the patient about adverse effects. Also stress the importance of having regular follow-up blood studies and of having his family observe and record his seizure activity to ensure proper treatment.

Pediatric pointers

Generalized seizures are common in children. In fact, between 75% and 90% of epileptic patients experience their first seizure before age 20. Many children between ages 3 months and 3 years experience generalized seizures associated with fever; some of these children later develop seizures without fever. Generalized seizures may also stem from inborn errors of metabolism, perinatal injury, brain infections, Reye's syndrome, Sturge-Weber syndrome, arteriovenous malformation, lead poisoning, hypoglycemia, and idiopathic causes. Rarely, the pertussis component of the DTP vaccine causes seizures.

SEIZURE, PSYCHOMOTOR

[Complex partial seizure, temporal lobe seizure]

A psychomotor seizure occurs when a focal seizure begins in the temporal lobe and causes a partial alteration of consciousness—usually confusion. A psychomotor seizure can occur at any age, but incidence usually increases during adolescence and adulthood. Two-thirds of patients also have generalized seizures.

Typically, an aura—usually a complex hallucination or illusion—precedes a psychomotor seizure. The hallucination may be audiovisual (images with sounds), auditory (abnormal or normal sounds or voices from the patient's past), or olfactory (unpleasant smells, such as rotten eggs or burning materials). Other types of auras include feelings of déjà vu, unfamiliarity with surroundings, or depersonalization. Some patients become fearful or anxious. Others have an unpleasant feeling in the epigastric region that rises toward the chest and throat or manifest lip smacking. The patient usually recognizes the aura and lies down before losing consciousness.

A period of unresponsiveness follows the aura. The patient may experience automatisms, appear dazed and wander aimlessly, perform inappropriate acts (such as undressing in public), be unresponsive, utter incoherent phrases or, rarely, go into a rage or tantrum. After the seizure, the patient is confused and drowsy and doesn't remember the seizure. Behavioral automatisms rarely last longer than 5 minutes, but postseizure confusion and amnesia may persist.

Between attacks, the patient may exhibit slow and rigid thinking, outbursts of anger and aggressiveness, tedious conversation, a preoccupation with naive philosophical ideas, diminished libido, mood swings, and paranoid tendencies.

History

If you witness a psychomotor seizure, never attempt to restrain the patient. Instead, lead him gently to a safe area. (*Exception:* Don't approach him if he's angry or violent.) You should calmly encourage the patient to sit down, and remain with him until he's fully alert. After the seizure, ask him if he experienced an aura. Record all your observations and findings.

Common medical causes

• *Brain abscess.* If the brain abscess is in the temporal lobe, psychomotor seizures commonly occur in the acute phase or after the abscess disappears. Related problems may include headache, nausea, vomiting, generalized seizures, and a decreased level of consciousness (LOC). The patient may also have central facial weakness, auditory receptive aphasia, hemiparesis, and ocular disturbances.

• *Head trauma.* Severe trauma to the temporal lobe (especially from a penetrating injury) can produce psychomotor seizures months or years later. The seizures may decrease in frequency and eventually stop. Head trauma also causes generalized seizures and behavior and personality changes.

• *Herpes simplex encephalitis.* The herpes simplex virus commonly attacks the temporal lobe, which may result in psychomotor seizures. Other features include fever, headache, coma, and generalized seizures.

• *Temporal lobe tumor.* Psychomotor seizures may be the first sign of this disorder. Other signs and symptoms include headache, pupillary changes, and mental dullness. Increased intracranial pressure may cause a decreased LOC, vomiting, and possible papilledema.

Special considerations

After the seizure, remain with the patient to reorient him to his surroundings and to protect him from injury. Keep him in bed until he's fully alert, and remove harmful objects. Offer emotional support to the patient and his family, and teach them how to cope with seizures.

Prepare the patient for diagnostic tests, such as EEG, a computed tomography scan, or magnetic resonance imaging.

Pediatric pointers

Psychomotor seizures in children may resemble absence seizures. They can result from birth injury, abuse, infections, or neoplasms. In about one-third of patients, their cause is unknown.

Repeated psychomotor seizures commonly lead to generalized seizures. The child may experience a slight aura, but it is rarely as definite as that seen in generalized tonic-clonic seizures.

SETTING-SUN SIGN
[Sunset eyes]

Setting-sun sign describes the position of an infant's or young child's eyes as a result of pressure on cranial nerves III, IV, and VI. Both eyes are forced downward, revealing an area of sclera above the irises; occasionally, the irises appear to be forced outward.

Setting-sun sign is a late and ominous sign of increased intracranial pressure (ICP). Typically, increased ICP results from space-occupying lesions such as tumors or from an accumulation of fluid in the brain's ventricular system, as occurs in hydrocephalus. It also results from intracranial bleeding or cerebral edema.

Setting-sun sign may be intermittent— for example, it may disappear when the infant is upright because this position slightly reduces ICP. The sign may be elicited in a normal infant under age 4 weeks by suddenly changing his head position. It can also be elicited in a normal infant up to age 9 months by placing a bright light before his eyes and removing it quickly.

History and physical examination

If you observe the setting-sun sign in an infant, evaluate the infant's neurologic status. Then obtain a brief history from the parents. Has the infant had a fall or even a minor trauma? When did this sign appear? Ask about early nonspecific signs of increasing ICP: Has the infant's sucking reflex diminished? Is he irritable, restless, or unusually tired? Does he cry when moved? Is his cry high pitched?

Now perform a physical examination, keeping in mind that neurologic responses are primarily reflexive during early infancy. Assess the infant's level of consciousness (LOC). Is he awake, irritable, or lethargic? Does he reach for a bright object or turn toward the sound of a music box? Observe his posture for normal flexion and extension or opisthotonos. Examine muscle tone, and observe for seizure automatisms.

Examine the infant's anterior fontanel for bulging, measure his head circumference, and observe his breathing pattern. (Cheyne-Stokes respirations may accompany increased ICP.) Also check his pupillary response to light: Unilateral or bilateral dilation occurs as ICP increases. Finally, elicit reflexes—diminished in increased ICP, especially Moro's reflex. Keep endotracheal (ET) intubation equipment available.

Medical causes

• *Increased ICP.* Transient or intermittent setting-sun sign commonly occurs late in increased ICP. The infant may have bulging, widened fontanels, increased head circumference, and widened sutures. He may also exhibit a decreased LOC, behavioral changes, high-pitched cry, pupillary abnormalities, and impaired motor movement. Other findings include increased systolic pressure, widened pulse pressure, bradycardia, changes in breathing pattern, vomiting, and seizures as ICP increases.

Special considerations

Care of the infant with setting-sun sign includes monitoring of vital signs and neurologic status. Elevate the head of the crib, and monitor intake and output. Monitor ICP, restrict fluids, and insert an I.V. line to administer diuretics and corticosteroids. For severely increased ICP, ET intubation and mechanical hyperventilation may be required to reduce serum carbon dioxide levels and constrict cerebral vessels. Barbiturate coma or hypothermia therapy may be required to lower metabolic rate.

Try to maintain a calm environment. When the infant is crying, comfort him to help prevent stress-related ICP elevations. Encourage the parents' help, and offer emotional support.

SHALLOW RESPIRATIONS

Respirations are shallow when a diminished volume of air enters the lungs during inspiration. In an effort to obtain enough air, the patient with shallow respirations usually breathes at an accelerated rate. However, as he tires or as his muscles weaken, this compensatory increase in respirations diminishes, leading to inadequate gas exchange and such signs as dyspnea, cyanosis, confusion, agitation, loss of consciousness, and tachycardia.

Shallow respirations may develop suddenly or gradually and may last briefly or become chronic. They're a key sign of respiratory distress and neurologic deterioration. Causes include inadequate central respiratory control over breathing, neuromuscular disorders, increased re-

MEASURING LUNG VOLUMES

Use a Wright respirometer to measure tidal volume (the amount of air inspired with each breath) and minute volume (the volume of air inspired in a minute— or tidal volume multiplied by respiratory rate). You can connect the respirometer to an intubated patient's airway via an endotracheal tube (shown here) or a tracheostomy tube. If the patient isn't intubated, connect it to a face mask, making sure the seal over the patient's mouth and nose is airtight.

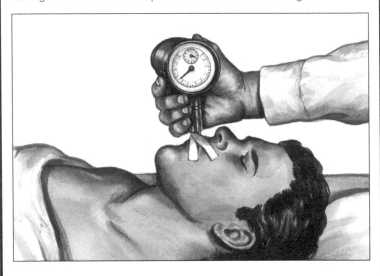

sistance to airflow into the lungs, respiratory muscle fatigue or weakness, voluntary alterations in breathing, and decreased activity from prolonged bed rest.

Emergency interventions

 If you observe shallow respirations, be alert for impending respiratory failure or arrest. Is the patient severely dyspneic? Agitated or frightened? Look for signs of airway obstruction. If the patient is choking, perform a series of four back blows, then four abdominal thrusts, to try to expel the foreign object. Use suction if secretions occlude the patient's airway.

If the patient is also wheezing, check for stridor, nasal flaring, and use of accessory muscles. Administer oxygen with a face mask or a handheld resuscitation bag. Attempt to calm the patient. Administer I.V. epinephrine.

If the patient loses consciousness, insert an artificial airway and prepare for endotracheal intubation and ventilatory support. Measure his tidal volume and minute volume with a Wright respirometer to determine the need for mechanical ventilation. (See *Measuring lung volumes.*) Check arterial blood gas (ABG) levels, heart rate, and blood pressure. Tachycardia, increased or decreased blood pressure, poor minute volume, and deteriorating ABGs signal the need for intubation and mechanical ventilation.

History and physical examination

If the patient isn't in severe respiratory distress, begin with the history. Ask about chronic illness and any surgery or trauma. Has he had a tetanus booster in the past 10 years? Does he have asthma, allergies, or a history of heart failure or vascular disease? Does he have chronic respiratory disorders or infections, or neurologic or neuromuscular disease? Does he smoke? Obtain a medication history, too, and explore the possibility of drug abuse.

Ask about the patient's shallow respirations: When did they begin? How long do they last? What makes them subside? What aggravates them? Ask about changes in appetite, weight, activity level, and behavior.

Begin the physical examination by assessing the patient's level of consciousness (LOC) and his orientation to time, person, and place. Observe spontaneous movements, and test muscle strength and deep tendon reflexes. Next, inspect the chest for deformities or abnormal movements such as intercostal retractions. Inspect the extremities for cyanosis and digital clubbing.

Now, palpate for expansion and diaphragmatic tactile fremitus, and percuss for hyperresonance or dullness. Auscultate for diminished, absent, or adventitious breath sounds and for abnormal or distant heart sounds. Do you note any peripheral edema? Finally, examine the abdomen for distention, tenderness, or masses.

Common medical causes

● *Adult respiratory distress syndrome.* Initially, this life-threatening syndrome produces rapid, shallow respirations and dyspnea—sometimes after the patient appears stable. Hypoxemia leads to intercostal and suprasternal retractions, diaphoresis, and fluid accumulation, causing rhonchi and crackles. As hypoxemia worsens, the patient has increased breathing difficulty, restlessness, apprehension, decreased LOC, cyanosis, and possibly tachycardia.

● *Amyotrophic lateral sclerosis (ALS).* Respiratory muscle weakness in this disorder causes progressive shallow respirations. Exertion may result in increased weakness and respiratory distress. ALS initially produces upper extremity muscle weakness and wasting that, within several years, affect the trunk, neck, tongue, and muscles of the larynx, pharynx, and lower extremities. Associated signs and symptoms include muscle cramps and atrophy, hyperreflexia, slight spasticity of the legs, coarse fasciculations of the affected muscle, impaired speech, and difficulty chewing and swallowing.

● *Asthma.* In this disorder, bronchospasm and hyperinflation of the lungs cause rapid, shallow respirations. In adults, mild persistent signs and symptoms may worsen during severe attacks. Related respiratory effects include wheezing, rhonchi, a dry cough, dyspnea, prolonged expirations, intercostal and supraclavicular retractions on inspiration, nasal flaring, and use of accessory muscles. Chest tightness, tachycardia, diaphoresis, and flushing or cyanosis may occur.

● *Atelectasis.* Decreased lung expansion or pleuritic pain causes sudden onset of rapid, shallow respirations. Other signs and symptoms may include a dry cough, dyspnea, tachycardia, anxiety, cyanosis, and diaphoresis. Examination reveals dullness to percussion, decreased breath sounds and vocal fremitus, inspiratory lag, and substernal or intercostal retractions.

● *Bronchiectasis.* Increased secretions obstruct airflow in the lungs, leading to shallow respirations and a productive cough with copious, foul-smelling, mucopurulent sputum (a classic finding). Other findings include hemoptysis, wheezing, rhonchi, coarse crackles during inspiration, and late-stage clubbing. The patient may complain of weight loss, fatigue, weakness and dyspnea on exertion, fever, malaise, and halitosis.

● *Coma.* Rapid, shallow respirations result from neurologic dysfunction or restricted chest movement.

● *Emphysema.* Increased breathing effort causes muscle fatigue, leading to chronic shallow respirations. The patient may also display dyspnea, anorexia, malaise, tachypnea, diminished breath sounds, cyanosis, pursed-lip breathing, accessory muscle use, barrel chest, chronic productive cough, and clubbing (a late sign).

● *Flail chest.* In this disorder, decreased air movement results in rapid, shallow respirations, paradoxical chest wall motion from rib instability, tachycardia, hypotension, ecchymoses, cyanosis, and pain over the affected area.

● *Guillain-Barré syndrome.* Progressive ascending paralysis causes rapid or progressive onset of shallow respirations. Muscle weakness begins in the lower limbs and extends finally to the face. Associated findings include paresthesia, dysarthria, diminished or absent corneal reflex, nasal speech, dysphagia, ipsilateral loss of facial muscle control, and flaccid paralysis.

● *Multiple sclerosis.* Muscle weakness causes progressive shallow respirations. Early features may include diplopia, blurred vision, and paresthesia. Other possible findings are nystagmus, constipation, paralysis, spasticity, hyperreflexia, intention tremor, ataxic gait, dysphagia, dysarthria, urinary dysfunction, impotence, and emotional lability.

● *Myasthenia gravis.* Progression of this disorder causes respiratory muscle weakness marked by shallow respirations, dyspnea, and cyanosis. Other effects include fatigue, weak eye closure, ptosis, diplopia, and difficulty chewing and swallowing.

● *Pleural effusion.* In this disorder, restricted lung expansion causes shallow respirations, beginning suddenly or gradually. Other findings include nonproductive cough, weight loss, dyspnea, and pleuritic chest pain. Examination reveals pleural friction rub, tachycardia, tachypnea, decreased chest motion, flatness to percussion, egophony, decreased or absent breath sounds, and decreased tactile fremitus.

● *Pneumothorax.* This disorder causes sudden onset of shallow respirations and dyspnea. Related effects are tachycardia; tachypnea; sudden, sharp, severe chest pain (commonly unilateral) worsening with movement; nonproductive cough; cyanosis; accessory muscle use; asymmetrical chest expansion; anxiety; restlessness; hyperresonance or tympany on the affected side; subcutaneous crepitation; decreased vocal fremitus; and diminished or absent breath sounds on the affected side.

● *Pulmonary edema.* Pulmonary vascular congestion causes rapid, shallow respirations. Early signs and symptoms include dyspnea on exertion, paroxysmal nocturnal dyspnea, and a nonproductive cough. Clinical features also include tachycardia, tachypnea, dependent crackles, and a ventricular gallop. Severe pulmonary edema produces more rapid and labored respirations; widespread crackles; a productive cough with frothy, bloody sputum; worsening tachycardia; arrhythmias; cold, clammy skin; cyanosis; hypotension; and thready pulse.

● *Pulmonary embolism.* This disorder causes sudden, rapid, shallow respirations and severe dyspnea with anginal or pleuritic chest pain. Other clinical features include tachycardia, tachypnea, a nonproductive cough or a productive cough with blood-tinged sputum, low-grade fever, restlessness, diaphoresis, pleural friction rub, crackles, diffuse wheezing, dullness to percussion, decreased breath sounds, and signs of circulatory collapse. Less common findings are massive hemoptysis, chest splinting, leg edema, and (with a large embolus) cyanosis, syncope, and neck vein distention.

Other causes

• *Drugs.* Narcotics, sedatives and hypnotics, tranquilizers, neuromuscular blockers, magnesium sulfate, and anesthetics can produce slow, shallow respirations.

• *Surgery.* After abdominal or thoracic surgery, pain associated with chest splinting and decreased chest wall motion may cause shallow respirations.

Special considerations

Prepare the patient for diagnostic tests: ABG analysis, pulmonary function tests, chest X-rays, or bronchoscopy.

Position the patient as nearly upright as possible to ease his breathing. (Help a postoperative patient splint his incision while coughing.) If he's taking a drug that depresses respirations, follow all precautions, and monitor him closely. Ensure adequate hydration, and use humidification as needed to thin secretions and to relieve inflamed, dry, or irritated airway mucosa. Administer humidified oxygen, bronchodilators, mucolytics, expectorants, or antibiotics.

Have the patient cough and deep-breathe every hour to clear secretions and to counteract possible hypoventilation. Turn him frequently. He may require chest physiotherapy, incentive spirometry, or intermittent positive-pressure breathing.

Pediatric pointers

In children, shallow respirations commonly indicate a life-threatening condition. Airway obstruction can occur rapidly; if it does, administer back blows or chest thrusts but *not* abdominal thrusts, which can damage internal organs.

Causes of shallow respirations in infants and children may include idiopathic (infant) respiratory distress syndrome, acute epiglottitis, diphtheria, aspiration of a foreign body, croup, acute bronchiolitis, cystic fibrosis, and bacterial pneumonia.

Observe the child to detect apnea. As needed, use humidification and suction,

and administer supplemental oxygen. Give parenteral fluids to ensure adequate hydration. Chest physiotherapy may be required.

SKIN, CLAMMY

Clammy skin—moist, cool, and commonly pale—is a sympathetic nervous system response to stress, which triggers release of the hormones epinephrine and norepinephrine. These hormones cause cutaneous vasoconstriction and secretion of cold sweat from eccrine glands, particularly on the palms, forehead, and soles.

Clammy skin typically accompanies shock, acute hypoglycemia, anxiety reactions, arrhythmias, and heat exhaustion. It also occurs as a vasovagal reaction to severe pain associated with nausea, anorexia, epigastric distress, hyperpnea, tachypnea, weakness, confusion, tachycardia, and pupillary dilation or a combination of these findings. Marked bradycardia and syncope may follow. (See *Clammy skin: Know how to respond,* page 528.)

History and physical examination

If you detect clammy skin, remember that rapid evaluation and intervention are paramount. For example, ask about a history of insulin-dependent diabetes mellitus or cardiac disorders. Is the patient currently taking any medications, especially antiarrhythmics? Is he experiencing pain, chest pressure, nausea, or epigastric distress? Does he feel weak? Does he have a dry mouth? Diarrhea or increased urination?

Next, examine the pupils for dilation. Also check for abdominal distention and increased muscle tension.

CLAMMY SKIN: KNOW HOW TO RESPOND

Be alert for clammy skin. Why? Because it commonly accompanies emergency conditions, such as shock, acute hypoglycemia, and arrhythmias. To know what to do, review these typical clinical situations.

You detect clammy skin in a patient who appears anxious and restless.	You detect clammy skin and possible tremors in a patient who appears irritable and anxious and reports persistent hunger.	You detect clammy skin in a patient with changes in mental status such as confusion.
▼		▼
Quickly take his vital signs, noting tachypnea, tachycardia, hypotension, and a weak, irregular pulse. If present:	▼	Quickly take his vital signs, noting hypotension and changes in pulse rate and rhythm. If present:
	Quickly take his vital signs, noting hypotension. If present:	
▼		▼
Suspect *shock.*	▼	Suspect *arrhythmias.*
	Suspect *acute hypoglycemia.*	
▼		▼
Place the patient in the supine position in bed. Elevate his legs 20 to 30 degrees to promote perfusion to vital organs.	▼	Insert an I.V. line and administer antiarrhythmic drugs. Also give supplemental oxygen, and begin cardiac monitoring.
	Immediately draw blood for glucose studies, and test a drop with a glucose monitor or a reagent strip. Insert an I.V. line, and give a 50-ml bolus of dextrose 50%. Also begin cardiac monitoring.	
▼		
Insert an I.V. line for administration of drugs, fluids, or blood. Also give supplemental oxygen, and begin cardiac monitoring.		

Common medical causes
• *Acute hypoglycemia.* Generalized cool, clammy skin or diaphoresis may accompany irritability, tremors, palpitations, hunger, headache, tachycardia, and anxiety. Central nervous system disturbances may include blurred vision, diplopia, confusion, motor weakness, hemiplegia, or coma.

• *Cardiogenic shock.* Generalized cool, moist, pale skin accompanies confusion and restlessness, hypotension, tachycardia, tachypnea, narrowing pulse pressure, cyanosis, and oliguria.

- *Arrhythmias.* Cardiac arrhythmias may produce generalized cool, clammy skin, mental status changes, dizziness, and hypotension.

- *Heat exhaustion.* In the acute stage, generalized cold, clammy skin accompanies an ashen gray appearance, headache, confusion, syncope, giddiness, and a normal or subnormal temperature. The patient may have a rapid and thready pulse, nausea, vomiting, tachypnea, oliguria, thirst, muscle cramps, and hypotension.

- *Hypovolemic shock.* In this common form of shock, generalized pale, cold, clammy skin accompanies subnormal body temperature, hypotension with narrowing pulse pressure, tachycardia, tachypnea, and rapid, thready pulse. Other findings are flat neck veins, prolonged capillary refill time, decreased urine output, confusion, and decreased level of consciousness.

- *Septic shock.* The cold shock stage causes generalized cold, clammy skin. Associated findings include rapid and thready pulse, severe hypotension, persistent oliguria or anuria, and respiratory failure.

Special considerations

Take the patient's vital signs frequently, and monitor urine output. If clammy skin occurs with an anxiety reaction or pain, you should offer the patient emotional support, administer pain medication and provide a quiet environment.

Pediatric pointers

Infants in shock will not have clammy skin because of their immature sweat glands.

SKIN, MOTTLED

Mottled skin is patchy discoloration indicating primary or secondary changes of the deep, middle, or superficial dermal blood vessels. It can result from hematologic, immune, or connective tissue disorders; chronic occlusive arterial disease; dysproteinemias; immobility; exposure to heat or cold; or shock. Or it can be a normal reaction such as the diffuse mottling (cutis marmorata) that occurs when exposure to cold causes venous stasis in cutaneous blood vessels.

Mottling that occurs with other signs and symptoms usually affects the extremities, indicating restricted blood flow. For example, livedo reticularis, a characteristic network pattern of reddish blue discoloration, occurs when vasospasm of the middermal blood vessels slows local blood flow in dilated superficial capillaries and small veins. Shock causes mottling from systemic vasoconstriction.

History and physical examination

Mottled skin may indicate an emergency condition requiring rapid evaluation and intervention. (See *Mottled skin: Know how to respond,* page 530.) However, if the patient isn't in distress, ask if the mottling began suddenly or gradually. What precipitated it? How long has he had it? Does anything make it go away? Does the patient have other symptoms, such as pain, numbness, or tingling in an extremity? If so, do they disappear with temperature changes?

Observe the patient's skin color, and palpate his arms and legs for skin texture, swelling, and temperature differences between extremities. Also palpate for the presence (or absence) of pulses and for their quality. Note breaks in the skin, muscle appearance, and hair distribution. Also assess motor and sensory function.

Common medical causes

- *Acrocyanosis.* In this rare disorder, anxiety or exposure to cold can cause vasospasm in small cutaneous arterioles. This results in persistent symmetrical

MOTTLED SKIN: KNOW HOW TO RESPOND

If your patient's skin is mottled at the elbows and knees, or all over, and is pale, cool, and clammy, he may be developing *hypovolemic shock.* Quickly take the patient's vital signs, and be sure to note tachycardia or a weak, thready pulse. Observe for flat neck veins. Does the patient appear anxious?

If you find these signs and symptoms, place the patient in the supine position in bed with his legs elevated 20 to 30 degrees. Administer oxygen by nasal cannula or face mask, and begin cardiac monitoring. Insert a large-bore I.V. line for rapid fluid administration, and prepare to insert a central line or a pulmonary artery catheter. Also prepare to catheterize the patient to monitor urine output.

Localized mottling in a pale, cool extremity that the patient says feels painful, numb, and tingling may signal *acute arterial occlusion.* Immediately check the patient's distal pulses: If they are absent or diminished, you will need to insert an I.V. line in an unaffected extremity, and prepare the patient for arteriography or immediate surgery.

blue and red mottling of the affected hands, feet, and nose.

● *Acute arterial occlusion.* Initial signs include temperature and color changes. Pallor may change to blotchy cyanosis and livedo reticularis. Color and temperature demarcation develop at the level of obstruction. Other effects include sudden onset of pain in the extremity, and possibly paresthesia, paresis, and a sensation of cold in the affected area. Examination reveals diminished or absent pulses, cool extremities, prolonged capillary refill time, pallor, and diminished reflexes.

● *Arteriosclerosis obliterans.* Atherosclerotic buildup narrows intra-arterial lumens, resulting in reduced blood flow through the affected artery. Obstructed blood flow to the extremities (usually the lower) produces such peripheral signs and symptoms as leg pallor, cyanosis, blotchy erythema, and livedo reticularis. Related findings include intermittent claudication (most common symptom), diminished or absent pedal pulses, and leg coolness. Other symptoms include coldness and paresthesia.

● *Buerger's disease.* This form of vasculitis produces unilateral or asymmetrical color changes and mottling, particularly livedo networking in the legs. It also typically causes intermittent claudication and erythema along extremity blood vessels. During exposure to cold, the feet are cold, cyanotic, and numb; later they're hot, red, and tingling. Other findings include impaired peripheral pulses and peripheral neuropathy.

● *Cryoglobulinemia.* This necrotizing disorder causes patchy livedo reticularis, petechiae, and ecchymoses. Other findings include fever, chills, urticaria, melena, skin ulcers, epistaxis, Raynaud's phenomenon, eye hemorrhages, hematuria, and gangrene.

● *Hypovolemic shock.* Vasoconstriction from shock commonly produces skin mottling, initially in the knees and elbows. As shock worsens, mottling becomes generalized. Early signs include sudden onset of pallor, cool skin, restlessness, thirst, tachypnea, and slight tachycardia. As shock progresses, associated findings include cool, clammy skin; rapid, thready pulse; hypotension; narrowed pulse pressure; decreased urine output; subnormal temperature; confusion; and decreased level of consciousness.

- *Idiopathic or primary livedo reticularis.* Symmetrical, diffuse, initially asymptomatic mottling can involve the hands, feet, arms, legs, buttocks, and trunk. Initially, networking is intermittent and most pronounced on exposure to cold or stress; eventually, mottling persists even with warming.

- *Periarteritis nodosa.* Skin findings may include asymmetrical, patchy livedo reticularis, palpable nodules along the path of medium-sized arteries, erythema, purpura, muscle wasting, ulcers, gangrene, peripheral neuropathy, fever, weight loss, and malaise.

- *Polycythemia vera.* This hematologic disorder produces livedo reticularis, hemangiomas, purpura, rubor, ulcerative nodules, and scleroderma-like lesions. Other symptoms include headache, a vague feeling of fullness in the head, dizziness, vertigo, visual disturbances, dyspnea, and pruritus.

- *Systemic lupus erythematosus.* This connective tissue disorder can cause livedo reticularis, most commonly on the outer arms. Other signs and symptoms may include a butterfly rash, nondeforming joint pain and stiffness, photosensitivity, Raynaud's phenomenon, patchy alopecia, seizures, fever, anorexia, weight loss, lymphadenopathy, and emotional lability.

Other causes

- *Immobility.* Prolonged immobility may cause bluish, asymptomatic mottling, most noticeably in dependent extremities.

- *Thermal exposure.* Prolonged thermal exposure, as from a heating pad or hot-water bottle, may cause erythema abigne—a localized, reticulated, brown to red mottling.

Special considerations

Typically, mottled skin results from chronic conditions. Teach patients to avoid tight clothing and overexposure to cold or to heating devices, such as hot-water bottles and heating pads.

Pediatric pointers

Mottled skin in children stems from the same causes as in adults. A common cause in children is systemic vasoconstriction from shock.

SKIN, SCALY

Scaly skin results when cells of the uppermost skin layer (stratum corneum) desiccate and shed, causing excessive accumulation of loosely adherent flakes of normal or abnormal keratin. Normally, skin cell loss is imperceptible; the appearance of scale indicates increased cell proliferation secondary to altered keratinization.

Scaly skin varies in texture from fine and delicate to branny, coarse, or stratified. Scales are typically dry, brittle, and shiny, but they can be greasy and dull. Their color ranges from whitish gray, yellow, or brown to a silvery sheen.

Usually benign, scaly skin occurs in fungal, bacterial, and viral infections (cutaneous or systemic), in lymphomas, and in lupus erythematosus; it's common in inflammatory skin diseases. A form of scaly skin—generalized fine desquamation—commonly follows prolonged febrile illness, sunburn, or thermal burn. Red patches of scaly skin that appear or worsen in the winter result from dry skin (or from actinic keratosis, common in the elderly). Drugs also cause scaly skin. Aggravating factors include cold, heat, immobility, and frequent bathing.

History and physical examination

Obtain a history: How long has the patient had scaly skin, and has he had it before? Where did it appear first? Did a lesion or skin eruption such as erythema precede it? Has the patient used a topical skin product recently? How often does he bathe? Has he had joint pain, illness, or malaise recently? Ask the patient about work exposure to chemicals, use of prescribed drugs, and a family history of skin disorders. Find out what kinds of soap, cosmetics, skin lotion, and hair preparations he uses.

Now examine the entire skin surface. Is it dry, oily, moist, or greasy? Observe the general pattern of skin lesions, and record their location. Note their color, shape, and size. Are they thick or fine? Do they itch? Does the patient have other lesions besides scaly skin? Examine the mucous membranes of his mouth, lips, and nose, and inspect his ears, hair, and nails.

Common medical causes

● *Bowen's disease.* This common form of intraepidermal carcinoma causes painless, erythematous plaques that are raised and indurated with a thick, hyperkeratotic scale and, possibly, ulcerated centers.

● *Dermatitis. Exfoliative dermatitis* begins with rapidly developing generalized erythema. Desquamation with fine scales or thick sheets of all or most of the skin surface may cause life-threatening hypothermia. Other possible complications include high cardiac output failure and septicemia. Systemic signs and symptoms may include low-grade fever, chills, malaise, lymphadenopathy, and gynecomastia.

In *nummular eczematous dermatitis,* round, pustular lesions often ooze purulent exudate, itch severely, and rapidly become encrusted and scaly. Lesions appear on the extensor surfaces of the limbs, posterior trunk, and buttocks.

Seborrheic dermatitis begins with erythematous, scaly papules that progress to larger scaly plaques. This disorder primarily involves the center of the face, the chest, scalp, and possibly the genitals, axillae, and perianal region. Pruritus occurs with scaling.

● *Dermatophytosis. Tinea capitis* produces lesions with reddened, slightly elevated borders and a central area of dense scaling; these lesions may become inflamed and pus-filled (kerions). Patchy alopecia and itching may also occur. *Tinea pedis* causes scaling and blisters between the toes. The squamous type produces diffuse, fine, branny scaling. Adherent and silvery white, it's most prominent in skin creases and may affect the entire dorsum of the foot. *Tinea corporis* produces crusty lesions. As they enlarge, their centers heal, causing the classic ringworm shape.

● *Lymphoma.* Hodgkin's disease and malignant lymphoma commonly cause scaly rashes. *Hodgkin's disease* may cause scaling dermatitis with pruritus that begins in the legs and spreads to the entire body. Remission and recurrence are common. Small nodules and diffuse pigmentation are related signs. This disorder typically produces painless enlargement of the peripheral lymph nodes. Other signs and symptoms of lymphoma include fever, fatigue, weight loss, malaise, and hepatosplenomegaly.

Malignant lymphoma initially produces erythematous patches with some scaling that later become interspersed with nodules. Pruritus and discomfort are common; later, tumors and ulcers form. Progression produces nontender lymphadenopathy.

● *Parapsoriasis (chronic).* This disorder produces small or moderate-sized papules, with a thin, adherent scale, on the trunk, hands, and feet. Removal of the scale reveals a shiny brown surface.

● *Pityriasis. Pityriasis rosea*—an acute, benign, and self-limiting disorder—produces widespread scales. It begins with an erythematous, raised, oval herald patch anywhere on the body. A few days or weeks later, yellow-tan or erythematous patches with scaly edges erupt on the trunk and limbs and sometimes on the face, hands, and feet. Pruritus also occurs.

Pityriasis rubra pilaris, an uncommon disorder, initially produces seborrheic scaling on the scalp, progressing to the face and ears. Later, scaly red patches develop on the palms and soles, becoming diffuse, thick, fissured, hyperkeratotic, and painful. Lesions also appear on the hands, fingers, wrists, and forearms and then on wide areas of the trunk, neck, and limbs.

● **Psoriasis.** Silvery white, micaceous scales in this disorder cover erythematous plaques that have sharply defined borders. Psoriasis most commonly appears on the scalp, chest, elbows, knees, back, buttocks, and genitals. Associated signs and symptoms include nail pitting, pruritus, arthritis, and sometimes pain from dry, cracked, encrusted lesions.

● *Systemic lupus erythematosus.* This disorder produces a bright red maculopapular eruption, sometimes with scaling. Patches are sharply defined and involve the nose and malar regions of the face in a butterfly pattern—a primary sign. Similar characteristic rashes appear on other body surfaces; scaling occurs along the lower lip or anterior hair line. Other primary clinical features include photosensitivity and joint pain and stiffness. Vasculitis can occur—leading to infarctive lesions, necrotic leg ulcers, or digital gangrene—as well as Raynaud's phenomenon, patchy alopecia, and mucous membrane ulcers.

● *Tinea versicolor.* This benign fungal skin infection typically produces macular hypopigmented, fawn-colored, or brown patches of varying sizes and shapes. All are slightly scaly. Lesions commonly affect the upper trunk, arms, and lower abdomen, sometimes the neck and, rarely, the face.

Other causes

● *Drugs.* Many drugs can produce scaling patches, among them penicillin, sulfonamides, barbiturates, quinidine, diazepam, phenytoin, and isoniazid.

Special considerations

Teach the patient proper skin care, and suggest lubricating baths and emollients. If scaling results from treatment with corticosteroids, withhold the drug.

Prepare the patient for such diagnostic tests as a Wood's light examination, skin scraping, and skin biopsy.

Elder tip

 Dry, scaly skin on an elderly person is prone to ripping or tearing. Encourage your elderly patient to use lotion to protect and moisturize his skin and to use a gentle soap. Harsh soaps or daily use of soap can be drying. Advise him to avoid sharp or tight bracelets, belts, or other accessories with sharp edges that could cut the skin.

Pediatric pointers

In children, scaly skin may stem from infantile eczema, pityriasis rosea, epidermolytic hyperkeratosis, psoriasis, various forms of ichthyosis, atopic dermatitis, a viral infection (especially hepatitis B virus, which can cause Gianotti-Crosti syndrome), or an acute transient dermatitis. Desquamation may follow a febrile illness.

SKIN TURGOR, DECREASED

Skin turgor—the skin's elasticity—is determined by observing the time required for the skin to return to its normal position after being stretched or pinched. With decreased turgor, pinched skin "holds" for up to 30 seconds, then slowly returns to its normal contour. Skin turgor is commonly assessed over the arm or the sternum, areas normally free from wrinkles and wide variations in tissue thickness. (See *Evaluating skin turgor,* page 534.)

EXAMINATION TIP

EVALUATING SKIN TURGOR

To evaluate skin turgor in an adult, pick up a fold of skin over the sternum or the arm, as shown at left. (In an infant, roll a fold of loosely adherent skin on the abdomen between your thumb and forefinger.) Then release it. Normal skin will immediately return to its previous contour. In decreased skin turgor, the fold of skin will "hold," as shown at right, for up to 30 seconds.

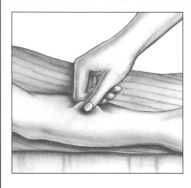
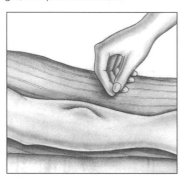

Decreased skin turgor results from dehydration, or volume depletion, which moves interstitial fluid into the vascular bed to maintain circulating blood volume, leading to slackness in the skin's dermal layer. It's a normal finding in the elderly and in people with rapid weight loss; it also occurs in disorders affecting the GI, renal, endocrine, and other systems.

History and physical examination

If your examination reveals decreased skin turgor, ask the patient about food and fluid intake—and fluid loss. Has he recently had prolonged fluid loss from vomiting, diarrhea, draining wounds, or increased urination? A recent fever with sweating? Is he taking diuretics? If so, how often?

Now take the patient's vital signs, noting if his systolic blood pressure while supine is abnormally low (90 mm Hg or less), if it drops 15 to 20 mm Hg or more when he stands, or if his pulse increases 10 beats/minute on standing or sitting. If you detect these signs of orthostatic hypotension or resting tachycardia, start an I.V. line for fluid administration.

Evaluate the patient's level of consciousness (LOC) for confusion and disorientation, and signs of profound dehydration. Inspect his oral mucosa, the furrows of the tongue (especially under the tongue), and the axillae for dryness. Also check his neck veins for flatness and monitor his urine output.

Common medical causes

• *Dehydration.* Decreased skin turgor commonly occurs in moderate to severe dehydration. Associated findings include dry oral mucosa, decreased perspiration, resting tachycardia, orthostatic hypotension, dry and furrowed tongue, increased thirst, weight loss, oliguria, fever, and fatigue. As dehydration worsens, other findings include enophthalmos, lethargy, weakness, confusion, delirium or obtundation, anuria, and shock. Hypotension persists even when the patient lies down.

Special considerations

Even a small deficit in body fluid may be critical in patients with diminished total body fluid—young children, the elderly, the obese, or those patients who've rapidly lost a large amount of weight.

To prevent skin breakdown in the dehydrated patient with poor skin turgor, a decreased LOC, and impaired peripheral circulation, turn the patient every 2 hours, and frequently massage his back and pressure points. Monitor the patient's intake and output, administer I.V. fluid replacement, and offer frequent oral fluids. Weigh the patient daily at the same time on the same scale. Be alert for urine output that falls below 30 ml/hour and for continued weight loss. Also closely monitor the patient for signs of electrolyte imbalance.

Elder tip

 Dehydration from fluid loss is always a concern in elderly people, especially in the summer. Ask your elderly patient if he has a functional fan or air conditioner for the hot weather, and find out if he knows how to use these appliances. Encourage neighbors and family members to arrange regular "check-in-times" to make sure the person is safely tolerating the heat. Advise the elderly patient to stay indoors during peak sun and heat hours, roughly between 10 a.m. and 2 p.m. Instruct him to take frequent rests during the day. Encourage fluid intake, keeping in mind any restrictions or diuretics ordered.

Pediatric pointers

Diarrhea secondary to gastroenteritis is the most common cause of dehydration in children, especially from birth to age 2.

SPLENOMEGALY

Because splenomegaly—an enlarged spleen—commonly occurs in many disorders, it isn't a diagnostic sign by itself. What's more, an enlarged spleen may occur in as many as 5% of normal adults. Usually, though, this sign points to infection, trauma, or hepatic, autoimmune, neoplastic, or hematologic disorders.

Because the spleen functions as the body's largest lymph node, splenomegaly can result from any process that triggers lymphadenopathy. For example, it may reflect reactive hyperplasia (a response to infection or inflammation), proliferation or infiltration of neoplastic cells, extramedullary hemopoiesis, phagocytic cell proliferation, increased blood cell destruction, or vascular congestion associated with portal hypertension.

Splenomegaly may be detected by *light* palpation under the left costal margin. (See *How to palpate for splenomegaly,* page 536.) Unfortunately, this technique isn't always advisable or effective. As a result, splenomegaly may need to be confirmed by a computed tomography or radionuclide scan.

Emergency interventions

 If the patient has a history of abdominal or thoracic trauma, do *not* palpate the abdomen because this may aggravate internal bleeding. Instead, examine for left upper quadrant pain and signs of shock, such as tachycardia and tachypnea. If you detect either one, suspect splenic rupture. Insert an I.V. line for emergency fluid and blood replacement and administer oxygen. Also catheterize the patient to evaluate urine output, and begin cardiac monitoring. Prepare the patient for surgery.

EXAMINATION TIP

HOW TO PALPATE FOR SPLENOMEGALY

Detecting splenomegaly requires skillful and gentle palpation to avoid ruptur-ing the enlarged organ. Follow these steps carefully:

• Place the patient in the supine po-sition, and stand at her right side. Place your left hand under the left costovertebral angle, and push light-ly to move the spleen forward. Then press your right hand gently under the left front costal margin.
• Have the patient take a deep breath and then exhale. As she ex-hales, move your right hand along the tissue contours under the ribs' border, feeling for the spleen's edge. The enlarged spleen should feel like a firm mass that bumps against your fingers. Remember to begin palpa-tion low enough in the abdomen to catch the edge of a massive spleen.
• Grade the splenomegaly as slight (1 to 4 cm below the costal margin), moderate (4 to 8 cm below the costal margin), or great (8 cm or more below the costal margin).
• Reposition the patient on her right side with her hips and knees flexed slightly to move the spleen forward. Then repeat the palpation procedure.

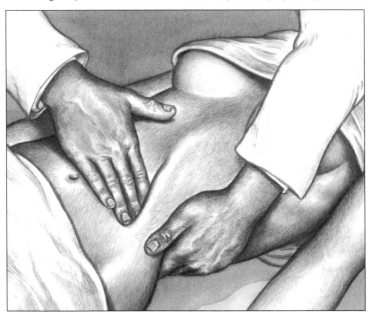

History and physical examination
If you detect splenomegaly during a rou-tine physical examination, begin by ex-ploring associated signs and symptoms.

Has the patient been unusually tired late-ly? Does he frequently have colds, sore throats, or other infections? Does he bruise easily? Ask about left upper quadrant pain, abdominal fullness, and early satiety. Finally, examine the patient's skin for pallor and ecchymoses. Palpate his axillae, groin, and neck for lymphadenopathy.

Common medical causes

● **Brucellosis.** In severe cases of this rare infection, splenomegaly is a major sign. Typically, brucellosis begins insidiously with fatigue, headache, backache, anorexia, and arthralgia. Later, it may cause hepatomegaly, lymphadenopathy, weight loss, and vertebral or peripheral nerve pain on pressure.

● **Cirrhosis.** About one-third of patients with advanced cirrhosis develop moderate to marked splenomegaly. Among other late findings are jaundice, hepatomegaly, leg edema, hematemesis, and ascites. Signs of hepatic encephalopathy—such as asterixis, fetor hepaticus, slurred speech, and decreased level of consciousness that may progress to coma—are also common. Besides jaundice, skin effects may include severe pruritus, poor tissue turgor, spider angiomas, palmar erythema, pallor, and signs of bleeding tendencies. Endocrine effects may include menstrual irregularities or testicular atrophy, gynecomastia, and loss of chest and axillary hair. The patient may also have fever and right upper abdominal pain that's aggravated by sitting up or leaning forward.

● **Felty's syndrome.** Splenomegaly is characteristic in this syndrome that occurs in chronic rheumatoid arthritis. Associated findings are joint pain and deformity, sensory or motor loss, rheumatoid nodules, lymphadenopathy, palmar erythema, and leg ulcers.

● **Histoplasmosis.** Acute disseminated histoplasmosis commonly produces splenomegaly and hepatomegaly. It may also cause lymphadenopathy, jaundice, fever, anorexia, emaciation, and signs and symptoms of anemia, such as weakness, fatigue, pallor, and malaise. Occasionally, the patient's tongue, palate,

epiglottis, and larynx become ulcerated, resulting in pain, hoarseness, and dysphagia.

● **Infectious mononucleosis.** A common sign of this disorder, splenomegaly is most pronounced during the second and third weeks of illness. Typically, it's accompanied by a triad of symptoms: sore throat, cervical lymphadenopathy, and fluctuating fever with an evening peak of 101° to 102° F (38.3° to 38.9° C). Occasionally, hepatomegaly, jaundice, and a maculopapular rash may also occur.

● **Leukemia.** Moderate to severe splenomegaly is an early sign of both acute and chronic leukemia. In chronic granulocytic leukemia, splenomegaly is sometimes painful. Accompanying it may be hepatomegaly, lymphadenopathy, fatigue, malaise, pallor, fever, gum swelling, bleeding tendencies, weight loss, anorexia, and abdominal, bone, and joint pain. Acute leukemia sometimes also causes dyspnea, tachycardia, and palpitations. In advanced disease, the patient may display confusion, headache, vomiting, seizures, papilledema, and nuchal rigidity.

● **Pancreatic cancer.** This cancer may cause moderate to severe splenomegaly if tumor growth compresses the splenic vein. Its other characteristics include abdominal or back pain, anorexia, nausea and vomiting, weight loss, GI bleeding, jaundice, pruritus, skin lesions, emotional lability, weakness, and fatigue. Palpation may reveal a tender abdominal mass and hepatomegaly, while auscultation reveals a bruit in the periumbilical area and left upper quadrant.

● **Polycythemia vera.** Late in this disorder, the spleen may become markedly enlarged, resulting in easy satiety, abdominal fullness, and left upper quadrant or pleuritic chest pain. Clinical features accompanying splenomegaly are widespread and numerous. The patient may have deep, purplish red oral mucous membranes, headache, dyspnea, dizziness, vertigo, weakness, and fatigue. He may also have finger and toe paresthesia, impaired mentation, tinnitus, blurred or double vision, scotoma, increased blood pressure, and intermittent claudication. Other signs and symptoms include pruritus, urticaria, ruddy cyanosis, epigastric distress, weight loss, hepatomegaly, and bleeding tendencies.

• *Sarcoidosis.* This granulomatous disorder may produce splenomegaly and hepatomegaly, possibly accompanied by vague abdominal discomfort. Its other findings vary with the affected body system but may include nonproductive cough, dyspnea, malaise, fatigue, arthralgia, myalgia, weight loss, lymphadenopathy, skin lesions, irregular pulse, impaired vision, dysphagia, and seizures.

• *Splenic rupture.* Splenomegaly may result from massive hemorrhage in this disorder. The patient may also have left upper quadrant pain, abdominal rigidity, and Kehr's sign.

• *Thrombotic thrombocytopenic purpura.* This disorder may produce splenomegaly and hepatomegaly accompanied by fever, generalized purpura, jaundice, pallor, vaginal bleeding, and hematuria. Other effects may include fatigue, weakness, headache, pallor, abdominal pain, and arthralgias. Eventually, the patient develops signs of neurologic deterioration and of renal failure.

Special considerations
Prepare the patient for diagnostic studies, such as the complete blood count and radionuclide and computed tomography scans of the spleen.

Pediatric pointers
Besides the causes of splenomegaly described above, the pediatric patient may develop splenomegaly in histiocytic disorders, congenital hemolytic anemia, Gaucher's disease, Niemann-Pick disease, hereditary spherocytosis, sickle cell disease, or beta-thalassemia (Cooley's anemia). Splenic abscess is the most common cause of splenomegaly in immunocompromised children.

STERTOROUS RESPIRATIONS

Characterized by a harsh, rattling, or snoring sound, stertorous respirations usually result from the vibration of relaxed oropharyngeal structures during sleep or coma, causing partial airway obstruction. Less commonly, these respirations result from retained mucus in the upper airway.

This common sign occurs in about 10% of normal individuals, especially middle-aged, obese men. It may be aggravated by use of alcohol or sedatives before bed, which increases oropharyngeal flaccidity, and by sleeping in the supine position, which allows the relaxed tongue to slip back into the airway. The major pathologic causes of stertorous respirations are obstructive sleep apnea and life-threatening upper airway obstruction associated with an oropharyngeal tumor or with uvular or palatal edema. This obstruction may also occur during the postictal phase of a generalized seizure when mucous secretions or a relaxed tongue blocks the airway.

Occasionally, stertorous respirations are mistaken for stridor, which is another sign of upper airway obstruction. However, stridor indicates laryngeal or tracheal obstruction, whereas stertorous respirations signal higher airway obstruction.

Emergency interventions
 If you detect stertorous respirations, check the patient's mouth and throat for edema, redness, and masses. If edema is marked, quickly take vital signs. Observe for signs and symptoms of respiratory distress, such as dyspnea, tachypnea, use of accessory muscles, intercostal muscle retractions, and cyanosis. Elevate the head of the bed

30 degrees to help ease breathing and reduce the edema. Then administer supplemental oxygen by nasal cannula or face mask, and prepare to intubate the patient, perform a tracheostomy, or provide mechanical ventilation. Insert an I.V. line for fluid and drug access, and begin cardiac monitoring.

If you detect stertorous respirations while the patient is sleeping, observe his breathing pattern for 3 to 4 minutes. Do noisy respirations cease when he turns on his side and recur when he assumes a supine position? Watch carefully for periods of apnea and note their length. When possible, question the patient's sleep partner about his snoring habits. Is she frequently awakened by the patient's snoring? Has she also observed the patient talk in his sleep or sleepwalk? Ask about signs of sleep deprivation, such as personality changes, headaches, daytime somnolence, or decreased mental acuity.

Common medical causes

● *Airway obstruction.* Regardless of its cause, partial airway obstruction may lead to stertorous respirations accompanied by wheezing, dyspnea, tachypnea and, later, intercostal retractions and nasal flaring. If the obstruction becomes complete, the patient abruptly loses his ability to talk and displays diaphoresis, tachycardia, and inspiratory chest movement but absent breath sounds. Severe hypoxemia rapidly ensues, resulting in cyanosis, loss of consciousness, and cardiopulmonary collapse.

● *Obstructive sleep apnea.* Loud and disruptive snoring is a major characteristic of this syndrome, which commonly affects the obese. Typically, the snoring alternates with periods of sleep apnea, which usually end with loud, gasping sounds. Alternating tachycardia and bradycardia may occur.

Episodes of snoring and apnea recur in a cyclic pattern throughout the night. Sleep disturbances, such as somnambulism and talking during sleep, may also occur. Some patients display hypertension and ankle edema. Most awaken in the morning with a generalized headache, feeling tired and unrefreshed. The most common complaint is excessive daytime sleepiness. Lack of sleep may cause depression, hostility, and decreased mental acuity.

Other causes

● *Endotracheal surgery, intubation, or suction.* These procedures may cause significant palatal or uvular edema, resulting in stertorous respirations.

Special considerations

Continue to monitor the patient's respiratory status carefully. Administer corticosteroids or antibiotics and cool, humidified oxygen to reduce palatal and uvular inflammation and edema.

Laryngoscopy and bronchoscopy (to rule out airway obstruction) or formal sleep studies may be necessary.

Pediatric pointers

In children, the most common cause of stertorous respirations is nasal or pharyngeal obstruction secondary to tonsillar or adenoid hypertrophy or the presence of a foreign body.

STOOL, CLAY-COLORED

Pale, putty-colored stools usually result from hepatic, gallbladder, or pancreatic disorders. Normally, bile pigments give the stool its characteristic brown color. However, hepatocellular degeneration or biliary obstruction may interfere with the formation or release of these pigments into the intestine, resulting in clay-colored stools. Commonly, these stools are associated with jaundice and dark urine.

History and physical examination

After noting when the patient first noticed clay-colored stools, explore associated signs and symptoms such as abdominal pain. Also ask about nausea and vomiting, fatigue, anorexia, weight loss, and dark urine. Does the patient have trouble digesting fatty foods or heavy meals? Does he bruise easily?

Next, review the patient's medical history for gallbladder, hepatic, or pancreatic disorders. Has he ever had biliary surgery? Has he recently undergone barium studies? (Barium lightens stool color for several days.) Also ask about antacid use; large amounts may lighten stool color. Note a history of alcoholism or exposure to other hepatotoxins.

After assessing the patient's general appearance, take his vital signs and check his skin and eyes for jaundice. Then examine the abdomen; inspect for distention and auscultate for hypoactive bowel sounds. Percuss and palpate for masses and rebound tenderness. Finally, obtain urine and stool specimens for laboratory analysis.

Common medical causes

● *Bile duct cancer.* A common presenting sign of this cancer, clay-colored stools may be accompanied by jaundice, pruritus, and weight loss. Upper abdominal pain and bleeding tendencies may also occur.

● *Biliary cirrhosis.* Clay-colored stools typically follow unexplained pruritus that worsens at bedtime, weakness, fatigue, weight loss, and vague abdominal pain; these features may be present for years. Associated findings include jaundice, hyperpigmentation, and signs of malabsorption, such as nocturnal diarrhea, steatorrhea, purpura, and bone and back pain resulting from osteomalacia. The patient may also have hepatomegaly, hematemesis, ascites, edema, and xanthomas on his palms, soles, and elbows.

● *Cholangitis (sclerosing).* Characterized by fibrosis of the bile ducts, this chronic inflammatory disorder may cause clay-colored stools, chronic or intermittent jaundice, pruritus, and right upper abdominal pain.

● *Cholelithiasis.* Stones in the biliary tract may cause clay-colored stools when they obstruct the common bile duct (choledocholithiasis). However, if the obstruction is intermittent, the stools may alternate between normal and clay color. Associated symptoms may include dyspepsia and—in sudden, severe obstruction—characteristic biliary colic. This right upper quadrant pain intensifies over several hours and may radiate to the epigastrium or shoulder blades. The pain is accompanied by tachycardia, restlessness, nausea, vomiting, upper abdominal tenderness, fever, chills, and jaundice.

● *Hepatic carcinoma.* Before clay-colored stools occur in this disorder, the patient usually has weight loss, weakness, and anorexia. Later, he may develop jaundice, right upper quadrant pain, hepatomegaly, ascites, dependent edema, and fever. A bruit, hum, or rubbing sound may be heard on auscultation if the carcinoma involves a large part of the liver.

● *Hepatitis.* In *viral hepatitis,* clay-colored stools signal the start of the icteric phase and are typically followed by jaundice within 1 to 5 days. Associated signs include mild weight loss and dark urine as well as continuation of some preicteric findings, such as anorexia and tender hepatomegaly. During the icteric phase, the patient may become irritable and develop right upper quadrant pain, splenomegaly, enlarged cervical lymph nodes, and severe pruritus. After jaundice disappears, the patient continues to experience fatigue, flatulence, abdominal pain or tenderness, and dyspepsia, although his appetite usually returns and hepatomegaly subsides. The posticteric phase generally lasts from 2 to 6 weeks, with full recovery in 6 months.

In cholestatic *nonviral hepatitis,* clay-colored stools occur with other signs of viral hepatitis.

Other causes
● *Biliary surgery.* This surgery may cause bile duct stricture, resulting in clay-colored stools.

Special considerations
Prepare the patient for diagnostic tests, such as liver enzyme and serum bilirubin levels, sonograms, computed tomography scan, and stool analysis.

Pediatric pointers
Clay-colored stools may occur in infants with biliary atresia.

STRIDOR

A loud, harsh, musical respiratory sound, stridor results from obstruction in the trachea or larynx. Usually heard during inspiration, this sign may also occur during expiration in severe upper airway obstruction. It may begin as low-pitched "croaking" and progress to high-pitched "crowing" as respirations become more vigorous.

Life-threatening upper airway obstruction can stem from foreign body aspiration, increased secretions, intraluminal tumor, localized edema or muscle spasms, and external compression by a tumor or aneurysm.

Emergency interventions
 If you hear stridor, quickly check the patient's vital signs and examine for other signs of partial airway obstruction—choking or gagging, tachypnea, dyspnea, shallow respirations, intercostal retractions, nasal flaring, tachycardia, cyanosis, and diaphoresis. (Recognize that abrupt cessation of stridor signals complete obstruction in which the patient has inspiratory chest movement but absent breath sounds. Unable to talk, he quickly becomes lethargic and loses consciousness.) If you detect any signs of airway obstruction, try to clear the airway with back blows or abdominal thrusts (Heimlich maneuver). Next, administer oxygen by nasal cannula or face mask, or prepare for intubation or emergency tracheostomy and mechanical ventilation. (See *Performing emergency ET intubation,* page 542.) Have equipment ready to suction any aspirated vomitus or blood through the endotracheal or tracheostomy tube. Connect the patient to a cardiac monitor and position him upright to ease his breathing.

History and physical examination
When the patient's condition permits, discuss his medical history with him or his family. First, find out when the stridor began. Has he had it before? Does he have an upper respiratory infection? If so, how long has he had it? Ask about a history of allergies, tumors, and respiratory and vascular disorders. Note recent exposure to smoke or noxious fumes or gases. Next, explore associated signs and symptoms. Does stridor occur with pain or cough?

Then examine the patient's mouth for excessive secretions, foreign matter, inflammation, and swelling. Assess his neck for swelling, masses, subcutaneous crepitation, or scars. Observe the patient's chest for delayed, decreased, or asymmetrical chest expansion. Auscultate for wheezing, rhonchi, crackles, rubs, and other abnormal breath sounds. Percuss for dullness, tympany, or flatness. Finally, note any burns or signs of trauma, such as ecchymoses and lacerations.

Common medical causes
● *Airway trauma.* Local trauma to the upper airway commonly causes acute obstruction, resulting in the sudden onset of stridor. Accompanying this sign are dysphonia, dysphagia, hemoptysis, cya-

PERFORMING EMERGENCY E.T. INTUBATION

For a patient with stridor, you may have to perform emergency endotracheal (ET) intubation to establish a patent airway and administer mechanical ventilation. Just follow these essential steps:

- Gather the necessary equipment.
- Explain the procedure to your patient.
- Place the patient flat on his back with a small blanket or pillow under his head. This position aligns the axis of the oropharynx, posterior pharynx, and trachea.
- Check the cuff on the ET tube for leaks.
- After intubation, inflate the cuff, using the minimal leak technique.
- Check tube placement by auscultating for bilateral breath sounds; observe the patient for chest expansion and feel for warm exhalations at the ET tube's opening.
- Insert an oral airway or bite block.

- Secure the tube and airway with tape applied to skin treated with compound benzoin tincture.
- Suction secretions from the patient's mouth and ET tube, as needed.
- Administer oxygen and/or initiate mechanical ventilation.
- After the patient is intubated, be sure to suction secretions at least every 2 hours and check cuff pressure once every shift (correcting any air leaks with the minimal leak technique).
- Prepare the patient for chest X-rays to check tube placement, and restrain and reassure him as needed.

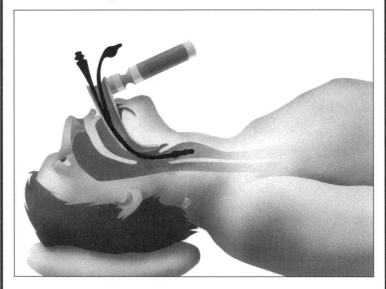

nosis, accessory muscle use, intercostal retractions, nasal flaring, tachypnea, progressive dyspnea, and shallow respirations. Palpation may reveal subcutaneous crepitation in the neck or upper chest.

• *Anaphylaxis.* In a severe allergic reaction, upper airway edema and laryngospasm cause stridor and other signs of respiratory distress: nasal flaring, wheezing, accessory muscle use, intercostal retractions, and dyspnea. The patient may also have nasal congestion and profuse, watery rhinorrhea. Typically, these respiratory effects are preceded by a feeling of impending doom or fear, weakness, diaphoresis, sneezing, nasal pruritus, urticaria, erythema, and angioedema. Common associated findings include chest or throat tightness, dysphagia, and possibly signs of shock, such as hypotension, tachycardia, and cool, clammy skin.

• *Aspiration of a foreign body.* Sudden stridor is characteristic in life-threatening aspiration of a foreign body. Related findings are abrupt onset of dry, paroxysmal coughing, gagging or choking, hoarseness, tachycardia, wheezing, dyspnea, tachypnea, intercostal muscle retractions, diminished breath sounds, cyanosis, and shallow respirations. The patient's expression is typically anxious and distressed.

• *Hypocalcemia.* In this disorder, laryngospasm can cause stridor. Other findings include paresthesia, carpopedal spasm, and positive Chvostek's and Trousseau's signs.

• *Inhalation injury.* Within 48 hours after inhalation of smoke or noxious fumes, the patient may develop laryngeal edema and bronchospasms, resulting in stridor. Associated signs and symptoms include singed nasal hairs, orofacial burns, coughing, hoarseness, sooty sputum, crackles, rhonchi, wheezing, and other signs of respiratory distress, such as dyspnea, accessory muscle use, intercostal retractions, and nasal flaring.

• *Mediastinal tumor.* Commonly asymptomatic at first, this tumor may eventually compress the trachea and bronchi, resulting in stridor. Its other effects include hoarseness, brassy cough, tracheal shift or tug, dilated neck veins, swelling of the face and neck, stertorous respirations, and suprasternal retractions on inspiration. The patient may also report dyspnea, dysphagia, and pain in the chest, shoulder, or arm.

• *Retrosternal thyroid.* This anatomic abnormality causes stridor, dysphagia, cough, hoarseness, and tracheal deviation. It can also cause signs of thyrotoxicosis.

Other causes

• *Diagnostic tests.* Bronchoscopy or laryngoscopy may precipitate laryngospasm and stridor.

• *Treatments.* After prolonged intubation, the patient may have laryngeal edema and stridor when the tube is removed. Neck surgery such as thyroidectomy may cause laryngeal paralysis and stridor.

Special considerations

Continue to monitor the patient's vital signs closely. Prepare him for diagnostic tests, such as arterial blood gas analysis and chest X-rays.

Pediatric pointers

Stridor is a major sign of airway obstruction in the pediatric patient. When you hear this sign, you must intervene quickly to prevent total airway obstruction. This emergency can happen more rapidly in a child because his airway is narrower than an adult's.

Causes of stridor include foreign body aspiration, croup, laryngeal diphtheria, pertussis, retropharyngeal abscess, and congenital abnormalities of the larynx.

Therapy for partial airway obstruction typically involves hot or cold steam in a mist tent or hood, parenteral fluids and electrolytes, and plenty of rest.

SYNCOPE

A common neurologic sign, syncope (or fainting) refers to transient loss of consciousness associated with impaired cerebral blood supply. It usually occurs abruptly and lasts for seconds to minutes. Typically, the patient lies motionless with his skeletal muscles relaxed but sphincter muscles controlled. However, the depth of unconsciousness varies; some patients can hear voices or see blurred outlines; others are unaware of their surroundings.

In many ways, syncope simulates death: The patient is strikingly pale with a slow, weak pulse, hypotension, and almost imperceptible breathing. If severe hypotension lasts for 15 to 20 seconds or more, the patient may also develop convulsive, tonic-clonic movements. However, in the majority of cases, confusion, headache, and drowsiness don't follow a syncope episode.

Syncope may result from cardiac and cerebrovascular disorders, hypoxemia, and postural changes in the presence of autonomic dysfunction. It may also follow vigorous coughing (tussive syncope) and emotional stress, injury, shock, or pain (vasovagal syncope, or common fainting). Hysterical syncope may also follow emotional stress but isn't accompanied by other vasodepressor effects.

Emergency interventions

 If you witness syncope, ensure a patent airway and take vital signs. Then place the patient in a supine position, elevate his legs, and loosen any tight clothing. Be alert for tachycardia, bradycardia, or an irregular pulse. Meanwhile, place him on a cardiac monitor to detect arrhythmias. Give oxygen and insert an I.V. line for drug administration if an arrhythmia appears.

Be ready to begin cardiopulmonary resuscitation. Cardioversion, defibrillation, or insertion of a temporary pacemaker may be required.

History and physical examination

If the patient reports syncope, collect information about the episode from him and his family. Did he feel weak, lightheaded, nauseous, or sweaty just before he fainted? Did he get up quickly from a chair or from lying down? During the syncope, did he have muscle spasms or incontinence? How long was he unconscious? When he regained consciousness, was he alert or confused? Did he have a headache? Has he had syncope before? If so, how often does it occur?

Next, take the patient's vital signs and examine him for any injuries that may have occurred during his fall.

Common medical causes

● *Aortic arch syndrome.* In addition to syncope, the patient may have weak or abruptly absent carotid pulses and unequal or absent radial pulses. Early signs and symptoms include night sweats, pallor, nausea, anorexia, weight loss, arthralgia, and Raynaud's phenomenon. He may also have hypotension in the arms, dizziness, paresthesia, intermittent claudication, bruits, visual disturbances, and neck, shoulder, and chest pain.

● *Aortic stenosis.* A cardinal late sign, syncope is accompanied by exertional dyspnea and anginal chest pain. Related findings include marked fatigue, orthopnea, paroxysmal nocturnal dyspnea, palpitations, and diminished carotid pulses. Typically, auscultation reveals atrial and ventricular gallops as well as a harsh, crescendo-decrescendo systolic ejection murmur that's loudest at the right sternal border of the second intercostal space.

● *Cardiac arrhythmias.* Any arrhythmia that decreases cardiac output and impairs cerebral circulation may cause syncope. Usually, other effects develop first, such as palpitations, pallor, confusion, diaphoresis, dyspnea, and hypotension. But in Adams-Stokes syndrome, syncope may occur without warning. During syncope, the patient has asystole, which may precipitate spasms and myoclonic jerks if prolonged. He also has an ashen gray pallor that progresses to cyanosis, incontinence, bilateral Babinski's reflex, and fixed pupils.

● *Hypoxemia.* Regardless of its cause, severe hypoxemia may produce syncope. Common related effects include confusion, tachycardia, restlessness, and incoordination.

● *Orthostatic hypotension.* Syncope occurs when the patient rises quickly from a recumbent position. Look for a drop of 10 to 20 mm Hg or more in systolic or diastolic blood pressure; also look for tachycardia, pallor, dizziness, blurred vision, nausea, and diaphoresis.

● *Transient ischemic attacks.* Marked by transient neurologic deficits, these attacks may produce syncope and decreased level of consciousness. Other findings vary with the affected artery but may include vision loss, nystagmus, aphasia, dysarthria, unilateral numbness, hemiparesis or hemiplegia, tinnitus, facial weakness, dysphagia, and staggering or uncoordinated gait.

Other causes
● *Drugs.* Quinidine may cause syncope—and possibly sudden death—associated with ventricular fibrillation. Prazosin may cause severe orthostatic hypotension and syncope, usually after the first dose. Occasionally, griseofulvin, levodopa, and indomethacin produce syncope, too.

Special considerations
Continue to monitor the patient's vital signs closely. Advise him to pace his activities, to rise slowly from a recumbent position, to avoid standing still for a prolonged time, and to sit or lie down as soon as he feels faint.

Pediatric pointers
Syncope is much less common in children than in adults. It may result from cardiac or neurologic disorders, allergy, or emotional stress.

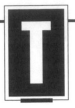

TACHYCARDIA

Easily detected by counting the apical, carotid, or radial pulse, tachycardia is a heart rate greater than 100 beats/minute. Usually, the patient also complains of palpitations or of his heart "racing." This common sign normally occurs in response to emotional or physical stress, such as excitement, exercise, pain, and fever. It may also result from use of stimulants, such as caffeine and tobacco. More important, though, tachycardia may be an early sign of a life-threatening disorder, such as cardiogenic, hypovolemic, or septic shock. It may also result from cardiovascular, respiratory, and metabolic disorders and from the effects of certain drugs, tests, and treatments. (See *What happens in tachycardia.*)

Emergency interventions

 After detecting tachycardia, first examine for reduced cardiac output, which may initiate or result from tachycardia. Take the patient's other vital signs and determine his level of consciousness (LOC). If the patient has increased or decreased blood pressure and is drowsy or confused, administer oxygen and begin cardiac monitoring. Insert an I.V. line to allow fluid and drug administration, and gather emergency resuscitation equipment.

History and physical examination

When the patient's condition permits, take a focused history. Find out if he has had palpitations before. If so, how were they treated? Explore associated symptoms. Is the patient dizzy or short of breath? Weak or fatigued? Is he experiencing chest pain? Next, ask about a history of trauma, diabetes, or cardiac, pulmonary, or thyroid disorders. Also obtain a drug history.

Now, inspect the patient's skin for pallor or cyanosis. Assess pulses, noting peripheral edema. Finally, auscultate the heart and lungs for abnormal sounds or rhythms.

Common medical causes

• *Adrenocortical insufficiency.* In this disorder, tachycardia commonly occurs with a weak pulse as well as progressive weakness and fatigue, which may become so severe that the patient requires bed rest. Other clinical features include abdominal pain, nausea and vomiting, altered bowel habits, weight loss, orthostatic hypotension, irritability, bronze skin, decreased libido, and syncope. Some patients report an enhanced sense of taste, smell, and hearing.

• *Adult respiratory distress syndrome (ARDS).* Besides tachycardia, ARDS causes crackles, rhonchi, dyspnea, tachypnea, nasal flaring, and grunting respirations. Other findings include cyanosis, anxiety, decreased LOC, and abnormal chest X-ray findings.

• *Anaphylactic shock.* In life-threatening anaphylactic shock, tachycardia and sudden hypotension develop within minutes after exposure to an allergen, such as penicillin or an insect sting. Typically, the patient is visibly anxious and has severe pruritus, perhaps with urticaria and a pounding headache. Other findings may include flushed and clammy skin, a cough, dyspnea, nausea, abdominal cramps, seizures, stridor, change or loss of voice associated with laryngeal edema, and urinary urgency and incontinence.

• **Anemia.** Tachycardia and bounding pulse are characteristic in anemia. Associated signs and symptoms include fatigue, pallor, dyspnea, and possibly bleeding tendencies. Auscultation may reveal an atrial gallop, a systolic bruit over the carotid arteries, and crackles.

• **Aortic insufficiency.** Accompanying tachycardia in this disorder are a "water-hammer" bounding pulse and a large, diffuse apical heave. In severe insufficiency, widened pulse pressure occurs. The hallmark of auscultation is a diastolic murmur that starts with the second heart sound; is decrescendo, high-pitched, and blowing; and is heard best at the left sternal border of the second and third intercostal space. Atrial or ventricular gallop, an early systolic murmur, an Austin Flint murmur (apical diastolic rumble), or Duroziez's murmur (heard over the femoral artery during systole and diastole) also may be heard. Other findings may include anginal chest pain, dyspnea, palpitations, strong abrupt carotid pulsations, pallor, and signs of heart failure, such as crackles and neck vein distention.

• **Aortic stenosis.** Typically, this valvular disorder causes tachycardia, a weak, thready pulse, and an atrial gallop. Its chief features, though, are exertional dyspnea, anginal chest pain, dizziness, and syncope. Aortic stenosis also causes a harsh, crescendo-decrescendo systolic ejection murmur that's loudest at the right sternal border of the second intercostal space. Other findings may include palpitations, crackles, and fatigue.

• **Cardiac arrhythmias.** Tachycardia may occur with a regular or irregular heart rhythm here. The patient may be hypotensive and report dizziness, palpita-

WHAT HAPPENS IN TACHYCARDIA

Tachycardia represents the heart's effort to deliver more oxygen to body tissues by increasing the rate at which blood passes through the vessels. This sign can reflect overstimulation within the sinoatrial node, the atrium, the atrioventricular node, or the ventricles.

Because heart rate affects cardiac output (cardiac output = heart rate x stroke volume), tachycardia can lower cardiac output by reducing ventricular filling time and stroke volume (the output of each ventricle at every contraction). As cardiac output plummets, arterial pressure and peripheral perfusion decrease. Tachycardia further aggravates myocardial ischemia by increasing the heart's demand for oxygen while reducing the duration of diastole—the period of greatest coronary flow.

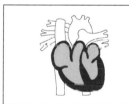

Normally, ventricular volume reaches 120 to 130 ml during diastolic filling.

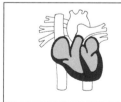

In tachycardia, decreased ventricular volume leads to hypotension and decreased peripheral perfusion.

tions, weakness, and fatigue. Depending on his heart rate, he may also have tachypnea, decreased LOC, and pale, cool, clammy skin.

• *Cardiac tamponade.* In life-threatening cardiac tamponade, tachycardia commonly occurs with pulsus paradoxus, dyspnea, and tachypnea. The patient is visibly anxious and restless with cyanotic, clammy skin and distended neck veins. He may have muffled heart sounds, pericardial friction rub, chest pain, hypotension, narrowed pulse pressure, and hepatomegaly.

• *Cardiogenic shock.* Although many features of cardiogenic shock appear in other types of shock, they're usually more profound here. Accompanying tachycardia are weak, thready pulse; narrowing pulse pressure; hypotension; tachypnea; cold, pale, clammy, and cyanotic skin; oliguria; restlessness; and altered LOC.

• *Chronic obstructive pulmonary disease (COPD).* Although the clinical picture varies widely in COPD, tachycardia is a common sign. Other characteristic findings include cough, tachypnea, dyspnea, pursed-lip breathing, accessory muscle use, cyanosis, diminished breath sounds, rhonchi, crackles, and wheezing. Clubbing and barrel chest are usually late findings.

• *Diabetic ketoacidosis.* This life-threatening disorder commonly produces tachycardia and a thready pulse. Its cardinal sign, though, is Kussmaul's respirations—abnormally rapid, deep breathing. Other signs and symptoms of acidosis may include fruity breath odor, orthostatic hypotension, generalized weakness, anorexia, nausea, vomiting, and abdominal pain. The patient's LOC may vary from lethargy to coma.

• *Heart failure.* Especially common in left-sided heart failure, tachycardia may be accompanied by a ventricular gallop, fatigue, dyspnea (exertional and paroxysmal nocturnal), orthopnea, and leg edema. Eventually, the patient develops widespread effects, such as palpitations, narrowed pulse pressure, hypotension, tachypnea, crackles, dependent edema, weight gain, slowed mental response, diaphoresis, pallor, and possibly oliguria. Late signs include hemoptysis, cyanosis, and marked hepatomegaly and pitting edema.

• *Hyperosmolar hyperglycemic nonketotic syndrome.* Rapidly deteriorating LOC is typically accompanied by tachycardia, hypotension, tachypnea, seizures, oliguria, and severe dehydration with poor skin turgor and dry mucous membranes.

• *Hypertensive crisis.* Life-threatening hypertensive crisis is characterized by tachycardia, tachypnea, diastolic blood pressure that exceeds 120 mm Hg, and systolic blood pressure that may exceed 200 mm Hg. Typically, the patient develops pulmonary edema with neck vein distention, dyspnea, and pink, frothy sputum. Related findings may include chest pain, severe headache, drowsiness, confusion, anxiety, tinnitus, epistaxis, muscle twitching, seizures, nausea, and vomiting. Focal neurologic signs such as paresthesia may also occur.

• *Hypoglycemia.* A common sign of hypoglycemia, tachycardia is accompanied by hypothermia, nervousness, trembling, fatigue, malaise, weakness, headache, hunger, nausea, diaphoresis, and moist, clammy skin. Central nervous system effects include blurred or double vision, motor weakness, hemiplegia, seizures, and decreased LOC.

• *Hypovolemic shock.* Slight tachycardia is an early sign of life-threatening hypovolemic shock. It may be accompanied by tachypnea, restlessness, thirst, and pale, cool skin. As shock progresses, the patient's skin becomes clammy and his pulse increasingly rapid and thready. He may also develop hypotension, narrowed pulse pressure, oliguria, subnormal body temperature, and decreased LOC.

- **Neurogenic shock.** Tachycardia or bradycardia may occur. Related effects include tachypnea, apprehension, oliguria, variable body temperature, decreased LOC, and warm, dry skin.
- **Orthostatic hypotension.** Tachycardia accompanies the characteristic signs and symptoms in this condition: dizziness, syncope, pallor, blurred vision, diaphoresis, and nausea.
- **Pneumothorax.** Life-threatening pneumothorax causes tachycardia and other signs and symptoms of distress, such as severe dyspnea and chest pain, tachypnea, and cyanosis. Related findings include dry cough, subcutaneous crepitation, absent or decreased breath sounds, and decreased vocal fremitus.
- **Pulmonary embolism.** In this disorder, tachycardia is usually preceded by sudden dyspnea and anginal or pleuritic chest pain. Common associated signs and symptoms include tachypnea, weak peripheral pulses, low-grade fever, restlessness, diaphoresis, and a dry cough or a cough with blood-tinged sputum.
- **Thyrotoxicosis.** Tachycardia is a classic feature of this thyroid disorder, as are an enlarged thyroid, nervousness, heat intolerance, weight loss despite increased appetite, diaphoresis, diarrhea, tremors, and palpitations. Although also considered characteristic, exophthalmos is sometimes absent.

Because thyrotoxicosis affects virtually every body system, its associated signs and symptoms are diverse and numerous. Some examples include full and bounding pulse, widened pulse pressure, dyspnea, anorexia, nausea, vomiting, altered bowel habits, hepatomegaly, and muscle weakness, fatigue, and atrophy. The patient's skin is smooth, warm, and flushed, while his hair is fine and soft and may gray prematurely or fall out. The female patient may have reduced libido and oligomenorrhea or amenorrhea; the male patient, reduced libido and gynecomastia.

Other causes

- **Diagnostic tests.** Cardiac catheterization and electrophysiologic studies may induce transient tachycardia.
- **Drugs and alcohol.** Various drugs affect the nervous system, circulatory system, or heart muscle, resulting in tachycardia. Examples of these include sympathomimetics, phenothiazines, anticholinergics (such as atropine), thyroid drugs, alpha-adrenergic blockers (such as phentolamine), acetylcholinesterase inhibitors (such as captopril), nitrates (such as nitroglycerin), and vasodilators (such as hydralazine and nifedipine). Excessive caffeine intake and alcohol intoxication may also cause tachycardia.
- **Surgery and pacemakers.** Cardiac surgery and pacemaker malfunction or wire irritation may cause tachycardia.

Special considerations

Continue to monitor the patient closely. If appropriate, prepare him for ambulatory electrocardiography. In addition, explain ordered diagnostic tests, such as blood work, pulmonary function studies, and a 12-lead electrocardiogram.

Pediatric pointers

When examining a child for tachycardia, be aware that normal heart rates for children are higher than those for adults. In children, tachycardia may result from many of the adult causes described above.

TACHYPNEA

A common sign of cardiopulmonary disorders, tachypnea is an abnormally fast respiratory rate—20 breaths/minute or more. Tachypnea may reflect the need to increase minute volume—the amount of air breathed each minute. Under these circumstances, it may be accompanied by an increase in tidal volume—the volume of air inhaled or exhaled per breath—resulting in hyperventilation. Tachypnea, however, may also reflect stiff lungs or overloaded ventilatory muscles, in which case, the tidal volume may actually be reduced.

Tachypnea may result from reduced arterial oxygen tension or arterial oxygen content, decreased perfusion, or increased oxygen demand. Heightened oxygen demand, for example, may result from fever, exertion, anxiety, and pain. Tachypnea is one of the earliest and most reliable signs of weaning intolerance. It may also occur as a compensatory response to metabolic acidosis and may result from pulmonary irritation, stretch receptor stimulation, or neurologic disorders that upset medullary respiratory control. Generally, respiratory rate increases by 4 breaths/minute for every 1° F (0.5° C) rise in body temperature.

Emergency interventions

 After detecting tachypnea, quickly evaluate cardiopulmonary status; check for cyanosis, chest pain, dyspnea, tachycardia, and hypotension. If the patient has paradoxical chest movement, suspect flail chest and immediately splint his chest with your hands or with sandbags. Then administer supplemental oxygen by nasal cannula or face mask and, if possible, place the patient in a semi-Fowler's position to help ease his breathing. Intubation and mechanical ventilation may be necessary if respiratory failure ensues. Also, insert an I.V. line for fluid and drug administration and begin cardiac monitoring.

History and physical examination

When the patient's condition permits, obtain a medical history. Find out when the tachypnea began. Did it follow activity? Has he had it before? Then have him describe associated signs and symptoms, such as diaphoresis and recent weight loss. Is he anxious about anything or does he have a history of anxiety attacks? Note whether he is taking drugs for pain relief. How effective are they?

Begin the physical examination by taking the patient's other vital signs, if you haven't already done so, and observing his overall behavior. Does he seem restless? Then auscultate the chest for abnormal heart and lung sounds. If he has a productive cough, record the color, amount, and consistency of sputum. Last, examine for jugular vein distention and check his skin for pallor, cyanosis, edema, and warmth or coolness.

Common medical causes

● *Adult respiratory distress syndrome (ARDS).* In this life-threatening disorder, tachypnea and apprehension may be the earliest features. Tachypnea gradually worsens as fluid accumulates in the patient's lungs, causing them to stiffen. It's accompanied by accessory muscle use, grunting expirations, suprasternal and intercostal retractions, and crackles and rhonchi. Eventually, ARDS produces hypoxemia, resulting in tachycardia, dyspnea, cyanosis, respiratory failure, and shock.

● *Anaphylactic shock.* In this type of shock, tachypnea develops within minutes after exposure to an allergen, such as penicillin or insect venom. Accompanying features include anxiety, pounding headache, skin flushing and intense pruritus, and possibly diffuse urticaria. The patient may have widespread edema, affecting the eyelids, lips, tongue, hands, feet, and genitalia. Other findings in this life-threatening shock are cool, clammy skin; rapid, thready pulse; cough; dyspnea; stridor; and change or loss of voice associated with laryngeal edema.

● *Aspiration of a foreign body.* Life-threatening upper airway obstruction may result from aspiration of a foreign body. In *partial obstruction,* the patient abruptly develops a dry, paroxysmal cough with rapid, shallow respirations. Other signs and symptoms include dyspnea, gagging or choking, intercostal retractions, nasal flaring, cyanosis, decreased or absent breath sounds, hoarseness, and stridor or coarse wheezes. Typically, the patient appears frightened and distressed. *Complete obstruction* may rapidly cause asphyxia and death.

• *Asthma.* Tachypnea is common in life-threatening asthmatic attacks, which commonly occur at night. These attacks usually begin with mild wheezing and a dry cough that progresses to mucus expectoration. Eventually, the patient becomes apprehensive and develops prolonged expirations, intercostal and supraclavicular retractions on inspiration, accessory muscle use, severe audible wheezing, rhonchi, flaring nostrils, tachycardia, diaphoresis, and flushing or cyanosis.

• *Bronchitis (chronic).* Mild tachypnea may occur in this form of chronic obstructive pulmonary disease, but it's not typically a major sign. Usually, chronic bronchitis begins with a dry, hacking cough that later produces copious sputum. Other characteristics include dyspnea, prolonged expirations, wheezing, scattered rhonchi, accessory muscle use, and cyanosis. Clubbing and barrel chest are late signs.

• *Cardiac arrhythmias.* Depending on the patient's heart rate, tachypnea may occur along with hypotension, dizziness, palpitations, weakness, and fatigue. The patient's level of consciousness (LOC) may be decreased.

• *Cardiac tamponade.* In life-threatening tamponade, tachypnea may accompany tachycardia, dyspnea, and pulsus paradoxus. Related findings include muffled heart sounds, pericardial friction rub, chest pain, hypotension, narrowed pulse pressure, and hepatomegaly. The patient is noticeably anxious and restless. His skin is clammy and cyanotic, and his neck veins are distended.

• *Cardiogenic shock.* Although signs of cardiogenic shock resemble signs of other types of shock, they're usually more severe. Besides tachypnea, the patient commonly has cold, pale, clammy, cyanotic skin; hypotension; tachycardia; narrowed pulse pressure; a ventricular gallop; oliguria; decreased LOC; and neck vein distention.

• *Emphysema.* This chronic pulmonary disorder commonly produces tachypnea accompanied by dyspnea on exertion. It may also cause anorexia, malaise, peripheral cyanosis, pursed-lip breathing, accessory muscle use, and chronic productive cough. Percussion yields a hyperresonant tone while auscultation reveals wheezing, crackles, and diminished breath sounds. Clubbing and barrel chest are late signs.

• *Flail chest.* Tachypnea usually appears early in this life-threatening disorder. Other findings include paradoxical chest wall movement, rib bruises and palpable fractures, localized chest pain, hypotension, and diminished breath sounds. The patient may also develop signs of respiratory distress, such as dyspnea and accessory muscle use.

• *Hyperosmolar hyperglycemic nonketotic syndrome.* Rapidly deteriorating LOC occurs with tachypnea, tachycardia, hypotension, seizures, oliguria, and signs of dehydration.

• *Hypovolemic shock.* An early sign of life-threatening hypovolemic shock, tachypnea is accompanied by cool, pale skin; restlessness; thirst; and mild tachycardia. As shock progresses, the patient's skin becomes clammy; his pulse, increasingly rapid and thready. Other findings include hypotension, narrowed pulse pressure, oliguria, subnormal body temperature, and decreased LOC.

• *Interstitial fibrosis.* In this disorder, tachypnea develops gradually and may become severe. Associated features may include dyspnea on exertion, pleuritic chest pain, a paroxysmal dry cough, crackles, late inspiratory wheezing, cyanosis, fatigue, and weight loss. Clubbing is a late sign.

NORMAL PEDIATRIC VITAL SIGNS

AGE	TEMPERATURE		PULSE RATE (beats/minute)
	FAHRENHEIT	CELSIUS	
Newborn	98.6° to 99.8°	37° to 37.7°	70 to 190
3 years	98.5° to 99.5°	36.9° to 37.5°	80 to 125
10 years	97.5° to 98.6°	36.3° to 37°	70 to 110
16 years	97.6° to 98.8°	36.4° to 37.1°	55 to 100

• *Lung abscess.* In this abscess, tachypnea is usually paired with dyspnea and accentuated by fever. However, the chief sign is a productive cough with copious, purulent, foul-smelling, and possibly bloody sputum. Other findings may include chest pain, halitosis, diaphoresis, chills, fatigue, weakness, anorexia, weight loss, and clubbing.

• *Mesothelioma (malignant).* Commonly related to asbestos exposure, this pleural mass initially produces tachypnea and dyspnea on mild exertion. Other classic symptoms are persistent, dull chest pain and aching shoulder pain that progresses to arm weakness and paresthesia. Later signs and symptoms include a cough, insomnia associated with pain, clubbing, and dullness over the malignant mesothelioma.

• *Neurogenic shock.* Tachypnea is characteristic in this life-threatening type of shock. It commonly occurs with apprehension, bradycardia or tachycardia, oliguria, fluctuating body temperature, and decreased LOC that may progress to coma. The patient's skin is warm, dry, and perhaps flushed. He may experience nausea and vomiting.

• *Pneumonia (bacterial).* A common sign in this infection, tachypnea is usually preceded by a painful, hacking, dry cough that rapidly becomes productive. Other signs and symptoms quickly follow, including high fever, shaking chills, headache, dyspnea, pleuritic chest pain, tachycardia, grunting respirations, nasal flaring, and cyanosis. Auscultation reveals diminished breath sounds and fine crackles, while percussion yields a dull tone.

• *Pneumothorax.* Tachypnea is a common sign of life-threatening pneumothorax. Typically, it's accompanied by severe, sharp, and commonly unilateral chest pain that's aggravated by chest movement. Associated signs and symptoms may include dyspnea, tachycardia, accessory muscle use, asymmetrical chest expansion, dry cough, cyanosis, anxiety, and restlessness. Examination of the affected lung reveals hyperresonance or tympany, subcutaneous crepitation, decreased vocal fremitus, and diminished or absent breath sounds. The patient with tension pneumothorax will also have a deviated trachea.

RESPIRATORY RATE (breaths/minute)	BLOOD PRESSURE (mm Hg)
30 to 80	systolic: 50 to 52 diastolic: 25 to 30 mean: 35 to 40
20 to 30	systolic: 78 to 114 diastolic: 46 to 78
16 to 22	systolic: 90 to 132 diastolic: 56 to 86
15 to 20	systolic: 104 to 108 diastolic: 60 to 92

• *Pulmonary edema.* An early sign of this life-threatening disorder, tachypnea is accompanied by dyspnea on exertion, paroxysmal nocturnal dyspnea and, later, orthopnea. Other features include a dry cough, crackles, tachycardia, and a ventricular gallop. In severe pulmonary edema, respirations become increasingly rapid and labored, tachycardia worsens, and crackles become more diffuse. The patient's cough also produces frothy, bloody sputum. Signs of shock—such as hypotension, thready pulse, and cold, clammy skin—may also occur.

• *Pulmonary embolism (acute).* Tachypnea occurs suddenly in pulmonary embolism and is usually accompanied by dyspnea. The patient may complain of anginal or pleuritic chest pain. Other common characteristics include tachycardia, a dry or productive cough with blood tinged sputum, low-grade fever, restlessness, and diaphoresis. Less common signs include massive hemoptysis, chest splinting, leg edema, and—with a large embolus—distended neck veins, cyanosis, and syncope. In addition, pleural friction rub, crackles, diffuse wheezing, dullness on percussion, diminished breath sounds, and signs of shock, such as hypotension and a weak, rapid pulse may be present.

• *Septic shock.* Early in septic shock, the patient usually has tachypnea accompanied by sudden fever, chills and, possibly, nausea, vomiting, and diarrhea. He may also have tachycardia and normal or slightly decreased blood pressure; his skin is flushed and warm, yet dry. As this life-threatening type of shock progresses, the patient may display anxiety; restlessness; decreased LOC; hypotension; cool, clammy, and cyanotic skin; rapid, thready pulse; thirst; and oliguria that may progress to anuria.

Other causes

• *Drugs.* Tachypnea may result from an overdose of salicylates.

Special considerations

Continue to monitor the patient's vital signs closely. Be sure to keep suction and emergency equipment nearby, and prepare to intubate the patient and to provide mechanical ventilation, if necessary.

Prepare the patient for diagnostic studies, such as arterial blood gas analysis, chest X-rays, and an electrocardiogram.

Pediatric pointers

When assessing for tachypnea, recognize that a child's normal respiratory rate varies with age. (See *Normal pediatric vital signs.*) If you detect tachypnea, you'll need to rule out the causes listed above. Then consider these pediatric causes: congenital heart defects, meningitis, metabolic acidosis, and cystic fibrosis. Keep in mind, though, that hunger and anxiety may also cause tachypnea.

THROAT PAIN
[Sore throat]

Throat pain refers to discomfort in any part of the pharynx: the nasopharynx, the oropharynx, or the hypopharynx. This common symptom ranges from a sensation of scratchiness to severe pain. It's commonly accompanied by ear pain because cranial nerves IX and X innervate the pharynx as well as the middle and external ear.

Throat pain may result from infection, trauma, allergy, neoplasms, and certain systemic disorders. It may also follow surgery and endotracheal intubation. Nonpathologic causes include dry mucous membranes associated with mouth breathing and laryngeal irritation associated with alcohol consumption, inhaling smoke or chemicals like ammonia, and vocal strain.

History and physical examination

Ask the patient when he first noticed the pain and have him describe it. Has he had throat pain before? Is it accompanied by fever, ear pain, or dysphagia? Review the patient's medical history for throat problems, allergies, and systemic disorders.

Next, carefully examine the pharynx, noting redness, exudate, or swelling. Examine the oropharynx, using a warmed metal spatula or tongue blade, and the nasopharynx, using a warmed laryngeal mirror or fiberoptic nasopharyngoscope. Laryngoscopic examination of the hypopharynx may be required. (If necessary, spray the soft palate and pharyngeal wall with a local anesthetic to prevent gagging.) Observe the tonsils for redness, swelling, or exudate, too. (See *Reviewing anatomy of the throat.*) In addition, obtain an exudate specimen for culture. Then examine the patient's nose, using a nasal speculum. Also check his ears—especially if he reports ear pain. Finally, palpate the neck and oropharynx for nodules or lymph node enlargement.

Common medical causes

• *Agranulocytosis.* In this disorder, sore throat may accompany other signs of infection, such as fever, chills, and headache. Typically, it follows progressive fatigue and weakness. Other findings may include nausea, vomiting, anorexia, and bleeding tendencies. Rough-edged ulcers with gray or black membranes may appear on the gums, palate, or perianal area.

• *Allergic rhinitis.* Occurring seasonally or year-round, this disorder may produce sore throat. The patient may also complain of nasal congestion with thin nasal discharge, postnasal drip, paroxysmal sneezing, decreased sense of smell, frontal or temporal headache, and itchy eyes, nose, and possibly throat. Examination reveals pale and glistening nasal mucosa with edematous nasal turbinates, watery eyes, reddened conjunctiva and eyelids and, possibly, swollen lids.

• *Bronchitis (acute).* This disorder may produce lower throat pain. Associated findings may include fever, chills, cough, and muscle and back pain. Auscultation reveals rhonchi, wheezing and, at times, crackles.

• *Common cold.* Sore throat may accompany cough, sneezing, nasal congestion, rhinorrhea, fatigue, headache, myalgia, and arthralgia.

• *Contact ulcers.* Common in men with stressful jobs, contact ulcers appear symmetrically on the posterior vocal cords, resulting in sore throat. The pain is aggravated by talking and may be accompanied by referred ear pain and, occasionally, hemoptysis. Typically, the patient also has a history of chronic throat clearing or acid reflux.

• *Foreign body.* A foreign body lodged in the palatine or lingual tonsil and pyriform sinus may produce localized throat

REVIEWING ANATOMY OF THE THROAT

The throat, or pharynx, is divided into three areas: the nasopharynx (the soft palate and posterior nasal cavity), the oropharynx (the area between the soft palate and upper edge of the epiglottis), and the hypopharynx (the area between the epiglottis and level of the cricoid cartilage). A disorder affecting any of these areas may cause sore throat. Pinpointing the causative disorder begins with accurate assessment of the throat structures illustrated here.

Frontal view

Cross-sectional view

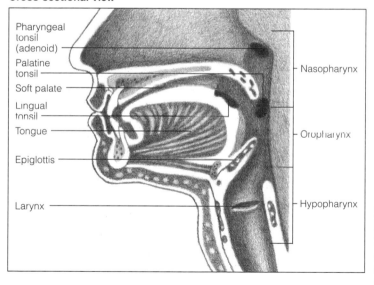

Pharyngeal tonsil (adenoid)
Palatine tonsil
Soft palate
Lingual tonsil
Tongue
Epiglottis
Larynx

Nasopharynx
Oropharynx
Hypopharynx

pain. The pain may persist after the foreign body is dislodged until mucosal irritation resolves.

- **Infectious mononucleosis.** Sore throat is one of the three classic findings in this infection. Other classic signs are cervical lymphadenopathy and fluctuating temperature with an evening peak of 101° to 102° F (38.3° to 38.9° C). Splenomegaly and hepatomegaly may also develop.

• *Influenza.* Patients with the flu commonly complain of sore throat, fever with chills, headache, weakness, malaise, muscle aches, cough, and occasionally hoarseness and rhinorrhea.

• *Laryngeal cancer.* In *extrinsic laryngeal cancer,* the chief symptom is pain or burning in the throat when drinking citrus juice or hot liquids, or a lump in the throat; in *intrinsic laryngeal cancer,* it's hoarseness that persists for more than 3 weeks. Later, clinical effects of metastases include dysphagia, dyspnea, a cough, enlarged cervical lymph nodes, and pain that radiates to the ear.

• *Necrotizing ulcerative gingivitis (acute).* Also known as trench mouth, this disorder usually begins abruptly with sore throat and tender gums that ulcerate and bleed. A gray exudate may cover the gums and pharyngeal tonsils. Related signs and symptoms include a foul taste in the mouth, halitosis, cervical lymphadenopathy, headache, malaise, and fever.

• *Peritonsillar abscess.* A complication of bacterial tonsillitis, this abscess typically causes severe throat pain that radiates to the ear. Accompanying the pain may be dysphagia, drooling, dysarthria, halitosis, fever with chills, malaise, and nausea. Usually, the patient tilts his head to the side of the abscess. Examination may also reveal a deviated uvula, trismus, and tender cervical lymphadenopathy.

• *Pharyngitis.* Whether bacterial, fungal, or viral, pharyngitis may cause sore throat and localized erythema and edema. *Bacterial pharyngitis* begins abruptly with unilateral sore throat. Associated signs and symptoms include dysphagia, fever, malaise, headache, abdominal pain, myalgia, and arthralgia. Inspection reveals an exudate on the tonsil or tonsillar fossae, uvular edema, soft palate erythema, and tender cervical lymph nodes.

Also known as thrush, *fungal pharyngitis* causes diffuse sore throat—commonly described as a burning sensation—accompanied by pharyngeal erythema and edema. White plaques mark the pharynx, tonsil, tonsillar pillars, base of the tongue, and oral mucosa; scraping these plaques uncovers a hemorrhagic base.

In *viral pharyngitis,* findings include diffuse sore throat, malaise, fever, and mild erythema and edema of the posterior oropharyngeal wall. The tonsils aren't inflamed, but the cervical lymph nodes may be enlarged.

• *Sinusitis (acute).* This disorder may cause sore throat with purulent nasal discharge and postnasal drip, resulting in halitosis. Other effects may include headache, malaise, cough, fever, and facial pain and swelling associated with nasal congestion.

• *Tongue carcinoma.* In this type of cancer, the patient experiences localized throat pain that may occur around a raised white lesion or ulcer. The pain may radiate to the ear and be accompanied by dysphagia.

• *Tonsillar carcinoma.* Sore throat is the presenting symptom in tonsillar carcinoma. Unfortunately, the carcinoma is usually quite advanced before this symptom appears. The pain radiates to the ear and is accompanied by a superficial ulcer on the tonsil or one that extends to the base of the tongue.

• *Tonsillitis.* In *acute tonsillitis,* mild to severe sore throat is usually the first symptom. The pain may radiate to the ears and be accompanied by dysphagia and headache. Related findings include malaise, fever with chills, halitosis, myalgia, arthralgia, and tender cervical lymphadenopathy. Examination reveals edematous, reddened tonsils with a purulent exudate.

Chronic tonsillitis causes mild sore throat, malaise, and tender cervical lymph nodes. The tonsils appear smooth, pink, and possibly enlarged, with a purulent debris in the crypts. Halitosis and a foul taste in the mouth are also common.

Unilateral or bilateral throat pain just above the hyoid bone occurs in *lingual tonsillitis*. The lingual tonsils appear red and swollen and are covered with exudate. Other findings include a muffled voice, dysphagia, and tender cervical lymphadenopathy on the affected side.

• *Uvulitis.* This inflammation may cause throat pain or a sensation of something in the throat. Usually, the uvula is swollen and red; however, in allergic uvulitis, it's pale.

Other causes

• *Treatments.* Endotracheal intubation and local surgery, such as tonsillectomy and adenoidectomy, commonly cause sore throat.

Special considerations

Provide analgesic sprays or lozenges to relieve throat pain. You should also prepare the patient for throat culture, complete blood count, and a Monospot test.

Pediatric pointers

In children, sore throat is a common complaint. It may result from many of the same disorders that affect adults. Other pediatric causes of sore throat include acute epiglottitis, herpangina, scarlet fever, acute follicular tonsillitis, and retropharyngeal abscess.

THYROID ENLARGEMENT

An enlarged thyroid can result from inflammation, physiologic changes, iodine deficiency, and thyroid tumors. Depending on the medical cause, hyperfunction or hypofunction may occur with resulting excess or deficiency, respectively, of the hormone thyroxine. If no infection is present, enlargement is usually slow and progressive. An enlarged thyroid that causes visible swelling in the front of the neck is called a goiter.

History and physical examination

The patient's history typically will reveal the cause of thyroid enlargement. Important data include a family history of thyroid disease, when the thyroid enlargement began, any previous irradiation of the thyroid or the neck, recent infections, and the use of thyroid replacement drugs.

Begin the physical examination by inspecting the patient's trachea for midline deviation. Although you can frequently see an enlarged gland, you should always palpate it. To palpate the thyroid gland, you will need to stand in front of or behind the patient. Give the patient a cup of water, and have him extend the neck slightly. Place the fingers of both hands on the patient's neck, just below the cricoid cartilage and just lateral to the trachea. Tell the patient to take a sip of water and swallow. The thyroid gland should rise as he swallows. Use the fingers to palpate laterally and downward to feel the whole thyroid gland. Palpate over the midline to feel the isthmus of the thyroid.

When palpating, be sure to note the size, shape, and consistency of the gland, and the presence or absence of nodules, which are abnormal rounded masses of tissue. Using a stethoscope, listen over the lateral lobes for a bruit. The bruit may be continuous and must be distinguished from a carotid bruit.

Common medical causes

• *Hypothyroidism.* This disease, which is most prevalent in women, usually results from a dysfunction of the thyroid gland, which may be due to surgery, irradiation therapy, chronic autoimmune thyroiditis (Hashimoto's disease), or inflammatory conditions, such as amyloidosis and sarcoidosis. Besides an enlarged thyroid, signs and symptoms may include weight gain despite anorexia; fatigue; cold intolerance; constipation; menorrhagia; slowed intellectual and motor activity; dry, pale, cool skin; dry sparse hair; and thick, brittle nails. Eventually, the face assumes a dull expression with periorbital edema.

• *Iodine deficiency.* Goiter may result from lack of iodine in the diet. If the goiter arises from a deficiency of iodine in the food or water of a particular area, it's called *endemic goiter.* Associated signs and symptoms of endemic goiter include dysphagia, dyspnea, and tracheal deviation.

• *Thyroiditis.* Thyroiditis, which is inflammation of the thyroid gland, may be acute or subacute. If thyroiditis is due to bacterial or viral infections, associated features may include fever and tenderness of the thyroid. Inflammation also may result from autoimmune reactions, as in *Hashimoto's thyroiditis.* Besides thyroid enlargement, autoimmune thyroiditis usually is asymptomatic. It is, however, the most common cause of spontaneous hypothyroidism.

• *Thyrotoxicosis.* Overproduction of thyroid hormone causes thyrotoxicosis. The most common form is *Graves' disease,* which may result from genetic or immunologic factors. Associated signs and symptoms include nervousness; heat intolerance; fatigue; weight loss despite increased appetite; diarrhea; sweating; palpitations; tremors; smooth, warm, flushed skin; fine, soft hair; exophthalmos; nausea and vomiting due to increased GI motility and peristalsis; and, in females, oligomenorrhea or amenorrhea.

• *Tumors.* An enlarged thyroid may be due to the added tissue of a malignant tumor or a nonmalignant tumor (such as an adenoma). A malignant tumor usually appears as a single nodule in the neck, whereas a nonmalignant tumor may appear as multiple nodules in the neck. Associated signs and symptoms may include hoarseness, loss of voice, and dysphagia.

Other causes

• *Goitrogens.* Certain drugs and compounds in foods decrease thyroxine production and cause goiters. Such agents include lithium, sulfonamides, phenylbutazone and para-aminosalicylic acid. Foods containing goitrogens include peanuts, cabbage, soybeans, strawberries, spinach, rutabagas, and radishes.

Special considerations

Prepare the patient with an enlarged thyroid for any scheduled tests, which may include needle aspiration, ultrasound, and radioactive thyroid scanning. Reassure the patient about his appearance. Prepare the patient for surgery or radiation therapy, if necessary.

The hypothyroid patient will need a warm room and moisturizing lotion for his skin. A gentle laxative and stool softener may help with constipation. Provide a high-bulk, low-calorie diet and encourage activity to promote weight loss. Warn the patient to report infection immediately. Monitor temperature until stable. After thyroid replacement begins, watch for signs and symptoms of hyperthyroidism, such as restlessness, sweating, and excessive weight loss. Avoid sedation when possible or reduce dosage because hypothyroidism delays metabolism of many drugs. Check arterial blood gas levels for indications of hypoxia and respiratory acidosis to determine whether the patient needs ventilatory assistance.

For thyroiditis patients, give antibiotics and watch for elevations in temperature, which may indicate developing resistance to antibiotics. Check vital signs, and examine the patient's neck for unusual swelling or redness. Provide a liquid diet if the patient has difficulty swallowing. Instruct the patient to watch for signs and symptoms of hypothyroidism, such as lethargy, restlessness, dry skin and sensitivity to cold. Also check for signs and symptoms of hyperthyroidism—such as nervousness, tremor, and weakness—which commonly occur in subacute thyroiditis.

If the patient has Graves' disease, proptosis may cause the eyes to become dry. The patient should be taught to use artificial tears frequently. The patient with severe hyperthyroidism (those with thyroid storm) will need close monitoring of temperature, volume status, heart rate, and blood pressure. If the hyperthyroid patient is on radioactive iodine therapy, tell him not to expectorate or cough freely after treatment because his saliva remains radioactive for 24 hours.

After thyroidectomy, check vital signs every 15 to 30 minutes until the patient's condition stabilizes. Be alert for signs of tetany secondary to accidental parathyroid injury during surgery. Keep 10% calcium gluconate available for I.V. use, if needed. Evaluate dressings frequently for excessive bleeding, and watch for signs of airway obstruction, such as difficulty in talking or increased swallowing. Keep tracheotomy equipment handy.

After thyroidectomy or radioactive destruction of the gland, explain to the patient that lifelong thyroid hormone replacement therapy is necessary. Tell him to watch for signs of overdose, such as nervousness and palpitations.

Pediatric pointers
Congenital goiter, a syndrome of infantile myxedema or cretinism, is characterized by mental retardation, growth failure, and other signs and symptoms of hypothyroidism. Early treatment can prevent mental retardation. Genetic counseling is important, as subsequent children are at risk.

TICS

A tic is an involuntary, repetitive movement of a specific group of muscles—usually those of the face, neck, shoulders, trunk, and hands. Typically, this sign occurs suddenly and intermittently. It may involve a single isolated movement, such as lip smacking, grimacing, blinking, sniffing, tongue thrusting, throat clearing, hitching up one shoulder, or protruding the chin. Or it may involve a complex set of movements. Mild tics, such as twitching of an eyelid, are especially common.

Usually, tics are psychogenic and may be aggravated by stress or anxiety. However, they're also associated with one rare affliction—Tourette syndrome. Psychogenic tics, though, commonly begin between ages 5 and 10 as voluntary, coordinated, and purposeful actions that the child feels compelled to perform to decrease anxiety. Unless the tics are severe, the child may be unaware of them. The tics may subside as the child matures, or they may persist into adulthood.

Tics differ from minor seizures in that tics aren't associated with transient loss of consciousness or amnesia.

History
Begin by asking the parents how long the child has had the tic. Can they identify any precipitating factors? Ask about stress in the child's life such as difficult schoolwork. Next, carefully observe the tic. Is it a purposeful or involuntary movement? Note whether it's localized or generalized and describe it in detail.

Common medical causes
• *Tourette syndrome.* This syndrome, which is thought to be largely a genetic disorder, typically begins between ages 2 and 15 with a tic that involves the face or neck. Symptoms include both motor and vocal tics that may involve the muscles of the shoulders, arms, trunk, and legs, and may occur with violent movement and outbursts of obscenities (coprolalia). The patient snorts, barks, and grunts and may emit explosive sounds such as hissing when he speaks. He may involuntarily repeat another person's

words (echolalia) or movements (echopraxia). At times, this syndrome subsides spontaneously or undergoes a prolonged remission, but it may persist throughout life.

Special considerations
Psychotherapy and administration of tranquilizers may be helpful in providing relief. Many patients with Tourette syndrome receive haloperidol, pimozide, or other antipsychotics to control tics.

TINNITUS

Tinnitus literally means ringing in the ears, although many other abnormal sounds fall under this term. For example, tinnitus may be described as the sound of escaping air, running water, or the inside of a seashell or as a sizzling, buzzing, or humming noise. Occasionally, it's described as a roaring or musical sound. This common symptom may be unilateral or bilateral and constant or intermittent. Although the brain can adjust to or suppress constant tinnitus, intermittent tinnitus may be so disturbing that some patients contemplate suicide as their only source of relief.

Tinnitus can be classified in several ways. *Subjective tinnitus* is heard only by the patient, while *objective tinnitus* is also heard by the observer who places a stethoscope near the patient's affected ear. *Tinnitus aurium* refers to noise that the patient hears in his ears; *tinnitus cerebri,* to noise that he hears in his head.

Tinnitus is usually associated with neural injury within the auditory pathway, resulting in altered, spontaneous firing of sensory auditory neurons. Commonly resulting from ear disorders, tinnitus may also stem from cardiovascular and systemic disorders and from the effects of certain drugs. Nonpathologic causes of tinnitus include acute anxiety and presbycusis. (See *Common causes of tinnitus.*)

History and physical examination
Ask the patient to describe the tinnitus, including its onset, pattern, pitch, location, and intensity. Ask whether it's accompanied by other symptoms, such as vertigo, headache, or hearing loss. Next, take a health history, including a complete drug history.

Using an otoscope, inspect the patient's ears and examine the tympanic membrane. To check for hearing loss, perform the Weber and Rinne tuning fork tests.

Also auscultate for bruits in the neck. Then compress the jugular or carotid artery to see if this affects the tinnitus. Finally, examine the nasopharynx for masses that might cause eustachian tube dysfunction and tinnitus.

Common medical causes
• *Acoustic neuroma.* An early symptom of this eighth cranial nerve tumor, unilateral tinnitus precedes unilateral sensorineural hearing loss and vertigo. Facial paralysis, headache, nausea, vomiting, and papilledema may also occur.

• *Atherosclerosis of the carotid artery.* In this disorder, the patient has constant tinnitus that can be stopped by applying pressure over the carotid artery. He also feels confused, weak, and unsteady when he rises in the morning or stands up quickly. Auscultation over the upper part of the neck, on the auricle, or near the ear on the affected side may detect a bruit. Palpation may reveal a weak carotid pulse.

• *Cervical spondylosis.* In this degenerative disorder, osteophytic growths may compress the vertebral arteries, resulting in tinnitus. Typically, a stiff neck and pain aggravated by activity produce tinnitus. Other features may include brief vertigo, nystagmus, hearing loss, and pain that radiates down the arms. Paresthesia or weakness may be present.

COMMON CAUSES OF TINNITUS

Usually, tinnitus results from disorders that affect the external, middle, or inner ear. Below are some of its more common causes and their locations.

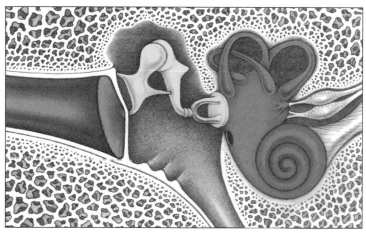

External ear
Ear canal obstruction
  by cerumen or a foreign body
Otitis externa
Tympanic membrane
  perforation

Middle ear
Ossicle dislocation
Otitis media
Otosclerosis

Inner ear
Acoustic neuroma
Atherosclerosis of the
  carotid artery
Labyrinthitis
Ménière's disease

● *Eustachian tube patency.* Normally, the eustachian tube remains closed, except during swallowing. However, persistent patency of this tube can cause tinnitus, audible breath sounds, loud and distorted voice sounds, and a sense of fullness in the ear. Examination with a pneumatic otoscope reveals movement of the tympanic membrane with respirations. At times, breath sounds can be heard with a stethoscope placed over the auricle.

● *Glomus jugulare or tympanicum tumor.* Usually, a pulsating sound is the first symptom of this tumor. Other early features include a reddish blue mass behind the tympanic membrane and progressive conductive hearing loss. Later,

total unilateral deafness is accompanied by ear pain and dizziness. Otorrhagia may also occur if the tumor breaks through the tympanic membrane.

● *Hypertension.* Bilateral, high-pitched tinnitus may occur in severe hypertension. Diastolic blood pressure exceeding 120 mm Hg may also cause severe, throbbing headache, restlessness, nausea, vomiting, blurred vision, seizures, and decreased level of consciousness.

● *Labyrinthitis (suppurative).* Here, tinnitus may accompany sudden, severe attacks of vertigo, unilateral or bilateral sensorineural hearing loss, nystagmus, dizziness, nausea, and vomiting.

● *Ménière's disease.* Most common in men between ages 55 and 65, this labyrinthine disease is characterized by attacks of low-pitched tinnitus, vertigo, and fluctuating sensorineural hearing loss. Usually, these attacks are unilateral and last from 10 minutes to several hours; they occur over a few days or weeks followed by a remission. Severe nausea, vomiting, diaphoresis, and nystagmus may also occur during attacks.

• *Noise.* Chronic exposure to noise, especially high-pitch sounds, may damage the ear's hair cells, causing tinnitus and a bilateral hearing loss. These symptoms may be temporary or permanent.

• *Ossicle dislocation.* Acoustic trauma—such as a slap on the ear—may cause ossicle dislocation. This may result in tinnitus and sensorineural hearing loss. Bleeding from the middle ear also may occur.

• *Otitis externa (acute).* Although not a major complaint here, tinnitus may result if debris in the external ear canal impinges on the tympanic membrane. More typical findings include pruritus, foul-smelling purulent discharge, and severe ear pain that's aggravated by manipulation of the tragus or auricle, teeth clenching, mouth opening, and chewing. Typically, the external ear canal appears red and edematous and may be occluded by debris, causing partial hearing loss.

• *Otitis media.* This infection may cause tinnitus and conductive hearing loss. However, its more typical features include ear pain, a red and bulging tympanic membrane, high fever, chills, and dizziness.

• *Otosclerosis.* In this disorder, the patient may describe ringing, roaring, or whistling tinnitus or a combination of these sounds. The patient may also report progressive hearing loss—which may lead to bilateral deafness—and vertigo.

• *Tympanic membrane perforation.* In this disorder, tinnitus and hearing loss go hand-in-hand. Tinnitus is usually the chief complaint in a small perforation; hearing loss, in a larger perforation. Typical-

ly, these symptoms develop suddenly and may occur with pain, vertigo, and a feeling of fullness in the ear.

Other causes

• *Drugs and alcohol.* An overdose of salicylates commonly causes reversible tinnitus. Quinine, alcohol, and indomethacin may also cause reversible tinnitus. Common drugs that may cause irreversible tinnitus include the aminoglycoside antibiotics (especially kanamycin, streptomycin, and gentamicin) and vancomycin.

Special considerations

Tinnitus usually cannot be treated successfully. To help the patient tolerate this symptom, you may have to provide vasodilators, tranquilizers, and antiseizure drugs, or encourage the use of biofeedback and tinnitus maskers. A tinnitus masker produces a band of noise measuring about 1,800 Hz, which will help block out tinnitus without interfering with hearing.

In addition, a hearing aid may be prescribed to amplify environmental sounds, thereby obscuring tinnitus. At times, a device that combines features of a masker and hearing aid may be used to block out tinnitus.

Pediatric pointers

An expectant mother's use of ototoxic drugs during the third trimester of pregnancy can cause labyrinthine damage in the fetus, resulting in tinnitus. This symptom also may occur in children with many of the disorders described above.

TRACHEAL DEVIATION

Normally, the trachea is located at the midline of the neck—except at the bifurcation, where it shifts slightly toward the right. Visible deviation from its normal position signals an underlying condition that can compromise pulmonary function and possibly cause respiratory distress. A hallmark of life-threatening tension pneumothorax, this sign occurs in disorders that produce mediastinal shift due to asymmetrical thoracic volume or pressure. A nonlesion pneumothorax can produce tracheal deviation to the ipsilateral side.

Elder tip

 In elderly people, tracheal deviation to the right commonly stems from an elongated, atherosclerotic aortic arch, but this deviation isn't considered abnormal.

Emergency interventions

 Be alert for signs and symptoms of respiratory distress (tachypnea, dyspnea, stridor, nasal flaring, accessory muscle use, asymmetrical chest expansion, restlessness, and anxiety). If possible, place the patient in semi-Fowler's position to aid respiratory excursion and improve oxygenation. Give supplemental oxygen, and intubate the patient if necessary. Insert an I.V. line for fluid and drug administration. In addition, palpate for subcutaneous crepitation in the neck and chest—a sign of tension pneumothorax. Chest tube insertion may be necessary to release trapped air or fluid and to restore normal intrapleural and intrathoracic pressure gradients.

History and physical examination

If the patient doesn't display signs of distress, ask about a history of pulmonary or cardiac disorders, trauma, or infection. If he smokes, determine how much. Ask about associated symptoms, especially breathing difficulty, pain, and cough. On inspection, the trachea is visibly deviated from its normal position at the midline of the neck. (See *Detecting slight tracheal deviation,* page 564.)

Common medical causes

- *Atelectasis.* Extensive lung collapse can produce tracheal deviation toward the affected side. Respiratory findings may include dyspnea, tachypnea, pleuritic chest pain, dry cough, dullness on percussion, decreased vocal fremitus and breath sounds, inspiratory lag, and substernal or intercostal retraction.

- *Hiatal hernia.* Intrusion of abdominal viscera into the pleural space causes tracheal deviation toward the unaffected side. The degree of attendant respiratory distress depends on the extent of herniation. Other effects may include pyrosis, regurgitation or vomiting, and chest or abdominal pain.

- *Kyphoscoliosis.* This disorder can cause rib cage distortion and mediastinal shift, producing tracheal deviation toward the compressed lung. Respiratory effects include dry coughing, dyspnea, and asymmetrical chest expansion. Backache and fatigue commonly occur.

- *Mediastinal tumor.* Commonly asymptomatic in its early stages, this tumor, when large, can press against the trachea and nearby structures, causing tracheal deviation and dysphagia. Other late findings may include stridor, dyspnea, brassy cough, hoarseness, and stertorous respirations with suprasternal retraction. The patient may experience shoulder, arm, or chest pain, and edema of the neck, face, or arm. His neck and chest wall veins may be dilated.

- *Pulmonary tuberculosis.* With a large cavitation, tracheal deviation toward the affected side accompanies asymmetrical chest excursion, dullness on percussion, increased tactile fremitus, amphoric breath sounds, and inspiratory crackles. Insidious early effects include fatigue, anorexia, weight loss, fever, chills, and night sweats. Productive cough, hemoptysis, pleuritic chest pain, and dyspnea develop as the disease progresses.

- *Retrosternal thyroid.* This anatomic abnormality can displace the trachea. The gland is felt as a movable neck mass

DETECTING SLIGHT TRACHEAL DEVIATION

Although gross tracheal deviation will be visible, detection of slight deviation requires palpation and perhaps even an X-ray. Try palpation first.

With the tip of your index finger, locate the patient's trachea by palpating between the sternocleidomastoid muscles. Then compare the trachea's position to an imaginary line drawn vertically through the suprasternal notch. Any deviation from midline is usually considered abnormal.

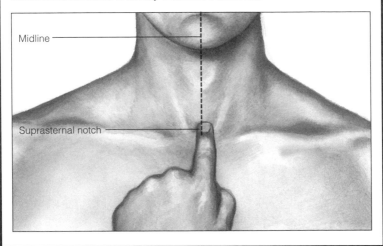

Midline

Suprasternal notch

above the suprasternal notch. Dysphagia, cough, hoarseness, and stridor commonly occur. Signs of thyrotoxicosis may be present.

• **Tension pneumothorax.** This acute, life-threatening condition produces tracheal deviation toward the unaffected side. It's marked by a sudden onset of respiratory distress with sharp chest pain, dry cough, severe dyspnea, tachycardia, wheezing, cyanosis, accessory muscle use, nasal flaring, air hunger, and asymmetrical chest movement. Restless and anxious, the patient may also have subcutaneous crepitation in the neck and upper chest, decreased vocal fremitus, decreased or absent breath sounds on the affected side, distended neck veins, and hypotension.

• **Thoracic aortic aneurysm.** This disorder usually causes the trachea to deviate to the right. Highly variable associated findings may include stridor, dyspnea, wheezing, brassy cough, hoarseness, and dysphagia. Edema of the face, neck, or arm may occur with distended chest wall and neck veins. Substernal, neck, shoulder, or lower back pain may occur, possibly with paresthesia or neuralgia.

Special considerations

Because tracheal deviation usually signals a severe underlying disorder that can cause respiratory distress at any time, monitor the patient's respiratory and cardiac status constantly, and make sure that emergency equipment is readily available. Prepare the patient for diagnostic tests, such as chest X-ray, electrocardiogram, and arterial blood gas analysis.

Pediatric pointers

Keep in mind that respiratory distress generally develops more rapidly in children than in adults.

TRACHEAL TUGGING
[Cardarelli's sign, Castellino's sign, Oliver's sign]

A visible recession of the larynx and trachea that occurs in synchrony with cardiac systole, tracheal tugging commonly results from an aneurysm or a tumor near the aortic arch and may signal dangerous compression or obstruction of major airways. The tugging movement, best observed with the patient's neck hyperextended, reflects abnormal transmission of aortic pulsations because of compression and distortion of the heart, esophagus, great vessels, airways, and nerves.

Emergency interventions

 If you observe tracheal tugging, examine the patient for signs and symptoms of respiratory distress, such as tachypnea, stridor, accessory muscle use, cyanosis, and agitation. If the patient is in distress, you should check airway patency. Administer oxygen, and prepare to intubate the patient, if necessary. Insert an I.V. line for fluid and drug access, and institute cardiac monitoring.

History and physical examination

If the patient isn't in distress, obtain a pertinent history. Ask about associated symptoms, especially pain, and about any history of cardiovascular disease, cancer, chest surgery, or trauma.

Now examine the patient's neck and chest for abnormalities. Palpate the neck

for masses, enlarged lymph nodes, abnormal arterial pulsations, and tracheal deviation. Percuss and auscultate the lung fields for abnormal sounds, and auscultate the heart for murmurs.

Common medical causes

- *Aortic arch aneurysm.* A large aneurysm can distort and compress surrounding tissues and structures, producing tracheal tugging. The cardinal symptom of this aneurysm is severe pain in the substernal area, sometimes radiating to the back or side of the chest. A sudden increase in pain may herald impending rupture—a medical emergency. Depending on the aneurysm's site and size, associated findings may include a visible pulsatile mass in the first or second intercostal space or suprasternal notch, a diastolic murmur of aortic regurgitation, and an aortic systolic murmur and thrill in the absence of any peripheral signs of aortic stenosis. Dyspnea and stridor may occur with hoarseness, dysphagia, brassy cough, and hemoptysis. Distended jugular veins may also occur along with edema of the face, neck, or arm. Compression of the left main bronchus can cause atelectasis of the left lung.

- *Hodgkin's disease.* Development of a tumor adjacent to the aortic arch can cause tracheal tugging. Initial signs and symptoms include usually painless cervical lymphadenopathy, sustained or remittent fever, fatigue, malaise, pruritus, night sweats, and weight loss. Swollen lymph nodes may become tender and painful. Later findings include dyspnea and stridor; dry cough; dysphagia; distended neck veins; edema of the face, neck, or arm; hepatosplenomegaly; hyperpigmentation, jaundice, or pallor; and neuralgia.

- *Malignant lymphoma.* Tracheal tugging may reflect anterior mediastinal lymphadenopathy or tumor development next to the aortic arch. The most common initial sign, though, is painless peripheral

TRACHEAL TUGGING: COMMON CAUSES AND ASSOCIATED FINDINGS

CAUSES	MAJOR ASSOCIATED SIGNS AND SYMPTOMS											
	Chest pain	Cough, brassy	Cough, crowing	Dyspnea	Edema of face, neck, or arm	Fever	Hemoptysis	Hoarseness	Lymphadenopathy	Murmur	Neck vein distention	Stridor
Aortic arch aneurysm	●	●		●	●		●	●		●	●	●
Hodgkin's disease				●	●	●			●		●	●
Malignant lymphoma			●	●	●	●			●		●	●
Thymoma	●			●	●			●			●	

lymphadenopathy. Other early findings include fever, fatigue, malaise, night sweats, and weight loss. Later findings include a crowing cough, dyspnea, stridor, dysphagia, distended neck veins, neck edema, hepatomegaly, and splenomegaly.

- *Thymoma.* This rare tumor can cause tracheal tugging if it develops in the anterior mediastinum. Cough, chest pain, dysphagia, dyspnea, hoarseness, a palpable neck mass, distended neck veins, and edema of the face, neck, or upper arm are common findings.

Special considerations

Prepare the patient for diagnostic procedures, which may include chest X-ray, computed tomography scan, lymphangiography, aortography, bone marrow biopsy, liver biopsy, echocardiography, and a complete blood count.

Place the patient in semi-Fowler's position to ease respiration. Administer cough suppressants. You also should give prescribed pain medications, but keep alert for signs of respiratory depression.

Pediatric pointers

In infants and children, tracheal tugging may indicate a mediastinal tumor, such as occurs in either Hodgkin's disease or malignant lymphoma. It may also be present in Marfan syndrome.

TREMORS

The most common involuntary muscle movement, tremors are regular rhythmic oscillations that result from alternating contraction of opposing muscle groups. They're typical signs of extrapyramidal or cerebellar disorders and can also result from certain drugs.

Tremors can be characterized by their location, amplitude, and frequency. They're classified as resting, intention, or postural. *Resting tremors* occur when an extremity is at rest and subside with movement. They include the classic pill-rolling tremor of Parkinson's disease. Conversely, *intention tremors* occur only with movement and subside with rest. *Postural (or action) tremors* appear when an extremity or the trunk is actively held in a particular posture or position. A common postural tremor is called an *essential tremor*.

Tremorlike movements such as asterixis (the characteristic flapping tremor seen in hepatic failure) may also be elicited. (See the entry "Asterixis.")

Stress or emotional upset tends to aggravate a tremor. Alcohol commonly diminishes postural tremors.

History and physical examination

Begin your examination by asking the patient about the tremor's onset (sudden or gradual) and about its duration, progression, and any aggravating or alleviating factors. Does the tremor interfere with his normal activities? Does the patient have other symptoms? Has he noticed any behavioral changes or memory loss (the patient's family or friends may provide more accurate information on this)?

Explore the patient's personal and family medical history for neurologic (especially seizures), endocrine, or metabolic disorders. Obtain a complete drug history, noting especially the use of phenothiazines. Also ask about alcohol use.

Assess the patient's overall appearance and demeanor, noting mental status. Test range of motion and strength in all major muscle groups while observing for chorea, athetosis, dystonia, and other involuntary movements. Check deep tendon reflexes and, if possible, observe the patient's gait.

Common medical causes

• *Alkalosis.* Severe alkalosis may produce a severe intention tremor, along with twitching, carpopedal spasms, agitation, diaphoresis, and hyperventilation. The patient may complain of dizziness, tinnitus, palpitations, and peripheral and circumoral paresthesia.

• *Benign familial essential tremor.* This disorder of early adulthood produces a bilateral essential tremor that typically begins in the fingers and hands and may spread to the head, jaw, lips, and tongue. Laryngeal involvement may result in a quavering voice.

• *Cerebellar tumor.* Intention tremor is a cardinal sign of this disorder; related findings include ataxia, nystagmus, incoordination, muscle weakness and atrophy, and hypoactive or absent deep tendon reflexes.

• *Hypercapnia.* Elevated partial pressure of carbon dioxide levels may result in a rapid, fine intention tremor. Other common findings include headache, fatigue, blurred vision, weakness, lethargy, and decreasing level of consciousness (LOC).

• *Hypoglycemia.* Acute hypoglycemia may produce a rapid, fine intention tremor accompanied by confusion, weakness, tachycardia, diaphoresis, and cold, clammy skin. Early patient complaints typically include mild generalized headache, profound hunger, nervousness, and blurred or double vision. The tremor may disappear as hypoglycemia worsens and hypotonia and decreased LOC become evident.

• *Multiple sclerosis (MS).* Intention tremor may be an early sign of MS. Like the disorder's other effects, it tends to wax and wane. Commonly, visual and sensory impairments are the earliest findings. Associated effects vary greatly and may include nystagmus, muscle weakness, paralysis, spasticity, hyperreflexia, ataxic gait, dysphagia, and dysarthria. Constipation, urinary frequency and urgency, incontinence, impotence, and emotional lability may also occur.

• *Parkinson's disease.* Tremors, a classic early sign of this degenerative disease, usually begin in the fingers and may eventually affect the foot, eyelids, jaw, lips, and tongue. The slow, regular, rhythmic resting tremor takes the form of flexion-extension or abduction-adduction of the fingers or hand, or pronation-supination of the hand. Flexion-extension of the fingers combined with abduction-adduction of the thumb yields the characteristic pill-rolling tremor.

Leg involvement produces flexion-extension foot movement. Lightly closing the eyelids causes them to flutter. The jaw may move up and down, and the lips may purse. The tongue, when protruded, may move in and out of the mouth in tempo with tremors elsewhere in the body. The rate of the tremor holds constant over time, but amplitude varies.

Other characteristic findings include cogwheel or lead-pipe rigidity, bradykinesia, propulsive gait with forward-leaning posture, monotone voice, masklike facies, drooling, dysphagia, dysarthria, and occasionally oculogyric crisis (eyes fix upward, with involuntary tonic movements) or blepharospasm (eyelids close completely).

• *Thalamic syndrome. Central midbrain syndromes* are heralded by contralateral ataxic tremors and other abnormal movements, along with Weber's syndrome (oculomotor palsy with contralateral hemiplegia), paralysis of vertical gaze, and stupor or coma. *Anteromedial-inferior thalamic syndrome* produces varying combinations of tremor, deep sensory loss, and hemiataxia. However, the main effect of this syndrome may be an extrapyramidal dysfunction, such as hemiballismus or hemichoreoathetosis.

• *Thyrotoxicosis.* Neuromuscular effects of this disorder include a rapid, fine intention tremor of the hands and tongue, along with clonus, hyperreflexia, and Babinski's reflex. Other common signs and symptoms include tachycardia, cardiac arrhythmias, palpitations, anxiety, dyspnea, diaphoresis, heat intolerance, weight loss despite increased appetite, diarrhea, an enlarged thyroid, and possibly exophthalmos.

• *Wernicke's disease.* Intention tremor is an early sign of this thiamine deficiency. Other features include ocular abnormalities (such as gaze paralysis and nystagmus), and ataxia, apathy, and confusion. Orthostatic hypotension and tachycardia may also develop in this disorder.

Other causes

• *Drugs.* Phenothiazines (particularly piperazine derivatives, such as fluphenazine) and other antipsychotics may cause resting and pill-rolling tremors. Infrequently, metoclopramide and metyrosine also cause these tremors. Lithium toxicity, sympathomimetics (such as terbutaline and pseudoephedrine), amphetamines, and phenytoin can all cause essential tremors that disappear with dose reduction.

Special considerations

Severe intention tremors may interfere with the patient's ability to perform activities of daily living. Assist the patient with these activities as necessary, and take precautions against injury during such activities as walking or eating.

Pediatric pointers

The normal newborn may display coarse tremors with stiffening—an exaggerated hypocalcemic startle reflex—in response to noises and chills. Pediatric-specific causes of pathologic tremor include cerebral palsy, fetal alcohol syndrome, and maternal drug addiction.

TUNNEL VISION
[Gunbarrel vision, tubular vision]

Resulting from severe constriction of the visual field that leaves only a small central area of sight, tunnel vision is typically described as the sensation of looking through a tunnel or gun barrel. It may be unilateral or bilateral and usually develops gradually. This abnormality results from chronic open-angle glaucoma and advanced retinal degeneration. Tunnel vision also can result from laser photocoagulation therapy, which aims to correct retinal detachment. Also a common complaint of malingerers, tunnel vision can be verified or discounted by visual field examination performed by an ophthalmologist.

History and physical examination

Ask the patient when he first noticed a loss of peripheral vision. Then have him describe the progression of vision loss. Next, ask the patient to describe in detail exactly what and how far he can see peripherally. You should explore the patient's personal and family history for ocular problems, especially progressive blindness that began at an early age.

To rule out malingering, observe the patient as he walks. A patient with severely limited peripheral vision may frequently bump into objects (and may even have bruises), whereas the malingerer will manage to avoid them.

If your examination findings suggest tunnel vision, you should refer the patient to an ophthalmologist for further evaluation.

Common medical causes

• *Chronic open-angle glaucoma.* In this insidious disorder, bilateral tunnel vision occurs late and slowly progresses to complete blindness. Other late findings include mild eye pain, halo vision, and reduced visual acuity (especially at night) that is uncorrectable with glasses.

• *Retinal pigmentary degeneration.* This group of hereditary disorders, such as retinitis pigmentosa, will produce an annular scotoma that progresses concentrically, causing tunnel vision and eventually resulting in complete blindness, usually by age 50. Typically, impaired night vision, the earliest symptom, appears in the first or second decade of life. Also, an ophthalmoscopic examination may reveal narrowed retinal blood vessels and a pale optic disk.

Special considerations

To protect the patient from injury, be sure to remove all potentially dangerous objects and orient him to his surroundings.

If tunnel vision is permanent, teach the patient to move his eyes from side to side when he walks to avoid bumping into objects. Because any visual impairment is frightening, remember to reassure the patient and clearly explain diagnostic procedures, such as tonometry, perimeter examination, and visual field testing.

Pediatric pointers

In children with retinitis pigmentosa, night blindness foreshadows tunnel vision, which usually doesn't develop until later in the disease process.

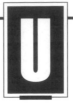

URETHRAL DISCHARGE

Urethral discharge comes from the urethral meatus and may be purulent, mucoid, or thin; sanguineous or clear; and scant or profuse. It usually develops suddenly, most commonly in men with a prostate infection.

History and physical examination
Ask the patient when he first noticed the discharge, and have him describe its color, consistency, and quantity. Does he have any pain on urination or difficulty initiating a urine stream? Ask him about other associated symptoms, such as fever, chills, and perineal fullness. Explore his history for any prostate problems, sexually transmitted diseases, and urinary tract infections. Ask the patient if he has had recent sexual contacts or a new sexual partner.

Inspect the patient's urethral meatus for inflammation and swelling. Using proper technique, obtain a culture specimen. Then obtain a urine specimen for urinalysis and possibly a three-glass urine specimen. You may have to palpate the male patient's prostate gland.

Common medical causes
• *Prostatitis.* *Acute prostatitis* is characterized by a purulent urethral discharge. Other initial signs and symptoms include sudden fever, chills, low back pain, myalgia, perineal fullness, and arthralgia. Urination becomes increasingly frequent and urgent, and the urine may appear cloudy.

Dysuria, nocturia, and some degree of urinary obstruction may also occur. A rectal examination to palpate the prostate is contraindicated if the patient has acute prostatitis.

Chronic prostatitis, although commonly asymptomatic, may produce a persistent urethral discharge that's thin, milky or clear, and sometimes sticky. The discharge appears at the meatus after a long interval between voidings—for example, in the morning. Associated effects include a dull ache in the prostate or rectum, sexual dysfunction, and urinary disturbances, such as frequency, urgency, and dysuria.
• *Reiter's syndrome.* In this self-limiting disorder that usually affects males, urethral discharge and other signs of acute urethritis occur 1 to 2 weeks after sexual contact. Arthritic and ocular symptoms and skin lesions usually develop within several weeks.
• *Urethritis.* This inflammatory disorder, which is commonly sexually transmitted (as in gonorrhea), generally produces a scant or profuse urethral discharge that's either thin and clear, mucoid, or thick and purulent. Other effects include itching and burning around the meatus, dysuria, and urinary hesitancy, urgency, and frequency.

Special considerations
Advise the patient with acute prostatitis to avoid sexual activity until his acute symptoms subside. However, encourage the patient with chronic prostatitis to engage in sexual activity frequently. To help relieve his symptoms, suggest that this patient take hot sitz baths several times

daily, drink more fluids, urinate frequently, and avoid caffeine, tea, and alcohol. Monitor him for urine retention.

Pediatric pointers
Carefully evaluate a child with urethral discharge for evidence of sexual and physical abuse.

URINARY FREQUENCY

Urinary frequency refers to increased incidence of the urge to void. Usually resulting from decreased bladder capacity, frequency is a cardinal sign of urinary tract infection (UTI), However, it can also stem from other urologic disorders, neurologic dysfunction, and pressure on the bladder from a nearby tumor or from organ enlargement (as in pregnancy).

Urinary frequency may be reported by the patient with polyuria—an increase in total daily urine output. (See the entry "Polyuria.")

History and physical examination
Ask the patient how many times a day he voids. How does this compare to his previous pattern of voiding? Ask about the onset and duration of the abnormal frequency and about any associated urinary symptoms, such as dysuria, urgency, incontinence, hematuria, or lower abdominal pain with urination. Also ask about any neurologic symptoms, such as muscle weakness, numbness, or tingling. Explore his medical history for UTIs, other urologic problems or recent urologic procedures, and neurologic disorders. Ask a male patient about a history of prostatic enlargement. Ask a female patient of childbearing age whether she is or could be pregnant.

Obtain a clean-catch midstream sample for urinalysis and culture and sensitivity tests. Then palpate the suprapubic area, abdomen, and flanks, noting any tenderness. Examine his urethral meatus for redness, discharge, or swelling. In a male patient, the doctor may palpate the prostate gland.

If the patient's history reveals symptoms or a history of neurologic disorders, perform a neurologic examination.

Common medical causes
• *Benign prostatic hyperplasia.* Prostatic enlargement causes urinary frequency, along with nocturia and, possibly, incontinence and hematuria. Initial effects are those of prostatism: reduced caliber and force of the urine stream, urinary hesitancy and tenesmus, a feeling of incomplete voiding, and occasionally urine retention. Assessment reveals bladder distention.

• *Bladder calculus.* Bladder irritation may lead to urinary frequency and urgency, dysuria, hematuria, and suprapubic pain from bladder spasms. The patient may have overflow incontinence if the calculus lodges in the bladder neck.

• *Diabetes insipidus.* Here, antidiuretic hormone deficiency typically results in periodic voiding of moderate to large amounts of urine. Diabetes insipidus can also produce polydipsia.

• *Diabetes mellitus.* Besides greater urinary frequency, other findings include nocturia, daytime polyuria, polydipsia, polyphagia, weight loss, fatigue, weakness and, possibly, signs of dehydration.

• *Prostatic cancer.* In advanced stages, urinary frequency may occur, along with hesitancy, dribbling, nocturia, dysuria, bladder distention, perineal pain, constipation, and a hard, irregularly shaped prostate.

• *Prostatitis.* *Acute prostatitis* commonly produces urinary frequency, along with urgency, dysuria, nocturia, and purulent urethral discharge. Other findings include fever, chills, low back pain, myalgia, arthralgia, and perineal fullness. Rectal examination to palpate the prostate is contraindicated in acute prostatitis. Clinical features of *chronic prostatitis* are usually the same as those of the acute form, but to a lesser degree.

• *Reproductive tract tumor.* A tumor in the female reproductive tract may compress the bladder, causing urinary frequency. Other findings vary but may include abdominal distention, menstrual disturbances, vaginal bleeding, weight loss, pelvic pain, and fatigue.

• *Spinal cord lesion.* Incomplete cord transection results in urinary frequency and urgency when voluntary control of sphincter function weakens. Added urologic effects may include hesitancy and bladder distention. Other effects occur below the level of the lesion and may include weakness, paralysis, sensory disturbances, hyperreflexia, and impotence.

• *Urethral stricture.* Bladder decompensation produces urinary frequency, urgency, and nocturia. Early signs include hesitancy, tenesmus, and reduced caliber and force of the urine stream. Eventually, overflow incontinence may occur.

• *Urinary tract infection.* Affecting the urethra, bladder, or kidneys, this common cause of urinary frequency also may produce urgency, dysuria, hematuria, cloudy urine, urethral discharge (in males), bladder spasms, or a feeling of warmth during urination.

Other causes

• *Diuretics.* These substances, which include caffeine, reduce the body's total volume of water and salt by increasing urine excretion. Excessive intake of coffee, tea and other caffeine-containing drinks will lead to urinary frequency.

• *Treatments.* Radiation therapy may cause bladder inflammation, leading to urinary frequency.

Special considerations

Prepare the patient for diagnostic tests, such as urinalysis, culture and sensitivity tests, imaging tests, ultrasonography, cystoscopy, cystometry, and a complete neurologic workup. If the patient's mobility is impaired, keep a bedpan or commode near his bed.

Pediatric pointers

UTI is a common cause of urinary frequency in children, especially girls. Congenital anomalies that can cause UTI include a duplicated ureter, congenital bladder diverticulum, and an ectopic ureteral orifice.

URINARY HESITANCY

Hesitancy—difficulty starting a urine stream—can result from a urinary tract infection (UTI), a partial lower urinary tract obstruction, a neuromuscular disorder, or use of certain drugs. Occurring at all ages and in both sexes, it's most common in older men with prostatic enlargement. It also occurs in women with gravid uterus, tumors in the reproductive system, such as uterine fibroids, or ovarian, uterine or vaginal carcinoma. Hesitancy usually arises gradually, commonly going unnoticed until urine retention causes bladder distention and discomfort.

History and physical examination

Ask the patient when he first noticed hesitancy and if he's ever had the problem before. Ask about other urinary problems, especially reduced force or interruption of the urine stream. Ask if he's ever been treated for a prostate problem or a UTI or obstruction. Obtain a drug history.

Inspect the urethral meatus for inflammation, discharge, and other abnormalities. Examine the anal sphincter and test sensation in the perineum. Obtain a clean-catch sample for urinalysis. In a male patient, the prostate gland will require palpation. A female patient will require a gynecologic examination.

Common medical causes

• *Benign prostatic hyperplasia.* Clinical features of this disorder depend on the extent of prostatic enlargement and the lobes affected. Characteristic early findings include urinary hesitancy, reduced caliber and force of urine stream, a feeling of incomplete voiding and, occasionally, urine retention. As the obstruction increases, urination becomes more frequent, with nocturia, urinary overflow, incontinence, bladder distention, and possibly hematuria.

• *Prostatic cancer.* In advanced cancer, urinary hesitancy may occur, accompanied by frequency, dribbling, nocturia, dysuria, bladder distention, perineal pain, and constipation.

• *Spinal cord lesion.* A lesion below the micturition center that has destroyed the sacral nerve roots causes urinary hesitancy, tenesmus, and constant dribbling from retention and overflow incontinence. Associated findings are urinary frequency and urgency, dysuria, and nocturia.

• *Urethral stricture.* Partial obstruction of the lower urinary tract secondary to trauma or infection produces urinary hesitancy, tenesmus, and decreased force and caliber of the urine stream. Urinary frequency and urgency, nocturia and, eventually, overflow incontinence may develop. Pyuria usually indicates accompanying infection.

• *Urinary tract infection.* Urinary hesitancy may be associated with this infection. Characteristic urinary changes include frequency, possible hematuria, dysuria, nocturia, and cloudy urine. Associated findings may include bladder spasms; costovertebral angle tenderness; suprapubic, low back, or flank pain; urethral discharge in males; and constitutional effects, such as fever, chills, malaise, nausea, and vomiting.

Other causes

• *Drugs.* Anticholinergics and drugs with anticholinergic properties (such as tricyclic antidepressants and some nasal decongestants and cold remedies) may cause urinary hesitancy. Hesitancy also may occur in patients recovering from general anesthesia.

Special considerations

Monitor the patient's voiding pattern, and frequently palpate for bladder distention. Apply local heat to the perineum or the abdomen to enhance muscle relaxation and aid urination. Also teach how to perform a clean, intermittent self-catheterization. Prepare him for tests, such as cystometrography or cystourethroscopy.

Pediatric pointers

The most common cause of urinary obstruction in male infants is posterior structures in the prostatic urethra. Infants with this problem may have a less forceful urine stream and may also present with fever due to a UTI, failure to thrive, or a palpable bladder.

URINARY INCONTINENCE

Incontinence, the uncontrollable passage of urine, results from either bladder abnormalities or neurologic disorders. A common urologic sign, incontinence may be transient or permanent, and may involve large volumes of urine or scant dribbling. It can be classified as stress, overflow, urge, or total incontinence.

Stress incontinence is intermittent leakage resulting from a sudden physical strain, such as a cough, sneeze, or quick movement. *Overflow incontinence* is a dribble resulting from urine retention, which fills the bladder and prevents it from contracting with sufficient force to expel a urine stream. *Urge incontinence* is the inability to suppress a sudden urge to urinate. *Total incontinence* is continuous leakage due to the bladder's inability to retain any urine.

History and physical examination

Ask the patient when he first noticed the incontinence and whether it began suddenly or gradually. Have him describe his typical urinary pattern: Does incontinence usually occur during the day or at night? Does he have any urinary control, or is he totally incontinent? If he sometimes urinates with control, ask him the usual times and amounts voided. Determine his normal fluid intake. Ask about other urinary problems, such as hesitancy, frequency, urgency, nocturia, and decreased force or interruption of the urine stream. Also ask if he's ever sought treatment for incontinence or found a way to deal with it himself.

Obtain a medical history, especially noting urinary tract infection, prostate conditions, spinal injury or tumor, cerebrovascular accident, or surgery involving the bladder, prostate, or pelvic floor.

After completing the history, have the patient empty his bladder. Inspect the urethral meatus for obvious inflammation or anatomic defect. Have female patients bear down; note any urine leakage. Gently palpate the abdomen for bladder distention, which signals urine retention. Perform a complete neurologic assessment, noting motor and sensory function and obvious muscle atrophy.

Common medical causes

• **Benign prostatic hyperplasia (BPH).** Overflow incontinence is common in this disorder as a result of urethral obstruction and urine retention. BPH begins with a group of symptoms known as prostatism: reduced caliber and force of urine stream, urinary hesitancy, and a feeling of incomplete voiding. As obstruction increases, urination becomes more frequent, with nocturia and, possibly, hematuria. Examination reveals bladder distention and an enlarged prostate.

• **Bladder cancer.** This disease commonly presents with urge incontinence and hematuria; obstruction by a tumor may produce overflow incontinence. The early stages can be asymptomatic. Other urinary complaints may include frequency, dysuria, nocturia, dribbling, and suprapubic pain from bladder spasms after voiding.

• **Cerebrovascular accident.** Urinary incontinence may be transient or permanent. Associated findings reflect the site and extent of the lesion and may include impaired mentation, emotional lability, behavioral changes, altered level of consciousness, and seizures. Headache, vomiting, visual deficits, and decreased visual acuity are possible. Sensorimotor effects may include contralateral hemiplegia, dysarthria, dysphagia, ataxia, apraxia, agnosia, aphasia, and unilateral sensory loss.

• **Diabetic neuropathy.** Autonomic neuropathy may cause painless bladder distention with overflow incontinence. Related findings may include episodic constipation or diarrhea, impotence and retrograde ejaculation, orthostatic hypotension, syncope, and dysphagia.

• **Multiple sclerosis (MS).** Urinary incontinence, urgency, and frequency are common urologic findings in MS. In most patients, visual problems and sensory impairment occur early. Other findings may include constipation, muscle weakness, paralysis, spasticity, hyperreflexia, intention tremor, ataxic gait, dysarthria, impotence, and emotional lability.

• **Prostatitis (chronic).** Urinary incontinence may occur as a result of urethral obstruction from an enlarged prostate. Other findings may include urinary frequency and urgency, dysuria, hematuria, bladder distention, persistent urethral discharge, dull perineal pain that may radiate, and decreased libido.

• **Spinal cord injury.** Complete cord transection above the sacral level causes flaccid paralysis of the bladder. Overflow incontinence follows rapid bladder distention. Other findings include paraplegia, sexual dysfunction, sensory loss, muscle atrophy, anhidrosis, and loss of reflexes distal to the injury.

CORRECTING INCONTINENCE WITH BLADDER RETRAINING

The incontinent patient typically feels frustrated, embarrassed, and sometimes hopeless. Fortunately, though, his problem can usually be corrected by bladder retraining—a program that aims to establish a regular voiding pattern. Here are some guidelines for establishing such a program.

• Before you start the program, assess the patient's intake pattern, voiding pattern, and behavior (for example, restlessness or talkativeness) before each voiding.
• Encourage the patient to use the toilet 30 minutes before he's usually incontinent. If this isn't successful, readjust the schedule. Once he's able to stay dry for 2 hours, increase the time between voidings by 30 minutes each day until he achieves a 3- to 4-hour voiding schedule.
• When your patient voids, make sure that the sequence of conditioning stimuli is always the same.
• Ensure that the patient has privacy while voiding—any inhibiting stimuli should be avoided.
• Keep a record of continence and incontinence for 5 days—this may reinforce your patient's efforts to remain continent.
• Remember, both your positive attitude and your patient's are crucial to

his successful bladder retraining.
• Make sure the patient is close to a bathroom or portable toilet. Leave a light on at night.
• If your patient needs assistance getting out of his bed or chair, promptly answer his call for help.
• Encourage him to wear his usual clothing as an indication that you're confident he can remain continent. Acceptable alternatives to diapers include condoms for the male patient and incontinence pads or panties for the female patient.
• Encourage him to drink 2 to 2½ qt (2 to 2.5 L) of fluid each day. Less fluid doesn't prevent incontinence but does promote bladder infection. Limiting his intake after 5 p.m., however, will help him remain continent during the night.
• Reassure your patient that episodes of incontinence don't signal a failure of the program. Encourage him to be patient and to persevere.

• *Urethral stricture.* Eventually, overflow incontinence may occur here.
• *Urinary tract infection.* Besides incontinence, this infection may produce urinary urgency, dysuria, hematuria, cloudy urine and, in males, urethral discharge. Bladder spasms or a feeling of warmth during urination may occur.

Other causes
• *Surgery.* Urinary incontinence may occur after prostatectomy as a result of urethral sphincter damage.

Special considerations
Prepare the patient for diagnostic tests, such as cystoscopy, cystometry, and a complete neurologic workup. Obtain a urine specimen.

Begin managing incontinence by implementing a bladder retraining program. (See *Correcting incontinence with bladder retraining.*) To prevent stress incontinence, teach the patient exercises to help strengthen the pelvic floor muscles. He may also benefit from alternative therapies such as biofeedback. (See *Biofeedback to correct incontinence,* page 576.)

BIOFEEDBACK TO CORRECT INCONTINENCE

Stress-related conditions such as incontinence (which involves muscle tone) have been treated successfully with biofeedback. This procedure is a type of relaxation therapy that uses electronic feedback devices to teach the patient to be aware of and to consciously control involuntary body functions, such as heart and respiratory rates, blood pressure, temperature, digestion, and muscle behavior.

Electrodes are applied to the perianal skin and lateral thigh and are then attached to a sequential light display mechanism. As the patient tightens his perianal and thigh muscles in an attempt to increase muscle tone, the light illuminates, offering immediate feedback. The device can also measure the strength and duration of the muscle exercises, allowing the patient's progress to be monitored.

If the patient's incontinence has a neurologic basis, monitor for urine retention, which may require periodic catheterizations. If appropriate, teach the patient self-catheterization techniques. A patient with permanent urinary incontinence may require surgical creation of a urinary diversion.

Pediatric pointers

Causes of incontinence in children include infrequent or incomplete voiding, which may also lead to urinary tract infection. Ectopic ureteral orifice is an uncommon congenital anomaly associated with incontinence. A complete diagnostic evaluation usually is necessary to rule out organic disease.

URINARY URGENCY

A sudden compelling urge to urinate, accompanied by bladder pain, is a classic symptom of urinary tract infection (UTI). As inflammation decreases bladder capacity, discomfort results from the accumulation of even small amounts of urine. Repeated, frequent voiding in an effort to alleviate this discomfort produces urine output of only a few milliliters at each voiding.

Urgency without bladder pain may point to an upper motor neuron lesion that has disrupted bladder control.

History and physical examination

Ask the patient about the onset of urinary urgency and whether he has ever experienced it before. Ask about other urologic symptoms, such as dysuria and cloudy urine, and about neurologic symptoms such as paresthesia. Examine medical history for recurrent or chronic UTIs or for surgery or procedures involving the urinary tract.

Obtain a clean-catch sample for urinalysis. Note urine character, color, and odor, and use a reagent strip to test for pH, glucose, and blood. Then palpate the suprapubic area and both flanks for tenderness. If the patient's history or symptoms suggest neurologic dysfunction, perform a neurologic examination.

Common medical causes

• **Bladder calculus.** Bladder irritation can lead to urinary urgency and frequency, dysuria, hematuria, and suprapubic pain from bladder spasms.

• **Multiple sclerosis (MS).** Urinary urgency can occur with or without the frequent UTIs that commonly accompany MS. Like MS's other variable effects, urinary urgency may wax and wane. Visual and sensory impairments are often the earliest findings. Others include urinary frequency, incontinence, constipation, muscle weakness, paralysis, spasticity, intention tremor, hyperreflexia, ataxic gait, dysphagia, dysarthria, impotence, and emotional lability.

● *Reiter's syndrome.* In this self-limiting syndrome that primarily affects males, urgency occurs with other symptoms of acute urethritis 1 to 2 weeks after sexual contact. Arthritic and ocular symptoms and skin lesions usually develop within several weeks.

● *Spinal cord lesion.* Urinary urgency can result from incomplete cord transection when voluntary control of sphincter function weakens. Other symptoms may include urinary frequency, difficulty initiating and inhibiting a urine stream, and bladder distention and discomfort. Neuromuscular effects distal to the lesion may include weakness, paralysis, hyperreflexia, sensory disturbances, and impotence.

● *Urethral stricture.* Bladder decompensation produces urinary urgency, frequency, and nocturia. Early signs include hesitancy, tenesmus, and reduced caliber and force of the urine stream. Eventually, overflow incontinence may occur.

● *Urinary tract infection.* Urinary urgency is commonly associated with UTIs. Other characteristic urinary changes include frequency, hematuria, dysuria, nocturia, and cloudy urine. Urinary hesitancy may also occur. Associated findings may include bladder spasms; costovertebral angle tenderness; suprapubic, low back, or flank pain; urethral discharge in males; and constitutional effects, such as fever, chills, malaise, nausea, and vomiting.

Other causes

● *Treatments.* Radiation therapy may irritate and inflame the bladder, causing urinary urgency.

Special considerations

Prepare the patient for the diagnostic workup, including a complete urinalysis, culture and sensitivity studies, and possibly neurologic tests.

Increase the patient's fluid intake, if not contraindicated, to dilute the urine and diminish the sensation of urgency. Administer antibiotics and urinary anesthetics (such as phenazopyridine), as ordered.

Pediatric pointers

In young children, urinary urgency may appear as a change in toilet habits, such as a sudden onset of bed-wetting or daytime accidents in a toilet-trained child. Urgency may also result from urethral irritation by bubble bath salts.

URINE CLOUDINESS

Cloudy, murky, or turbid urine reflects the presence of bacteria, mucus, leukocytes or erythrocytes, epithelial cells, fat, or phosphates (in alkaline urine). This sign is characteristic of urinary tract infection (UTI) but can also result from prolonged storage of a urine specimen at room temperature.

History and physical examination

Ask about symptoms of UTIs, such as dysuria, urinary urgency or frequency, or pain in the flank, lower back, or suprapubic area. Also ask about recurrent UTIs as well as recent surgery or treatment involving the urinary tract.

Obtain a urine sample to check for pus or mucus. (See *How to perform the three-glass urine test,* page 578.) Using a reagent strip, test for blood, glucose, and pH. Palpate the suprapubic area and flanks for tenderness.

If you detect cloudy urine in a patient with an indwelling urinary catheter, especially if he has a concurrent fever, re-

HOW TO PERFORM THE THREE-GLASS URINE TEST

If your male patient complains of urinary frequency and urgency, dysuria, flank or lower back pain, or other signs of urethritis, and if his urine specimen is cloudy, perform the three-glass urine test.

First ask him to void into three conical glasses labeled with numbers 1, 2, and 3. First-voided urine goes into glass #1; midstream urine goes into #2; and the remainder goes into glass #3. Tell the patient to avoid interrupting the stream of urine when shifting glasses, if possible.

Now observe each glass for pus and mucus shreds. Also note urine color and odor. Glass #1 will contain matter from the anterior urethra; glass #2 will contain bladder contents; and glass #3 will contain sediment from the prostate and seminal vesicles.

Some common findings are shown below. However, confirming the diagnosis requires microscopic examination and a bacteriology report.

	SPECIMEN I	SPECIMEN II	SPECIMEN III
Acute or sub-acute urethritis	Cloudy	Clear	Clear
Acute posterior urethritis	Cloudy	Clear or cloudy	Cloudy
Chronic anterior urethritis	Small shreds	Clear	Clear
Chronic posterior urethritis	Large shreds	Clear	Clear
Chronic urethritis (anterior and posterior)	Small and large shreds	Clear	Clear
Prostatitis	Clear or large shreds	Clear	Cloudy or large shreds
Cystitis and pyelonephritis	Cloudy	Cloudy	Cloudy

move the catheter immediately (or change it if the patient must have one in place).

Common medical causes

• *Urinary tract infection.* Cloudy urine is common in UTIs. Other urinary changes include urgency, frequency, hematuria, dysuria, nocturia and, in males, urethral discharge. Urinary hesitancy, bladder spasms, costovertebral angle tenderness, and suprapubic, lower back, or flank pain may occur. Other effects may include fever, chills, malaise, nausea, and vomiting.

Special considerations

Collect urine samples for urinalysis and culture and sensitivity tests. Increase the patient's fluid intake and administer antibiotics and urinary anesthetics (such as phenazopyridine). Continue checking the appearance of the patient's urine to monitor the effectiveness of therapy.

Pediatric pointers
Cloudy urine in children also points to UTI.

URICARIA
[Hives]

Urticaria is a vascular skin reaction characterized by the eruption of transient pruritic wheals—smooth, slightly elevated patches with well-defined erythematous margins and pale centers. It's produced by the local release of histamine or other vasoactive substances as part of a hypersensitivity reaction.

Acute urticaria evolves rapidly and usually has a detectable cause, commonly hypersensitivity to certain drugs, foods, insect bites, inhalants, or contactants, emotional stress, or environmental factors. Although individual lesions usually subside within 12 to 24 hours, new crops of lesions may erupt continuously, thus prolonging the attack.

Urticaria lasting longer than 6 weeks is classified as chronic. The lesions may recur for months or years, and the underlying cause is usually unknown. Occasionally, a diagnosis of psychogenic urticaria is made.

Angioedema, also known as giant urticaria, is characterized by the acute eruption of wheals involving the mucous membranes and, occasionally, the arms, legs, or genitalia.

Emergency interventions
 In acute cases of urticaria, quickly evaluate respiratory status and take vital signs. Start an I.V. infusion of dextrose 5% in water if you note any respiratory difficulty or signs of impending anaphylactic shock.

Also, as appropriate, give local epinephrine or apply ice to the affected site to decrease absorption through vasoconstriction. Clear and maintain the airway, give oxygen as needed, and institute cardiac monitoring. Have resuscitation equipment at hand, and be prepared to begin cardiopulmonary resuscitation. Intubation or a tracheostomy may be required.

History
If the patient is not in distress, obtain a complete history. Does the urticaria follow any seasonal pattern? Do certain foods or drugs seem to aggravate it? Does it seem to have any relationship to physical exertion? Is the patient routinely exposed to any chemicals on the job or at home? Obtain a detailed drug history, including prescription and over-the-counter drugs. Note any history of chronic or parasitic infections, skin disease, or GI disorders.

Common medical causes
● *Anaphylaxis.* This acute reaction is marked by the rapid eruption of diffuse urticaria and angioedema, with pinpoint to palm-size or larger wheals. Lesions are usually pruritic and stinging; paresthesia commonly precedes their eruption. Other acute findings include profound anxiety, weakness, diaphoresis, sneezing, shortness of breath, profuse rhinorrhea, nasal congestion, dysphagia, and warm, moist skin.
● *Hereditary angioedema.* In this autosomal-dominant disorder, cutaneous involvement is manifested by nonpitting, nonpruritic edema of an extremity or the face. Respiratory mucosal involvement can produce life-threatening acute laryngeal edema.
● *Lyme disease.* Although not diagnostic for this tick-borne disease, urticaria may result from the disorder's characteristic skin lesion (erythema chronicum migrans). Later effects may include constant malaise and fatigue, intermittent

headache, fever, chills, lymphadenopathy, neurologic and cardiac abnormalities, and arthritis.

Other causes
• *Drugs.* Many drugs can cause urticaria. Among the most common are aspirin, atropine, codeine, dextrans, immune serums, insulin, morphine, penicillin, quinine, sulfonamides, and vaccines.
• *Contrast media.* Radiographic contrast media commonly produce urticaria, especially when they're administered I.V.

Special considerations
To help relieve the patient's discomfort, apply a bland skin emollient or one containing menthol and phenol. Expect to give antihistamines, systemic corticosteroids or, if stress is a suspected contributing factor, tranquilizers. Tepid baths and cool compresses may also enhance vasoconstriction and decrease pruritus.

Teach the patient to avoid the causative stimulus, if identified.

Pediatric pointers
Pediatric causes of urticaria include acute papular urticaria (usually after insect bites), hereditary angioedema, and urticaria pigmentosa (rare).

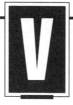

VAGINAL BLEEDING, POSTMENOPAUSAL

Postmenopausal vaginal bleeding—bleeding that occurs 6 months or more after menopause—is an important indicator of gynecologic cancer. But it can also result from infection, local pelvic disorders, estrogenic stimulation, atrophy of the endometrium, and physiologic thinning and drying of the vaginal mucous membranes. It usually occurs as slight, brown or red spotting either spontaneously or following coitus or douching, but it may also occur as oozing of fresh blood or as bright red hemorrhage. Many patients—especially those with a history of heavy menstrual flow—minimize the importance of this bleeding, delaying diagnosis.

History and physical examination
Determine the patient's current age and her age at menopause. Ask when she first noticed the abnormal bleeding. Then obtain a thorough obstetric and gynecologic history. When did she begin menstruating? Were her periods regular? If not, ask her to describe any menstrual irregularities. How old was she when she first had intercourse? How many sexual partners has she had? Has she had any children? Has she had fertility problems? If possible, obtain an obstetric and gynecologic history of the patient's mother, and ask about a family history of gynecologic cancer. Determine if the patient has any associated symptoms and if she's currently taking estrogen.

Observe the external genitalia, noting the character of any vaginal discharge and the appearance of the labia, vaginal rugae, and clitoris. Carefully palpate the patient's breasts and lymph nodes for nodules or enlargement. The patient may require pelvic and rectal examinations.

Common medical causes
• *Atrophic vaginitis.* When bloody staining occurs, it usually follows coitus or douching. Characteristic white vaginal discharge may be accompanied by pruritus, dyspareunia, and a burning sensation in the vagina and labia. Sparse pubic hair, a pale vagina with decreased rugae and small hemorrhagic spots, clitoral atrophy, and shrinking of the labia minora may also occur.
• *Cervical cancer.* Early invasive cervical cancer causes vaginal spotting or heavier bleeding, usually after coitus or douching but occasionally spontaneously. Related findings include persistent vaginal discharge and postcoital pain. As the cancer spreads, back and sciatic pain, leg swelling, anorexia, weight loss, and weakness may occur.
• *Cervical or endometrial polyps.* These small, pedunculated growths may cause spotting (possibly as a mucopurulent, pink discharge) after coitus, douching, or straining at stool. Many endometrial polyps are asymptomatic, however.
• *Endometrial hyperplasia or cancer.* Bleeding occurs early and can be brownish and scant or bright red and profuse; it commonly follows coitus or douching. Bleeding later becomes heavier, more

frequent, and longer in duration and may be accompanied by pelvic, rectal, lower back, and leg pain.

• *Ovarian tumors (feminizing).* Estrogen-producing ovarian tumors can stimulate endometrial shedding and cause heavy bleeding unassociated with coitus or douching. A palpable pelvic mass, increased cervical mucus, breast enlargement, and spider angiomas may be present.

• *Vaginal cancer.* Characteristic spotting or bleeding may be preceded by a thin, watery vaginal discharge. Bleeding may be spontaneous but usually follows coitus or douching. A firm, ulcerated vaginal lesion may be present; dyspareunia, urinary frequency, bladder and pelvic pain, rectal bleeding, and vulvar lesions may develop later.

Other causes

• *Drugs.* Excessive or prolonged estrogen administration is the most common drug cause of postmenopausal vaginal bleeding.

Special considerations

Prepare the patient for diagnostic tests, such as ultrasonography to outline a cervical or uterine tumor, endometrial biopsy or dilatation and fractional curettage to obtain tissue for histologic examination, testing for occult blood in the stool, and vaginal and cervical cultures to detect infection. Discontinue estrogens until a diagnosis is made.

VAGINAL DISCHARGE

Common in women of childbearing age, physiologic vaginal discharge is mucoid, clear or white, nonbloody, and odorless. Produced by the cervical mucosa and, to a lesser degree, by the vulvar glands, this discharge may occasionally be scant or profuse due to estrogenic stimulation and changes during the patient's menstrual cycle. However, a marked increase in discharge or a change in discharge color, odor, or consistency can signal disease. The discharge may result from infection, sexually transmitted disease, reproductive tract disease, fistulas, and use of certain drugs. (See *Common causes of vaginal discharge.*) In addition, the prolonged presence of a foreign body, such as a tampon or diaphragm, in the patient's vagina can cause irritation and an inflammatory exudate, as can frequent douching, feminine hygiene products, contraceptive products, bubble baths, and colored or perfumed toilet papers.

History and physical examination

Ask the patient to describe the onset, color, consistency, odor, and texture of her vaginal discharge. How does the discharge differ from her usual vaginal secretions? Is the onset related to her menstrual cycle? Also ask about associated symptoms, such as dysuria and perineal pruritus and burning. Does she have spotting after coitus or douching? Ask about recent changes in her sexual habits and hygiene practices. Is she or could she be pregnant? Next, ask if she has had vaginal discharge before or has ever been treated for a vaginal infection. If so, what treatment did she receive? Did she complete the course of medication? Ask about her current use of medications, especially antibiotics, oral estrogens, and contraceptives.

Examine the external genitalia and note the character of the discharge. Observe vulvar and vaginal tissues for redness, edema, and excoriation. Palpate the inguinal lymph nodes to detect tenderness or enlargement, and palpate the abdomen for tenderness. A pelvic examination may be required. Obtain vaginal discharge specimens for testing.

Common medical causes

• *Atrophic vaginitis.* In this disorder, a thin, scant, white vaginal discharge may

COMMON CAUSES OF VAGINAL DISCHARGE

The color, consistency, amount, and odor of your patient's vaginal discharge provide important clues about the underlying disorder. For quick reference, use this chart to match common characteristics of vaginal discharge to their possible causes.

CHARACTERISTICS	POSSIBLE CAUSES
Thin, scant, white discharge	Atrophic vaginitis
White, curdlike, profuse discharge with yeasty, sweet odor	Candidiasis
Yellow, mucopurulent, odorless or acrid discharge	*Chlamydia* infection
Thin, green or grayish white, foul-smelling discharge	*Gardnerella* vaginitis
Profuse, mucopurulent discharge, possibly foul-smelling	Genital warts
Yellow or green, foul-smelling discharge from the cervix or occasionally from Bartholin's or Skene's ducts	Gonorrhea
Chronic, watery, bloody, or purulent discharge, possibly foul-smelling	Gynecologic cancer
Frothy, greenish yellow, and profuse (or thin, white, and scant), foul-smelling discharge	Trichomoniasis

be accompanied by pruritus, burning, tenderness, and bloody spotting after coitus or douching. Sparse pubic hair, a pale vagina with decreased rugae and small hemorrhagic spots, clitoral atrophy, and shrinking of the labia minora may also occur.

• *Candidiasis.* Infection with *Candida albicans* causes a profuse, white, curdlike discharge with a yeasty, sweet odor. Onset is abrupt, usually just before menses. Exudate may be lightly attached to the labia and vaginal walls and is commonly accompanied by vulvar redness and edema. The inner thighs may be covered with a fine, red dermatitis. Intense labial itching and burning may also occur.

• *Chlamydia infection.* This infection causes a yellow, mucopurulent, odorless or acrid vaginal discharge. Other findings may include dysuria, dyspareunia, and vaginal bleeding after douching or coitus, especially following menses.

• *Gardnerella vaginitis.* This infection (by *Gardnerella vaginalis,* formerly called *Haemophilus vaginalis*) causes a thin, foul-smelling, green or grayish white discharge. It adheres to the vaginal walls and can be easily wiped away, leaving healthy-looking tissue. Pruritus, redness, and other signs of vaginal irritation may occur.

• *Genital warts.* Characteristic vulvar lesions can cause a profuse, mucopurulent vaginal discharge, which may be foul smelling if the warts are infected. Pruritus and erythema are common.

• **Gonorrhea.** Although 80% of women with gonorrhea are asymptomatic, others have a yellow or green, foul-smelling discharge that can be expressed from Bartholin's or Skene's ducts. Other findings include dysuria, urinary frequency and incontinence, and vaginal redness and swelling. Severe pelvic and lower abdominal pain and fever may develop.

• **Gynecologic cancer.** Endometrial or cervical cancer produces a chronic, watery, bloody or purulent vaginal discharge that may be foul smelling. Other findings include abnormal vaginal bleeding and, later, weight loss; pelvic, back, and leg pain; fatigue; and abdominal distention.

• **Trichomoniasis.** This infection can cause a foul-smelling discharge, which may be frothy, greenish yellow, and profuse or thin, white, and scant. Other findings may include pruritus; a red, inflamed vagina with tiny petechiae; dysuria and urinary frequency; and dyspareunia, postcoital spotting, menorrhagia, or dysmenorrhea. About 70% of patients are asymptomatic.

Other causes

• **Contraceptive creams and jellies.** These products can increase vaginal secretions.

• **Drugs.** Estrogen-containing drugs, including oral contraceptives, can cause increased mucoid vaginal discharge. Antibiotics such as tetracycline may increase the risk of a monilial vaginal infection and discharge.

• **Radiation therapy.** Irradiation of the reproductive tract can cause a watery, odorless vaginal discharge.

Special considerations

Teach the patient to keep her perineum clean and dry. Also tell her to avoid wearing tight-fitting clothing and nylon underwear, and instead to wear cotton-crotched underwear and pantyhose. If appropriate, suggest that the patient douche with a solution of 5 tbs of white vinegar to 2 qt (2 L) of warm water to help relieve her discomfort.

If the patient has a vaginal infection, tell her to continue taking the prescribed medication even if her symptoms clear or she menstruates. Also advise her to avoid intercourse until her symptoms clear, and then to have her partner use condoms until she completes her course of medication.

Pediatric pointers

Female newborns who have been exposed to maternal estrogens in utero may have a white mucous vaginal discharge for the first month after birth; a yellow mucous discharge indicates a pathologic condition. In the older child, a purulent, foul-smelling, and possibly bloody vaginal discharge commonly results from a foreign object placed in the vagina.

VERTIGO

Vertigo is an illusion of movement in which the patient feels that he's revolving in space (subjective vertigo) or that his surroundings are revolving around him (objective vertigo). He may complain of feeling pulled sideways, as though drawn by a magnet.

A common symptom, vertigo usually begins abruptly and may be temporary or permanent, mild or severe. It may worsen when the patient moves and subside when he lies down. It's commonly confused with dizziness—a sensation of imbalance and light-headedness that is nonspecific. However, unlike dizziness, vertigo is commonly accompanied by nausea, vomiting, nystagmus, and tinnitus or hearing loss. Although the patient's limb coordination is unaffected, vertiginous gait may occur.

Vertigo may result from neurologic or otologic disorders that affect the equilibratory apparatus (the vestibule, semicircular canals, eighth cranial nerve, vestibular nuclei in the brain stem and their temporal lobe connections, and eyes). However, this symptom may also result from alcohol intoxication, hyperventilation, postural changes (benign postural vertigo), and the effects of certain drugs, tests, and procedures.

History and physical examination

Ask your patient to describe the onset and duration of his vertigo, being careful to distinguish this symptom from dizziness. Does he feel that he's moving or that his surroundings are moving around him? How often do the attacks occur? Do they follow position changes, or are they unpredictable? Find out if the patient can walk during an attack, if he leans to one side, and if he has ever fallen. Ask if he experiences motion sickness and if he prefers one position during an attack. Obtain a recent drug history and note any evidence of alcohol abuse.

Perform a neurologic assessment, focusing particularly on eighth cranial nerve function. Observe the patient's gait and posture for abnormalities.

Common medical causes

• *Acoustic neuroma.* This tumor of the eighth cranial nerve causes mild, intermittent vertigo and unilateral sensorineural hearing loss. Other findings include tinnitus, postauricular or suboccipital pain, and—with cranial nerve compression—facial paralysis.

• *Benign positional vertigo.* In this disorder, debris in a semicircular canal produces vertigo on head position change, which lasts a few minutes. It is usually temporary and can be effectively treated with positional maneuvers.

• *Brain stem ischemia.* This condition produces sudden, severe vertigo that may become episodic and later persistent. Associated findings include ataxia, nausea, vomiting, increased blood pressure, tachycardia, nystagmus, and lateral deviation of the eyes toward the side of the lesion. Hemiparesis and paresthesia may also occur.

• *Head trauma.* Persistent vertigo, occurring soon after injury, accompanies spontaneous or positional nystagmus and, if the temporal bone is fractured, hearing loss. Associated findings include headache, nausea, vomiting, and decreased level of consciousness (LOC). Behavioral changes, diplopia or visual blurring, seizures, motor or sensory deficits, and signs of increased intracranial pressure may also occur.

• *Herpes zoster.* Infection of the eighth cranial nerve produces sudden onset of vertigo accompanied by facial paralysis, hearing loss in the affected ear, and herpetic vesicular lesions in the auditory canal.

• *Labyrinthitis.* Severe vertigo begins abruptly with this inner ear infection. Vertigo may occur in a single episode or may recur over months or years. Associated findings may include nausea, vomiting, progressive sensorineural hearing loss, and nystagmus.

• *Ménière's disease.* In this disease, labyrinthine dysfunction causes abrupt onset of vertigo, lasting minutes, hours, or days. Unpredictable episodes of severe vertigo and unsteady gait may cause the patient to fall. During an attack, any sudden motion of the head or eyes can precipitate nausea and vomiting.

• *Multiple sclerosis (MS).* Episodic vertigo may occur early and become persistent. Other early findings include diplopia, visual blurring, and paresthesia. MS may also produce nystagmus, constipation, muscle weakness, paralysis, spasticity, hyperreflexia, intention tremor, and ataxia.

• *Seizures.* Temporal lobe seizures may produce vertigo, usually associated with other symptoms of partial complex seizures.

Other causes

• *Diagnostic tests.* Caloric testing (irrigating the ears with warm or cold water) can induce vertigo.

• *Drugs and alcohol.* High or toxic doses of certain drugs or alcohol may produce vertigo. These drugs include salicylates, aminoglycosides, antibiotics, quinine, and oral contraceptives.

• *Surgery and other procedures.* Middle ear surgery may cause vertigo that lasts for several days. In addition, administration of overly warm or cold ear drops or irrigating solutions may cause vertigo.

Special considerations

Place the patient in a comfortable position, and monitor his vital signs and LOC. Keep the side rails up if he's in bed, or help him to a chair if he's standing when vertigo occurs. Darken the room and keep him calm. Administer drugs to control nausea and vomiting, and meclizine or dimenhydrinate to decrease labyrinthine irritability.

Prepare the patient for diagnostic tests, such as electronystagmography and X-rays of the middle and inner ears.

Pediatric pointers

Ear infection is a common cause of vertigo in children. Vestibular neuritis may also cause this symptom.

VESICULAR RASH

A vesicular rash is a scattered or linear distribution of vesicles—sharply circumscribed lesions filled with clear, cloudy, or bloody fluid. The lesions, which are usually less than 0.5 cm in diameter, may occur singly or in groups. They sometimes occur with bullae—fluid-filled lesions larger than 0.5 cm in diameter.

A vesicular rash may be mild or severe and temporary or permanent. It can result from infection, inflammation, or allergic reactions.

History and physical examination

Ask your patient when the rash began, how it spread, and whether it has appeared before. Did other skin lesions precede eruption of the vesicles? Obtain a thorough drug history. If the patient has used any topical medication, what type did he use and when was it last applied? Also ask about associated signs and symptoms. Find out if he has a family history of skin disorders, and ask about allergies, recent infections, insect bites, and exposure to allergens.

Examine the patient's skin, noting if it's dry, oily, or moist. Observe the general distribution of the lesions and record their exact location. Note the color, shape, and size of the lesions, and check for crusts, scales, scars, macules, papules, or wheals. Palpate the vesicles or bullae to determine if they're flaccid or tense. Slide your finger across the skin to see if the outer layer of epidermis separates easily from the basal layer (Nikolsky's sign).

Common medical causes

• *Burns.* Thermal burns that affect the epidermis and part of the dermis commonly cause vesicles and bullae, with erythema, swelling, pain, and moistness.

• *Dermatitis.* In *contact dermatitis,* a severe hypersensitivity reaction produces an eruption of small vesicles surrounded by redness and marked edema. The vesicles may ooze, scale, and cause severe pruritus.

Dermatitis herpetiformis, which usually occurs in men between ages 20 and 50, produces chronic inflammatory eruptions marked by vesicular, papular, bullous, pustular, or erythematous lesions. Usually, the rash is symmetrically distributed on the buttocks, shoulders, extensor surfaces of the elbows and knees, and sometimes the face, scalp, and neck. Other symptoms include severe pruritus, burning, and stinging.

In *nummular eczematous dermatitis,* groups of pinpoint vesicles and papules appear on erythematous or pustular lesions that are nummular (coinlike) or annular (ringlike). The pustular lesions commonly ooze a purulent exudate, itch severely, and rapidly become crusted and scaly. Two or three lesions may develop on the hands, but the lesions usually develop on the extensor surfaces of the limbs and on the buttocks and posterior trunk.

• *Erythema multiforme.* This acute inflammatory skin disease is heralded by a sudden eruption of erythematous macules, papules and, occasionally, vesicles and bullae. The characteristic rash appears symmetrically over the hands, arms, feet, legs, face, and neck and tends to reappear. Vesicles and bullae may also erupt on the eyes and genitalia. Usually, though, vesiculobullous lesions appear on the mucous membranes—especially the lips and buccal mucosa—where they rupture and ulcerate, producing a thick, yellow or white exudate. Bloody, painful crusts, a foul-smelling oral discharge, and difficulty chewing may develop. Lymphadenopathy may also occur.

• *Herpes simplex.* This common viral infection produces groups of vesicles on an inflamed base, usually on the lips and lower face. In about 25% of cases, the genital region is affected. Vesicles are preceded by itching, tingling, burning, or pain; develop singly or in groups; are 2 to 3 mm in size; and do not coalesce. Eventually, they rupture, forming a painful ulcer followed by a yellowish crust.

• *Herpes zoster.* A vesicular rash is preceded by erythema and, occasionally, by a nodular skin eruption and unilateral, sharp, shooting chest pain that mimics a myocardial infarction. About 5 days later, the lesions erupt and commonly spread unilaterally over the thorax or vertically over the arms and legs. The pain becomes burning. Vesicles dry and scab about 10 days after eruption. Associated findings include fever, malaise, pruritus, and paresthesia or hyperesthesia of the involved area. Occasionally, herpes zoster involves the cranial nerves, producing facial palsy, hearing loss, dizziness, loss of taste, eye pain, and impaired vision.

• *Insect bites.* Vesicles appear on red hivelike papules and may become hemorrhagic.

• *Pemphigoid (bullous).* Generalized pruritus or an urticarial or eczematous eruption may precede the classic bullous rash. Bullae are large, tense, and irregular, and usually form on an erythematous base. They usually appear on the lower abdomen, groin, inner thighs, and forearms.

Pemphigus vulgaris may be acute and rapidly progressive, or chronic. The bullae may be tender or painful and large or small, and are usually flaccid. When they rupture, denuded skin exudes a clear, bloody, or purulent discharge. Commonly, the bullae first erupt in a specific location, such as the mouth or scalp and, eventually, become widespread. Nikolsky's sign and pruritus may be present.

• *Pompholyx.* This common, recurrent disorder produces symmetrical vesicular lesions that can become pustular. The pruritic lesions appear on the palms more commonly than on the soles and may be accompanied by minimal erythema.

• *Porphyria cutanea tarda.* Bullae—especially on areas exposed to sun, friction, trauma, or heat—result from abnormal porphyrin metabolism. Photosensitivity is also a common sign. Papulovesicular lesions evolving into erosions or ulcers and scars may appear. Chronic skin changes include hyperpigmentation or hypopigmentation, hypertrichosis, and sclerodermoid lesions. Urine is pink to brown.

• *Scabies.* Small vesicles erupt on an erythematous base and may be at the end of a threadlike burrow. Burrows are a few

DRUGS THAT MAY CAUSE TOXIC EPIDERMAL NECROLYSIS

Various drugs can trigger toxic epidermal necrolysis (TEN)—a rare but potentially fatal immune reaction characterized by a vesicular rash. TEN produces large, flaccid bullae that rupture easily, exposing extensive areas of denuded skin. The resulting loss of fluid and electrolytes—along with widespread systemic involvement—can lead to such life-threatening complications as pulmonary edema, shock, renal failure, sepsis, and disseminated intravascular coagulation.

Here's a list of some drugs that can cause TEN:

- allopurinol
- aspirin
- barbiturates
- chloramphenicol
- chlorpropamide
- gold salts
- nitrofurantoin
- penicillin
- phenolphthalein
- phenylbutazone
- phenytoin
- primidone
- sulfonamides
- tetracycline.

millimeters long, with a swollen nodule or red papule that contains the itch mite. Pustules and excoriations may also occur. Men may develop burrows on the glans, shaft, and scrotum; women may develop burrows on the nipples. Both sexes may develop burrows on the wrists, elbows, axilla, and waistline. Associated pruritus worsens with inactivity and warmth and at night.

- *Tinea pedis.* This fungal infection causes vesicles and scaling between the toes and, possibly, scaling over the entire sole. Severe infection causes inflammation, pruritus, and difficulty walking.

- *Toxic epidermal necrolysis.* In this immune reaction to drugs or other toxins, vesicles and bullae are preceded by a diffuse erythematous rash and followed by large-scale epidermal necrolysis and desquamation. Large, flaccid bullae develop after mucous membrane inflammation, a burning sensation in the conjunctivae, malaise, fever, and generalized skin tenderness. The bullae rupture easily, exposing extensive areas of denuded skin. (See *Drugs that may cause toxic epidermal necrolysis.*)

Special considerations

Any skin eruption that covers a large area may cause substantial fluid loss through the vesicles, bullae, or other weeping lesions. If necessary, start an I.V. to replace fluids and electrolytes. Keep the patient's environment warm and free from drafts, cover him with sheets or blankets as necessary, and take his rectal temperature every 4 hours because increased fluid loss and increased blood flow to inflamed skin may lead to hyperthermia.

Obtain cultures to determine the causative organism. Use universal precautions until infection is ruled out. Tell the patient to wash his hands often and not to touch the lesions. Be alert for any signs of secondary infection. Give the patient antibiotics and apply corticosteroid or antimicrobial ointment to the lesions.

Pediatric pointers

Vesicular rashes in children are caused by staphylococcal infections (staphylococcal scalded skin syndrome is a life-threatening infection occurring in infants), varicella, hand-foot-and-mouth disease, and miliaria rubra.

VIOLENT BEHAVIOR

Marked by sudden loss of self-control, violent behavior refers to the use of physical force to violate, injure, or abuse an object or a person. This behavior may also be self-directed. It may result from organic and psychiatric disorders and from the effects of drugs.

History and physical examination

During your evaluation, determine if the patient has a history of violent behavior. Is he intoxicated or suffering symptoms of alcohol or drug withdrawal? Does he have a history of family violence, including corporal punishment and child or spouse abuse? (See *Understanding family violence,* page 590.)

Watch for clues indicating that the patient is losing control and may become violent. Has he exhibited abrupt behavioral changes? Is he unable to sit still? Increased activity may indicate an attempt to discharge aggression. Does he suddenly cease activity (suggesting the calm before the storm)? Does he make verbal threats or angry gestures? Is he jumpy, extremely tense, or laughing? Such intensifying of emotion may herald loss of control.

If your patient's violent behavior is a new development, he may have an organic disorder. Obtain a medical history and perform a physical examination. Watch for a sudden change in his level of consciousness. Disorientation, failure to recall recent events, or display of tics, jerks, tremors, or asterixis all suggest an organic disorder.

Common medical causes

• *Organic disorders.* Many disorders may cause violent behavior due to metabolic and neurologic dysfunction. Common causes include epilepsy, brain tumor, encephalitis, head injury, endocrine disorders, metabolic disorders (such as uremia and calcium imbalance), and severe physical trauma.

• *Psychiatric disorders.* Violent behavior occurs as a protective mechanism in response to a perceived threat in psychotic disorders such as schizophrenia. A similar response may occur in personality disorders, such as antisocial or borderline personality.

Other causes

• *Drugs and alcohol.* Various drugs, such as lidocaine and procaine penicillin, may cause violent behavior as an adverse effect. Alcohol abuse or withdrawal, hallucinogens, amphetamines, and barbiturate withdrawal may also cause violent behavior.

Special considerations

Violent behavior is most prevalent in emergency rooms, critical care units, and crisis and acute psychiatric units. Natural disasters and accidents also increase the potential for violent behavior, so be on guard in these situations.

If your patient becomes violent or potentially violent, your goal is to remain composed and to establish environmental control. First, protect yourself. Remain at a distance from the patient, call for assistance, and don't overreact. Remain calm, and make sure you have enough personnel for a show of force to subdue or restrain the patient if necessary. Encourage the patient to move to a quiet location—free from noise, activity, and people—to avoid frightening or stimulating him further. Reassure him, explain what's happening, and tell him that he's safe.

If the patient makes violent threats, take them seriously, and inform those at whom the threats are directed. Administer psychotropic medications as ordered.

Remember, your own attitudes can affect your ability to care for a violent patient. If you feel fearful or judgmental, ask another staff member for help.

UNDERSTANDING FAMILY VIOLENCE

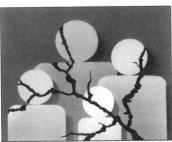

Effectively managing a violent patient requires an understanding of the roots of his behavior. For example, his behavior may be spawned by a family history of corporal punishment or child or spouse abuse. It may also be associated with drug or alcohol abuse and fixed family roles that stifle growth and individuality.

What causes family violence? Social scientists suggest that it stems from cultural attitudes fostering violence and from the frustration and stress associated with overcrowded living conditions and poverty. Albert Bandura, a social learning theorist, believes that individuals learn violent behavior by observing and imitating other family members who vent their aggressive feelings through verbal abuse and physical force. (They also learn from television and the movies, especially when the violent hero gains power and recognition.) Members of families with these characteristics may have an increased potential for violent behavior, initiating a cycle of violence that passes from generation to generation.

Elder tip

Dependent elders are most at risk for abuse and neglect, usually by a close relative. Such treatment may stem from learned violent behavior, high levels of stress, or an inability to cope properly. When you examine an elderly person, try to do so in private. Be on the lookout for signs of mistreatment, such as multiple cuts or bruises, especially on the upper arms, back, buttocks, and thighs. Rope burns or contractures can indicate prolonged restraint. Pressure sores in various stages of healing may be a sign of dehydration or malnourishment.

Ask the abused person if he feels safe or mistreated at home. Assess the scope of support he receives from family and friends. Teach the family about the aging process so they know what to expect. Encourage the use of outside resources, such as home health or respite care programs.

Keep in mind that the patient's safety is your priority. Aside from arranging for medical and psychiatric treatment where appropriate, you may need to consider alternative placement if safety is a continued risk. Become familiar with your state laws, state and county agencies, and institutional protocols for reporting abuse. Be sure to document your assessment thoroughly and accurately.

Pediatric pointers

Adolescents and younger children commonly make threats resulting from violent dreams or fantasies or unmet needs. Adolescents who exhibit extreme violence can be from families with a history of physical or psychological abuse. These children may display violent behavior toward their peers, siblings, and pets.

VISION LOSS

Vision loss—the inability to perceive visual stimuli—can occur suddenly or gradually and be temporary or permanent. The deficit can range from a slight vision impairment to total blindness. It may result from ocular, neurologic, and systemic disorders as well as from trauma and reactions to certain drugs.

History and physical examination

Sudden vision loss can signal an ocular emergency. (See *Managing sudden vision loss,* page 592.) Don't touch the eye if the patient has perforating or penetrating ocular trauma.

If the patient's vision loss occurred gradually, ask him if the vision loss affects one eye or both, and all or only part of the visual field. Ask the patient if he has experienced photosensitivity, and ask him about the location, intensity, and duration of any eye pain. In addition, you should obtain an ocular history and a family history of eye problems or systemic diseases that may lead to eye problems, such as hypertension; diabetes mellitus; thyroid, rheumatic, or vascular disease; infections; and cancer.

Carefully inspect both eyes, noting edema, foreign bodies, drainage, or conjunctival or scleral redness. Observe whether lid closure is complete or incomplete, and check for ptosis. Using a flashlight, examine the cornea and iris for scars, irregularities, and foreign bodies. Observe the size, shape, and color of the pupils, and test the direct and consensual light reflex and the effect of accommodation. Evaluate extraocular muscle function by testing the six cardinal fields of gaze. Assess the extent of vision loss by testing visual acuity in each eye.

Common medical causes

- *Amaurosis fugax.* In this disorder, recurrent attacks of unilateral vision loss may last from a few seconds to a few minutes. Vision is normal at other times. Transient unilateral weakness, hypertension, and elevated intraocular pressure in the affected eye may also occur.
- *Cataract.* Typically, painless and gradual visual blurring precedes vision loss. As the cataract progresses, the pupil turns milky white.
- *Concussion.* Immediately or shortly after blunt head trauma, vision may be blurred, double, or lost. Vision loss is usually temporary. Other findings may include headache, anterograde and retrograde amnesia, transient loss of consciousness, nausea, vomiting, dizziness, irritability, confusion, lethargy, and aphasia.
- *Diabetic retinopathy.* Retinal edema and hemorrhage lead to visual blurring, which may progress to blindness.
- *Endophthalmitis.* Typically, this intraocular infection follows penetrating trauma, I.V. drug use, or intraocular surgery, causing possibly permanent unilateral vision loss; a sympathetic inflammation may affect the other eye.
- *Glaucoma.* This disorder produces gradual visual blurring that may progress to total blindness. *Acute angle-closure glaucoma* is an ocular emergency that may produce blindness within 3 to 5 days. Signs and symptoms include rapid onset of unilateral inflammation and pain, pressure over the eye, moderate pupil dilation, nonreactive pupillary response, a cloudy cornea, reduced visual acuity, photophobia, and perception of blue or red halos around lights. Nausea and vomiting may also occur.

Chronic angle-closure glaucoma has a gradual onset and usually produces no symptoms, although blurred or halo vision may occur. If untreated, it progresses to blindness and extreme pain.

Chronic open-angle glaucoma is usually bilateral, with an insidious onset and

MANAGING SUDDEN VISION LOSS

Sudden vision loss can signal central retinal artery occlusion or acute angle-closure glaucoma—ocular emergencies that require immediate intervention. If your patient reports sudden vision loss, summon an ophthalmologist immediately for an emergency examination, and perform these interventions.

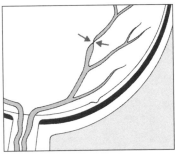

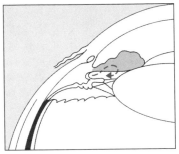

For a patient with suspected central retinal artery occlusion, perform light massage over his closed eyelid. Increase his carbon dioxide level by administering a set flow of oxygen and carbon dioxide through a Venturi mask. Or have the patient rebreathe in a paper bag to retain exhaled carbon dioxide. These steps will dilate the artery and, possibly, restore blood flow to the retina.

For a patient with suspected acute angle-closure glaucoma, measure intraocular pressure with a tonometer. (You can also estimate intraocular pressure without a tonometer by placing your fingers over the patient's closed eyelid. A rock-hard eyeball usually indicates increased intraocular pressure.) Expect to administer timolol drops and I.V. acetazolamide to help decrease intraocular pressure.

a slowly progressive course. It causes peripheral vision loss, aching eyes, halo vision, and reduced visual acuity (especially at night).

• *Ocular trauma.* Following eye injury, sudden unilateral or bilateral vision loss may occur. Vision loss may be total or partial, and permanent or temporary. The eyelids may be reddened, edematous, and lacerated; and intraocular contents may be extruded.

• *Optic atrophy.* Degeneration of the optic nerve, optic atrophy can develop spontaneously or follow inflammation or edema of the nerve head, causing irreversible loss of the visual field with changes in

color visions. Pupillary reactions are sluggish, and optic disk pallor is evident.

• *Optic neuritis.* An umbrella term for inflammation, degeneration, or demyelinization of the optic nerve, optic neuritis usually produces temporary but severe unilateral vision loss. Pain around the eye occurs, especially with movement of the globe. This may occur with visual field defects and a sluggish pupillary response to light. Ophthalmoscopic examination commonly reveals hyperemia of the optic disk, blurred disk margins, and filling of the physiologic cup.

• *Pituitary tumor.* As a pituitary adenoma grows, blurred vision progresses to hemianopia and, possibly, unilateral blindness. Double vision, nystagmus, ptosis, limited eye movement, and headaches may also occur.

• *Retinal artery occlusion (central).* This painless ocular emergency causes sudden, unilateral vision loss, which may be partial or complete. Pupil examination reveals a sluggish direct pupillary response and a normal consensual response. Permanent blindness may occur within hours.

• *Retinal detachment.* Depending on the degree and location of detachment, painless vision loss may be gradual or sudden and total or partial. Macular involvement will cause total blindness. With partial vision loss, the patient may describe visual field defects or a shadow or curtain over the visual field, as well as visual floaters.

• *Retinal vein occlusion (central).* Most common in geriatric patients, this painless disorder causes a unilateral decrease in visual acuity with variable vision loss. Intraocular pressure may be elevated in both eyes.

• *Senile macular degeneration.* Occurring in elderly patients, this disorder causes painless blurring or loss of central vision. Vision loss may proceed slowly or rapidly, eventually affecting both eyes. Visual acuity may be worse at night.

• *Stevens-Johnson syndrome.* Corneal scarring from associated conjunctival lesions produces marked vision loss. Purulent conjunctivitis, eye pain, and difficulty opening the eyes occur. Additional findings may include widespread bullae, fever, malaise, cough, drooling, inability to eat, sore throat, chest pain, vomiting, diarrhea, myalgias, arthralgias, hematuria, and possibly signs of renal failure.

• *Temporal arteritis.* Vision loss and visual blurring with a throbbing, unilateral headache characterize this disorder. Other findings include malaise, anorexia, weight loss, weakness, low-grade fever, generalized muscle aches, and confusion.

• *Vitreous hemorrhage.* In this condition, sudden unilateral vision loss may result from intraocular trauma, ocular tumors, or systemic disease (especially diabetes, hypertension, sickle cell anemia, or leukemia). Visual floaters and partial vision with a reddish haze may occur. The patient's vision loss may be permanent.

Other causes

• *Drugs.* Chloroquine therapy may cause gradual vision loss that continues even after the drug is discontinued; prolonged use causes irreversible vision loss. Phenylbutazone may cause vision loss and increased susceptibility to retinal detachment. Digitalis glycoside derivatives, indomethacin, ethambutol, quinine sulfate, and methanol toxicity may also cause vision loss.

Special considerations

Any degree of vision loss is extremely frightening to your patient. To ease his fears, orient him to his environment, and announce your presence each time you approach him. If the patient reports photophobia, darken the room and suggest that he wear sunglasses during the day.

Obtain cultures of any drainage, and instruct him not to touch the unaffected eye with anything that has come in contact with the affected eye. Tell him to wash his hands often and to avoid rubbing his eyes. If necessary, prepare him for surgery.

Pediatric pointers

Children who complain of slowly progressive vision loss may have an optic nerve glioma (a slow-growing, usually benign tumor) or retinoblastoma (a malignant tumor of the retina). Congenital rubella and syphilis may cause vision loss in infants. Retrolental fibroplasia may cause vision loss in premature infants. Other congenital causes of vision loss include Marfan syndrome, retinitis pigmentosa, and amblyopia.

VISUAL BLURRING

This common symptom refers to the loss of visual acuity with indistinct visual details. It may result from eye injury, neurologic and eye disorders, or disorders with vascular complications such as diabetes mellitus. Visual blurring may also result from mucus passing over the cornea, refractive errors, improperly fitted contact lenses, or the effects of drugs.

History and physical examination
If your patient has visual blurring accompanied by sudden, severe eye pain, a history of trauma, or sudden vision loss, order an ophthalmologic examination. If the patient has a penetrating or perforating eye injury, don't touch the eye.

If the patient isn't in distress, ask him how long he has had the visual blurring. Does it occur only at certain times? Ask about associated symptoms, such as pain or discharge. If visual blurring followed injury, obtain details of the accident, and ask if vision was impaired immediately after the injury. Obtain a medical and drug history.

Inspect the patient's eye, noting lid edema, drainage, or conjunctival or scleral redness. Also note an irregularly shaped iris, which may indicate previous trauma, and excessive blinking, which may indicate corneal damage. Assess for pupillary changes, and test visual acuity in both eyes. (See *Testing visual acuity.*)

Common medical causes
• *Brain tumor.* Visual blurring may occur with a brain tumor. Associated findings may include decreased level of consciousness (LOC), headache, apathy, behavioral changes, memory loss, decreased attention span, dizziness, and confusion. A tumor can also cause aphasia, seizures, ataxia, and signs of hormonal imbalance. Its later effects are papilledema, vomiting, increased systolic blood pressure, widened pulse pressure, and decorticate posture.
• *Cataract.* This painless disorder causes gradual visual blurring. Other effects include halo vision (an early symptom), visual glare in bright light, progressive vision loss, and a gray pupil that later turns milky white.
• *Cerebrovascular accident (CVA).* Brief attacks of bilateral visual blurring may precede or accompany a CVA. Associated findings may include decreased LOC, contralateral hemiplegia, dysarthria, dysphagia, ataxia, unilateral sensory loss, and apraxia. CVA may also cause agnosia, aphasia, homonymous hemianopia, diplopia, disorientation, memory loss, and poor judgment. Other features include urine retention or incontinence, constipation, personality changes, emotional lability, headache, vomiting, and seizures.
• *Concussion.* Immediately or shortly after blunt head trauma, vision may be blurred, double, or temporarily lost. Other findings include changes in LOC and behavior.
• *Corneal abrasions.* Visual blurring may occur with severe eye pain, photophobia, redness, and excessive tearing.
• *Corneal foreign bodies.* Visual blurring may accompany a foreign body sensation, excessive tearing, photophobia, intense eye pain, miosis, conjunctival injection, and a dark corneal speck.
• *Dislocated lens.* Dislocation of the lens, especially beyond the line of vision, causes visual blurring and (with trauma) redness.
• *Eye tumor.* If the tumor involves the macula, visual blurring may be the presenting symptom. Related findings include varying visual field losses.
• *Glaucoma.* In *acute angle-closure glaucoma,* an ocular emergency, unilateral visual blurring and severe pain begin suddenly. Other findings include halo vision; a moderately dilated, nonreactive pupil; conjunctival injection; a cloudy

EXAMINATION TIP

TESTING VISUAL ACUITY

To test visual acuity in a literate patient over age 6, use a Snellen letter chart. Have the patient sit or stand 20′ (6 m) from the chart. Then tell him to cover his left eye and read aloud the smallest line of letters that he can see. Record the fraction assigned to that line (the numerator indicates distance from the chart; the denominator indicates the distance at which a normal eye can read the chart). Normal vision is 20/20. Repeat the test with the patient's right eye covered.

If your patient can't read the largest letter from a distance of 20′,

have him approach the chart until he can read it. Then, record the distance between him and the chart as the numerator of the fraction. For example, if he can see the top line of the chart at a distance of 3′ (1 m), record the test result as 3/200.

To test children ages 3 to 6 and illiterate patients, use a Snellen symbol chart. Follow the same procedure as for the Snellen letter chart, but ask the patient to indicate the direction of the E's fingers as you point to each symbol.

Snellen letter chart

20/200	**E**	200 FT / 61 M **1**
20/200	**F P**	100 FT / 30.5 M **2**
20/70	**T O Z**	70 FT / 21.3 M **3**
20/50	**L P E D**	50 FT / 15.2 M **4**
20/40	**P E C F D**	40 FT / 12.2 M **5**
20/30	**E D F C Z P**	30 FT / 9.14 M **6**
20/25	**F E L O P Z D**	25 FT / 7.62 M **7**
20/20	**D E F P O T E C**	20 FT / 6.10 M **8**
20/15	L E F O D P C T	15 FT / 4.57 M **9**
20/13	F D P L T C E O	13 FT / 3.96 M **10**
20/10	P E Z O L C F T D	10 FT / 3.05 M **11**

Snellen symbol chart

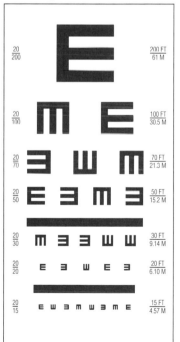

cornea; and decreased visual acuity. Severely elevated intraocular pressure may cause nausea and vomiting.

In *chronic angle-closure glaucoma,* transient visual blurring and halo vision may precede pain and blindness.

● *Hypertension.* This disorder may cause visual blurring and a constant morning headache that decreases in severity during the day. If diastolic blood pressure exceeds 120 mm Hg, the patient may report a severe, throbbing headache. Associated findings may include restlessness, confusion, nausea, vomiting, seizures, and decreased LOC.

● *Hyphema.* Blunt eye trauma with hemorrhage into the anterior chamber causes visual blurring. Other effects include moderate pain, diffuse conjunctival injection, visible blood in the anterior chamber, ecchymoses, eyelid edema, and a hard eye.

● *Iritis.* Acute iritis causes sudden visual blurring, moderate to severe eye pain, photophobia, conjunctival injection, and a constricted pupil.

● *Optic neuritis.* Inflammation, degeneration, or demyelinization of the optic nerve usually causes an acute attack of visual blurring and vision loss. Related findings include scotomas and eye pain. Ophthalmoscopic examination reveals hyperemia of the optic disk, large vein distention, blurred disk margins, and filling of the physiologic cup.

● *Retinal detachment.* Sudden visual blurring may be the initial symptom of this disorder. Blurring worsens, accompanied by visual floaters and recurring flashes of light. Progressive detachment increases vision loss.

● *Retinal vein occlusion (central).* This disorder causes gradual unilateral visual blurring and varying degrees of vision loss.

● *Senile macular degeneration.* This retinal disorder may cause visual blurring (initially worse at night) and slowly or rapidly progressive vision loss.

● *Temporal arteritis.* Most common in women over age 60, this disorder causes sudden blurred vision accompanied by vision loss and a throbbing unilateral headache in the temporal or frontotemporal region. Prodromal symptoms include malaise, anorexia, weight loss, weakness, low-grade fever, and generalized muscle aches. Other findings include confusion; disorientation; swollen, nodular, tender temporal arteries; and erythema of overlying skin.

● *Vitreous hemorrhage.* Sudden unilateral visual blurring and varying vision loss occur with this condition. Visual floaters or dark streaks may also occur.

Other causes

● *Drugs.* Visual blurring may stem from the effects of cycloplegics, guanethidine, reserpine, clomiphene, phenylbutazone, thiazide diuretics, antihistamines, anticholinergics, and phenothiazines.

Special considerations

Prepare the patient for diagnostic tests, such as tonometry, slit-lamp examination, X-rays of the skull and orbit and, if a neurologic lesion is suspected, a computed tomography scan. As necessary, teach him how to instill ophthalmic medication. If visual blurring leads to permanent vision loss, provide emotional support, orient him to his surroundings, and provide for his safety. If necessary, prepare him for surgery.

Pediatric pointers

Visual blurring in children may stem from congenital syphilis, congenital cataracts, refractive errors, eye injuries or infections, and increased intracranial pressure. Refer the child to an ophthalmologist if appropriate.

Test vision in school-age children as you would in adults; test children ages 3 to 6 with the Snellen symbol chart. Test toddlers with Allen cards, each illustrated with a familiar object such as an animal. Ask the child to cover one eye and identify the objects as you flash them. Then ask him to identify them as you gradually back away. Record the maximum distance at which he can identify at least three pictures.

VISUAL FLOATERS

Visual floaters are particles of blood or cellular debris that move about in the vitreous. As these enter the visual field, they appear as spots or dots. Chronic floaters may occur normally in elderly or myopic patients. However, the sudden onset of visual floaters commonly signals retinal detachment, an ocular emergency.

Emergency interventions

 Sudden onset of visual floaters may signal retinal detachment. Does the patient also see flashing lights or spots in the affected eye? Is he experiencing a curtainlike loss of vision? If so, notify an ophthalmologist immediately. Restrict the patient's eye movements until the diagnosis is made.

History and physical examination

If the patient's condition permits, obtain a drug and allergy history. Ask about any nearsightedness (a predisposing factor), use of corrective lenses, eye trauma, or other eye disorders. Also ask about a history of granulomatous disease, diabetes mellitus, or hypertension, which may have predisposed him to retinal detachment, vitreous hemorrhage, or uveitis. If appropriate, inspect his eyes for signs of injury, such as bruising or edema, and determine his visual acuity.

Common medical causes

• *Retinal detachment.* Floaters and light flashes appear suddenly in the portion of the visual field where the retina is detached. As the retina detaches further (a painless process), gradual vision loss oc-

curs, likened to a cloud or curtain falling in front of the eyes. Ophthalmoscopic examination reveals a gray, opaque, detached retina with an indefinite margin. Retinal vessels appear almost black.

• *Uveitis (posterior).* This disorder may cause visual floaters accompanied by gradual eye pain, photophobia, blurred vision, and conjunctival injection.

• *Vitreous hemorrhage.* Rupture of retinal vessels produces a shower of red or black dots or a red haze across the visual field. Vision is suddenly blurred in the affected eye, and visual acuity may be greatly reduced.

Special considerations

Encourage bed rest and provide a calm environment. Depending on the cause, the patient may require eye patches, surgery, and corticosteroids or other drug therapy. If bilateral eye patches are necessary—as with retinal detachment—you will need to ensure the patient's safety. You should identify yourself when you approach the patient and orient him to time frequently. Provide sensory stimulation, such as a radio or tape player. Place pillows or towels behind the patient's head to maintain the appropriate patient position. Be sure to warn him not to touch or rub his eyes and to avoid straining or sudden movements.

Pediatric pointers

Visual floaters in children usually follow trauma that causes retinal detachment or vitreous hemorrhage. However, they may also result from vitreous debris, a benign congenital condition with no other signs or symptoms.

VOMITING

Vomiting is the forceful expulsion of gastric contents through the mouth. Characteristically preceded by nausea, vomiting results from a coordinated sequence of abdominal muscle contractions and reverse esophageal peristalsis.

A common sign of GI disorders, vomiting also occurs with fluid and electrolyte imbalances, infections, and metabolic, endocrine, labyrinthine, central nervous system (CNS), and cardiac disorders. It can also result from drug therapy, surgery, and radiation.

Vomiting occurs normally during the first trimester of pregnancy, but its subsequent development may signal complications. It can also result from stress, anxiety, pain, alcohol intoxication, overeating, or ingestion of distasteful foods or liquids.

History and physical examination

Ask your patient to describe the onset, duration, and intensity of his vomiting. What started the vomiting? What makes it subside? If possible, collect, measure, and inspect the character of the vomitus. (See *Identifying causes of vomiting.*) Explore any associated complaints, particularly nausea, abdominal pain, anorexia and weight loss, changes in bowel habits or stools, excessive belching or flatus, and bloating or fullness.

Obtain a medical history, noting GI, endocrine, and metabolic disorders; recent infections; and cancer, including chemotherapy or radiation therapy. Ask about current medication use and alcohol consumption. If the patient is a female of childbearing age, ask if she is or could be pregnant.

Inspect the abdomen for distention, and auscultate for bowel sounds and bruits. Palpate for rigidity and tenderness, and test for rebound tenderness. Next, palpate and percuss the liver for enlargement. Assess other body systems as appropriate.

During the examination, keep in mind that projectile vomiting *unaccompanied* by nausea may indicate increased intracranial pressure (ICP), a life-threatening emergency. If this occurs in a patient with CNS injury, you should quickly check his vital signs. Be alert for widened pulse pressure or bradycardia.

Common medical causes

- *Adrenal insufficiency.* Common GI findings in the disorder include vomiting, nausea, anorexia, and diarrhea. Other findings include weakness, fatigue, weight loss, bronze skin, hypotension, and weak, irregular pulse.
- *Appendicitis.* Vomiting and nausea may follow or accompany abdominal pain. Pain typically begins as vague epigastric or periumbilical discomfort and rapidly progresses to severe, stabbing pain in the right lower quadrant. Associated findings usually include abdominal rigidity and tenderness, anorexia, constipation or diarrhea, fever, tachycardia, and malaise.
- *Cholecystitis (acute).* In this disorder, nausea and mild vomiting commonly follow severe upper quadrant pain that may radiate to the back or shoulders. Associated findings include abdominal tenderness and, possibly, rigidity and distention, fever, and diaphoresis.
- *Cholelithiasis.* Nausea and vomiting accompany severe right upper quadrant or epigastric pain following ingestion of fatty foods. Other findings include abdominal tenderness and guarding, flatulence, belching, epigastric burning, pyrosis, tachycardia, and restlessness.
- *Cirrhosis.* Insidious early symptoms of cirrhosis typically include nausea and vomiting, anorexia, aching abdominal pain, and constipation or diarrhea. Later findings include jaundice, hepatomegaly, and abdominal distention.
- *Electrolyte imbalances.* Nausea and vomiting commonly occur in electrolyte disturbances, such as hyponatremia, hypernatremia, hypokalemia, and hypercalcemia. Other effects may include arrhythmias, tremors, seizures, anorexia, malaise, and weakness.
- *Food poisoning.* Certain toxins, such as *Salmonella,* cause vomiting, nausea, and diarrhea.

• *Gastric cancer.* This rare cancer may produce mild nausea, vomiting (possibly of mucus or blood), anorexia, upper abdominal discomfort, and chronic dyspepsia. Fatigue, weight loss, melena, and altered bowel habits are also common.

• *Gastritis.* Nausea and vomiting of mucus or blood are common here, especially after ingestion of alcohol, aspirin, spicy foods, or caffeine. Epigastric pain, belching, and fever may occur.

• *Gastroenteritis.* This disorder causes nausea, vomiting (generally of undigested food), diarrhea, and abdominal cramping. Fever, malaise, hyperactive bowel sounds, and abdominal pain and tenderness may also occur.

• *Heart failure.* Nausea and vomiting may occur, especially in right-sided heart failure. Associated findings include tachycardia, ventricular gallop, fatigue, dyspnea, crackles, peripheral edema, and jugular vein distention.

• *Hepatitis.* Vomiting commonly follows nausea as an early sign of viral hepatitis. Fatigue, myalgia, arthralgia, headache, photophobia, anorexia, pharyngitis, cough, and fever also occur early.

• *Hyperemesis gravidarum.* Unremitting nausea and vomiting that last beyond the first trimester characterize this disorder of pregnancy. Vomitus contains undigested food, mucus, and small amounts of bile early in the disorder; later, it has a coffee-ground appearance. Associated findings include weight loss, headache, and delirium.

• *Increased ICP.* Projectile vomiting that *isn't* preceded by nausea is a sign of increased ICP. The patient may exhibit a decreased level of consciousness and Cushing's triad (bradycardia, hypertension, and respiratory pattern changes). He may also have headache, widened pulse pressure, impaired motor movement, visual disturbances, and pupillary changes.

• *Intestinal obstruction.* Nausea and vomiting (bilious or fecal) generally occur with obstruction, especially of the

---

IDENTIFYING CAUSES OF VOMITING

When you collect a sample of the patient's vomitus, observe it carefully for clues to the underlying disorder. Here's what different types of vomitus may indicate:

• bile-stained (greenish) vomitus: obstruction below the pylorus, as from a duodenal lesion

• bloody vomitus: if bright red, upper GI bleeding, as from gastritis or peptic ulcer; if dark red, bleeding from esophageal or gastric varices

• brown vomitus with a fecal odor: intestinal obstruction or infarction

• burning, bitter-tasting vomitus: excessive hydrochloric acid in gastric contents

• coffee-ground vomitus: digested blood from slowly bleeding gastric or duodenal lesion

• undigested food: gastric outlet obstruction, as from gastric tumor or ulcer.

---

upper small intestine. Abdominal pain is usually episodic and colicky but can become severe and steady. Constipation occurs early in large intestinal obstruction and late in small intestinal obstruction. Obstipation, however, may signal complete obstruction. Bowel sounds are typically high-pitched and hyperactive in partial obstruction; hypoactive or absent in complete obstruction. Abdominal distention and tenderness also occur, possibly with visible peristaltic waves and a palpable abdominal mass.

• *Labyrinthitis.* Nausea and vomiting commonly occur with this acute inner ear inflammation. Other findings include severe vertigo, progressive hearing loss, nystagmus, and possibly otorrhea.

• *Migraine headache.* Nausea and vomiting are prodromal symptoms, with fatigue, photophobia, light flashes, increased noise sensitivity, and possibly partial vision loss and paresthesia.

• *Motion sickness.* Nausea and vomiting may be accompanied by headache, dizziness, fatigue, diaphoresis, and dyspnea.

• *Pancreatitis (acute).* Vomiting, usually preceded by nausea, is an early sign of pancreatitis. Associated findings include steady, severe epigastric or left upper quadrant pain that may radiate to the back, abdominal tenderness and rigidity, hypoactive bowel sounds, and fever. Tachycardia, restlessness, hypotension, skin mottling, and cold, sweaty extremities may occur in severe cases.

• *Peritonitis.* Nausea and vomiting usually accompany acute abdominal pain in the area of inflammation. Other findings may include high fever with chills; tachycardia; hypoactive or absent bowel sounds; abdominal distention and tenderness; weakness; pale, cold skin; diaphoresis; hypotension; signs of dehydration; and shallow respirations.

• *Preeclampsia.* Nausea and vomiting are common in this disorder of pregnancy. Rapid weight gain, epigastric pain, generalized edema, elevated blood pressure, oliguria, severe frontal headache, and blurred or double vision also occur.

• *Renal and urologic disorders.* Cystitis, pyelonephritis, calculi, and other disorders of this system can cause vomiting. Accompanying findings reflect the specific disorder.

Other causes

• *Drugs.* Drugs that commonly cause vomiting include antineoplastic agents, opiates, ferrous sulfate, levodopa, oral potassium, chloride replacements, estrogens, sulfasalazine, antibiotics, quinidine, anesthetic agents, and overdoses of digitalis glycosides and theophylline.

• *Radiation and surgery.* Radiation therapy may cause nausea and vomiting if it disrupts the gastric mucosa. Postoperative nausea and vomiting are common, especially after abdominal surgery.

Special considerations

Draw blood to determine fluid, electrolyte, and acid-base balance. (Prolonged vomiting can cause dehydration, electrolyte imbalances, and metabolic alkalosis.) Have the patient breathe deeply to ease his nausea and help prevent further vomiting. Keep his room fresh and clean smelling by removing bedpans and emesis basins promptly after use. Elevate his head or position him on his side to prevent aspiration of vomitus. Continuously monitor vital signs and intake and output (including vomitus and liquid stools). If necessary, administer I.V. fluids or have the patient sip clear liquids to maintain hydration.

Because pain can precipitate or intensify nausea and vomiting, administer pain medications promptly. If possible, give these by injection or suppository to prevent exacerbating associated nausea. If you administer antiemetics, be alert for abdominal distention and hypoactive bowel sounds, which may indicate gastric retention. If this occurs, insert a nasogastric tube.

Pediatric pointers

In a newborn, pyloric obstruction may cause projectile vomiting, whereas Hirschsprung's disease may cause fecal vomiting. Intussusception may lead to vomiting of bile and fecal matter in an infant or toddler. Because an infant may aspirate vomitus as a result of his immature cough and gag reflexes, position him on his side or abdomen and clear any vomitus immediately.

VULVAR LESIONS

Vulvar lesions are cutaneous lumps, nodules, papules, vesicles, and ulcers that result from benign or malignant tumors, dystrophies, dermatoses, or infection. They can appear anywhere on the vulva and may go undetected until a gynecologic examination. Usually, however, the patient notices lesions because of associated symptoms, such as pruritus, dysuria, or dyspareunia. (See *Recognizing common vulvar lesions,* page 602.)

History and physical examination

Ask the patient when she first noticed a vulvar lesion, and find out about associated features, such as swelling, pain, tenderness, itching, or discharge. Does she have lesions elsewhere on her body? Ask about signs and symptoms of systemic illness, such as malaise, fever, or rash on other body areas. Is the patient sexually active? Could she have been exposed to a sexually transmitted disease?

In addition, examine the lesion, do a pelvic examination, and obtain cultures.

Common medical causes

• *Basal cell carcinoma.* Occurring mostly in postmenopausal women, this nodular tumor has a central ulcer and a raised, rolled border. Typically asymptomatic, the tumor may occasionally cause pruritus, bleeding, discharge, and a burning sensation.

• *Benign cysts. Epidermal inclusion cysts,* the most common vulvar cysts, appear primarily on the labia majora and are usually round and asymptomatic. *Bartholin's duct cysts* are usually tense, nontender, and palpable. They appear on the posterior labia minora and may cause minor discomfort during intercourse or, when large, difficulty with intercourse or even walking. *Bartholin's abscess,* infection of a Bartholin's duct cyst, causes gradual pain and tenderness and possibly vulvar swelling, redness, and deformity.

• *Benign vulvar tumors.* Cystic or solid benign vulvar tumors are usually asymptomatic.

• *Chancroid.* This rare, sexually transmitted disease causes painful vulvar lesions. Headache, malaise, and a fever up to 102.2° F (38.9° C) may occur, with enlarged, tender inguinal lymph nodes.

• *Genital warts.* This sexually transmitted disease produces painless warts on the vulva, vagina, and cervix. Warts start as tiny red or pink swellings that grow and become pedunculated. Multiple swellings with a cauliflower appearance are common. Other findings include pruritus, erythema, and a profuse, mucopurulent vaginal discharge.

• *Gonorrhea.* Vulvar lesions, which usually are confined to Bartholin's glands, may develop along with pruritus, a burning sensation, pain, and a greenish yellow vaginal discharge, but most patients are asymptomatic. Other findings, if any, may include dysuria and urinary incontinence; vaginal redness, swelling, and engorgement; and severe pelvic and lower abdominal pain.

• *Granuloma inguinale.* Initially, a single painless macule or papule appears on the vulva, ulcerating into a raised, beefy red lesion with a granulated, friable border. Other painless and possibly foul-smelling lesions may occur on the labia, vagina, or cervix. These become infected and painful, and regional lymph nodes enlarge and may become tender. Systemic effects include fever, weight loss, and malaise.

• *Herpes simplex (genital).* In this disorder, fluid-filled vesicles appear on the cervix and, possibly, on the vulva, labia, perianal skin, vagina, or mouth. The vesicles, initially painless, may rupture and develop into extensive, shallow, painful ulcers, with redness, marked edema, and tender inguinal lymph nodes. Other findings may include fever, malaise, and dysuria.

• *Hyperplastic dystrophy.* Vulvar lesions may be well delineated or poorly defined; localized or extensive; and red, brown, white, or both red and white. However, intense pruritus, possibly with vulvar pain and dyspareunia, is the cardinal symptom. In *lichen sclerosus,* a type of vulvar dystrophy, vulvar skin has a parch-

RECOGNIZING COMMON VULVAR LESIONS

Various disorders can cause vulvar lesions. Sexually transmitted diseases account for most vulvar lesions in premenopausal women, whereas vulvar tumors and cysts account for most lesions in women ages 50 to 70. The illustrations below will help you recognize some of the most common lesions.

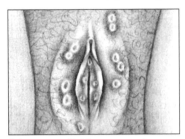

Primary genital herpes produces multiple ulcerated lesions surrounded by red halos.

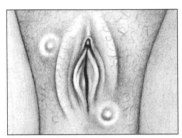

Primary syphilis produces chancres, which appear as ulcerated lesions with raised borders.

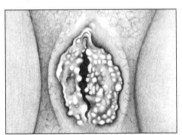

Squamous cell carcinoma produces a large, granulomatous-appearing ulcer.

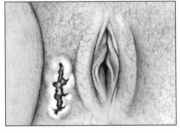

Basal cell carcinoma produces an ulcerated lesion with raised, rolled edges.

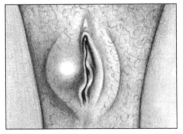

Epidermal inclusion cysts produce a round lump that usually appears on the labia majora.

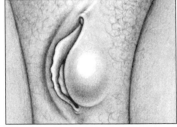

Bartholin's duct cysts produce a tense, nontender, palpable lump that usually appears on the labia minora.

mentlike appearance. Fissures may develop between the clitoris and urethra or other vulvar areas.

• *Lymphogranuloma venereum.* This bacterial infection commonly presents with a single, painless papule or ulcer on the posterior vulva that heals in a few days. Inguinal lymphadenopathy develops about 2 weeks later. Other findings may include fever, chills, headache, anorexia, myalgias, arthralgias, weight loss, and perineal edema.

• *Squamous cell carcinoma. Invasive carcinoma* occurs primarily in postmenopausal women and may produce vulvar pruritus and a vulvar lump. As the tumor enlarges, it may encroach on the vagina, anus, and urethra. *Carcinoma in situ* usually occurs in premenopausal women, producing a vulvar lesion that may be white or red, raised, well defined, moist, crusted, and isolated.

• *Syphilis.* Chancres, the primary vulvar lesions of this sexually transmitted disease, may appear on the vulva, vagina, or cervix 10 to 90 days after initial contact. Usually painless, they start as papules that then erode, with indurated, raised edges and clear bases. Condylo-

mata lata, highly contagious secondary vulvar lesions, are raised, gray, flat topped, and commonly ulcerated. Other findings include headache, malaise, anorexia, weight loss, fever, nausea, vomiting, generalized lymphadenopathy, a sore throat, and a maculopapular, pustular, or nodular rash.

Special considerations

Expect to administer systemic antibiotics, antiviral agents, topical corticosteroids, topical testosterone, or an antipruritic agent. Show the patient how to give herself a sitz bath to promote healing and comfort. If she has a sexually transmitted disease, encourage her to inform her sexual partners and persuade them to be treated. Advise her to avoid sexual contact until the lesions are no longer contagious.

Pediatric pointers

Vulvar lesions in children may result from sexual abuse or congenital syphilis or gonorrhea.

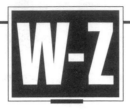

WEIGHT GAIN, EXCESSIVE

Weight gain occurs when ingested calories exceed body requirements for energy, causing increased adipose tissue storage. It can also occur when fluid retention causes edema. When weight gain results from overeating, emotional factors—most commonly anxiety, guilt, and depression—and social factors may be the primary causes.

Among the elderly, weight gain commonly reflects a sustained food intake in the presence of the normal, progressive fall in basal metabolic rate. Among women, a progressive weight gain occurs with pregnancy, whereas a periodic weight gain usually occurs with menstruation.

Weight gain, a primary symptom of many endocrine disorders, also occurs with conditions that limit activity, especially cardiovascular and pulmonary disorders. It can also result from drug therapy that increases appetite or causes fluid retention and from cardiovascular, hepatic, and renal disorders that cause edema.

History and physical examination

Determine your patient's previous patterns of weight gain and loss. Does he have a family history of obesity, thyroid disease, or diabetes mellitus? Assess his eating and activity patterns. Has his appetite increased? Does he exercise regularly or at all? Next, ask about associated symptoms. Has he experienced visual disturbances, hoarseness, paresthesia, or increased urination and thirst? Has he become impotent? If the patient is female, has she had menstrual irregularities or experienced weight gain during menstruation?

Form an impression of the patient's mental status. Is he anxious or depressed? Does he respond slowly? Is his memory poor? What medications is he currently using?

During your physical examination, measure skinfold thickness to estimate fat reserves. (See *Evaluating nutritional status*, pages 606 and 607.) Note fat distribution and the presence of localized or generalized edema. Inspect for other abnormalities, such as abnormal body hair distribution or hair loss and dry skin. Take and record the patient's vital signs.

Common medical causes

• *Acromegaly.* This disorder causes moderate weight gain. Other findings include coarsened facial features, prognathism, enlarged hands and feet, increased sweating, oily skin, deep voice, back and joint pain, lethargy, sleepiness, and heat intolerance. Occasionally, hirsutism may occur.

• *Diabetes mellitus.* The increased appetite associated with this disorder may lead to weight gain, although weight loss sometimes occurs instead. Other findings may include fatigue, polydipsia, polyuria, nocturia, weakness, polyphagia, and somnolence.

• *Heart failure.* Despite anorexia, weight gain may result from edema. Other typical findings include paroxysmal nocturnal dyspnea, orthopnea, and fatigue.

● **Hypercortisolism.** Excessive weight gain, usually over the trunk and the back of the neck (buffalo hump), characteristically occurs in this disorder. Other cushingoid features include slender extremities, moon face, weakness, purple striae, emotional lability, and increased susceptibility to infection. Gynecomastia may occur in men; hirsutism, acne, and menstrual irregularities, in women.

● **Hyperinsulinism.** This disorder increases appetite, leading to weight gain. Emotional lability, indigestion, weakness, diaphoresis, tachycardia, visual disturbances, and syncope also occur.

● **Hypogonadism.** Weight gain is common in this disorder. *Prepubertal hypogonadism* causes eunuchoid body proportions with relatively sparse facial and body hair and a high-pitched voice. *Postpubertal hypogonadism* causes loss of libido, impotence, and infertility.

● **Hypothalamic dysfunction.** Such conditions as Laurence-Moon-Biedl and Morgagni-Stewart-Morel syndromes cause a voracious appetite with subsequent weight gain, along with altered body temperature and sleep rhythms.

● **Hypothyroidism.** In this disorder, weight gain occurs despite anorexia. Related signs and symptoms include fatigue; cold intolerance; constipation; menorrhagia; slowed intellectual and motor activity; dry, pale, cool skin; dry, sparse hair; and thick, brittle nails. Myalgia, hoarseness, hypoactive deep tendon reflexes, bradycardia, and abdominal distention may occur. Eventually, the face assumes a dull expression with periorbital edema.

● **Nephrotic syndrome.** In this syndrome, weight gain results from edema. In severe cases, anasarca develops—increasing body weight up to 50%. Related effects include abdominal distention, orthostatic hypotension, and lethargy.

● **Pancreatic islet cell tumor.** This disorder causes excessive hunger, which leads to weight gain. Other findings include emotional lability, weakness, malaise, fatigue, restlessness, diaphoresis, palpitations, tachycardia, visual disturbances, and syncope.

● **Preeclampsia.** In this disorder, rapid weight gain (exceeding the normal weight gain of pregnancy) may accompany nausea and vomiting, epigastric pain, elevated blood pressure, and blurred or double vision.

● **Sheehan's syndrome.** Most common in women who experience severe obstetric hemorrhage, this syndrome may cause weight gain.

Other causes

● **Drugs.** Corticosteroids, phenothiazines, and tricyclic antidepressants cause weight gain from fluid retention and increased appetite. Other drugs that can lead to weight gain include oral contraceptives, which cause fluid retention; cyproheptadine, which increases appetite; and lithium, which can induce hypothyroidism.

Special considerations

Psychological counseling may be necessary for patients with weight gain, particularly when it results from emotional problems or when uneven weight distribution alters body image. If the patient is obese or has a cardiopulmonary disorder, any exercises should be monitored closely.

Pediatric pointers

Weight gain in children can result from endocrine disorders such as hypercortisolism. Other causes include inactivity caused by Prader-Willi syndrome, Werdnig-Hoffmann disease, Down syndrome, late stages of muscular dystrophy, and severe cerebral palsy.

Nonpathologic causes include poor eating habits, sedentary recreations, and emotional problems, especially among adolescents. Regardless of the cause, dis-

EVALUATING NUTRITIONAL STATUS

If your patient has lost or gained an excessive amount of weight, you can help assess his nutritional status by measuring his skinfold thickness and midarm circumference and by calculating his midarm muscle circumference. Skinfold measurements reflect adipose tissue mass (subcutaneous fat accounts for about 50% of the body's adipose tissue). Midarm measurements reflect both skeletal muscle and adipose tissue mass. Gather these measurements as described on the next page. Then express them as a percentage of standard by using this formula:

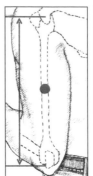

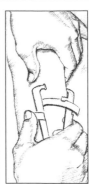

$$\frac{\text{actual measurement}}{\text{standard measurement}} \times 100 = \underline{\quad}\%$$

Standard anthropometric measurements vary according to age and sex. The abridged chart below lists standard arm measurements for adult men and women.

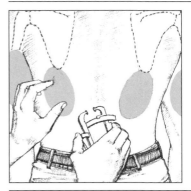

TEST		STANDARD
Triceps skinfold	Men	12.5 mm
	Women	16.5 mm
Midarm circum-ference	Men	29.3 cm
	Women	28.5 cm
Midarm muscle circumference	Men	25.3 cm
	Women	23.2 cm

A triceps or subscapular skinfold measurement < 60% of the standard value indicates severe depletion of fat reserves; a measurement between 60% and 90%, moderate to mild depletion; > 90%, significant fat reserves. A midarm circumference of < 90% of the standard value indicates caloric deprivation; > 90% adequate or ample muscle and fat. A midarm muscle circumference of < 90% indicates protein depletion; > 90%, adequate or ample protein reserves.

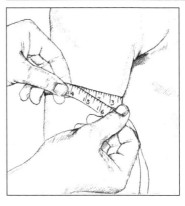

courage fad diets and provide a balanced weight loss program.

WEIGHT LOSS, EXCESSIVE

Weight loss can reflect decreased food intake, decreased food absorption, increased metabolic requirements, or a combination of the three. Its causes include endocrine, neoplastic, GI, and psychiatric disorders; nutritional deficiencies; infections; and neurologic lesions that cause paralysis and dysphagia. However, weight loss may accompany conditions that prevent sufficient food intake, such as painful oral lesions, ill-fitting dentures, and loss of teeth. It may be the metabolic sequela of poverty, fad diets, excessive exercise, and certain drugs.

Weight loss may occur as a late sign in such chronic diseases as congestive heart failure and renal disease. In these diseases, however, it's the result of anorexia. (See the entry "Anorexia.")

History and physical examination
Begin with a thorough dietary history because weight loss almost always is caused by inadequate caloric intake. If the patient hasn't been eating properly, try to determine why. Ask him about previous weight and if the recent loss was intentional. Be alert to lifestyle or occupational changes that may be a source of anxiety or depression. For example, has he recently become separated or divorced? Has he recently changed jobs?

Inquire about recent changes in bowel habits, such as diarrhea or bulky, floating stools. Has the patient had nausea, vomiting, or abdominal pain, which may indicate a GI disorder? Has he had excessive thirst, excessive urination, or heat intolerance, which may signal an endocrine disorder? Take a careful drug his-

---

To measure the triceps skinfold, locate the midpoint of the patient's upper arm, using a nonstretch tape measure. Mark the midpoint with a felt-tip pen (near right). Then grasp the skin with your thumb and forefinger about ⅜″ (1 cm) above the midpoint. Place the calipers at the midpoint and squeeze them for about 3 seconds (far right). Record the measurement registered on the handle gauge to the nearest 0.5 mm. Take two more readings and average all three to compensate for any measurement error.

To measure the subscapular skinfold, use your thumb and forefinger to grasp the skin just below the angle of the scapula, in line with the natural cleavage of the skin. Apply the calipers and proceed as you would when measuring the triceps skinfold. Both subscapular and triceps skinfold measurements are reliable measurements of fat loss or gain during hospitalization.

To measure midarm circumference, return to the midpoint you marked on the patient's upper arm. Use a tape measure to determine the circumference at this point. This measurement reflects both skeletal muscle and adipose tissue mass and helps evaluate protein and calorie reserves.
To calculate midarm muscle circumference, multiply the triceps skinfold thickness (in centimeters) by 3.143, and subtract this figure from the midarm circumference. Midarm muscle circumference reflects muscle mass alone, providing a more sensitive index of protein reserves.

tory, noting especially any use of diet pills and laxatives.

Carefully check the patient's height and weight, and ask about his previous weight. Take his vital signs and note his general appearance: Is he well nourished? Do his clothes fit? Is muscle wasting evident?

Now examine the patient's skin for turgor and abnormal pigmentation, especially around the joints. Does he have pallor or jaundice? Examine his mouth, including the condition of his teeth or dentures. Look for signs of infection or irritation on the roof of the mouth, and note any hyperpigmentation of the buccal mucosa. Also check the patient's eyes for exophthalmos and his neck for swelling, and evaluate his lungs for adventitious sounds. Inspect his abdomen for signs of wasting, and palpate for masses, tenderness, and an enlarged liver.

Common medical causes

• *Acromegaly.* This psychogenic disorder, most common in young women, is characterized by a severe, self-imposed weight loss ranging from 10% to 50% of premorbid weight, which typically was normal or not more than 5 lb (2.3 kg) over ideal weight. Related findings include skeletal muscle atrophy, loss of fatty tissue, hypotension, constipation, dental caries, susceptibility to infection, blotchy or sallow skin, cold intolerance, hairiness on the face and body, dryness or loss of scalp hair, and amenorrhea. The patient usually demonstrates restless activity and vigor and may also have a morbid fear of becoming fat. Self-induced vomiting or self-administration of laxatives or diuretics may lead to dehydration or to metabolic alkalosis or acidosis.

• *Cancer.* Weight loss is a common sign of cancer. Other findings reflect the type, location, and stage of the tumor, and generally include fatigue, pain, nausea, vomiting, anorexia, abnormal bleeding, and a palpable mass.

• *Crohn's disease.* Weight loss occurs with chronic cramping abdominal pain and anorexia. Other signs and symptoms may include diarrhea (possibly bloody) or constipation, nausea, fever, tachycardia, abdominal tenderness and guarding, hyperactive bowel sounds, abdominal distention, and pain. Perianal lesions and a palpable mass in the right or left lower quadrant may also be present.

• *Cryptosporidiosis.* Weight loss may occur in this opportunistic protozoan infection. Other findings include profuse watery diarrhea, abdominal cramping, flatulence, anorexia, malaise, fever, nausea, vomiting, and myalgia.

• *Depression.* Weight loss may occur in severe depression, along with insomnia or hypersomnia, anorexia, apathy, fatigue, and feelings of worthlessness. Indecisiveness, incoherence, and suicidal thoughts or behavior may also occur.

• *Diabetes mellitus.* Weight loss may occur with this disorder, despite increased appetite. Other findings include polydipsia, weakness, fatigue, and polyuria with nocturia.

• *Esophagitis.* Painful inflammation of the esophagus leads to temporary avoidance of eating and subsequent weight loss. Intense pain in the mouth and anterior chest occurs, along with hypersalivation, dysphagia, tachypnea, and hematemesis. If a stricture develops, dysphagia and weight loss will recur.

• *Gastroenteritis.* Malabsorption and dehydration cause weight loss in this disorder. The loss may be sudden in acute viral infections or reactions, or gradual in parasitic infection. Other findings include poor skin turgor, dry mucous membranes, tachycardia, hypotension, diarrhea, abdominal pain and tenderness, hyperactive bowel sounds, nausea, vomiting, fever, and malaise.

• *Leukemia.* *Acute leukemia* causes progressive weight loss accompanied by severe prostration; high fever; swollen, bleeding gums; and bleeding tendencies. Dyspnea, tachycardia, palpitations, and abdominal or bone pain may also occur. As the disease progresses, neurologic symptoms may eventually develop.

Chronic leukemia, which occurs insidiously in adults, causes progressive weight loss with malaise, fatigue, pallor, enlarged spleen, bleeding tendencies, anemia, skin eruptions, anorexia, and fever.

● *Lymphoma.* *Hodgkin's disease* and *malignant lymphoma* cause gradual weight loss. Associated findings include fever, fatigue, night sweats, malaise, hepatosplenomegaly, and lymphadenopathy. Scaly rashes and pruritus may develop.

● *Stomatitis.* Inflammation of the oral mucosa (usually red, swollen, and ulcerated) in this disorder causes weight loss due to decreased eating. Associated findings include fever, increased salivation, malaise, mouth pain, anorexia, and swollen, bleeding gums.

● *Thyrotoxicosis.* In this disorder, increased metabolism causes weight loss. Other characteristic signs and symptoms include nervousness, heat intolerance, diarrhea, increased appetite, palpitations, tachycardia, diaphoresis, fine tremor, and possibly an enlarged thyroid and exophthalmos. A ventricular or atrial gallop may be heard.

Other causes

● *Drugs.* Amphetamines and inappropriate dosage of thyroid preparations commonly lead to weight loss. Laxative abuse may cause a malabsorptive state that leads to weight loss. Chemotherapeutic agents cause stomatitis, which, when severe, causes weight loss.

Special considerations

Refer your patient for psychological counseling if weight loss negatively affects his body image. If the patient has a chronic disease, administer hyperalimentation or tube feedings to maintain nutrition and to prevent edema, poor healing, and muscle wasting. Take daily calo-

rie counts and weigh him weekly. Consult a dietitian, if necessary.

Pediatric pointers

In infants, weight loss may be caused by failure-to-thrive syndrome. In children, severe weight loss may be the first indication of diabetes mellitus. Chronic, gradual weight loss occurs in children with marasmus—nonedematous protein-calorie malnutrition. Weight loss may also occur as a result of child abuse or neglect, infections causing high fevers, GI disorders causing vomiting and diarrhea, or celiac disease.

WHEEZING
[Sibilant rhonchi]

Wheezes are adventitious breath sounds with a high-pitched, musical, squealing, creaking, or groaning quality. When they originate in the large airways, they can be heard by placing an unaided ear over the chest wall or at the mouth. When they originate in smaller airways, they can be heard by placing a stethoscope over the anterior or posterior chest. Unlike crackles and rhonchi, wheezes can't be cleared by coughing.

Prolonged wheezing usually occurs during expiration, when bronchi are shortened and narrowed. Causes of airway narrowing include bronchospasm; mucosal thickening or edema; partial obstruction from a tumor, a foreign body, or secretions; and extrinsic pressure, as in tension pneumothorax or goiter. With airway obstruction, wheezing occurs during inspiration.

Emergency interventions

 If you detect wheezing, determine the degree of the patient's respiratory distress. (See *Evaluating breath sounds,* pages 610 and 611.) Is he responsive? Is he restless, con-

EXAMINATION TIP

EVALUATING BREATH SOUNDS

Diminished or absent breath sounds indicate some interference with air flow. If pus, fluid, or air fills the pleural space, breath sounds will be quieter than normal. If a foreign body or secretions obstruct a bronchus, breath sounds will be diminished or absent over distal lung tissue. Increased thickness of the chest wall, such as with a patient who is obese or extremely muscular, may cause breath sounds to be decreased or inaudible. Absent breath sounds typically indicate loss of ventilation power.

When air passes through narrowed airways or through moisture, or when the membranes lining the chest cavity become inflamed, adventitious breath sounds will be heard. These include crackles, rhonchi, wheezes, and pleural friction rubs. Usually, these sounds indicate pulmonary disease.

Follow the auscultation sequences shown here to assess the patient's breath sounds. Have the patient take full, deep breaths, and compare sound variations from one side to the other. Note the location, timing, and character of any abnormal breath sounds.

Anterior

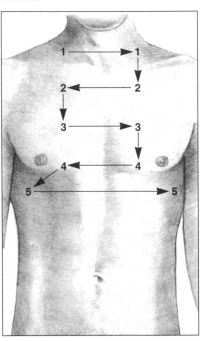

---

fused, anxious, or afraid? Are his respirations abnormally fast, slow, shallow, or deep? Are they irregular? Can you hear wheezing through his mouth? Does he have increased use of accessory muscles; increased chest wall motion; intercostal, suprasternal, or supraclavicular retractions; stridor; or nasal flaring? Take his other vital signs, noting hypotension or hypertension and an irregular, weak, rapid, or slow pulse. Help him relax, and administer humidified oxygen by face mask. Suction him, and encourage coughing and slow, deep breathing. Have intubation and emergency resuscitation equipment readily available. Call the respiratory therapy department to supply intermittent positive pressure breathing (IPPB) and nebulization treatments with bronchodilators. Insert an I.V. line to allow for administration of fluids and drugs, such as diuretics, steroids, bronchodilators, and sedatives.

History and physical examination
If the patient isn't in respiratory distress, obtain a history. What provokes his wheezing? Does he have asthma or allergies? Does he smoke or have a history of pulmonary, cardiac, or circulatory

Posterior

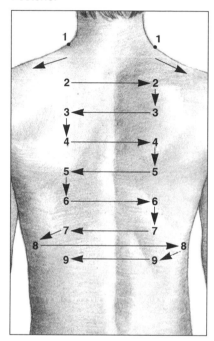

Left lateral

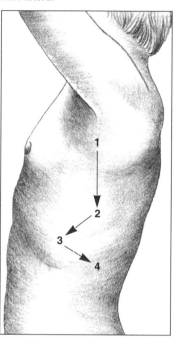

disorders? Does he have cancer? Ask about recent surgery, illness, or trauma, or changes in appetite, weight, exercise tolerance, or sleep patterns. Obtain a drug history. If he has a cough, ask how it sounds, when it starts, and how often it occurs. Does he have paroxysms of coughing? Is his cough dry, sputum producing, or bloody?

Ask the patient about chest pain. If he reports pain, determine its quality, onset, duration, intensity, and radiation. Does it increase with breathing, coughing, or certain positions?

Examine the patient's nose and mouth for congestion, drainage, or signs of infection such as halitosis. If he produces sputum, obtain a sample for examination. Check for cyanosis, pallor, clamminess, masses, tenderness, swelling, distended neck veins, and enlarged lymph nodes. Inspect his chest for abnormal configuration and asymmetrical motion, and determine if the trachea is midline. Percuss for dullness or hyperresonance, and auscultate for crackles, rhonchi, or pleural friction rubs. Note absent or hypoactive breath sounds, abnormal heart

ALTERNATIVE THERAPY

RELIEVING ASTHMA WITH QIGONG

Qigong, a traditional Chinese therapy that emphasizes preventive self-care by optimizing body systems, has been used to treat asthma. Blending therapeutic exercise, acupressure, meditation, breath regulation, and deep relaxation, qigong (pronounced chi-kung) stimulates the flow of energy throughout the body. This flow of energy is thought to enhance oxygen delivery to the tissues, to improve immune function, and to produce a relaxed state in the body.

sounds, gallops, murmurs, arrhythmias, bradycardia, or tachycardia.

Common medical causes

● *Anaphylaxis.* This allergic reaction can cause tracheal edema or bronchospasm, resulting in severe wheezing and stridor. Initial symptoms include fright, weakness, sneezing, dyspnea, nasal pruritus, urticaria, erythema, and angioedema. Respiratory distress occurs with nasal flaring, accessory muscle use, and intercostal retractions. Other findings include nasal edema and congestion, chest or throat tightness, dysphagia, and profuse, watery rhinorrhea. Cardiac effects include arrhythmias and hypotension.

● *Aspiration of a foreign body.* Partial obstruction by a foreign body produces sudden onset of wheezing and possibly stridor, gagging, hoarseness, and a dry, paroxysmal cough. Other findings include tachycardia, dyspnea, decreased breath sounds, and possibly cyanosis. A retained foreign body may cause inflammation leading to fever, pain, and swelling.

● *Aspiration pneumonitis.* In this disorder, wheezing may accompany tachypnea, marked dyspnea, cyanosis, tachycardia, fever, productive (eventually purulent) cough, and pink, frothy sputum.

● *Asthma.* Wheezing is an initial and cardinal sign of asthma. It's heard at the mouth during expiration. An initially dry cough later becomes productive with thick mucus. Other findings include apprehension, prolonged expiration, intercostal and supraclavicular retractions, rhonchi, accessory muscle use, nasal flaring, and tachypnea. Asthma also produces tachycardia, diaphoresis, and flushing or cyanosis.

● *Bronchial adenoma.* This insidious disorder produces unilateral, possibly severe wheezing. Common features are chronic cough and recurring hemoptysis. Symptoms of airway obstruction may occur later.

● *Bronchiectasis.* Excessive mucous commonly causes intermittent and localized or diffuse wheezing. A copious, foul-smelling, mucopurulent cough is classic. It's accompanied by hemoptysis, rhonchi, and coarse crackles. Weight loss, fatigue, weakness, dyspnea on exertion, fever, malaise, halitosis, and late-stage clubbing may also occur.

● *Bronchitis (chronic).* This disorder causes wheezing that varies in severity, location, and intensity. Associated findings include prolonged expiration, coarse crackles, scattered rhonchi, and a hacking cough that later becomes productive. Other effects include dyspnea, accessory muscle use, barrel chest, tachypnea, clubbing, edema, weight gain, and cyanosis.

● *Bronchogenic carcinoma.* Obstruction may cause localized wheezing. Typical findings include a productive cough, dyspnea, hemoptysis (initially blood-tinged sputum, possibly leading to massive hemorrhage), anorexia, and weight loss. Upper extremity edema and chest pain may also occur.

• *Emphysema.* Mild to moderate wheezing may occur in this form of chronic obstructive pulmonary disease. Related findings include dyspnea, malaise, tachypnea, diminished breath sounds, peripheral cyanosis, pursed-lip breathing, anorexia, and malaise. Accessory muscle use, barrel chest, a chronic productive cough, and clubbing may also occur.

• *Pulmonary coccidioidomycosis.* This disorder may cause wheezing and rhonchi along with cough, fever, chills, pleuritic chest pain, headache, weakness, malaise, anorexia, and macular rash.

• *Pulmonary edema.* Wheezing may occur with this life-threatening disorder. Other symptoms include coughing, exertional and paroxysmal nocturnal dyspnea and, later, orthopnea. Examination reveals tachycardia, tachypnea, dependent crackles, and a diastolic gallop. Severe pulmonary edema produces rapid, labored respirations; diffuse crackles; a productive cough with frothy, bloody sputum; arrhythmias; cold, clammy, cyanotic skin; hypotension; and thready pulse.

• *Pulmonary tuberculosis.* In late stages, fibrosis causes wheezing. Common findings include a mild to severe productive cough with pleuritic chest pain and fine crackles, night sweats, anorexia, weight loss, fever, malaise, dyspnea, and fatigue. Other features are dullness to percussion, increased tactile fremitus, and amphoric breath sounds.

• *Tracheobronchitis.* Auscultation may detect wheezing, rhonchi, and crackles. The patient also has a cough, slight fever, sudden chills, muscle and back pain, and substernal tightness.

Special considerations

Prepare the patient for diagnostic tests, such as chest X-rays, arterial blood gas analysis, and sputum culture.

Ease the patient's breathing by placing him in semi-Fowler's position and repositioning him frequently. If appropriate, encourage increased activity to promote drainage and prevent pooling of secretions. Encourage regular deep breathing and coughing. Perform pulmonary physiotherapy as necessary.

Administer antibiotics to treat infection, bronchodilators to relieve bronchospasm and maintain patent airways, steroids to reduce inflammation, and mucolytics and expectorants to increase the flow of secretions. Provide humidification to thin secretions. Encourage the patient to drink fluids to liquefy secretions and prevent dehydration.

If the patient has asthma, he may benefit from a Chinese therapy known as qigong. (See *Relieving asthma with qigong.*)

Pediatric pointers

Children are especially susceptible to wheezing because their small airways allow rapid obstruction. Primary causes of wheezing include bronchospasm, mucosal edema, and accumulation of secretions. These may occur with such disorders as cystic fibrosis, aspiration of a foreign body, acute bronchiolitis, and pulmonary hemosiderosis.

APPENDIX AND INDEX

UNCOMMON SIGNS AND SYMPTOMS

This appendix supplements the main text of *Handbook of Signs & Symptoms,* which provides detailed coverage of about 250 signs and symptoms that are familiar, diagnostically significant, or indicative of an emergency. The appendix, in contrast, provides the definition and common causes of about 250 less familiar, accessory, or nonspecific signs and symptoms. For elicited signs, such as Chaddock's sign, it also includes the technique for evoking the patient's response.

The appendix also covers selected pediatric signs, such as low-set ears and Allis' sign; psychiatric symptoms, such as delusions and hallucinations; and nail and tongue signs, such as nail plate hypertrophy and tongue discoloration.

A

Aaron's sign • Pain in the chest or abdominal area that's elicited by applying gentle but steadily increasing pressure over McBurney's point. A positive sign indicates appendicitis.

adipsia • Abnormal absence of thirst. This sign commonly occurs in hypothalamic injury or tumor, head injury, bronchial tumor, and cirrhosis.

agnosia • Inability to recognize and interpret sensory stimuli. *Auditory agnosia* refers to the inability to recognize familiar sounds; *visual agnosia,* the inability to recognize familiar objects by sight; and *gustatory agnosia,* the inability to recognize familiar tastes. *Astereognosis, or tactile agnosia,* is the inability to recognize objects by touch or feel. *Anosmia* is the inability to recognize familiar smells. *Autotopagnosia* is the inability to recognize body parts. *Anosognosia* refers to the denial or lack of awareness of a disease or defect (especially paralysis). Agnosias stem from lesions that affect the association areas of the parietal sensory cortex. They're common sequelae of cerebrovascular accident.

Allis' sign • In an adult: relaxation of the fascia lata between the iliac crest and greater trochanter due to fracture of the neck of the femur. To detect this sign, place a finger over the area between the iliac crest and greater trochanter and press firmly. If your finger sinks deeply into this area, you've detected Allis' sign. In an infant: unequal leg lengths due to hip dislocation. To detect this sign, place the infant on his back with his pelvis flat. Then flex both legs at the knee and hip with the feet even. Next, compare the height of the knees. If they differ, suspect hip dislocation in the shorter leg.

alopecia • Hair loss that usually occurs on the scalp. Alopecia typically develops gradually and may be diffuse or patchy. It can be classified as scarring or nonscarring. Scarring alopecia is permanent and results from hair follicle destruction; nonscarring alopecia is temporary and results from hair follicle damage.

ambivalence • Simultaneous existence of conflicting feelings about a person, idea, or object. It causes uncertainty or indecisiveness about which course to follow. Severe, debilitating ambivalence can occur in schizophrenia.

Allis' sign

615

anesthesia • Absence of cutaneous sensation of touch, temperature, and pain. This sensory loss may be partial or total, unilateral or bilateral. To detect anesthesia, ask the patient to close his eyes. Then touch him and ask him to specify the location. If the patient's verbal skills are immature or poor, watch for movement or changes in facial expression in response to your touch.

anhidrosis • An abnormal deficiency of sweat, which can be generalized (complete) or localized (partial). Generalized anhidrosis can lead to life-threatening impairment of thermoregulation. Anhidrosis may result from neurologic or skin disorders, the use of certain drugs, or congenital, atrophic or traumatic changes to sweat glands.

anisocoria • A difference of 0.5 to 2 mm in pupil size. Anisocoria occurs normally in about 2% of people, in whom the pupillary inequality remains constant over time and despite changes in light. However, if anisocoria results from fixed dilation or constriction of one pupil or slowed or impaired constriction of one pupil in response to light, it may indicate neurologic disease.

anosmia • Absence of the sense of smell. Temporary anosmia may result from any condition that irritates and causes swelling of the nasal mucosa and obstructs the olfactory area of the nose, such as heavy smoking, rhinitis, or sinusitis, or from inhaling irritants, such as cocaine or acid fumes.

apathy • Absence or suppression of emotion or interest in the external environment and personal affairs. This indifference can result from many disorders—chiefly neurologic, psychological, respiratory, and renal—as well as from alcohol and drug use or abuse. It's associated with many chronic disorders that cause personality changes and depression. In fact, apathy may be an early indicator of a serious disorder such as a brain tumor.

aphonia • Inability to produce speech sounds. This sign may result from overuse of the vocal cords, disorders of the larynx or laryngeal nerves, psychological disorders, or muscle spasm.

apraxia • Inability to perform purposeful movements in the absence of weakness, sensory loss, poor coordination, or lack of comprehension or motivation. It usually indicates a lesion in the cerebral hemisphere. Apraxia is classified as *ideational, ideomotor,* or *akinetic,* depending on the stage at which voluntary movement is impaired.

arthralgia • Joint pain. This symptom may have no pathologic importance or may indicate such disorders as arthritis or systemic lupus erythematosus.

asthenocoria • Slow dilation or constriction of the pupils in response to light changes. Photophobia may be present if constriction occurs slowly. Asthenocoria occurs in adrenal insufficiency.

asynergy • Impaired coordination of muscles or organs that normally function harmoniously. This extrapyramidal symptom stems from disorders of the basal ganglia and cerebellum.

anisocoria

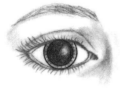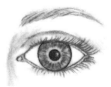

athetosis • An extrapyramidal sign characterized by slow, continuous, and twisting, involuntary movements that involve the face, neck, and distal extremities, such as the forearm, wrist, and hand. Athetosis worsens during stress and voluntary activity, may subside during relaxation, and disappears with sleep. It usually develops during childhood as a result of hypoxia at birth, kernicterus, or genetic disorders; in adults, it usually stems from vascular or neoplastic lesions, degenerative disease, drug toxicity, or hypoxia.

atrophy • Shrinkage or wasting away of a tissue or organ because of a reduction in the size or number of its cells. Its etiology may be physiologic, as seen in ovary, brain, and skin atrophy, or pathologic, as seen in neurologic disorders or spleen, liver, and thyroid abnormalities. This symptom is normally observed using inspection and palpation.

attention span decrease • Inability to focus selectively on a task while ignoring extraneous stimuli. Anxiety, emotional upset, and any dysfunction of the central nervous system may decrease a person's attention span.

autistic behavior • Exaggerated self-centered behavior marked by a lack of responsiveness to other people. It's characterized by highly personalized speech and actions that are not meaningful to an observer. For example, the patient may rock his body or repeatedly bang his head against the floor or wall.

B

Ballet's sign • Ophthalmoplegia, or paralysis of the external ocular muscles. The patient displays no control of voluntary eye movement but has normal reflexive movement and pupillary light reflexes. This sign is an indicator of thyrotoxicosis.

Bárány's symptom • With warm water irrigation of the ear, rotary nystagmus toward the irrigated side; with cold water irrigation, rotary nystagmus away from the irrigated side. Absence of this symptom indicates labyrinthine dysfunction.

Barlow's sign • An indicator of congenital dislocation of the hip, detected in the first 6 weeks of life. To elicit this sign, place the infant supine with his hips flexed 90 degrees and his knees fully flexed. Place your palm over the infant's knee, your thumb in the femoral triangle opposite the lesser trochanter, and your index finger over the greater trochanter. Bring the hip into midabduction while gently exerting posterior and lateral pressure with your thumb, and posterior and medial pressure with your palm. If you detect a click of the femoral head as it dislocates across the posterior lip of the acetabular socket, you've elicited this sign.

barrel chest • Rounded configuration of the chest in which the anteroposterior diameter enlarges to approximate the transverse diameter. The diaphragm is depressed and the sternum is pushed forward with the ribs attached in a horizontal, not angular, fashion. Typically a late sign of chronic obstructive pulmonary disease, barrel chest results from augmented lung volumes due to chronic airflow obstruction.

Barré's pyramidal sign • Inability to hold the lower legs still with the knees flexed. To detect this sign, place the patient prone and flex his knees 90 degrees. Then ask him to hold his lower legs still. If he can't maintain this position, you've observed this sign of pyramidal tract disease.

Barré's sign • Delayed contraction of the iris, seen in mental deterioration.

Beau's lines • Transverse white linear depressions on the fingernails. These lines may develop after any severe illness or toxic reaction. Other common

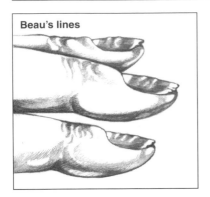

Beau's lines

causes include malnutrition, nail bed trauma, and coronary artery occlusion.

Beevor's sign • Upward movement of the umbilicus upon contraction of the abdominal muscles. To detect this sign, place the patient in the supine position and ask him to sit up. If his umbilicus moves upward, you've observed this sign—an indicator of paralysis of the lower rectus abdominis muscles, which is associated with lesions at T10.

Bell's sign • Reflexive upward and outward deviation of the eyes that occurs when the patient attempts to close his eyes. It occurs on the affected side in Bell's palsy and indicates that the defect is supranuclear.

Bezold's sign • Swelling and tenderness of the mastoid area. This sign, which indicates mastoiditis, results from

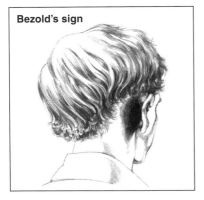

Bezold's sign

formation of an abscess beneath the sternocleidomastoid muscle.

blepharoclonus • Excessive blinking of the eyes. This extrapyramidal sign occurs with disorders of the basal ganglia and cerebellum.

blocking • A cognitive disturbance resulting in interruption of a stream of speech or thought. It usually occurs in midsentence or before completion of a thought. In most cases, the patient is unable to explain the interruption. Blocking may occur in normal individuals but usually occurs in schizophrenics.

Bonnet's sign • Pain on adduction of the thigh, seen in sciatica.

bradykinesia • Slowness of all voluntary movement and speech, believed to result from insufficient dopamine in the neurons of the brain stem region. Bradykinesia is commonly associated with parkinsonism or extrapyramidal or cerebellar disorders. It can also result from the use of certain drugs. Bradykinesia usually occurs in people over age 50, but it may also occur in children who have suffered hypoxic accidents. Associated findings include tremor and muscle rigidity.

breath sounds, decreased or absent • Diminished loudness or absence of breath sounds, detected by auscultation. This symptom may reflect reduced airflow to a lung segment caused by a tumor, foreign body, mucus plug, or mucosal edema. It may also reflect hyperinflation of the lungs due to emphysema or an asthmatic attack. Or it may indicate air or fluid in the pleural cavity from a pneumothorax, hemothorax, pleural effusion, atelectasis, or empyema. In an obese or extremely muscular patient, breath sounds may be diminished or inaudible because of increased thickness of the chest wall.

Broadbent's sign • Visible retraction of the left posterior chest wall near the 11th and 12th ribs, occurring during systole. To detect this sign, inspect the chest wall while standing at the patient's right side. Position a strong light so that it casts rays tangential to the skin. While auscultating the heart, watch for retraction of the skin and muscles and determine its timing in the cardiac cycle. Broadbent's sign may occur in extensive adhesive pericarditis.

buffalo hump • Accumulation of cervicodorsal fat, which may indicate hypercortisolism or Cushing's syndrome.

C

café-au-lait spots • Flat, light brown, uniformly hyperpigmented macules on the skin surface. These spots, which usually appear before age 10, are an important indicator of neurofibromatosis and other congenital melanotic disorders.

catatonia • Marked inhibition or excitation in motor behavior, occurring in psychotic disorders. *Catatonic stupor* refers to extreme inhibition of spontaneous activity or movement. *Catatonic excitement* refers to extreme psychomotor agitation.

Chaddock's sign • *Chaddock's toe sign:* Extension of the great toe and fanning of the other toes. To elicit this sign, firmly stroke the side of the patient's foot just distal to the lateral malleolus. A positive sign indicates pyramidal tract disorders.

Chaddock's wrist sign: Flexion of the wrist and extension of the fingers. To elicit this sign, stroke the ulnar surface of the patient's forearm near the wrist. A positive sign occurs on the affected side in hemiplegia. Although Chaddock's sign is a pathologic finding in children and adults, it occurs normally in infants up to age 7 months.

cherry red spot • The choroid appearing as a red circular area surrounded by an abnormal gray-white retina. This sign is viewed through the fovea cen-

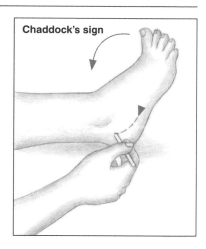

Chaddock's sign

tralis of the eye with an ophthalmoscope. It appears in infantile cerebral sphingolipidosis—for example, in over 90% of children with Tay-Sachs disease.

chorea • Brief, unpredictable bursts of rapid, jerky motion that interrupt normal coordinated movement. These movements are seldom repetitive but tend to appear purposeful and usually involve the face, head, lower arms, and hands. Chorea indicates dysfunction of the extrapyramidal system and is the first sign of Huntington's disease.

circumstantiality • Speech in which the main point is obscured by minute detail. Although the speaker may recognize his main point and return to it after many digressions, the listener may fail to recognize it. Circumstantiality commonly occurs in compulsive disorders, organic brain disorders, and schizophrenia.

Claude's hyperkinesis sign • Increased reflex activity of the paretic muscles, elicited by painful stimuli.

Cleeman's sign • Slight linear depression or wrinkling of the skin superior to the patella. This sign usually indicates a femoral fracture with overriding bone fragments.

clenched fist sign • Placement of a clenched fist against the chest. This gesture may be performed by patients with angina pectoris when they're asked to indicate the location of their pain. It conveys the constricting, oppressive quality of substernal pain.

clicks • Brief, high-frequency heart sounds auscultated during systole or diastole. *Ejection clicks* occur soon after the first heart sound and are believed to result from sudden distention of a dilated pulmonary artery or aorta or from forceful opening of the pulmonic or aortic valve. Associated with increased pulmonary resistance and hypertension, clicks occur most commonly in septal defects or patent ductus arteriosus. To detect ejection clicks best, have the patient sit upright or lie down; then auscultate his heart with the diaphragm of the stethoscope. *Systolic clicks* occur most often in mid-to-late systole and characterize mitral valve prolapse. To detect systolic clicks, auscultate over the mitral valve with the diaphragm of the stethoscope.

clonus • Abnormal response of a muscle to stretching. Clonus is a sign of damage to nerve fibers that carry impulses to a particular muscle from the motor cortex. A muscle that is stretched usually responds by contracting once and then relaxing. In clonus, stretching sets off a series of contractions of the muscle or muscles in rapid succession. Clonic muscle contractions are also a feature of generalized tonic-clonic seizures.

cognitive dysfunction • Inability to perceive, organize, and interpret sensory stimuli or to think and solve problems. This symptom may arise from various causes, including central nervous system disturbances, extrapyramidal conditions, systemic illness, endocrine diseases, and deficiency states, or from an unknown etiology, as in chronic fatigue syndrome.

Comolli's sign • Triangular swelling over the scapula that matches its shape. This sign indicates a scapular fracture.

compulsion • Repetitive behavior in which the individual recognizes the irrationality of his actions but is unable to stop them. An example is constant handwashing. Compulsions occur in obsessive-compulsive disorders and occasionally in schizophrenia.

confabulation • Fabrication to cover gaps in memory. Confabulation is usually seen in alcoholism and Korsakoff's syndrome.

conjunctival injection • Nonuniform redness of the conjunctiva from hyperemia associated with inflammation. The redness may be diffuse, localized, or peripheral or it may encircle a clear cornea. It usually results from bacterial or viral conjunctivitis, but it can also signal a serious ocular disorder such as trachoma, which if untreated can lead to blindness.

conjunctival paleness • Lack of color in the tissues inside the eyelid. Although the conjunctiva is a transparent mucous membrane, the portion lining the eyelids normally appears pink or red because it overlies the vasculature of the inner lid. Pale conjunctivae indicate anemia. To detect this sign, separate the eyelids widely by applying gentle pressure against the orbit of the eye. Ask the patient to look up, down, and to each side.

conversion • An alteration in physical activity or function that resembles an organic disorder but lacks an organic cause. Occurring without voluntary control, conversion is generally considered symbolic of psychological conflict and usually occurs in conversion disorders.

Coopernail's sign • Ecchymoses on the perineum, scrotum, or labia, indicating pelvic fracture.

Cowen's sign • A jerky, consensual pupillary light reflex. To detect this sign, observe for constriction and dilation of one pupil while the other is stimulated by increased and decreased light.

crowing respirations • Slow, deep inspirations accompanied by a high-pitched crowing sound—the characteristic whoop of the paroxysmal stage of pertussis.

Cruveilhier's sign • Swelling in the groin associated with an inguinal hernia. To detect this sign, ask the patient to flex one knee slightly while you insert your index finger in the inguinal canal on the same side. When your finger is inserted as deeply as possible, ask the patient to cough. If a hernia is present, you'll feel a mass of tissue that meets your finger and then withdraws.

Cullen's sign • Irregular, bluish hemorrhagic patches on the skin around the umbilicus and occasionally around abdominal scars. Cullen's sign indicates massive hemorrhage after trauma or rupture in such disorders as duodenal ulcer, ectopic pregnancy, abdominal aneurysm, gallbladder or common bile duct obstruction, or acute hemorrhagic pancreatitis. This sign usually appears gradually; blood travels from a retroperitoneal organ or structure to the periumbilical area, where it diffuses through subcutaneous tissues. The extent of discoloration depends on the extent of bleeding (it may be difficult to detect in a dark-skinned patient). In time, the bluish discoloration fades to greenish yellow and then yellow before disappearing.

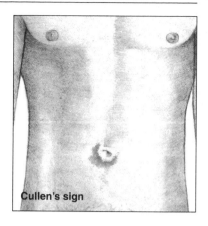
Cullen's sign

D

Dalrymple's sign • Abnormally wide palpebral fissures associated with retraction of the upper eyelids. To detect this sign of thyrotoxicosis, observe the eyes while the patient focuses on a fixed point or ask him to close his eyes. The patient may blink infrequently, noticeably restrict lid movement, and be unable to close his eyes completely.

Darier's sign • Whealing and itching of the skin upon rubbing the macular lesions of urticaria pigmentosa (mastocytosis). To elicit this sign, vigorously rub the pigmented macules with the blunt end of a pen or a similar blunt object. Red, pruritic, palpable wheals around the macules—a positive Darier's sign—appear after the release of histamine when mast cells are irritated.

Delbet's sign • Adequate collateral circulation to the distal portion of a limb associated with aneurysmal occlusion of the main artery. To detect this sign, check pulses, color, and temperature in the affected limb. If you find absent pulses but normal color and temperature, you've detected Delbet's sign.

delirium • Acute confusion characterized by restlessness, agitation, incoherence and, commonly, hallucinations. Delirium typically develops suddenly and lasts for a short period. It's a common effect of drug and alcohol abuse, metabolic disorders, and high fever. Delirium may also follow head trauma or seizure.

delusion • A persistent false belief held despite invalidating evidence. A *delusion of grandeur*, which may occur in schizophrenia and bipolar disorders, is an exaggerated belief in one's importance, wealth, or talent. The patient may take a powerful figure, such as

Napoleon, as his persona. In a *paranoid delusion,* which may occur in schizophrenia and paranoid disorders, the patient believes that he or someone close to him is the victim of an attack, a conspiracy, or harrassment. In a *somatic delusion,* which may occur in psychotic disorders, the patient believes that his body is diseased or distorted.

Demianoff's sign • Lumbar pain caused by stretching the sacrolumbar muscle. To elicit this sign, place the patient supine on the examining table and raise his extended leg. Lumbar pain that prevents him from lifting the leg high enough to form a 10-degree angle to the table—a positive Demianoff's sign—occurs in lumbago.

denial • An unconscious defense mechanism used to ward off distressing feelings, thoughts, wishes, or needs. Denial occurs in normal and pathologic mental states. In terminal illness, it represents the first stage of the response to dying.

depersonalization • Perception of the self as strange or unreal. For example, a person may report feeling as if he's observing himself from a distance. This symptom occurs in patients with schizophrenia and depersonalization disorders and in normal individuals during periods of great stress or anxiety.

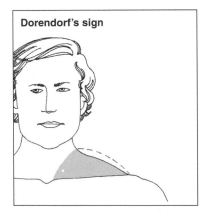

Dorendorf's sign

Dorendorf's sign • Fullness at the supraclavicular groove. This sign may occur in an aneurysm of the aortic arch.

drooling • The flow of saliva from the mouth, resulting from a failure to swallow or retain saliva or from excess salivation. It may stem from facial muscle paralysis, weakness that prevents mouth closure, neuromuscular disorders, pain, or the effects of drugs or toxins that induce salivation.

Duchenne's sign • Inward movement of the epigastrium during inspiration. This sign may indicate diaphragmatic paralysis or accumulation of fluid in the pericardium.

Dugas' sign • An indicator of a dislocated shoulder. To detect this sign, ask the patient to place the hand from the affected side onto his opposite shoulder and to move his elbow toward his chest. The inability to perform this maneuver—a positive Dugas' sign—indicates dislocation.

Duroziez's sign • A double murmur heard over a large peripheral artery. To detect this sign, auscultate over the femoral artery, alternately compressing the vessel proximally and then distally. If you hear a systolic murmur with proximal compression and a diastolic murmur with distal compression, you've detected Duroziez's sign—an indicator of aortic insufficiency.

dyspareunia • Painful or difficult coitus. Although it commonly accompanies pelvic disorders, this symptom may also result from diminished vaginal secretions associated with aging, the effects of drugs, or psychological factors.

E

echolalia • *In an adult:* repetition of another's words or phrases with no comprehension of their meaning. This sign occurs in schizophrenia and frontal lobe disorders.

In a child: an imitation of sounds or words produced by others.

ectropion • Eyelid eversion, which may affect the lower eyelid or both lids, exposing the palpebral conjunctiva. If the lacrimal puncta are everted, the eye cannot drain properly and tearing occurs. Ectropion may occur gradually as part of the aging process or as a result of injury or paralysis of the facial nerve.

enophthalmos • Backward displacement of the eye into the orbit. This sign most commonly follows trauma but may also result from severe dehydration or eye disorders.

entropion • Eyelid inversion, which typically affects the lower lid but may also affect the upper lid. The eyelashes may touch and irritate the cornea. Usually associated with aging, entropion may also stem from chemical burns, mechanical injuries, spasm of the orbicular muscle, pemphigoid, Stevens-Johnson syndrome, or trachoma.

epicanthal folds • Vertical skin folds that partially or fully obscure the inner canthus of the eye. These folds may make the eyes appear crossed because the pupil lies closer to the inner canthus than to the outer canthus. Epicanthal folds are a normal characteristic in many young children and Asians. They also occur as a familial trait in other ethnic groups and as an acquired trait in elderly people. However, the presence of epicanthal folds along with oblique palpebral fissures in non-Asian children indicates Down syndrome.

Erben's reflex • Slowing of the pulse when the head and trunk are forcibly bent forward. This sign may indicate vagal excitability.

Erb's sign • In tetany, increased irritability of motor nerves, detected by electromyography. Erb's sign also refers to dullness on percussion over the sternum's manubrium in acromegaly.

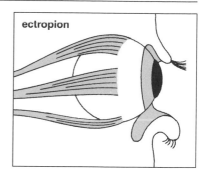

ectropion

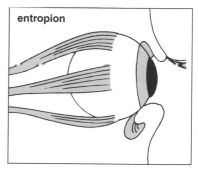

entropion

eructation • Belching, which occurs when gas or acidic fluid arises from the stomach, producing a characteristic sound. This sign sometimes results from GI disorders, but it usually stems from swallowing air or ingesting gas-producing food.

Escherich's sign • Contraction of the lips, tongue, and masseters, occurring in tetany. To elicit Escherich's sign, percuss the inner surface of the lips or the tongue.

euphoria • A feeling of great happiness or well-being. When euphoria doesn't accompany enlightening experiences or superb achievements, it may reflect bipolar disorders, organic brain disease, or use of such drugs as heroin, cocaine, and amphetamines.

Ewart's sign • Bronchial breathing heard on auscultation and dullness heard on percussion below the angle of the left scapula. These compression signs commonly occur in pericardial effusion.

extensor thrust reflex • Leg extension upon stimulation of the sole of the foot; a normal reflex in newborn infants. This reflex is mediated at the spinal cord level and should disappear after age 6 months.

To elicit the extensor thrust reflex, place the infant supine with his leg flexed; then stimulate the sole of the foot. If the extensor thrust reflex is present, the leg will slowly extend. In premature infants, this reflex may be weak. Its persistence beyond age 6 months indicates anoxic brain damage. Its recurrence in a child signals a central nervous system lesion or injury.

F

facial pain • This symptom may result from various neurologic, vascular, or infectious disorders, or it may be referred to the face in disorders of the ear, nose, paranasal sinuses, teeth, neck, and jaw. Its most common causes are trigeminal neuralgia and tic douloureux.

Fajersztajn's crossed sciatic sign • In sciatica, pain on the affected side caused by lifting the extended opposite leg. To elicit this sign, place the patient in the supine position and have him flex his unaffected hip, keeping his knee extended. Flexion at the hip will cause pain on the affected side by stretching the irritated sciatic nerve.

fan sign • Spreading of the toes after firmly stroking the foot; a component of Babinski's reflex.

flatulence • A sensation of gaseous abdominal fullness that can result from GI disorders, abdominal surgery, or excessive intake of certain foods. This symptom reflects slowed intestinal motility (which hampers the passage of gas), excessive swallowing of air, or increased intraluminal gas production.

flexor withdrawal reflex • Knee flexion upon stimulation of the sole of the foot; a normal reflex in newborn infants. This reflex is mediated at the spinal cord level and should disappear after age 6 months.

To elicit this reflex, place the infant in the supine position, extend his legs, and pinch the sole of his foot. Normally, an infant less than 6 months old will respond with slow, uncontrolled flexion of the knee. (This reflex may be weak in premature infants.) Its persistence beyond age 6 months may indicate anoxic brain damage. Its recurrence signals a central nervous system lesion or injury.

flight of ideas • Continuous speech that commonly appears pressured and is characterized by abrupt topic changes. In contrast to *loose association,* a listener can discern the connection between topics based on word similarities or sounds. This sign characteristically occurs in the manic phase of a bipolar disorder.

foot drop • Plantar flexion of the foot with toes bent toward the instep. This sign results from weakness or paralysis of the dorsiflexion muscles of the foot and ankle, which is characteristic of certain peripheral nerve or motor neuron disorders. It may also result from prolonged immobility.

Fränkel's sign • In tabes dorsalis, the excessive range of passive motion at the hip joint stemming from decreased tone in the surrounding muscles.

G

Gallant's reflex • Movement of the pelvis toward the stimulated side when the back is stroked laterally to the spinal column. Normally present at birth, this reflex disappears by age 2 months. To elicit this reflex, place the infant prone on the examining table or on your hand. Then, using a pin or your finger, stroke his back laterally to the midline. Normally, the infant responds by moving the pelvis toward the stimulated side, indicating integrity of the spinal cord from T1 to S1. An absent, irregular, or asymmetrical reflex may indicate a spinal cord lesion.

Gifford's sign • Resistance to everting the upper eyelid, seen in thyrotoxicosis. To detect this sign, attempt to raise the eyelid and evert it over a blunt object.

glabella reflex • Persistent blinking in response to repeated light tapping on the forehead between the eyebrows. This reflex occurs in Parkinson's disease, presenile dementia, and diffuse tumors of the frontal lobes.

Goldthwait's sign • Pain elicited by maneuvers of the leg, pelvis, and lower back to differentiate irritation of the sacroiliac joint from irritation of the lumbosacral or sacroiliac articulation. To elicit this sign, place the patient in the supine position and put one hand under the small of his back. With your other hand, raise the patient's leg. If he reports pain, suspect sacroiliac joint irritation. If he reports no pain, place your hand under his lower back and apply pressure. If he reports pain, suspect irritation of the lumbosacral or sacroiliac articulation.

Gowers' sign • *In an adult:* irregular contraction of the iris, occurring when the eye is illuminated. This sign can be detected in certain stages of tabes dorsalis.
In a child: the characteristic maneuver used to rise from the floor or a low sitting position to compensate for proximal muscle weakness in Duchenne's or Becker's muscular dystrophy. (See the entry "Gait, waddling.")

Graefe's sign • An inability of the upper eyelid to follow the eye's downward movements; a cardinal sign of thyrotoxicosis. To test for this sign, hold a finger, penlight, or other target above the patient's eye level, then move it downward and observe eyelid movement as the eyes follow the target. Graefe's sign is demonstrated when a rim of sclera ap-

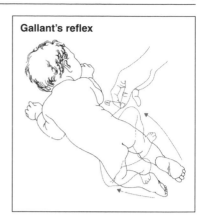

Gallant's reflex

pears between the upper lid margin and the iris when the eyes are lowered, when one lid closes more slowly than the other, or when both lids close slowly and incompletely with jerky movements.

grasp reflex • Flexion of the fingers when the palmar surface is touched and of the toes when the plantar surface is touched. This reflex is normal in infants; it develops at approximately 26 to 28 weeks' gestational age but may be weak until term. An absent, weak, or asymmetrical grasp reflex during the neonatal period may indicate paralysis, central nervous system depression, or injury.
To elicit this reflex, place a finger in each of the infant's palms. His reflexive grasping should be symmetrical and strong enough at term to allow him to be lifted. Elicit toe flexion by gently touching the ball of the foot. In an adult, the grasp reflex is an *abnormal* finding, indicating a premotor cortex disorder.

Grey Turner's sign • A bruiselike discoloration of the flank skin. This sign appears 6 to 24 hours after onset of retroperitoneal hemorrhage in acute pancreatitis.

grief • Deep anguish or sorrow typically felt upon the loss of a loved one, a job, a goal, or an ideal. In patients with terminal illness, grief typically precedes acceptance of dying. Unlike depression, grief proceeds in stages and often resolves with the passage of time.

Griffith's sign • Lagging motion of the lower eyelids during upward rotation of the eyes, seen in thyrotoxicosis. To detect this sign, ask the patient to focus on a steadily rising point, such as your moving finger. If the lower lid doesn't follow eye motion smoothly, you've observed this sign.

Guilland's sign • Quick, energetic flexion of the hip and knee in response to pinching the contralateral quadriceps muscle. This sign indicates meningeal irritation.

gum swelling • This common sign may result from an increase in the size of existing gum cells (hypertrophy) or from an increase in their number (hyperplasia). Possible causes include nutritional deficiencies, certain systemic disorders, and hormonal changes during pregnancy.

H

halitosis • Unpleasant, disagreeable, or offensive breath odor. Certain types are characteristic of certain disorders. (See the entries "Breath with ammonia odor," "Breath with fecal odor," "Breath with fruity odor," and "Fetor hepaticus.")

hallucination • A sensory perception without corresponding external stimuli. Hallucinations may occur in depression, schizophrenia, bipolar disorder, organic brain disorders, and drug-induced and toxic conditions.

An *auditory hallucination* is the perception of nonexistent sounds—typically voices but occasionally music or other sounds. Occurring in schizophrenia, this is the most common type of hallucination.

An *olfactory hallucination*—a perception of nonexistent odors from the patient's own body or from some other person or object—is typically associated with somatic delusions. It occurs most often in temporal lobe lesions and sometimes in schizophrenia.

A *tactile hallucination* is the perception of nonexistent tactile stimuli, generally described as something crawling on or under the skin. It occurs mainly in toxic conditions and addiction to certain drugs. Formication—the sensation of insects crawling on the skin—most commonly occurs in alcohol withdrawal syndrome and cocaine abuse.

A *visual hallucination* is the perception of nonexistent images of people, flashes of light, or other scenes. It occurs most often in acute, reversible organic brain disorders but may also occur in drug and alcohol intoxication, schizophrenia, febrile illness, and encephalopathy.

A *gustatory hallucination* is the perception of nonexistent, usually unpleasant tastes.

harlequin sign • A benign, erythematous color change that occurs primarily in low-birth-weight infants. This reddening of one longitudinal half of the body appears when the infant is placed on either side for a few minutes. When he's placed on his back, the sign usually disappears immediately but it may persist up to 20 minutes.

Heberden's nodes • Painless, irregular bony enlargements of the distal finger joints that develop on one or both sides of the dorsal midline, affecting one or more fingers but not the thumb. This sign is usually caused by osteoarthritis and occurs in more than half of patients with this disorder.

hemorrhage, subungual • Bleeding under the nail plate. Hemorrhagic lines, called splinter hemorrhages, run proximally from the distal edge and are an indicator of subacute bacterial endocarditis and trichinosis. Large hemorrhagic areas usually reflect nail bed injury.

hiccups • Involuntary spasmodic contraction of the diaphragm followed by a sudden closing of the glottis. The characteristic sound of hiccups reflects the vibration of closed vocal cords as air suddenly rushes into the lungs. Usually benign and transient, hiccups typically subside spontaneously; however, in a patient with a neurologic disorder, they may indicate increasing intracranial pressure or extension of a brain stem lesion.

Hill's sign • A femoral systolic pulse pressure 60 to 100 mm Hg higher in the right leg than in the right arm. Hill's sign may indicate severe aortic insufficiency. To detect this sign, place the patient in the supine position and take blood pressure readings, first in the right arm and then in the right leg, noting the difference.

hirsutism • Excessive growth of dark, coarse body hair in females stemming from excessive androgen production. It may result from endocrine abnormalities or idiopathic causes.

Hoehne's sign • Absence of uterine contractions during delivery, despite repeated doses of oxytocic drugs. This sign indicates a ruptured uterus.

Hoffmann's sign • Flexion of the terminal phalanx of the thumb and the second and third phalanx of another finger when the nail of the index, middle, or ring finger is snapped. A bilateral or strongly unilateral response suggests a pyramidal tract disorder such as spastic hemiparesis. To elicit this sign, dorsiflex the patient's wrist, have him flex his fingers, and then snap the nail of his index, middle, or ring finger.

Hoffmann's sign also refers to increased sensitivity of sensory nerves to electrical stimulation, as in tetany.

hyperacusis • Abnormally acute hearing resulting from increased irritability of the auditory neural mechanism.

hyperesthesia • Increased cutaneous sensitivity to touch, temperature, or pain.

hypernasality • A voice quality reflecting excessive expiration of air through

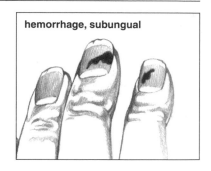

hemorrhage, subungual

the nose during speech. This sign is commonly associated with dysarthria and sometimes with swallowing defects. The sudden onset of hypernasality may indicate a neuromuscular disorder. This sign may also accompany cleft palate, abnormal nasopharyngeal size, and partial or complete velar paralysis. To detect this sign, ask the patient to extend vowel sounds first with the nostrils open, then closed (pinched). A significant shift in tone may indicate hypernasality.

hyperpigmentation • Excessive skin coloring, which usually reflects overproduction, abnormal location, or maldistribution of the pigment melanin. It usually results from exposure to sunlight but can also stem from metabolic, endocrine, neoplastic, and inflammatory disorders; genetic defects; use of certain drugs; and chemical poisoning.

hypoesthesia • Decreased cutaneous sensitivity to touch, temperature, or pain.

hypopigmentation • A decrease in normal skin, hair, mucous membrane, or nail color resulting from a deficiency, absence, or abnormal degradation of the pigment melanin.

I

idea of reference • A delusion that other people, statements, actions, or events have a meaning specific to oneself. This delusion occurs in schizophrenia and paranoid states.

illusion • A misperception of external stimuli—usually visual or auditory—for example, the sound of the wind being perceived as a voice. Illusions occur normally as well as in schizophrenia and toxic states.

J

Janeway's lesions • Slightly raised but usually flat, irregular, nontender, small erythematous lesions (1 to 4 mm in diameter) on the palms and soles. They blanch with pressure and with elevation of the affected extremity; in rare cases, they form a diffuse rash over the trunk and extremities. They disappear spontaneously. Once a common finding in infective endocarditis, Janeway's lesions may reflect an immunologic reaction to the infecting organisms (usually bacteria). They're rare today because the disease is now detected and managed at an earlier stage.

Jellinek's sign • Brownish pigmentation on the eyelids, usually more prominent on the upper lid than on the lower one. This sign appears in Graves' disease.

K

Kanavel's sign • An area of tenderness in the palm, caused by inflamma-

tion of the tendon sheath of the little finger. To detect this sign, apply pressure to the palm proximal to the metacarpophalangeal joint of the little finger.

Kashida's sign • Hyperesthesia and muscle spasms produced by application of heat or cold. This sign occurs in tetany.

Keen's sign • Increased ankle circumference in Pott's fracture of the fibula. To detect this sign, measure the ankles at the malleoli and compare their circumferences.

Koplik's spots • Small red spots with bluish white centers on the lingual and buccal mucosa, characteristic of measles. The measles rash usually erupts 1 to 2 days after this sign appears.

Kussmaul's respirations • An abnormal breathing pattern characterized by deep, rapid sighing respirations, generally associated with metabolic acidosis.

Kussmaul's sign • Distention of the jugular veins on inspiration, occurring in constrictive pericarditis and mediastinal tumor. Kussmaul's sign also refers to a paradoxical pulse, seizures, and coma that result from absorption of toxins.

L

Langoria's sign • Relaxation of the extensor muscles of the thigh and hip joint resulting from an intracapsular fracture of the femur. To elicit this sign, place the patient in a prone position and then press firmly on the gluteus maximus and hamstring muscles on both sides, noting greater muscle relaxation on the affected side. (The muscles are soft and spongy.)

large for gestational age • Neonatal weight that exceeds the 90th percentile for the infant's gestational age. The high-birth-weight neonate is at increased risk for birth trauma, respirato-

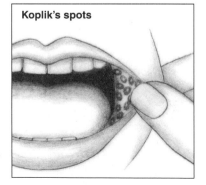

Koplik's spots

ry distress, hypocalcemia, hypoglycemia, and polycythemia.

Lasègue's sign • Pain upon passive
leg movement that distinguishes hip
joint disease from sciatica. To elicit this
sign, place the patient in the supine position, raise one leg, and bend the knee
to flex the hip joint. Pain with this movement indicates hip joint disease. With
the hip still flexed, slowly extend the
knee. Pain with this movement results
from stretching an irritated sciatic
nerve, indicating sciatica.

lead-pipe rigidity • Diffuse muscle stiffness occurring, for example, in Parkinson's disease.

Leichtenstern's sign • Pain upon gentle tapping of the bones of an extremity.
This sign occurs in cerebrospinal meningitis. The patient may wince, draw
back suddenly, or cry out loudly.

Lichtheim's sign • An inability to
speak that's associated with subcortical
aphasia. However, the patient can indicate with his fingers the number of syllables in the word he wants to say.

lid lag • Inability of the upper eyelid to
follow the eye's downward movements;
a cardinal sign of thyrotoxicosis.

Linder's sign • Pain upon neck flexion,
indicating sciatica. To elicit this sign,
place the patient in a supine or sitting
position with his legs fully extended.
Then passively flex his neck, noting if
he experiences pain in the lower back
or the affected leg as a result of stretching the irritated sciatic nerve.

Lloyd's sign • Referred loin pain elicited by deep percussion over the kidney.
This sign is associated with renal calculi.

loose association • A cognitive disturbance marked by absence of a logical
link between spoken statements. It occurs in schizophrenia, bipolar disorders, and other psychotic disorders.

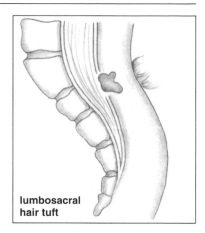

**lumbosacral
hair tuft**

low-set ears • A position of the ears in
which the superior helix lies lower than
the eyes. This sign appears in several
genetic syndromes, including Down,
Apert's, Turner's, Noonan's, and Pot-
ter's, and may also appear in other congenital abnormalities.

Ludloff's sign • Inability to raise the
thigh while sitting, along with edema
and ecchymosis at the base of Scar-
pa's triangle (the depressed area just
below the fold of the groin). Occurring
in children, this sign indicates traumatic
separation of the epiphyseal growth
plate of the greater trochanter.

lumbosacral hair tuft • Abnormal
growth of hair over the lower spine,
possibly accompanied by skin depression or discoloration. This sign may
mark the site of spina bifida occulta or
spina bifida cystica.

M

Macewen's sign • A "cracked pot"
sound heard on light percussion with
one finger over an infant's or young
child's anterior fontanel. An early indicator of hydrocephalus, this sign may
also occur in cerebral abscess.

Maisonneuve's sign • Hyperextension
of the wrist in Colles' fracture. This sign

results when a fracture of the lower radius causes posterior displacement of the distal fragment.

malaise • Listlessness, weariness, or absence of a sense of well-being. This nonspecific symptom may begin suddenly or gradually and may precede characteristic signs of an illness by several days or weeks. Malaise may reflect the metabolic alterations that precede or accompany infectious, endocrine, or neurologic disorders.

malingering • Exaggeration or simulation of symptoms to avoid an unpleasant situation or to gain attention or some other goal.

mania • An alteration in mood characterized by increased psychomotor activity, euphoria, flight of ideas, and pressured speech. It occurs most often in the manic phase of bipolar disorders.

Mannkopf's sign • Elevated pulse rate upon application of pressure over a painful area. This sign can help distinguish real pain from simulated pain.

Marcus Gunn's pupillary sign • Paradoxical dilation of a pupil in response to afferent visual stimuli. This sign results from an optic nerve lesion or severe retinal dysfunction. However, visual loss in the affected eye is minimal. To detect this sign, darken the room and instruct the patient to focus on a distant object. Shine a bright beam of light into the unaffected eye, and observe for bilateral pupillary constriction. Then shine the light into the affected eye; you'll observe brief bilateral dilation. Next, return the light beam to the unaffected eye; you'll observe prompt and persistent bilateral pupillary constriction.

masklike facies • A total loss of facial expression, resulting from bradykinesia—usually due to extrapyramidal damage. The rate of eye blinking drops to 1 to 4 blinks per minute, producing a characteristic "reptilian" stare. Although a neurologic disorder is the most common cause, masklike facies can also

result from certain systemic diseases and from the effects of certain drugs and toxins.

Mayo's sign • In deep anesthesia, relaxation of the muscles controlling the lower jaw.

Mean's sign • Lagging eye motion when the patient looks upward. In this sign of Graves' disease, the globe of the eye moves more slowly than the upper lid.

moon face • A distinctive facial adiposity that usually indicates hypercortisolism due to ectopic or excessive pituitary production of adrenocorticotropic hormone, adrenal adenoma or carcinoma, or long-term glucocorticoid therapy. Characteristics include marked facial roundness, a double chin, prominent upper lip, and full supraclavicular fossae.

Moro's reflex • An infant's generalized response to a loud noise or sudden movement. This reflex usually disappears by about age 3 months. Its persistence after age 6 months may indicate brain damage.
To elicit this reflex, make a sudden loud noise near the infant, or carefully hold his body with one hand while allowing his head to drop a few centimeters with the other hand. In a complete response, the infant's arms extend and abduct, and his fingers open; then his arms adduct and flex over his chest in a grasping motion. The infant may also extend his hips and legs and cry briefly. A bilaterally equal response is normal; an asymmetrical response may indicate a fractured clavicle or brachial nerve damage. The absence of a response may indicate hearing loss or severe central nervous system depression.

Murphy's sign • The arrest of inspiratory effort when gentle finger pressure beneath the right subcostal arch and below the margin of the liver causes pain during deep inspiration. This classic (but not always present) sign of acute cholecystitis may also occur in hepatitis.

muscle rigidity • Muscle tension, stiffness, and resistance to passive movement. This extrapyramidal symptom occurs in disorders affecting the basal ganglia and cerebellum, such as Parkinson's disease, Wilson's disease, Hallervorden-Spatz disease in adults, and kernicterus in infants.

myalgia • Diffuse muscle pain, usually accompanied by malaise, occurring in many infectious diseases, including brucellosis, dengue, influenza, leptospirosis, measles, and poliomyelitis. Myalgia also occurs in arteriosclerosis obliterans, fibrositis, fibromyositis, Guillain-Barré syndrome, hyperparathyroidism, hypoglycemia, hypothyroidism, muscle tumor, myoglobinuria, myositis, and renal tubular acidosis. In addition, various drugs may cause myalgia, including amphotericin B, chloroquine, clofibrate, and corticosteroids.

N

nail changes, periungual • Inflammatory reaction to acute bacterial or yeast infection. Periungual telangiectases are usually associated with collagen diseases.

nail plate discoloration • A change in the color of the nail plate or bed, resulting from infection or drugs. Blue-green discoloration may occur with *Pseudomonas* infection; brown or black, with fungal infection or fluorosis; and bluish gray, with excessive use of silver salts.

nail plate hypertrophy • Thickening of the nail plate resulting from the accumulation of irregular keratin layers. This condition is commonly associated with fungal infections of the nails or chronic irritation, although it can be hereditary.

nail separation • Separation of the nail plate from the nail bed. This sign occurs primarily in nail injury or infection

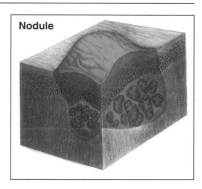

Nodule

but is also seen in psoriasis, in thyrotoxicosis, and as a drug reaction.

nasal obstruction • This symptom may result from inflammatory, neoplastic, endocrine, and metabolic disorders as well as from structural abnormalities and traumatic injuries. It may cause discomfort, alter the sense of smell and taste, and cause voice changes. Although commonly benign, nasal obstruction may herald basilar skull fracture or malignant tumors.

neuralgia • Severe paroxysmal pain, usually brief, over an area innervated by specific nerve fibers. The cause of neuralgia is unknown in many cases, but it may be precipitated by pressure, cold, movement, or stimulation of a trigger zone. Neuralgia may be accompanied by vasomotor symptoms, such as sweating or tearing.

Nicoladoni's sign • Bradycardia resulting from finger pressure on an artery proximal to an arteriovenous fistula.

night blindness • Impaired vision in the dark, especially after entering a darkened room or while driving at night. This symptom of choroidal and retinal degeneration occurs in various ocular disorders. It also may be an early indicator of vitamin A deficiency.

nodules • Small, solid, circumscribed masses of differentiated tissue that may or may not be raised, detected on palpation.

O

obsession • A persistent, usually disturbing thought or image that can't be eliminated by reason or logic. It's associated with obsessive-compulsive disorder and occasionally schizophrenia.

obturator sign • Pain in the right hypogastric region, occurring with flexion of the right leg at the hip, with the knee bent and internally rotated. It indicates irritation of the obturator muscle.

In children, this sign may signal acute appendicitis because the appendix lies rectocecally over the obturator muscle.

orbicularis sign • Inability to close one eye at a time, occurring in hemiplegia.

orofacial dyskinesia • Abnormal involuntary movements involving muscles of the face, mouth, tongue, eyes, and occasionally the neck. This sign may be unilateral or bilateral, and constant or intermittent. It may result from hemifacial spasm disease or the effects of certain drugs, but it's commonly idiopathic. This sign is believed to result from pressure on the facial nerves due to an extrapyramidal lesion or a chemical imbalance.

orthotonos • A form of tetanic spasm producing a rigid, straight line of the neck, limbs, and body.

Osler's nodes • Tender, raised, pea-sized, red or purple lesions that erupt on the palms, soles, and especially the pads of the fingers and toes. They're a rare but reliable sign of infective endocarditis and are pathognomonic of the subacute form. However, these nodes usually develop after other telling signs and symptoms and disappear spontaneously within several days. How and why they develop is uncertain; they may result from emboli caught in peripheral capillaries or may reflect an immunologic reaction to the causative organism. Osler's nodes must be distinguished from the even less common Janeway's lesions—small, painless, erythematous lesions that erupt on the palms and soles.

ostealgia • Bone pain associated with such disorders as osteomyelitis.

otorrhagia • Bleeding from the ear associated with a tumor, a severe infection, or an injury affecting the auricle, external canal, tympanic membrane, or temporal bone.

P

palmar crease abnormalities • An abnormal line pattern on the palms, resulting from faulty embryonic development between the second and fourth months of gestation. This pattern may occur normally but usually appears in Down syndrome as a single transverse crease formed by fusion of the proximal and distal palmar creases (called the *simian crease*). It also appears in Turner's syndrome and congenital rubella syndrome.

paradoxical respirations • An abnormal breathing pattern marked by paradoxical movement of an injured portion of the chest wall—it contracts on inspiration and bulges on expiration. This ominous sign is characteristic of flail chest—a thoracic injury involving multiple free-floating, fractured ribs.

paranoia • Extreme suspiciousness related to delusions of persecution by another person, group, or institution. This symptom may occur in schizophrenia, drug-induced or toxic states, or paranoid disorders.

Pastia's sign • Petechiae appearing along skin creases in such areas as the antecubital fossa, the groin, and the wrists. They accompany the rash of scarlet fever as a response to the erythrogenic toxin produced by scarlatinal strains of group A streptococci.

Perez's sign • Crackles auscultated over the lungs when a seated patient raises and lowers his arms. This sign commonly occurs in fibrous mediastinitis and may also occur in aortic arch aneurysm.

phobia • An irrational and persistent fear of an object, situation, or activity. Occurring in phobic disorders, it may interfere with normal functioning. Typical manifestations include faintness, fatigue, palpitations, diaphoresis, nausea, tremor, and panic.

pica • Craving and ingestion of normally inedible substances, such as plaster, charcoal, clay, wool, ashes, paint, or dirt. In children, the most commonly affected group, pica typically results from nutritional deficiencies. In adults, it may reflect a psychological disturbance. Depending on the substance eaten, pica can lead to poisoning and GI disorders.

Plummer's sign • Inability to ascend stairs or step onto a chair, as occurs in Graves' disease.

pneumaturia • The passage of gas in the urine while voiding. Causes include a fistula between the bowel and bladder, sigmoid diverticulitis, rectosigmoid cancer, and gas-forming urinary tract infections.

Pool-Schlesinger sign • In tetany, muscle spasm of the forearm, hand and fingers or of the leg and foot. To detect this sign, forcefully abduct and elevate the patient's arm with his forearm extended or forcefully flex the patient's extended leg at the hip. Spasm results from tension on the brachial plexus or the sciatic nerve.

postnasal drip • A sinus or nasal discharge that flows behind the nose and into the throat. It typically results from infection, allergies, or environmental irritants.

Prehn's sign • Relief of pain with elevation and support of the scrotum, occurring in epididymitis. This sign differentiates epididymitis from testicular torsion. Both disorders produce severe pain, tenderness, and scrotal swelling.

pressured speech • Verbal expression that is accelerated, difficult to interrupt, and at times unintelligible. This sign may accompany flight of ideas in the manic phase of a bipolar disorder.

Prévost's sign • Conjugate deviation of the head and eyes in hemiplegia. Typically, the eyes gaze toward the affected hemisphere.

prognathism • An enlarged, protuberant jaw associated with normal mandible condyles and temporomandibular joints. This sign most commonly appears in acromegaly.

pulsus bisferiens • A hyperdynamic, double-beating pulse characterized by two systolic peaks separated by a midsystolic dip. Both peaks may be equal or one may be larger; usually though, the first peak is taller or more forceful than the second. The first peak (percussion wave) is believed to be the pulse pressure and the second (tidal wave), reverberation from the periphery. This sign occurs in conditions in which a large volume of blood is rapidly ejected from the left ventricle, such as aortic insufficiency. The pulse can be palpated in peripheral arteries or observed on an arterial pressure wave recording.

To detect pulsus bisferiens, *lightly* palpate the carotid, brachial, radial, or femoral artery while listening to the heart sounds to determine if the two palpable peaks occur during systole. If they do, you'll feel the double pulse between the first and second heart sounds.

purple striae • Thin, purple streaks on the skin that characteristically occur in hypercortisolism along with other cushingoid signs, such as buffalo hump and moonface. Striae usually result from excessive use of glucocorticoid drugs.

pyrosis • A substernal burning sensation that rises in the chest and may ra-

Rumpel-Leede sign

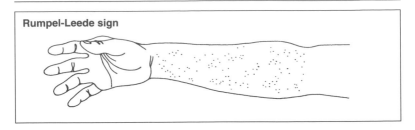

diate to the neck or throat; commonly known as heartburn. Caused by reflux of gastric contents into the esophagus, pyrosis is commonly accompanied by regurgitation. It usually develops after meals or when the patient lies down, bends over, lifts heavy objects, or exercises vigorously; it may worsen with swallowing and improves when the patient sits upright or takes antacids.

Q

Quinquaud's sign • Trembling of the fingers, in alcoholism. To detect this sign, have the patient spread his hand, flex his fingers at the metacarpophalangeal joints, and touch your palm with his fingers at a 90-degree angle to your hand.

R

rectal pain • Discomfort that arises in the anal-rectal area, commonly a symptom of anorectal disorders. This pain may result from or be aggravated by diarrhea, constipation, or passage of hardened stools. It may also be aggravated by intense pruritus and continued scratching associated with drainage of mucus, blood, or fecal matter that irritates the skin and nerve endings.

rectal tenesmus • Spasmodic contraction of the anal sphincter with a persistent urge to defecate and involuntary, ineffective straining. This symptom occurs in inflammatory bowel disorders, such as ulcerative colitis and Crohn's disease, and in rectal tumors. Often painful, rectal tenesmus usually accom-

panies passage of small amounts of blood, pus, or mucus.

regression • Return to a behavioral level appropriate to an earlier developmental age. This defense mechanism may occur in various psychiatric and organic disorders.

repression • The unconscious retreat from awareness of unacceptable ideas or impulses. This defense mechanism may occur normally or may accompany psychiatric disorders.

Romberg's sign • An inability to maintain balance when standing erect with the feet together and eyes closed. This sign indicates a vestibular or proprioceptive disorder or a disorder of the spinal tracts that carry proprioceptive information. Insufficient vestibular or proprioceptive information causes an inability to execute precise movements and maintain balance without visual cues.

Rotch's sign • Dullness on percussion over the right lung at the fifth intercostal space. This sign occurs in pericardial effusion.

Rovsing's sign • Pain in the right lower quadrant upon palpation and quick withdrawal of the fingers in the left lower quadrant. This referred rebound tenderness suggests appendicitis.

Rumpel-Leede sign • Extensive petechiae distal to a tourniquet placed around the upper arm, indicating capillary fragility in scarlet fever or severe thrombocytopenia. To elicit this sign, place a tourniquet around the upper arm for 5 to 10 minutes and observe for distal petechiae.

S

salivation, decreased • Diminished production or excretion of saliva (also known as dry mouth or xerostomia). This sign usually results from mouth breathing but can also stem from salivary duct obstruction, Sjögren's syndrome, the use of anticholinergics and other drugs, or radiation effects. It can even result from vigorous exercise or autonomic stimulation—for example, by fear.

salivation, increased • This uncommon symptom may result from GI disorders, especially of the esophagus. It also accompanies certain systemic disorders and may result from the effects of drugs and toxins or from difficulty swallowing. (See the entry "Dysphagia.")

salt craving • A compensatory response to the body's failure to adequately conserve sodium, probably as a result of adrenal dysfunction. Such dysfunction can reduce aldosterone levels, thereby impairing reabsorption and increasing excretion of sodium.

Seellgmüller's sign • In facial neuralgia, pupillary dilation on the affected side.

Siegert's sign • Short, inwardly curved little fingers, typically appearing in Down syndrome.

Signorelli's sign • Extreme tenderness on palpation of the retromandibular point; associated with meningitis.

Simon's sign • Incoordination of the movements of the diaphragm and thorax, occurring early in meningitis.

skin, bronze • The result of excess circulating melanin, a bronze skin tone that tends to appear at pressure points—such as the knuckles, elbows, toes, and knees—and in creases on the palms and soles; eventually, it may extend to the buccal mucosa and gums before covering the entire body. Sun exposure deepens the bronze color of exposed areas, but this effect fades. In fair-skinned people, the bronze tone can range from light to dark. It also varies with the underlying disorder. Bronze skin is a classic sign of adrenal insufficiency.

spasmodic torticollis • Intermittent or continuous spasms of the shoulder and neck muscles that turn the head to one side. Often transient and idiopathic, this sign can occur in extrapyramidal disorders. It can also occur in patients with shortened neck muscles. (See the entry "Dystonia.")

spider angioma • A fiery red vascular lesion with an elevated central body, branching spiderlike legs, and a surrounding flush. Ranging from a few millimeters to several centimeters in diameter, spider angiomas usually appear on the face and neck and may occur singly or in multiples. On palpation, they may be slightly warmer than the surrounding skin and may have a pulsating central body. This sign is usually associated with cirrhosis but may also occur in the second to third month of pregnancy and in elderly people.

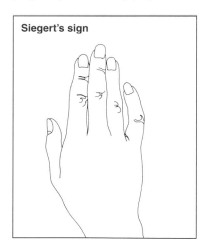

Siegert's sign

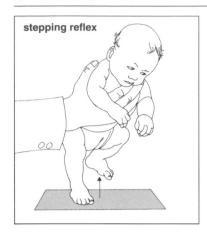

stepping reflex

age 1. To elicit this response, place your finger in the infant's mouth. Rhythmic sucking movements are normal; weak or absent sucking movements may indicate elevated intracranial pressure.

T

tangentiality • Speech characterized by tedious detail that prevents the speaker from ever reaching the point of the statement. This sign occurs in schizophrenia and organic brain disorders.

taste abnormality • This sign encompasses several types of taste impairment: *ageusia* (complete loss of taste), *hypogeusia* (partial loss of taste), *dysgeusia* (distorted sense of taste), and *cacogeusia* (unpleasant or even revolting sense of taste). Any factor that interrupts transmission of taste stimuli to the brain, such as trauma, infection, vitamin or mineral deficiency, neurologic or oral disorders, and the effects of drugs, may cause taste abnormalities. Aging and heavy smoking may also play a role.

tearing increase • Excessive production of tears (also known as lacrimation) due to stimulation of the lacrimal glands. *Psychic lacrimation* is usually a response to emotional or physical stress such as pain. *Neurogenic lacrimation* is triggered by reflex stimulation associated with ocular trauma, inflammation, or exposure to environmental irritants (such as strong light, wind, or airborne allergens); it may also accompany eyestrain, yawning, vomiting, and laughing.

testicular pain • Unilateral or bilateral pain localized in or around the testicle and possibly radiating along the spermatic cord and into the lower abdomen. This pain usually results from trauma, infection, or torsion. Its onset is typically sudden and severe; however, its intensity can vary from sharp pain accompanied by nausea and vomiting to a

spine sign • Resistance to anterior flexion of the spine, resulting from pain in poliomyelitis.

spoon nails • Malformation of the nails characterized by a concave outer surface instead of the normal convex surface. This sign commonly occurs in severe hypochromic anemia but occasionally may be hereditary.

Stellwag's sign • Incomplete and infrequent blinking, usually related to exophthalmos in Graves' disease.

stepping reflex • In neonates, spontaneous stepping movements that simulate walking. This reciprocal flexion and extension of the legs is normal and disappears after about age 4 weeks. To elicit this sign, hold the infant erect with the soles of his feet touching a hard surface. In contrast, scissoring movements with persistent extension and crossing of the legs or asymmetrical stepping is abnormal, possibly indicating central nervous system damage.

sucking reflex • Involuntary circumoral sucking movements in response to stimulation. Present at about 26 weeks' gestational age, this reflex is initially weak and not synchronized with swallowing. It persists through infancy, becoming more discriminating during the first few months and disappearing by

chronic, dull ache. In a child, sudden onset of severe testicular pain is a urologic emergency. Assume testicular torsion is the cause until disproven. If a young male complains of abdominal pain, always carefully examine the scrotum because abdominal pain commonly precedes testicular pain in testicular torsion.

Thornton's sign • Severe flank pain resulting from nephrolithiasis.

thrill • A palpable sensation resulting from the vibration of a loud murmur or from turbulent blood flow in an aneurysm. Thrills are associated with heart murmurs of grade IV to VI and may be palpable over major arteries. (See the entries "Bruits" and "Murmurs.")

tibialis sign • Involuntary dorsiflexion and inversion of the foot upon brisk, voluntary flexion of the patient's knee and hip, occurring in spastic paralysis of the lower limb.

To detect this sign, place the patient in the supine position and have him flex his leg at the hip and knee so that his thigh touches his abdomen. Or you can place the patient prone, and have him flex his leg at the knee so that his calf touches his thigh. If this sign is present, you may observe dorsiflexion of the great toe or of all the toes as the foot dorsiflexes and inverts. Normally, plantar flexion of the foot occurs with this action.

Tommasi's sign • Absence of hair on the posteroexternal aspect of the leg, occurring in males with gout.

tongue enlargement • An increase in the tongue's size, causing it to protrude from the mouth. Causes include Down syndrome, acromegaly, lymphangioma, Beckwith's syndrome, and congenital micrognathia. An enlarged tongue can also stem from cancer of the tongue, amyloidosis, and neurofibromatosis.

tongue fissures • Shallow or deep grooving on the dorsum of the tongue. Usually a congenital defect, tongue fis-

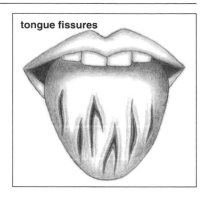

tongue fissures

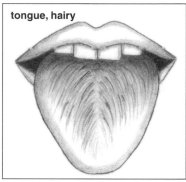

tongue, hairy

cures occur normally in about 10% of the population. Deep fissures may promote collection of food particles, leading to chronic inflammation and tenderness.

tongue, hairy • Hypertrophy and elongation of the tongue's filiform papillae. Normally white, the papillae may turn yellow, brown, or black from bacteria, food, tobacco, coffee, or dyes in drugs and food. Hairy tongue may also result from antibiotic therapy, irradiation of the head and neck, chronic debilitating disorders, and habitual use of mouthwashes containing oxidizing or astringent agents.

tongue, magenta, cobblestone • Swelling and hyperemia of the tongue, resulting in rows of elevated fungiform and filiform papillae that give the tongue a magenta-colored or cobblestone appearance. Magenta tongue is usually a sign of vitamin B_2 (riboflavin) deficiency.

tongue, red • Patchy or uniform redness (ranging from pink to magenta) of the tongue, which may be swollen and smooth, rough, or fissured. This sign usually indicates glossitis due to emotional stress or nutritional disorders, such as pernicious anemia, Plummer-Vinson syndrome, pellagra, sprue, or a deficiency of folic acid or vitamin B.

tongue, smooth • Absence or atrophy of the filiform papillae, causing a smooth (patchy or uniform), glossy, red tongue. This primary sign of undernutrition results from anemia and vitamin B deficiency.

tongue swelling • Edema of the tongue, most commonly associated with pernicious anemia, pellagra, hypothyroidism, and allergic angioneurotic edema.

tongue ulcers • Circumscribed necrotic lesions on the dorsum, margin, tip, and inferior surface of the tongue. Ulcers most commonly result from biting, chewing, or burning of the tongue. They may also stem from type 1 herpes simplex virus, tuberculosis, histoplasmosis, or cancer of the tongue.

tongue, white • A uniform white coating or plaques on the tongue. Lesions associated with a white tongue may be premalignant or malignant and may require a biopsy. *Necrotic white lesions*—collections of cells, bacteria, and debris—are painful and can be scraped from the tongue. They commonly appear in children with candidiasis or thermal burns. *Keratotic white lesions*—thickened, keratinized patches—usually produce no symptoms and can't be scraped from the tongue. These lesions commonly result from alcohol use and local irritation from tobacco smoke or other substances.

tonic neck reflex • Extension of the limbs on the side to which the head is turned and flexion of the opposite limbs. In neonates, this normal reflex appears between 28 and 32 weeks' gestational age, diminishes as voluntary muscle control increases, and disappears by age 3 or 4 months. The absence or persistence of this reflex may indicate central nervous system damage. To elicit this response, place the infant in the supine position; then turn his head to one side.

tooth discoloration • Bluish yellow or gray teeth may result from hypoplasia of the dentin and pulp, nerve damage, or caries. Yellow teeth may indicate caries. Mottling and staining suggest fluorine excess or the effects of certain drugs, such as tetracycline. Tooth discoloration (and small tooth size) may also occur in osteogenesis imperfecta.

transference • Unconscious transferral of feelings and attitudes originally associated with important figures, such as parents, to another. Used therapeutically in psychoanalysis, transference can also occur in other settings and relationships.

Trendelenburg's test • A demonstration of valvular incompetence of the saphenous vein and inefficiency of the communicating veins at different levels. To perform this test, raise the patient's legs above the heart level until the veins empty; then rapidly lower them. If the valves are incompetent, the veins immediately distend.

trismus • Prolonged and painful spasms of the lower jaw muscles, commonly known as lockjaw. Trismus is a characteristic early sign of tetanus, but it can also result from drug therapy. A milder form may accompany neuromuscular involvement in other disorders, or infection or disease of the jaw, teeth, parotid glands, or tonsils.

Trousseau's sign • In tetany, carpopedal spasm upon ischemic compression of the upper arm. To elicit this sign, apply a blood pressure cuff to the patient's arm; then inflate the cuff to a pressure between the patient's diastolic and systolic readings, maintaining it for 4 minutes. The patient's hand and fingers assume the "obstetrical hand" position, with wrist and metacarpophalangeal joints flexed, interphalangeal joints extended, and fingers and thumb adducted. (See the entry "Carpopedal spasm.")

twitching • Nonspecific intermittent contraction of muscles or muscle bundles. (See the entries "Fasciculations" and "Tics.")

U

uremic frost • A fine white powder, believed to be urate crystals, that covers the skin and is a characteristic sign of end-stage renal failure or uremia. Urea compounds and other waste substances that can't be excreted by the kidneys in urine are excreted in sweat and remain as powdery deposits on the skin when the sweat evaporates. The frost typically appears on the face, neck, axillae, groin, and genitalia.

urinary tenesmus • Persistent, ineffective, painful straining to empty the bladder. This symptom results from irritation of nerve endings in the bladder mucosa due to infection or an indwelling catheter.

V

vaginal bleeding abnormalities • Passage of blood from the vagina at times other than menses. This sign may indicate abnormalities of the uterus, cervix, ovaries, fallopian tubes, or vagina. It may also indicate an abnormal pregnancy. (See also the entries "Menorrhagia," "Metrorrhagia," and "Vaginal bleeding, postmenopausal.")

venous hum • A functional or innocent murmur heard above the clavicles throughout the cardiac cycle. Loudest during diastole, it may be low-pitched, rough, or noisy. It's best heard by applying the bell of the stethoscope to the medial aspect of the right supraclavicular area, with the patient seated upright, or by placing the stethoscope bell in the second or third parasternal interspaces, with the patient standing upright.

A venous hum is a common and normal finding in children and pregnant women, but it can also occur in hyperdynamic states, such as anemia and thyrotoxicosis. The hum commonly accompanies a thrill or, possibly, a high-pitched whine. Unlike an intracardiac murmur or a thyroid bruit, it disappears with jugular vein compression and waxes and wanes with head-turning.

WX

Weill's sign • In infantile pneumonia, absence of expansion in the subclavicular area of the affected side on inspiration.

Westphal's sign • Absence of the knee jerk reflex, occurring in tabes dorsalis.

Wilder's sign • Subtle twitching of the eyeball on medial or lateral gaze. This early sign of Graves' disease is discernible as a slight jerk of the eyeball when the patient changes the direction of his gaze.

wrist drop • A weakness in which the hand remains in a flexed position because of paresis of the extensor muscles of the hand, wrist, and fingers. This weakness may be mild or severe, and temporary or permanent; it may occur unilaterally and suddenly in a radial nerve injury, or bilaterally and gradually in neurologic disorders, such as myasthenia gravis, Guillain-Barré syndrome, and multiple sclerosis.

YZ

yawning, excessive • Persistent involuntary opening of the mouth, accompanied by attempted deep inspiration. In the absence of sleepiness, excessive yawning may indicate cerebral hypoxia.

INDEX

A

i refers to an illustration; t refers to a table.

i refers to an illustration; t refers to a table.

i refers to an illustration; t refers to a table.

i refers to an illustration; t refers to a table.

Muscle spasticity, 381-384
  development of, 382i
Muscle strain, arm pain in, 49
Muscle strength, testing,
  385-386i
Muscle trauma, muscle spasms
  in, 381
Muscle wasting, 376-379
Muscle weakness, 384,
  387-388
Muscular dystrophy, waddling
  gait in, 266-267
Music therapy for Alzheimer's
  patients, 134
Myalgia, 631
Myasthenia gravis
  chest expansion, asymmetri-
    cal, in, 116
  diplopia in, 188
  dysarthria in, 195
  dysphagia in, 204
  dyspnea in, 208
  fatigue in, 244
  muscle weakness in, 387
  paralysis in, 438
  ptosis in, 469
  shallow respirations in, 526
Mydriasis, 388-390
Myeloma, back pain in, 62
Myeloproliferative disorders,
  purpura in, 495
Myocardial infarction
  anxiety in, 40
  arm pain in, 49
  atrial gallop in, 269
  blood pressure decrease in,
    72
  blood pressure increase in,
    76-77
  bradycardia in, 85
  chest pain in, 121
  diaphoresis in, 181-182
  dyspnea in, 208
  jaw pain in, 334
Myoclonus, 390-391
Myotonic dystrophy, sluggish
  pupils in, 492
Myringitis
  otorrhea in, 427
  pruritus in, 462
Myxedema
  edema, generalized, in,
    217-218
  facial edema in, 223
Myxoma, murmur in, 373, 376

N

Nail changes, periungual, 631
Nail plate discoloration, 631
Nail plate hypertrophy, 631
Nail separation, 631
Nasal discharge, 505-507
Nasal flaring, 392-393

Nasal fracture, epistaxis in,
  227
Nasal obstruction, 631
Nasal speculum, 506i
Nasal tumors, rhinorrhea in,
  507
Nasogastric tubes, 297i
Nasopharyngeal cancer, hear-
  ing loss in, 292
Nausea, 393-396
Neck pain, 396-400
  associated findings in,
    398-399t
  causes of, 398-399t
  therapeutic touch for, 400
Neck sprain, neck pain in, 399
Necrotizing vasculitis, papular
  rash in, 433
Negative oculocephalic reflex.
  See Doll's eye sign, ab-
  sent.
Neoplasms, fever in, 249
Neoplasms of the arm, arm
  pain in, 50
Nephrotic syndrome
  edema, generalized, in,
    218-219
  facial edema in, 223
  weight gain, excessive, in,
    605
Nerve trauma, muscle weak-
  ness in, 387
Neuralgia, 631
Neurofibromatosis, generalized
  tonic-clonic seizures in,
    520-521
Neurogenic claudication, 327
Neurogenic shock
  blood pressure decrease in,
    72
  tachycardia in, 549
  tachypnea in, 552
Neurologic tests, back pain
  and, 63
Neuromuscular failure, apnea
  in, 46
Neuropathy, miosis in, 366
Nicoladoni's sign, 631
Night blindness, 631
Nipple discharge, 400-402
  eliciting, 401i
Nipple inversion, 403i
Nipple retraction, 402-404,
  403i
Nocardiosis, productive cough,
  in, 151
Nocturia, 404-405
Nocturnal myoclonus, insom-
  nia in, 324
Nodule, 435i, 631, 631i
Noise, tinnitus in, 562
North American blastomyco-
  sis, productive cough in,
  151

Nosebleed. See Epistaxis.
Nuchal rigidity, 406-407
Nutritional deficiencies
  confusion in, 134
  purpura in, 495
Nutritional status, evaluating,
  606-607i
Nystagmus, 407-409
  classifying, 408i

O

Obesity, hepatomegaly in, 312
Obsession, 632
Obsessive-compulsive disor-
  ders, anxiety in, 40
Obstructive uropathy, flank
  pain in, 253
Obturator sign, 632
Occipital lobe lesion, hemi-
  anopia in, 306
Occlusive vascular disease, leg
  pain in, 343
Ocular deviation, 410-412
  characteristics of, 411t
Ocular laceration, eye pain in,
  239
Ocular muscle dystrophy,
  ptosis in, 469
Ocular trauma
  ptosis in, 469
  vision loss in, 592
Oculomotor nerve palsy
  mydriasis in, 389
  pupils, nonreactive, in, 490
Oligomenorrhea, 412-414
Oliguria, 414-418
  development of, 416-417i
Oliver's sign. See Tracheal tugging.
Olivopontocerebellar atrophy,
  ataxia in, 54
Olivopontocerebellar degeneration, dysarthria in, 195
Ophthalmalgia, 237-240
Ophthalmoplegic migraine,
  diplopia in, 188
Opisthotonos, 418-420
  recognizing, 419i
Optic atrophy, vision loss in,
  592
Optic nerve meningioma,
  exophthalmos in, 234
Optic neuritis
  eye pain in, 239
  scotoma in, 510
  vision loss in, 592
  visual blurring in, 596
Oral cavity tumor, dysphagia
  in, 204
Orange-peel skin, 443-444,
  444i
Orbicularis sign, 632

i refers to an illustration; t refers to a table.

i refers to an illustration; t refers to a table.

i refers to an illustration; t refers to a table.

i refers to an illustration; t refers to a table.

i refers to an illustration; t refers to a table.